a LANGE medical book

Basic
Histology

ninth edition

a LANGE medical book

Basic
Histology

ninth edition

Luiz Carlos Junqueira, MD
Professor Emeritus
University of São Paulo, Brazil
Honorary Research Associate in Biology
Harvard College, Boston
Formerly Research Associate
Medical School, University of Chicago

José Carneiro, MD
Dean and Professor of Histology & Embryology
Institute of Biomedical Sciences, University of São Paulo, Brazil
Formerly Research Associate, Department of Anatomy
Medical School, McGill University, Montreal, Canada
Formerly Visiting Associate Professor, Department of Anatomy
Medical School, University of Virginia, Charlottesville, Virginia

Robert O. Kelley, PhD
Associate Vice Chancellor for Research and
Executive Associate Dean of the Graduate College
Professor of Biological Sciences and Anatomy & Cell Biology
University of Illinois at Chicago

APPLETON & LANGE
Stamford, Connecticut

Original title: Histologia Basica, 8th ed. © 1995 by Editora Guanabara Koogan S.A., Rio de Janeiro, Brazil

Many of the illustrations in this book were prepared with financial aid from the Fundação de Amparo à Pesquisa do Estado de São Paulo, and National Research Council (CNPq).

99 00 01 02 / 10 9 8 7 6 5 4 3 2

Prentice Hall International (UK) Limited, *London*
Prentice Hall of Australia Pty. Limited, *Sydney*
Prentice Hall Canada, Inc., *Toronto*
Prentice Hall Hispanoamericana, S.A., *Mexico*
Prentice Hall of India Private Limited, *New Delhi*
Prentice Hall of Japan, Inc., *Tokyo*
Simon & Schuster Asia Pte. Ltd., *Singapore*
Editora Prentice Hall do Brasil Ltda., *Rio de Janeiro*
Prentice Hall, *Upper Saddle River, New Jersey*

ISSN: 0891–2106
ISBN: 0–8385–0590–2

Acquisitions Editor: David A. Barnes
Development Editor: Amanda M. Suver
Production Editor: Jeanmarie Roche
Associate Art Manager: Maggie Belis Darrow
Copy Editor: Mary McKenney
Illustrators: Teshin Associates

PRINTED IN THE UNITED STATES OF AMERICA

ISBN 0-8385-0590-2

90000

9 780838 505908

Contents

Preface

The ninth edition of *Basic Histology* continues to be a concise, well-illustrated exposition of the basic facts and interpretation of microscopic anatomy. The authors of this text recognize that students of biologic structure share a common goal—namely, to better understand how *structure* and function are integrated in the molecules, cells, tissues, and organs of a living creature. Histology is that branch of science which centers on the biology of cells and tissues within an organism and, as such, serves as the foundation on which pathology and pathophysiology are built. In this edition, we continue to emphasize the relationships and concepts that inextricably link cell and tissue structure with their functions as they constitute the fabric of a living organism.

In revising *Basic Histology,* our intent is to provide our readers with the most contemporary and useful text possible. We do this in two ways: by describing the most important recent developments in the sciences basic to histology and by recognizing that our readers are faced with the task of learning an ever-increasing number of facts in an ever-decreasing period of time. Because of this, every attempt has been made to present the information as concisely as possible and organize it in a way that will facilitate learning.

INTENDED AUDIENCE

This text is designed for students in professional schools of medicine, veterinary medicine, dentistry, nursing, and allied health sciences. It will also provide a useful, ready reference to both undergraduate students of microscopic anatomy and others in the structural biosciences.

ORGANIZATION

Because the study of histology requires a firm foundation in cell biology, *Basic Histology* begins with an accurate, up-to-date description of the structure and function of cells and their products and a brief introduction into the molecular biology of the cell.

This foundation is followed by a description of the four basic tissues of the body, emphasizing how cells become specialized to perform the specific functions of these tissues.

Finally, we devote individual chapters to each of the organs and organ systems of the human body. Here, the emphasis on spatial arrangements of the basic tissues provides the key to understanding the functions of each organ. Again, we emphasize cell biology as the most fundamental approach to the study of structure and function.

As a further aid to learning, numerous photomicrographs and electron micrographs amplify the text and remind the reader of the laboratory basis of the study of histology. In addition, we place particular emphasis on diagrams, three-dimensional illustrations, and charts to summarize morphologic and functional features of cells, tissues, and organs.

NEW TO THIS EDITION

- All chapters have been revised to reflect new findings and interpretations, and the emphasis on human histology has been further strengthened.

- The chapter on microscopy and techniques includes new information on methods that permit analysis of molecules, cells, and tissues.
- New information on the molecular biology of the genome and its regulation is included in the chapter on the nucleus.
- New information on the organization and molecular composition of the extracellular matrix has been included in the chapter on connective tissue.
- New micrographs of resin-embedded specimens provide clearer detail of cell and tissue organization.
- A discussion of the mechanisms of signal transduction in intercellular communication that adds to the student's understanding of tissue organization has been included in the chapter on the cell.
- The chapter on nerve tissue and the nervous system has been extensively rewritten to include contemporary concepts and information regarding neurons and glial cells and their interactions.
- The chapter on the immune system has been further revised to include current information and to organize that material into a readily assimilated body of knowledge.
- Existing diagrams have been revised and several new diagrams and figures have been added to enhance the usefulness of the text.
- Color has been used to highlight key points in illustrations and the principal issues in selected sections of the text.
- Clinical correlations in each chapter further illustrate the direct application of basic histologic information to the diagnosis, prognosis, pathobiology, and clinical aspects of disease. They, too, are highlighted in color in each chapter.

ACKNOWLEDGMENTS

We wish to thank all the biomedical scientists and educators who provided information and micrographs that added to the usefulness of this edition, especially Professor Juan Mota (Immune System) and Professor Cesar Timo-Jaria (Nerve Tissue). We also extend our appreciation to the staff of Appleton & Lange—John Butler, Amanda Suver, Maggie Darrow, Jeanmarie Roche, and Mary McKenney—for editorial support and assistance.

We are pleased to announce that Italian, Spanish, Dutch, Indonesian, Japanese, Turkish, Korean, German, Serbo-Croatian, French, Portuguese, and Greek translations of *Basic Histology* are now available.

Luiz Carlos Junqueira, MD
José Carneiro, MD
Robert O. Kelley, PhD
June, 1998

Histology & Its Methods of Study

1

Histology (Gr. *histo,* web or tissue, + *logos,* study) is the study of cells and the extracellular matrix of tissues. The small size of cells and matrix components makes histology dependent on the use of and improvements in microscopes. Advances in chemistry, physiology, immunology, and pathology—and the interactions among these fields—contribute to a better knowledge of tissue biology. Integration of knowledge in these fields has resulted in histochemistry, histophysiology, immunohistochemistry, and histopathology, all of which help students develop a better understanding of tissue biology.

Familiarity with the tools and methods of any branch of science is essential for a proper understanding of the subject. Here, we review some of the more common methods used to study cells and tissues and the principles involved in these methods: units of measurement, preparation of tissues for examination, microscopy, histochemistry, problems in interpretation of tissue sections, autoradiography, examination of living cells and tissues, isolation and study in vitro of pure cell strains, and cell fractionation. The most important units of measurement used in histology are given in Table 1–1.

PREPARATION OF TISSUES FOR MICROSCOPIC EXAMINATION

The most common procedure used in the study of tissues is the preparation of histologic sections that can be studied with the aid of the light microscope. Under the light microscope, tissues are examined via transillumination. Since tissues and organs are usually too thick for transillumination, they must be sectioned to obtain thin, translucent sections. In some cases, very thin layers of tissues or transparent membranes of living animals (eg, the mesentery, the tail of a tadpole, the wall of a hamster's cheek pouch) can be observed in the microscope without first sectioning the tissue. It is then possible to study these structures for long periods and under varying physiologic or experimental conditions. If a permanent preparation is desired, small fragments of these thin structures can be fixed, spread on a glass slide, stained, mounted with resin, and examined under the microscope. In most cases, however, tissues must be sliced into thin sections before they can be examined. These sections are precisely cut, using fine cutting instruments called **microtomes** (Figure 1–1), from tissues previously prepared for sectioning (see Table 1–2).

The ideal microscope tissue preparation would be preserved with suitable chemicals so that the tissue on the slide would have the same structure and molecular composition as it had in the body. This is sometimes possible but—as a practical matter—seldom feasible, and artifacts from the preparation process are almost always present.

Fixation

To avoid tissue digestion by enzymes (autolysis) or bacteria and to preserve the physical structure, pieces of organs should be promptly and adequately treated before or as soon as possible after removal from the animal's body. This treatment—**fixation**—usually consists of submerging the tissues in stabilizing or cross-linking agents or perfusing them with these substances to preserve as much as possible of their morphologic and molecular characteristics.

The chemical substances used to preserve tissues are called **fixatives.** One of the best fixatives for routine light microscopy is a buffered isotonic solution of 4% formaldehyde. The chemistry of the process involved in fixation is complex and not well understood. Formaldehyde and glutaraldehyde, another widely used fixative, are known to react with the amine groups (NH_2) of tissue proteins. In the case of glutaraldehyde, the fixing action is reinforced by the fact that it is a dialdehyde and can cross-link proteins.

In view of the high resolution afforded by the electron microscope, greater care in fixation is necessary to preserve ultrastructural detail. Toward that end, a double fixation procedure, using a buffered glutaraldehyde solution followed by a second fixation in buffered osmium tetroxide, has become a standard procedure in preparations for fine structural studies. The effect of osmium tetroxide is to preserve and stain lipids and proteins.

Table 1–1. Units of measurement used in light and electron microscopy.

Système International (SI) Unit	Symbol and Value
Micrometer	$\mu m = 0.001$ mm, 10^{-6} m
Nanometer	nm = 0.001 μm, 10^{-9} m

Embedding

To obtain thin sections with the microtome, tissues must be infiltrated after fixation with embedding substances that impart a rigid consistency to the tissue. Embedding materials include paraffin and plastic resins. Paraffin is used routinely for light microscopy; resins are used for both light and electron microscopy.

The process of embedding, or tissue impregnation, is usually preceded by two main steps: **dehydration** and **clearing.** The water is first extracted from the fragments to be embedded by bathing them successively in a graded series of mixtures of ethanol and water (usually from 70% to 100% ethanol). The ethanol is then replaced with a solvent miscible with the embedding medium. (In paraffin embedding, the solvent used is xylene.) As the tissues become infiltrated with the solvent, they usually become transparent (clearing). Once the tissue is impregnated with the solvent, it is placed in plastic resin at room temperature or in melted paraffin in the oven, usually at 58–60 °C. The heat causes the solvent to evaporate, and the space becomes filled with paraffin. Tissues to be embedded with plastic resin are also dehydrated in ethanol and subsequently infiltrated with plastic solvents. These solvents are later replaced by plastic solutions that are hardened by means of cross-linking polymerizers. Plastic embedding avoids the shrinking effect of the high temperatures needed for paraffin embedding and gives much better results.

The small blocks containing the tissues are sectioned by the microtome's steel or glass blade to a thickness of 1–10 μm. The sections are floated on

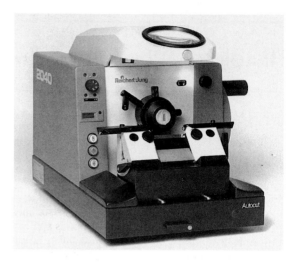

Figure 1–1. Microtome for sectioning resin- and paraffin-embedded tissues. Rotation of the drive wheel—seen with a handle on the right side of the instrument—moves the tissue-block holder up and down. Each turn of the drive wheel advances the specimen holder a controlled distance, generally 1.0–10 μm, and the embedded tissue passes over the knife edge, which cuts the sections. The sections adhere to each other, producing a ribbon of sections that is collected and affixed to a slide. (Courtesy of Cambridge Instruments.)

warm water and transferred to glass slides. Immersion of tissues in solvents such as xylene dissolves the tissue lipids, which is an undesirable effect when these compounds are to be studied. To avoid loss of lipids, a **freezing microtome** has been devised in which the tissues are hardened at low temperatures to provide the rigidity necessary to permit sectioning. The freezing microtome—and its more elaborate and efficient successor, the cryostat (Gr. *kryos,* cold, + *statos,* standing)—permit sections to be obtained quickly without going through the embedding procedure described above. Because these instruments al-

Table 1–2. Typical sequence of procedures in preparing tissues for observation under the light microscope. Following embedding in paraffin blocks, the tissues can be sectioned with a microtome (Figure 1–1).

Stage	Purpose	Duration
1. Fixation	To preserve tissue morphology and molecular composition	About 12 h, according to the fixative and the size of the piece of tissue
2. Dehydration in graded concentrated ethyl alcohol (70% up to 100% alcohol)	To replace tissue water with organic solvents	6–24 h
3. Clearing in benzene, xylene, or toluene	To impregnate the tissues with a paraffin or a plastic resin solvent	1–6 h
4. Embedding in melted paraffin at 60 °C or plastic resin at room temperature	Paraffin or resin penetrates all intercellular spaces and even into the cells, making the tissues more resistant to sectioning	1–3 h

low rapid study of specimens during surgical procedures, they are routinely used in hospitals. They are also effective in the histochemical study of very sensitive enzymes or small molecules, since freezing does not inactivate most enzymes, and it hinders the diffusion of small molecules.

Staining

With few exceptions, most tissues are colorless, so observing them unstained in the light microscope is difficult. Methods of staining tissues have therefore been devised that not only make the various tissue components conspicuous but also permit distinctions to be made between them. The dyes used stain tissue components more or less selectively. Most of these dyes behave like acidic or basic compounds and have a tendency to form electrostatic (salt) linkages with ionizable radicals of the tissues. Tissue components that stain more readily with basic dyes are termed **basophilic** (Gr. *basis,* base, + *phileo,* to love); those with an affinity for acid dyes are termed **acidophilic.**

Examples of basic dyes are toluidine blue and methylene blue. Hematoxylin behaves like a basic dye, ie, it stains the basophilic tissue components. The main tissue components that ionize and react with basic dyes do so because of acids in their composition (nucleoproteins, glycosaminoglycans, and acid glycoproteins). Acid dyes (eg, orange G, eosin, acid fuchsin) stain the acidophilic components of tissues such as mitochondria, secretory granules, and collagen.

Of all dyes, the combination of **hematoxylin and eosin (H&E)** is the most commonly used. Hematoxylin stains the cell nucleus and other acidic structures (such as RNA-rich portions of the cytoplasm) blue. In contrast, eosin stains the cytoplasm red and collagen pink. Many other dyes are used in different histologic procedures. Although they are useful in visualizing the various tissue components, they usually provide no insight into the chemical nature of the tissue being studied. In addition to tissue staining with dyes, impregnation with such metals as silver and gold is a common method, especially in studies of the nervous system.

LIGHT MICROSCOPY

Conventional light, phase contrast, polarizing, confocal, and fluorescence microscopy are all based on the interaction of photons and tissue components.

With the light microscope, stained preparations are usually examined by means of transillumination. The microscope is composed of both mechanical and optical parts. The mechanical components are illustrated in Figure 1–2. The optical components consist of three systems of lenses: condenser, objective, and ocular. The **condenser** collects and focuses the illumination to produce a cone of light that illuminates

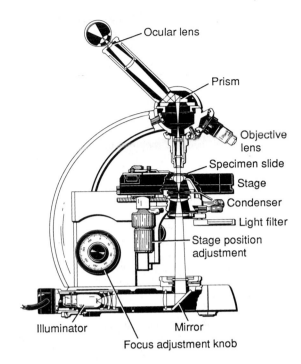

Figure 1–2. Schematic drawing of a light microscope showing its main components and the pathway of light from the source (substage lamp) to the eye of the observer. (Courtesy of Carl Zeiss Co.)

the object to be observed. The **objective** lens enlarges and projects the illuminated image of the object in the direction of the ocular lens. The **ocular** lens further magnifies this image and projects it onto the viewer's retina or a photographic plate. The total magnification is obtained by multiplying the magnifying power of the objective and ocular lenses.

Resolution

The critical factor in obtaining a crisp, detailed image with the microscope is its **resolving power,** that is, the smallest distance between two particles at which they can be seen as separate objects. The maximal resolving power of the light microscope is approximately 0.1 μm; this power permits good images magnified 1000–1500 times. Objects smaller than 0.1 μm cannot be distinguished with this instrument.

The quality of the image—its clarity and richness of detail—depends on the microscope's resolving power. The **magnification** is independent of its resolving power and is of value only when accompanied by high resolution. The resolving power of a microscope depends mainly on the quality of its objective lens. The ocular lens only enlarges the image obtained by the objective; it does not improve resolution.

Highly sensitive video cameras enhance the power of the light microscope and facilitate cre-

ation of digitized images that can be fed into computers for quantitative image analysis.

The frontiers of light microscopy have been redefined by the use of video cameras highly sensitive to light. With these silicon-intensified cameras and image-enhancement programs, objects that may not be visible when viewed directly through the ocular may be made visible in the video screen. These video systems are also useful for studying living cells for long periods of time, because they use low-intensity light and thus avoid the cellular damage that can result from intense illumination.

The electronic images from video cameras can be easily digitized and adapted to the specific requirements of an experiment through computer programming. For example, contrast enhancement is an important computer-assisted technique that may reward the investigator with a structural image not immediately seen when the specimen is observed directly in the microscope.

PHASE CONTRAST MICROSCOPY

Unstained biologic specimens are usually transparent and difficult to view in detail, since all parts of the specimen have almost the same optical density. Phase contrast microscopy, however, uses a lens system that produces visible images from transparent objects (Figure 1–3).

The principle on which phase contrast microscopy is based is the fact that light changes its speed and direction when passing through cellular and extracellular structures with different refractive indices. These changes cause the structures to appear lighter or darker relative to each other. Differential interference (Nomarski) optics (as shown in Figure 1–3C) produces an apparently three-dimensional image of living cells and tissues.

POLARIZING MICROSCOPY

When normal light passes through a **polarizing filter,** it exits vibrating in only one direction. If a second filter is placed in the microscope above the first one, with its main axis perpendicular to the first filter, no light passes through, resulting in a dark-field effect. If, however, tissue structures containing oriented molecules (such as cellulose, collagen, microtubules, and microfilaments) are located between the two Polaroid filters, their repetitive, oriented molecular structure allows them to rotate the axis of the light emerging from the polarizer. Consequently, they appear as bright structures against a dark background (Figures 5–12, 8–9, and 10–3). The ability to rotate the direction of vibration of polarized light is called **birefringence** and is a feature of crystalline substances or substances containing oriented molecules.

CONFOCAL MICROSCOPY

Confocal microscopy uses lasers and computers to produce three-dimensional images of living cells and tissue slices. Because of the way in which the image is produced, the investigator can visually dissect through the specimen, observing structures above or below others. Storing information from each visual plane of the section in a computer allows a three-dimensional image to be reconstructed.

FLUORESCENCE MICROSCOPY

When certain fluorescent substances are irradiated by light of a proper wavelength, they emit light with a longer wavelength. In fluorescence microscopy, tissue sections are usually irradiated with ultraviolet light so that the emission is in the visible portion of the spectrum. The fluorescent substances appear as brilliant, shiny particles on a dark background. For this method, the microscope has a strong ultraviolet light source, and special filters that eliminate ultraviolet light are placed after the objective lens to protect the observer's eyes.

Fluorescent compounds that have an affinity for cell macromolecules are used as fluorescent stains. Acridine orange, which can combine with DNA and RNA, is an example. When observed in the fluorescence microscope, the DNA–acridine orange complex emits a yellowish-green light, and the RNA–acridine orange complex emits a reddish-orange light. It is thus possible to identify and localize nucleic acids in the cells (Figure 1–4).

Fluorescence spectroscopy is a method of analyzing the light emitted by a fluorescent compound in a microspectrophotometer. It can be used to characterize several compounds present in cells and is of particular importance in the study of catecholamines. The development of fluorescent probes (substances that react specifically with cell components) has permitted highly sensitive assays for various substances within cells.

ELECTRON MICROSCOPY

Both transmission and scanning electron microscopy are based on the interaction of electrons and tissue components.

The electron microscope is an imaging system that permits high resolution (0.1 nm). In practice, however, a resolution of 1 nm in tissue sections is considered satisfactory. This by itself permits enlargements to be obtained up to 400 times greater than those achieved with light microscopes.

The electron microscope functions on the principle that a beam of electrons can be deflected by electromagnetic fields in a manner similar to light deflec-

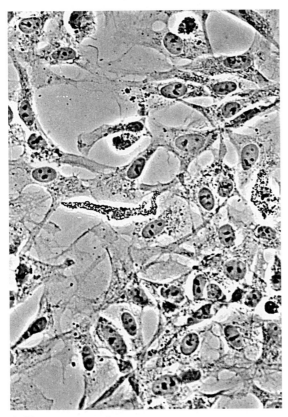

A. Phase contrast microscopy

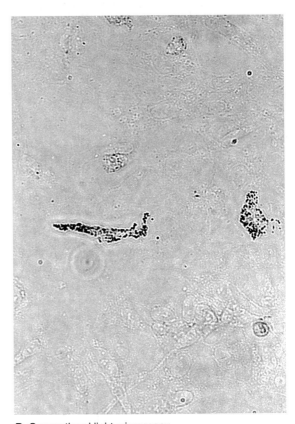

B. Conventional light microscopy

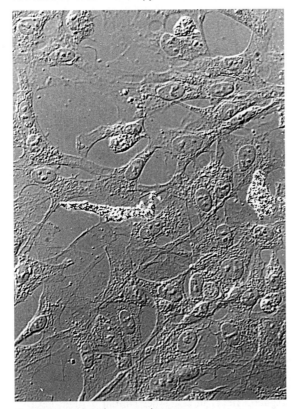

C. Differential interference microscopy

Figure 1–3. Cultured neural crest cells seen with different optical techniques. Unstained cells photographed with a phase contrast microscope (**A**), with a conventional light microscope (**B**), and using Nomarski differential interference microscopy (**C**). (Use the two pigmented cells for orientation in each image.) × 300. (Courtesy of S Rogers.)

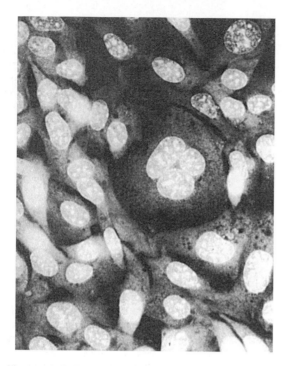

Figure 1–4. Photomicrograph of kidney cell culture transformed by infection with simian virus 40, stained with acridine orange, and photographed with the fluorescence (shown as white in the photo) appearing in the regions containing DNA (nucleus); a reddish-orange color (shown as gray) is characteristic of the RNA-rich cytoplasm. A giant cell is in the center. × 1000. (Courtesy of A Geraldes and JMV Costa.)

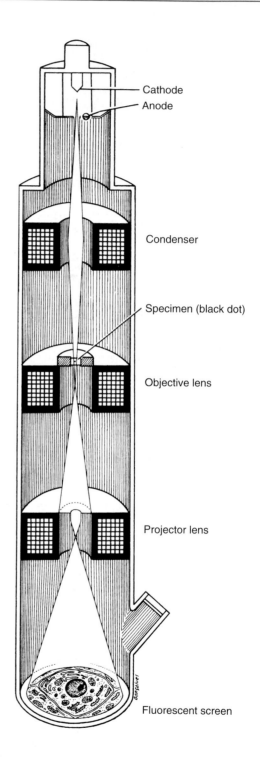

Figure 1–5. Pathway of the electron beam in the electron microscope. The ultrathin section is placed just over the objective electromagnetic lens. The image is projected onto a fluorescent screen and observed directly or through a 10 × magnifying optical system.

tion in glass lenses. Electrons are produced by high-temperature heating of a metallic filament (cathode) in a vacuum. The emitted electrons are then submitted to a potential difference of approximately 60–100 kV or more between the cathode and the anode (Figure 1–5). The anode is a metallic plate with a small hole in its center. Electrons are accelerated from the cathode to the anode. Some of these particles pass through the central opening in the anode, forming a constant stream (or beam) of electrons. The beam is deflected by electromagnetic lenses in a way roughly analogous to what occurs in the optical microscope. Thus, the condenser focuses the beam at the object plane and the objective lens forms an image of the object. The image obtained is further enlarged by one or two projecting lenses and is finally seen on a fluorescent screen or is projected onto photographic plates (Figures 1–5 and 1–6).

Because electron microscopy requires a much thinner section (0.02–0.1 μm), embedding is performed with a hard epoxy plastic. The blocks thus obtained are so hard that glass or diamond knives are usually necessary to section them. Since the electron beam in the microscope cannot penetrate glass, the

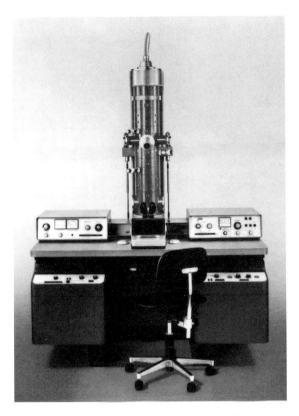

Figure 1–6. Photograph of the Zeiss model EM 10 electron microscope. (Courtesy of Carl Zeiss Co.)

extremely thin sections are collected on small metal grids. Those portions of the section spanning the holes in the mesh of the grid can be examined in the microscope.

Cryofracture (freeze fracture), which is sometimes used with electron microscopy, allows the examination of tissues without the need for fixation and embedding. Although the technique is not artifact-free, there are fewer artifacts than with other methods, and because cellular membranes are often split open, details of their internal structure can also be seen.

SCANNING ELECTRON MICROSCOPY

A variant of electron microscopy, scanning electron microscopy, permits pseudo–three-dimensional views of the surfaces of cells, tissues, and organs. The very narrow (10-nm) electron beam is moved sequentially from point to point across the surface to be examined. At each point, the primary electron beam interacts with a thin metal coating previously applied to the specimen and produces reflected or emitted electrons. The electron signal fluctuation is captured by a detector that modulates the brightness of a cath-

ode ray tube whose electron beam is being moved (scanned) in synchrony with the primary electron beam of the microscope. The resulting photographs are easily understood, since they present a view that appears to be illuminated from above, just as our ordinary macroscopic world is filled with highlights and shadows caused by illumination from above. Scanning electron micrographs are shown in Figures 14–19, 16–14, 16–17, and 17–18.

PROBLEMS IN THE INTERPRETATION OF TISSUE SECTIONS

While studying and interpreting stained tissue sections in microscope preparations, one should remember that the observed product is the end result of a series of processes that considerably distort the image observable in living tissue, mainly through shrinkage. This shrinkage is produced mainly by the heat (60 °C) needed for paraffin embedding; it is virtually eliminated when specimens are embedded in resin. As a consequence of these processes, the spaces frequently seen between cells and other tissue components are artifacts. Furthermore, there is a tendency to think in terms of only two dimensions when examining thin sections, when the structures from which the sections are made actually have three dimensions. To understand the architecture of an organ, one must study sections made in different planes and to reason accordingly (Figure 1–7).

Another difficulty in the study of microscope preparations is the impossibility of differentially staining all tissue components on only one slide. It is therefore necessary to examine several preparations stained by different methods before a general idea of the composition and structure of any type of tissue can be obtained.

AUTORADIOGRAPHY

Autoradiography permits the localization of radioactive substances in tissues by means of the effect of emitted radiation on photographic emulsions. Silver bromide crystals present in the emulsion act as microdetectors of radioactivity. In autoradiography, tissue sections from animals previously treated with radioactive compounds are covered with photographic emulsion and stored in a lightproof box in a refrigerator. After various exposure times the slides are developed photographically and examined. All silver bromide crystals hit by radiation are reduced to small black granules of elemental silver, which reveal the existence of radioactivity in the tissue structures in close proximity to these granules. This procedure can be used in both light and electron microscopy (Figure 1–8).

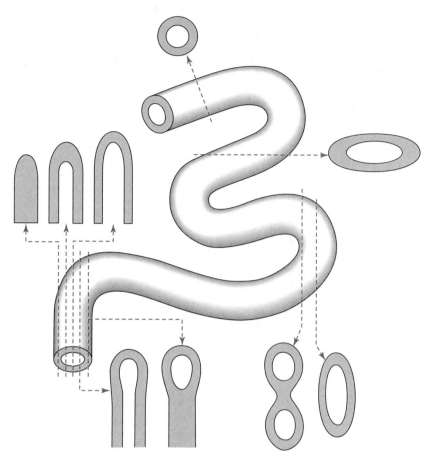

Figure 1–7. Some of the aspects a tube-shaped organ might exhibit when sectioned. The arrows indicate what is seen under the microscope in each particular section plane.

By localizing radioactivity in tissue components it is possible to obtain data on the sequence of events occurring in tissues. Thus, if a radioactive protein precursor (amino acid) is given to a protein-synthesizing cell, its pathway can be followed in the cell after varying periods of time. Furthermore, the intensity of the process is proportional to the number of granules formed over the tissue components.

EXAMINATION OF LIVING CELLS & TISSUES

Cell- and tissue-culture techniques permit direct analysis of cell behavior. Cells and tissues are grown in chemically defined synthetic media to which growth factors, hormones, and serum components are frequently added.

In preparing cultures, cells are usually dispersed mechanically or by previous treatment with enzymes, such as trypsin or collagenase. Once isolated, the cells can be cultivated either in a suspension or spread out on a culture plate to which they can adhere as a single layer of cells (Figure 1–9).

Cell culture has also been used for the study of the metabolism of normal and cancerous cells. This technique is also useful in the study of parasites that grow only within cells, such as viruses, mycoplasma, and some protozoa. The use of extracellular matrix components such as collagens and laminin and the addition of hormones and growth factors greatly increase the survival of cells in vitro. Thanks to these improvements in culture technology, most cell types can now be maintained in the laboratory, an important step in the study of pure cultures of one cell type. Most cells obtained from normal tissues have a finite, genetically programmed life span. Certain changes, however (mainly related to oncogenes; see Chapter 3), can promote cell immortality, a process called **transformation,** which may be a first step in a normal cell's becoming a cancer cell.

In cytogenetic research, tissue cultures are used to study mitoses and chromosomes in human cells. De-

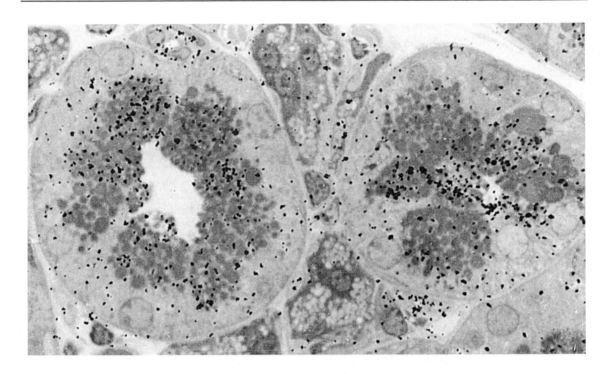

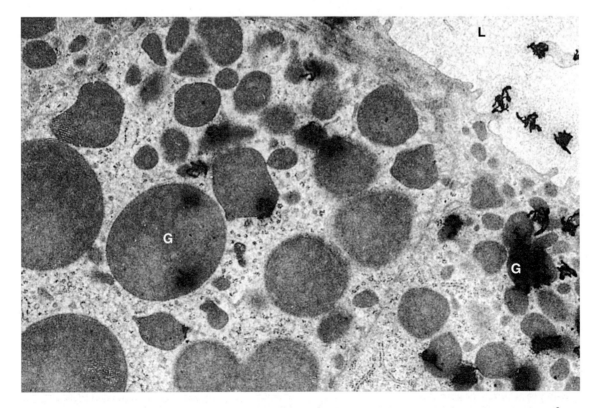

Figure 1–8. Autoradiographs from the submandibular gland of a mouse injected 8 hours before being killed with ^{3}H fucose. **Top:** Photomicrograph showing black silver grains indicating radioactive regions in the cells. Most radioactivity is in the granules of the cells of the granular ducts of the gland. × 500. **Bottom:** The same cells in an electron micrograph. Observe the silver grains that, in this enlargement, appear as coiled structures localized mainly over the granules (G) and in the tubular lumen (L). × 9000. (Courtesy of TG Lima and A Haddad.)

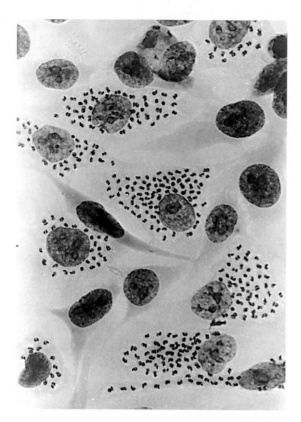

Figure 1–9. Photomicrograph of chicken fibroblasts grown in tissue culture and infected by *Trypanosoma cruzi.* × 340. (Courtesy of S Yoneda.)

termination of human karyotypes (the number and morphology of an individual's chromosomes) is accomplished by the short-term cultivation of blood lymphocytes or of skin fibroblasts.

> In examining these cells during mitotic division in tissue cultures, one can detect anomalies in the number and morphology of the chromosomes. These anomalies have been shown to be related and are diagnostic of numerous diseases collectively called **genetic disorders.**

In addition, cell culture is central to contemporary techniques of molecular biology and recombinant DNA technology.

CELL FRACTIONATION

Cell fractionation is the physical process by which centrifugal force is used to separate organelles and cellular components as a function of their sedimentation coefficients. The sedimentation coefficient of a particle depends on its size, form, and density and on the viscosity of the medium. By means of differential centrifugation, cellular organelles can be isolated and their chemical composition and functions determined in vitro.

Differential centrifugation is achieved by subjecting a suspension of cellular components, obtained by disrupting the cells in a process called **homogenization,** to the action of different centrifugal forces as shown in Figure 1–10. This process results in the production of pure fractions containing different organelles that can be biochemically studied and analyzed for purity in the electron microscope (Figure 1–11). Isolation of cellular components by differential centrifugation allows detailed study of cellular components obtained in a relatively pure state; eg, nuclei, nucleoli, mitochondria, rough endoplasmic reticula, ribosomes, secretory granules, and pigment granules.

HISTOCHEMISTRY & CYTOCHEMISTRY

The terms **histochemistry** and **cytochemistry** are used mainly to indicate methods for localizing different substances in tissue sections. Several procedures are used to obtain this type of information, most of them based on specific chemical reactions or on high-affinity interactions between macromolecules. Both methods usually produce insoluble colored or electron-dense compounds that enable the localization of specific substances by means of light or electron microscopy. Several ions (eg, iron, phosphate) have been localized in tissue (Figure 1–12) with these methods. The identification of organic molecules through chemical reactions is discussed below.

Nucleic Acids

DNA can be identified and quantified in cell nuclei using the Feulgen reaction, which produces a red color in the presence of DNA. The reaction for both DNA- and RNA-induced basophilia can be abolished by previous digestion of sections with DNase or RNase, however.

Proteins

Although chemical methods do not permit localization of specific proteins in cells and tissues, the immunohistochemical methods presented later in this chapter can do so. Specific enzymes, such as RNase, DNase, collagenase, and elastase, that digest cell and tissue components are used extensively to analyze the distribution of certain cell and tissue elements.

Polysaccharides & Oligosaccharides

Polysaccharides in the body occur either in a free state or combined with proteins and lipids. In the combined state, they constitute an extremely complex heterogeneous group. A ubiquitous polysaccharide in the body, not bound to a protein or lipid, is

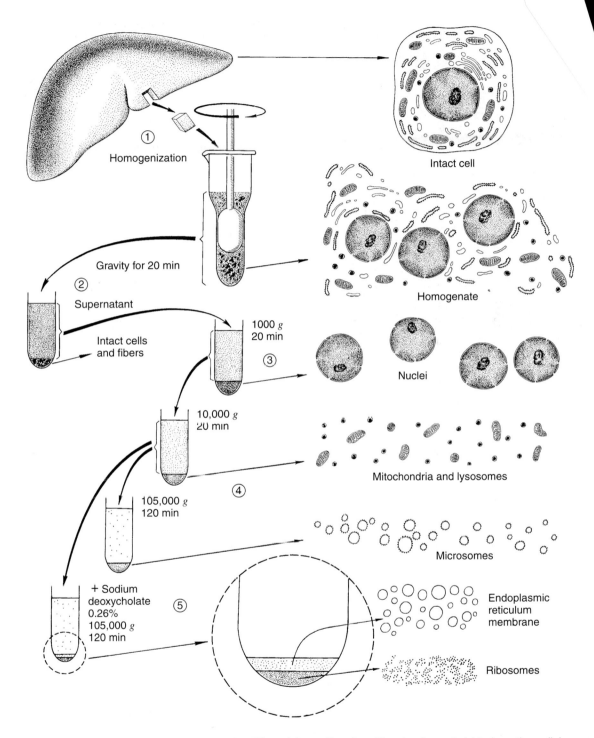

Figure 1–10. Isolation of cell constituents by differential centrifugation. The drawings at right show the cellular organelles at the bottom of each tube after centrifugation. Centrifugal force is expressed by *g*, which is equivalent to the force of gravity. (**1**) Small fragments of an organ are processed in a homogenizer, where a glass rod breaks cell membranes, liberating the cellular components into an inert sucrose or soluble plastic solution. (**2**) The suspension rests and large intact tissue remnants form a sediment. (**3**) The supernatant is centrifuged with weak force to create a sediment of the denser particles (nuclei). (**4**) By repeating this operation and increasing the centrifugal force in each step, it is possible to isolate mitochondria, lysosomes, rough endoplasmic reticulum (RER), etc. (**5**) With the addition of a detergent (deoxycholate) to the RER fraction and the addition of a very strong centrifugal force, it is possible to obtain pure ribosomes. (Redrawn and reproduced, with permission, from Bloom W, Fawcett DW: *A Textbook of Histology,* 9th ed. Saunders, 1968.)

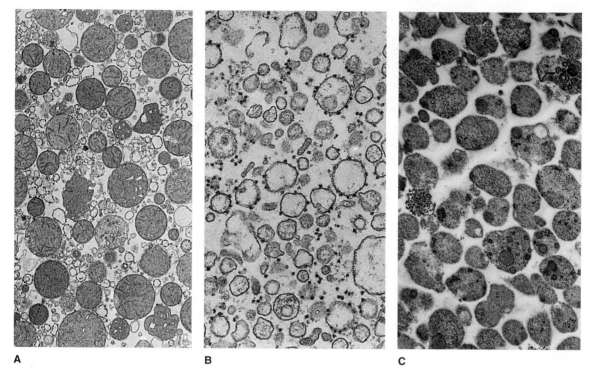

A   **B**   **C**

Figure 1–11. Electron micrographs of three cell fractions isolated by density gradient centrifugation. **A:** Mitochondrial fraction, contaminated with microsomes. × 13,000. **B:** Microsomal fraction. × 42,500. **C:** Lysosomal fraction. × 25,000. (Courtesy of P Baudhuin.)

glycogen, which can be demonstrated by the periodic acid–Schiff (PAS) reaction. The PAS reaction, based on the oxidative action of periodic acid (HIO_4) on 1,2-glycol groups present in the glucose residues, gives rise to aldehyde groups that react with Schiff's reagent, producing a new complex compound with a purple or magenta color. This can be seen in the light microscope; such substances are called PAS-positive. Since other PAS-positive substances occur in cells, the specificity of this reaction depends on pretreatment with a glycogenolytic enzyme (eg, salivary amylase). Structures that stain intensely with the PAS reaction but fail to do so after pretreatment with amylase contain glycogen. By this method, the presence of glycogen can be demonstrated in normal liver and striated muscle.

A variety of strongly anionic, unbranched long-chain polysaccharides containing aminated monosaccharides (amino sugars) constitute the **glycosaminoglycans.** These substances contain chains of repeating disaccharide units containing an N-acetylated hexosamine coupled to uronic acid. Complexes of covalently bound glycosaminoglycans inserted at regular intervals along a protein core constitute the proteoglycans. In proteoglycans, which are significant constituents of connective tissue matrices (see Chapters 5 and 7), the carbohydrate moieties constitute the major component of the molecule.

The general term **glycoconjugates** is used for the wide variety of sugar-containing macromolecules in the body and is applied to glycoproteins and glycolipids as well as proteoglycans. Glycoproteins differ from proteoglycans in several major ways: Their molecules are generally smaller than those of proteoglycans; their carbohydrate moieties contain fewer sugar residues. These moieties are usually termed **oligosaccharides** rather than polysaccharides. The oligosaccharide chains of glycoproteins are often branched, whereas the polysaccharides of proteoglycans are more likely to be unbranched. In addition, the glycoprotein oligosaccharides are characterized by wide variability in the types and order of the individual sugars in the chain, while the polysaccharides of proteoglycans generally are much less diverse.

Glycoproteins such as thyroglobulin (present in the thyroid gland) and gonadotropins of the pituitary contain a high proportion of protein. Other glycoproteins with a low protein content, such as those produced by some epithelial cells, are identified as mucous substances that have a protective and lubricating function. Some glycoproteins (eg, neutral glycoproteins) contain no acidic groups; others (eg, acid mu-

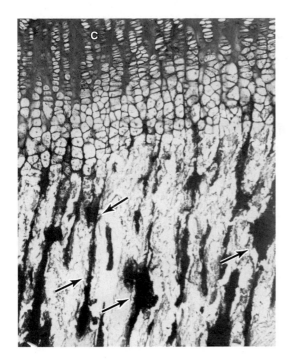

Figure 1–12. Photomicrograph of a section from the epiphysis of a bone treated with silver nitrate and subsequently reduced by hydroquinone. The black precipitate in the ossified tissue (arrows) indicates the presence of calcium phosphate. Nonreacting cartilage tissue (C) lies in the upper portion of the section. × 120.

cous substances) have limited amounts of carboxy sulfate radicals. In contrast to glycoproteins, glycoaminoglycans and acidic glycoproteins are strongly anionic because of their high content of carboxyl and sulfate groups. For this reason, they react strongly with the alcian blue dye (Figure 1–13). Neutral glycoproteins can be identified in tissue sections by the fact that they react with PAS but are not digested by incubation with a glycogenolytic enzyme. Using specific enzymes that digest proteoglycans and some glycoprotein components allows these substances to be distinguished in tissue sections.

Glycolipids are characteristic constituents of most cell membranes and are significant components of the plasma membranes of nerve cells (eg, gangliosides, cerebrosides). The carbohydrate moieties of glycolipids are oligosaccharides that are similar to those of glycoproteins.

Lipids

Lipids are best revealed with dyes that are more soluble in lipids than in the medium in which the dye is dissolved. In this process, frozen sections are immersed in alcoholic solutions saturated with the appropriate dye. The stain then migrates from the alco-

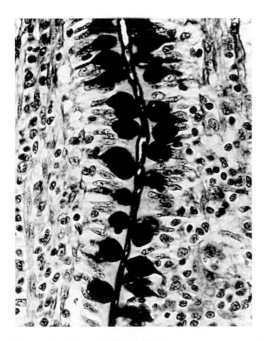

Figure 1–13. Photomicrograph of an intestinal villus stained by alcian blue. Staining is intense in the goblet cells because of their high content of acidic glycoproteins. × 400.

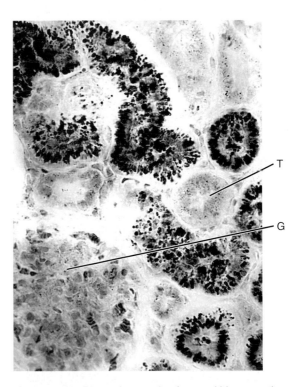

Figure 1–14. Photomicrograph of a rat kidney section treated by the Gomori method for acid phosphatase. The lysosomes stain intensely as dark granules in proximal convoluted tubule cells. The glomeruli (G) and other tubular cells (T) do not have enzymatic activity. × 400.

hol to the cellular lipid droplets. The dyes most commonly used for this purpose are Sudan IV and Sudan black; they confer red and black colors, respectively, on the lipids. Additional methods used for the localization of cholesterol and its esters, phospholipids, and glycolipids are useful in diagnosing metabolic diseases in which there are intracellular accumulations of different kinds of lipids.

> Many histochemical procedures are used frequently in laboratory diagnosis: Perls' reaction for iron, the PAS-amylase and alcian blue reactions for glycogen and glycosaminoglycans, and the reactions for lipids are routinely used in biopsies of tissue taken from patients with diseases that result in the storage of iron (eg, hemochromatosis, hemosiderosis), glycogen (glycogenosis), glycosaminoglycans (mucopolysaccharidosis), and sphingolipids (sphingolipidosis) in tissues.

Enzymes

Several histochemical methods are used to reveal and identify enzymes. Most enzymatic histochemical procedures are based on the production of intensely stained or electron-dense precipitates at the site of enzymatic activity. Three examples of enzymes that can be shown by either the light or the electron microscope are described below.

A. Acid Phosphatase: The Gomori method of demonstrating acid phosphatase activity consists of incubating formalin-fixed tissue sections in a solution containing sodium glycerophosphate and lead nitrate buffered to pH 5.0. The enzyme hydrolyzes the glycerophosphate, liberating phosphate ions that react with lead nitrate to produce an insoluble, electron-dispersing, colorless precipitate of lead phosphate at the site of the enzymatic activity. In a second step, the preparation is immersed in a solution of ammonium sulfide that reacts with the lead phosphate to produce a black precipitate of lead sulfide. This method permits the localization of this enzyme's activity and is frequently used to demonstrate **lysosomes,** cytoplasmic organelles that contain acid phosphatase (Figures 1–14 and 1–15). The ammonium sulfide step is omitted when the tissue is to be examined in the electron microscope.

B. Dehydrogenases: These enzymes remove

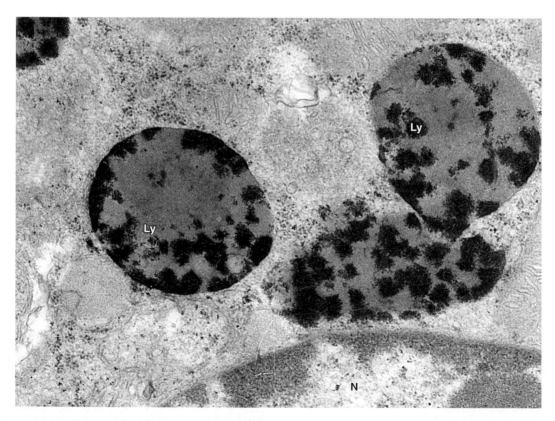

Figure 1–15. Electron micrograph of a rat kidney cell previously treated by the Gomori method for acid phosphatase. The three dark, rounded structures above the nucleus (N) are lysosomes (Ly). The dense heterogeneous precipitate within these structures is lead phosphate, which scatters the electrons. The information in this electron micrograph is equivalent to that in the light micrograph illustrated in Fig 1–14. × 25,000. (Courtesy of E Katchburian.)

hydrogen from one substrate and transfer it to another. There are many dehydrogenases in the body; they play an important role in several metabolic processes and can be distinguished by the substrate on which they act. The histochemical demonstration of dehydrogenases consists of incubating nonfixed tissue sections in a substrate solution containing tetrazole, a weakly colored soluble H^+ acceptor. The enzyme transports hydrogen from the substrate to the tetrazole and reduces it to an intensely colored insoluble compound called **formazan,** which precipitates at the site of the enzymatic activity. By this method, succinate dehydrogenase—a key enzyme in the citric acid (Krebs) cycle—can be localized in mitochondria (Figure 1–16).

C. Peroxidase: Peroxidase, which is present in several types of cells, promotes the oxidation of certain substrates with the transfer of hydrogen ions to hydrogen peroxide, forming molecules of water.

In this method, sections of adequately fixed tissue are incubated in a solution containing hydrogen peroxide and 3,3'-*d*iamino*azob*enzidine (DAB). The latter compound is oxidized in the presence of peroxidase, resulting in an insoluble, black, electron-dense precipitate that permits the localization of peroxidase activity in optical and electron microscopes. Since

the enzyme is extremely active, it produces an appreciable amount of insoluble precipitate in a short time, making this procedure a very sensitive histochemical assay. The DAB method is probably one of the most commonly used techniques of histochemistry, since it detects both the peroxidase activity in blood cells (important in the diagnosis of leukemias) and the peroxidase used as a label in lectin histochemistry, immunocytochemistry, and in hybridization methods.

IMMUNOCYTOCHEMISTRY

High-affinity interactions between macromolecules are the basis of such important techniques as lectin histochemistry, immunohistochemistry, and in situ hybridization.

These methods permit the study of the presence and activity of specific macromolecules in cells and tissues. In addition, these interactions are reversible and do not depend on classic chemical bonds. The

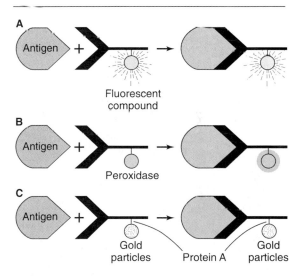

Figure 1–17. Three current methods of labeling and identifying specific proteins by immunocytochemistry. **A:** The antibody is coupled with a fluorescent compound, such as fluorescein isothiocyanate or rhodamine. After incubation, the sections containing the antigen exposed to the labeled antibody solution are studied in the fluorescence microscope. **B:** The antibody is coupled with peroxidase. After the antigen-antibody reaction, the section is submitted to the histochemical method for peroxidase and studied with the light or electron microscope (see text). **C:** The antibody is coupled with gold particles previously bound to protein A. This protein reacts with and labels the antibody. Preparations obtained by this method can also be studied by light and electron microscopy. The gold-particle–protein-A method is currently one of the most efficient and precise immunocytochemical methods.

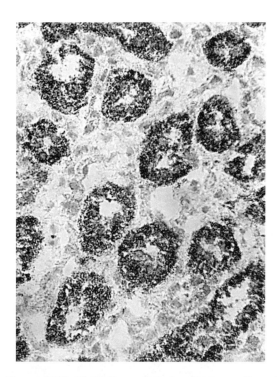

Figure 1–16. Photomicrograph of a frozen section of fresh, nonfixed kidney previously incubated in succinate plus monotetrazole. The dark precipitate seen in the tubules indicates the activity of succinate dehydrogenase. × 400. (Courtesy of AGE Pearse.)

best-studied example is the antigen-antibody interaction. High-affinity interactions are also used to locate segments of nucleic acids (hybridization) and specific carbohydrate moieties (lectin binding). Other high-affinity interactions provide molecular probes for macromolecules (eg, phalloidin interacts with actin in microfilaments).

Methods using labeled antibodies have proved most useful in localizing specific proteins and certain other macromolecules such as nucleic acids and polysaccharides. These tests are based on the reaction of the body when exposed to foreign substances called **antigens** or **immunogens.** The body responds by producing proteins—**antibodies**—that react specifically and bind strongly to the antigen and thus neutralize the foreign substance. Antibodies are proteins of the globulin group (immunoglobulins) that appear in plasma and tissue fluids after antigen injection. Their production enables the organism to oppose invasion by foreign microorganisms and to eliminate certain proteins and other foreign matter not recognized as self. Immunocytochemistry is based on the coupling of immunoglobulins to substances that render them visible in the microscope without causing a loss of the antibody's biologic activity. Since the labeled immunoglobulins bind only to their antigens, these compounds permit localization of specific antigens in tissue specimens. When a tissue section containing certain antigens is incubated in a solution containing labeled antibodies to these antigens, the antibodies bind specifically to the antigens, whose location can then be seen with either the light or electron microscope.

Methods of Labeling Antibodies

Three methods of labeling antibodies are frequently used (Figure 1–17).

- **Coupling with a fluorescent compound**—This permits the identification of the site of specific antigens by using a fluorescence microscope (Figures 1–17A and 1–18).
- **Coupling with an enzyme**—This permits detection of the labeled antibody by means of conventional enzyme cytochemistry. The enzyme most often used is peroxidase, which can be detected by the method described above by using either the light or electron microscope (Figures 1–17B and 1–19).
- **Coupling with a colored electron-scattering compound that can be detected in light and electron microscopes**—Gold particles that can be

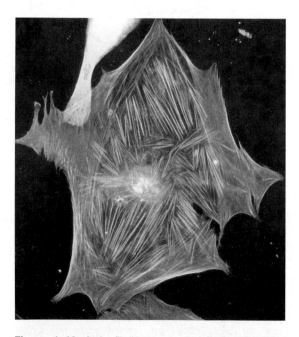

Figure 1–18. Actin fibrils composed of aggregates of actin filaments in the cytoplasm of a cultured human fibroblast preincubated in fluorescent actin antibody. × 1767. (Reproduced, with permission, from E Lazarides: J Cell Biol 1975;65:549.)

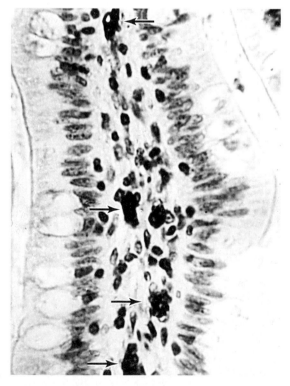

Figure 1–19. Photomicrograph of an intestinal villus showing macrophages stained by the immunoperoxidase method by using antilysozyme antibodies (arrows). × 400.

easily observed in both types of microscopy are at present the most commonly used label (Figures 1–17C, 1–20, and 21–15).

Methods of Localizing Antigens

There are both direct and indirect methods for antigen localization by immunocytochemistry (Figure 1–21).

- **Direct method**—Sections of a tissue suspected of containing an antigen (protein x) are incubated with a labeled antibody to x, and the antibody will specifically combine with x. The excess antibody is washed off, and the tissue is processed according to the methods outlined above. The location of the antigen is then detected with the fluorescence microscope (Figure 1–21A).

- **Indirect method**—Antibodies to protein x are produced in an animal, eg, a rabbit. Rabbit immunoglobulins are, in turn, capable of inducing an antibody response in another animal, such as a sheep or a goat, thus producing an anti-antibody (anti-immunoglobulin). A tissue section containing protein x is incubated with unlabeled rabbit anti-x antibodies. After washing, labeled rabbit anti-antibodies are added, and the location of protein x can be seen using a microscopic technique appropriate for the label. This method (Figure 1–21B) has an advantage in that the technique is considerably more sensitive than the direct method (Figure 1–21A).

Several variations of immunocytochemical methods have been developed that permit both specificity and sensitivity. The gold-particle–protein-A method (Figure 1–20) has been widely used and has contributed significantly to research in cell biology and to the improvement of medical diagnostic procedures. Table 1–3 shows some of the routine applications of immunocytochemical procedures in clinical practice.

HYBRIDIZATION TECHNIQUES

The central challenge in modern cell biology is to understand the workings of the cell in molecular detail. This goal requires techniques that permit analysis of the molecules involved in the process of infor-

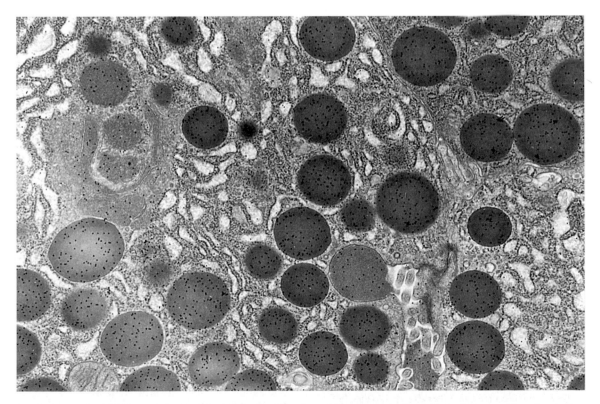

Figure 1–20. Section of a pancreatic acinar cell stained by the gold-particle–protein-A method after previous incubation with antiamylase antibody. The gold particles appear as very small black dots over the mature secretory granules and forming granules in the Golgi complex. (Courtesy of M Bendayan.)

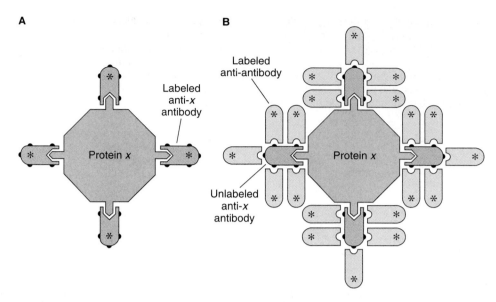

Figure 1–21. The direct (**A**) and indirect (**B**) techniques of immunocytochemistry. In the direct technique, a labeled anti-*x* antibody binds to an antigen present in the cells. In this case, each antigen molecule binds a few antibody molecules. In the first step of the indirect technique, unlabeled anti-*x* antibody is bound to the antigen; in the second step, the labeled anti-antibody then binds to the anti-*x* antibody. Because each anti-*x* antibody binds several molecules of labeled anti-antibody, the indirect procedure is more sensitive than the direct method.

mation flow from DNA to protein. These techniques include **Southern analysis,** which characterizes and quantifies the presence of DNA of a specific gene in the presence of all other genes in a eukaryotic organism; **Northern analysis,** which identifies and quanti-

Table 1–3. Partial list of the most commonly used proteins (antigens) important for the immunocytochemical diagnosis and subsequent treatment of disease.

Antigens	Diagnosis
Intermediate filament proteins Cytokeratins	Undifferentiated tumors of epithelial origin, carcinomas, adenocarcinomas
Glial fibrillary acid protein	Tumors of some glial cells
Vimentin	Tumors of connective tissue
Desmin	Muscle tumors
Other proteins Virtually all protein or polypeptide hormones	Protein or polypeptide hormone–producing tumors
Carcinoembryonic antigen (CEA)	Glandular tumors, mainly of the digestive tract and breast
Prostate-specific antigen	Prostate gland tumors
Steroid hormone receptors	Breast duct–cell tumors
Antigens produced by viruses	Specific virus infections

fies specific messenger RNA (mRNA) transcripts in the presence of all RNA transcripts expressed within a single cell type; and **Western analysis,** which detects a single protein species from among all other proteins expressed in a single cell or tissue. Southern and Northern analyses are based on the high affinity between complementary sequences of nucleic acids (**hybridization**). Western analysis is based on the high affinity and specificity between antibodies and antigens.

Nucleic acid hybridization is the technique that allows the identification of specific sequences of DNA or RNA based on the ability of single-stranded segments of these nucleic acids to bind specifically to previously labeled, known, complementary single-stranded nucleic acid sequences. These sequences, produced in the laboratory, are called **probes** and are usually labeled by radioisotopes or by the coupling of their nucleotides with biotin. The isotope-labeled probe can then be detected using autoradiography, and the biotin-labeled probe can be identified by its high affinity for avidin. Avidin was previously coupled with peroxidase, and in a further step, the peroxidase is detected by means of the DAB method currently used in immunohistochemistry.

When applied directly to cells and tissues, hybridization is called **in situ hybridization** (Figure 1–22). Through in situ hybridization one can localize specific DNA sequences (such as genes) or RNA. This technique can be applied to tissue sections,

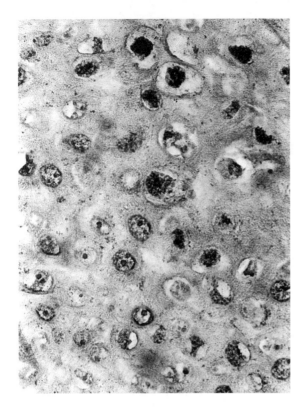

Figure 1–22. Photomicrograph of a section of human epithelial tumor (condyloma) in which in situ hybridization with the DNA of the human papilloma virus type II (HPVII) was performed. Observe dark staining in several nuclei; this indicates the presence of the virus genome in this tumor, suggesting its possible participation in the genesis of the tumor. (Courtesy of JE Levi.)

smears, or chromosomes of squashed mitotic cells, and it permits the localization of specific DNA (eg, cellular or viral genes) or gene expression, through the presence of mRNA in whole cells or cell components. The technique is highly specific and is routinely used in research, clinical diagnosis, and forensic medicine.

LECTIN HISTOCHEMISTRY

Lectins are proteins derived mainly from plant seeds that bind to cell-surface carbohydrates with high affinity and specificity. Different lectins bind to specific sequences of sugar residues. They bind to cell-surface glycoproteins, proteoglycans, and glycolipids and are widely used to characterize membrane molecules containing specific sequences of sugar residues. Lectins are usually labeled with peroxidase to make possible their identification and location by means of histochemical techniques for peroxidase.

REFERENCES

Alberts B et al: *Molecular Biology of the Cell,* 3rd ed. Garland, 1994.

Baak, JPA, *Manual of Quantitative Pathology in Cancer Diagnosis and Prognosis.* Springer-Verlag, 1991.

Bancroft JD, Stevens A: *Theory and Practice of Histological Techniques,* 2nd ed. Churchill Livingstone, 1990.

Bendayan M: Protein A–gold electron microscopic immunocytochemistry. Methods, applications and limitations. J Electron Microsc Techn 1984;1:243.

Cuello ACC: *Immunocytochemistry.* Wiley, 1983.

Darnell J, Lodish H, Baltimore D: *Molecular Cell Biology,* 2nd ed. Sci Am Books, 1990.

Everhart TE, Hayes TL: The scanning electron microscope. Sci Am 1972;226:54.

Hayat MA: *Stains and Cytochemical Methods.* Plenum. 1993.

James J: *Light Microscopic Techniques in Biology and Medicine.* Martinus Nijhoff, 1976.

Murray RK et al: *Harpers Biochemistry,* 22nd ed. Appleton & Lange, 1990.

Pease AGE: *Histochemistry: Theoretical and Applied,* 4th ed. Churchill Livingstone, 1980.

Rogers AW: *Techniques of Autoradiography,* 3rd ed. Elsevier, 1979.

Spencer M: *Fundamentals of Light Microscopy.* Cambridge Univ Press, 1982.

Stolinski C, Breathnack AS: *Freeze-Fracture Replication of Biological Tissues.* Academic Press, 1975.

Stoward PJ, Polak JM (editors): *Histochemistry: The Widening Horizons of Its Applications in Biological Sciences.* Wiley, 1981.

Wischnitzer S: *Introduction to Electron Microscopy.* Pergamon, 1981.

2

The Cytoplasm

Cells are the structural units of all living organisms. There are two fundamentally different types of cells, but so many biochemical similarities exist between them that some investigators have postulated that one group evolved from the other.

The **prokaryotic** (Gr. *pro,* before, + *karyon,* nucleus) cell is found only in bacteria. These cells are small (1–5 μm long), usually have a cell wall outside the plasmalemma, and lack a nuclear envelope separating the genetic material (DNA) from other cellular constituents. In addition, prokaryotes have no histones (specific basic proteins) bound to their DNA and usually no membranous organelles.

In contrast, **eukaryotic** (Gr. *eu,* good, + *karyon*) cells are larger and have a distinct nucleus surrounded by a nuclear envelope (Figure 2–1). Histones are associated with the genetic material, and numerous membrane-limited organelles are found in the cytoplasm. This book is concerned almost exclusively with eukaryotic cells.

CELLULAR DIFFERENTIATION

During the process of evolution, the cells of metazoa gradually became modified and specialized, resulting in increased functional efficiency. Through phylogenetic development, undifferentiated primitive cells that performed several functions, each with little efficiency, were transformed into a variety of differentiated cells able to perform some specific functions with much greater efficiency. This process of cell specialization is known as **cell differentiation.**

Cell differentiation is also an important process during the development of embryos. For example, muscle cell precursors elongate into spindle-shaped cells that synthesize and accumulate myofibrillar proteins. The resulting cell efficiently converts chemical energy into contractile force.

Morphologic modifications during differentiation are accompanied by chemical changes. In the example given, formation of the muscle cell results from the synthesis of several specific proteins, such as actin and myosin. The main cellular functions performed by specialized cells in the body are listed in Table 2–1.

Cells are not always restricted to a single activity and frequently perform two or more specialized functions. For example, intestinal epithelial cells both absorb nutrients and synthesize digestive enzymes, such as disaccharidases and peptidases (see Chapter 15).

CELL ECOLOGY

Cells, like all living creatures, respond and adapt to their environment. Since the body experiences considerable environmental diversity (eg, normal and pathological conditions), it is not surprising that the same cell type can be found exhibiting different characteristics and behaviors in different regions and circumstances. Thus, macrophages and neutrophils (both of which are phagocytic defense cells) will shift from oxidative metabolism to glycolysis in an anoxic, inflammatory environment. Because of their diverse library of receptors, breast fibroblasts and uterine smooth muscle cells are exceptionally sensitive to female sex hormones. In contrast, cartilage and bone cells are sensitive to local biochemical stimuli. Cells that appear to be structurally similar may react in different ways because they have different families of receptors for signaling molecules (such as hormones and extracellular matrix macromolecules).

CELL COMPONENTS

The cell is composed of two basic parts: **cytoplasm** (Gr. *kytos,* cell, + *plasma,* thing formed) and **nucleus** (L. *nux,* nut). Individual cytoplasmic components are usually not clearly distinguishable in common hematoxylin-and-eosin–stained preparations; the nucleus, however, appears intensely stained dark blue or black (see Figure 4–1).

Cytoplasm

The outermost component of the cell, separating the cytoplasm from its extracellular environment, is

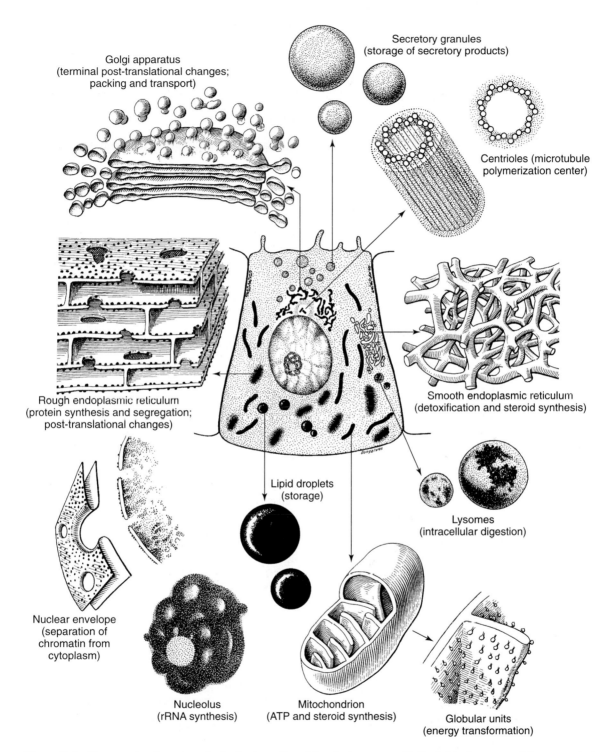

Figure 2–1. Diagram showing a hypothetical eukaryotic cell (**center**) as seen with the light microscope. It is surrounded by its various structures as seen with the electron microscope. (Redrawn and reproduced, with permission, from Bloom W, Fawcett DW: *A Textbook of Histology,* 9th ed. Saunders, 1968.)

Table 2–1. Cellular functions in some specialized cells.

Function	Specialized Cell(s)
Movement	Muscle cell
Conductivity	Nerve cell
Synthesis and secretion of enzymes	Pancreatic acinar cells
Synthesis and secretion of mucous substances	Mucous-gland cells
Synthesis and secretion of steroids	Some adrenal gland, testis, and ovary cells
Ion transport	Cells of the kidney and salivary gland ducts
Intracellular digestion	Macrophages and some white blood cells
Transformation of physical and chemical stimuli into nervous impulses	Sensory cells
Metabolite absorption	Cells of the intestine, kidney, etc

the **plasma membrane** (**plasmalemma**). The cytoplasm itself is composed of a matrix, or **cytosol,** in which are embedded several membrane-bound components, called **organelles,** plus **deposits** of carbohydrates, lipids, and pigments.

The cytoplasm of eukaryotic cells is divided into several distinct compartments by membranes that regulate the intracellular traffic of ions and molecules. These compartments concentrate enzymes and the respective substrates, thus increasing the efficiency of the cell.

Plasma Membrane

All eukaryotic cells are enveloped by a limiting membrane composed of phospholipids, cholesterol, proteins, and oligosaccharides covalently linked to other phospholipid and protein molecules. The cell, or plasma, membrane functions as a selective barrier that regulates the passage of certain materials into and out of the cell and facilitates the transport of specific molecules. One important role of the cell membrane is to keep constant the intracellular milieu, which is different from the extracellular fluid. Membranes also carry out a number of specific recognition and regulatory functions (to be discussed later), playing an important role in the interactions of the cell with its environment.

Membranes range from 7.5 to 10 nm in thickness and consequently are visible only in the electron microscope. Electron micrographs reveal that the plasmalemma—and, for that matter, all other organellar membranes—exhibit a trilaminar structure after fixation in osmium tetroxide (Figure 2–2). Because all membranes have this appearance, the three-layered structure has been designated the **unit membrane** (Figure 2–3). The three layers seen in the electron microscope are apparently produced by the deposit of reduced osmium on the hydrophilic groups present on each side of the lipid bilayer.

Membrane phospholipids, such as phosphatidylcholine (lecithin) and phosphatidylethanolamine (cephalin), consist of two long, nonpolar (hydrophobic) hydrocarbon chains linked to a charged (hydrophilic) head group. Cholesterol is also a constituent of cell membranes. Within the membrane, phospholipids are most stable when organized into a double layer with their hydrophobic (nonpolar) chains directed toward the center of the membrane and their hydrophilic (charged) heads directed outward (Figure 2–2). The lipid composition of each half of the bilayer is different. For example, in red blood cells (erythrocytes), phosphatidylcholine and sphingomyelin are more abundant in the outer half of the membrane, whereas phosphatidylserine and phosphatidylethanolamine are more concentrated in the inner half. Some of the lipids, known as glycolipids, possess oligosaccharide chains that extend outward from the surface of the cell membrane and thus contribute to the lipid asymmetry (Figures 2–4A and 2–5).

Proteins, which are a major molecular constituent

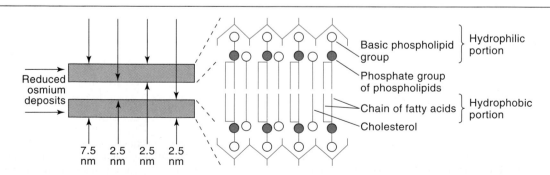

Figure 2–2. The ultrastructure and molecular organization (**right**) of the cell membrane. The dark lines at left represent the two dense layers observed in the electron microscope; these are caused by the deposit of osmium in the hydrophilic portions of the phospholipid molecules.

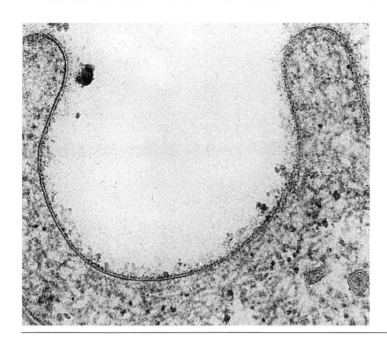

Figure 2–3. Electron micrograph of a section of the surface of an epithelial cell, showing the unit membrane with its two dark lines enclosing a clear band. The granular material on the surface of the membrane is the cell coat. × 100,000.

of membranes (about 50% w/w in the plasma membrane), can be divided into two groups. **Integral proteins** are directly incorporated within the lipid bilayer, whereas **peripheral proteins** exhibit a looser association with membrane surfaces. The loosely bound peripheral proteins can be easily extracted from cell membranes with salt solutions, whereas integral proteins can be extracted only by drastic methods that use detergents. Some integral proteins span the membrane one or more times, from one side to the other. Accordingly, they are called **one-pass** or **multipass transmembrane proteins** (Figure 2–5).

Freeze-fracture electron-microscope studies indicate that many integral proteins are distributed as globular molecules intercalated among the lipid molecules (Figure 2–4B). Some of these proteins are only partially embedded in the lipid bilayer, so that they may protrude from either the outer or inner surface. Other proteins are large enough to extend across the two lipid layers and protrude from both membrane surfaces (transmembrane proteins). The carbohydrate moieties of glycoproteins and glycolipids project from the external surface of the plasma membrane; they are important components of specific molecules called **receptors** that participate in important interactions such as cell adhesion, recognition, and response to protein hormones. As with lipids, the distribution of membrane proteins is different in the two surfaces of the cell membranes. Therefore, all membranes in the cell are asymmetric.

Integration of the proteins within the lipid bilayer is mainly the result of hydrophobic interactions between the lipids and nonpolar amino acids present on the outer shell of the integral proteins. Some integral proteins are not bound rigidly in place and are able to move within the plane of the cell membrane (Figure 2–6). Under certain circumstances, these proteins can accumulate at one region of the plasma membrane, occasionally forming a localized aggregation of proteins. This process, called **capping,** has been observed in some cell types and is controlled by cytoskeletal actin microfilaments and other proteins. However, unlike lipids, most membrane proteins are restricted in their lateral diffusion by attachment to the cytoskeletal components. In most epithelial cells, the tight junctions (see Chapter 4) prevent lateral diffusion of transmembrane proteins and even the diffusion of membrane lipids of the outer leaflet.

The mosaic disposition of membrane proteins, in conjunction with the fluid nature of the lipid bilayer, constitutes the basis of the **fluid mosaic model** for membrane structure shown in Figure 2–4A. Membrane proteins are synthesized in the rough endoplasmic reticulum; their molecules are completed in the Golgi apparatus; and they are transported in vesicles to the cell surface (Figure 2–7).

The plasma membrane is the site where materials are exchanged between the cell and its environment. Some ions, such as Na^+, K^+, and Ca^{2+}, are transported across the cell membrane through integral membrane proteins, using energy from the breakdown of adenosine triphosphate (ATP). Mass transfer of material also occurs through the plasma membrane. This bulk uptake of material is known as **endocytosis** (Gr. *endon,* within, + *kytos*). The corresponding name for release of material in bulk is

A. Carbohydrate chains bound to lipids and proteins

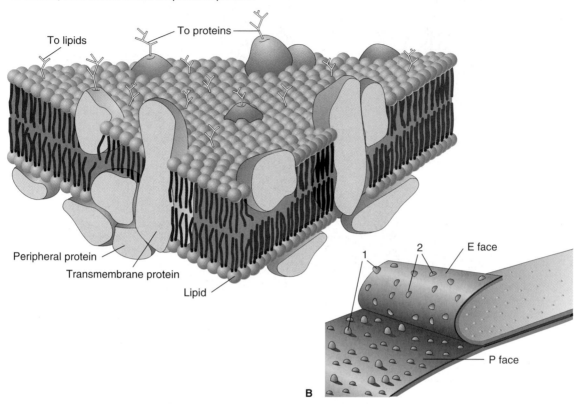

B

Figure 2–4. A: The fluid mosaic model of membrane structure. The membrane consists of a phospholipid double layer with proteins inserted in it (integral proteins) or bound to the cytoplasmic surface (peripheral proteins). Integral membrane proteins are firmly embedded in the lipid layers. Some of these proteins completely span the bilayer and are called transmembrane proteins, whereas others are embedded in either the outer or inner leaflet of the lipid bilayer. The dotted line in the integral membrane protein is the region where hydrophobic amino acids interact with the hydrophobic portions of the membrane. Many of the proteins and lipids have externally exposed oligosaccharide chains. **B:** Membrane cleavage occurs when a cell is frozen and fractured (cryofracture). Most of the membrane particles (**1**), are proteins or aggregates of proteins that remain attached to the half of the membrane adjacent to the cytoplasm (P, or protoplasmic, face of the membrane). Fewer particles are found attached to the outer half of the membrane (E, or extracellular, face). For every protein particle that bulges on one surface, a corresponding depression (**2**) appears in the opposite surface. Membrane splitting occurs along the line of weakness formed by the fatty acid tails of membrane phospholipids, since only weak hydrophobic interactions bind the halves of the membrane along this line. (Modified and reproduced, with permission, from Krstić RV: *Ultrastructure of the Mammalian Cell.* Springer-Verlag, 1979.)

exocytosis. However, at the molecular level, exocytosis and endocytosis are different processes that utilize different protein molecules; one is not the exact reverse of the other.

A. Fluid-Phase Pinocytosis: In fluid-phase pinocytosis, small invaginations of the cell membrane form and entrap extracellular fluid and anything in solution in the fluid. **Pinocytotic vesicles** (about 80 nm in diameter) pinch off from the cell surface (Figure 4–18), and most eventually fuse with lysosomes (see the section on lysosomes later in this chapter). In the lining cells of capillaries (endothelial cells), however, pinocytotic vesicles may move to the surface opposite their origin. There they fuse with the

plasma membrane and release their contents onto the cell surface, thus accomplishing bulk transfer of material across the cell (Figure 11–4).

B. Receptor-Mediated Endocytosis: Receptors for many substances, such as low-density lipoproteins and protein hormones, are located at the cell surface. The receptors are either originally widely dispersed over the surface or aggregated in special regions called **coated pits.** Binding of the ligand (a molecule with high affinity for a receptor) to its receptor causes widely dispersed receptors to accumulate in coated pits. The coating on the cytoplasmic surface of the membrane is composed of several polypeptides, the major one being clathrin (molecular

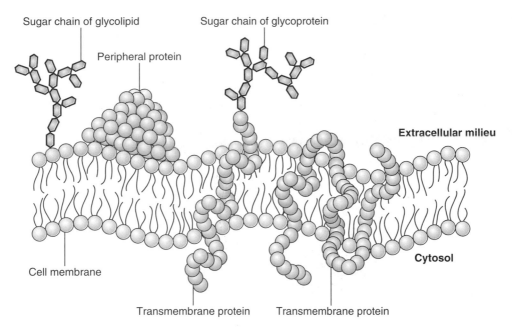

Figure 2–5. Schematic drawing of the molecular structure of the plasma membrane. Note the one-pass and multipass transmembrane proteins. The drawing shows a peripheral protein in the external face of the membrane, but the proteins are present mainly in the cytoplasmic face, as shown in Figure 2–4. (Redrawn and reproduced, with permission, from Junqueira LC, Carneiro J: *Biologia Celular e Molecular,* 6th ed. Editora Guanabara, 1997.)

mass 180 kDa). These proteins form a lattice composed of pentagons and hexagons very similar in arrangement to the struts in a geodesic dome. The coated pit invaginates and pinches off from the cell membrane, forming a coated vesicle that carries the ligand and its receptor into the cell.

The coated vesicles soon lose their clathrin coat and fuse with **endosomes,** a system of vesicles and tubules located in the cytosol near the cell surface (early endosomes) or deeper in the cytoplasm (late endosomes). Together they constitute the **endosomal compartment.** Whether early and late endosomes are separate compartments or one is a precursor of the other is still an open question. The membrane of all endosomes contains ATP-driven H^+ pumps that acidify their interior. The clathrin molecules separated from the coated vesicles are moved back to the cell membrane to participate in the formation of new coated pits.

Molecules penetrating the endosomes may take more than one pathway. Receptors that are separated from their ligands by the acidic pH of the endosome may return to the cell membrane to be reused. For example, low-density lipoprotein receptors are recycled several times. The ligands usually are transferred to late endosomes. However, some ligands are returned to the extracellular milieu to be used again. An example of this activity is the iron transporting protein transferrin.

C. Phagocytosis: Phagocytosis literally means

"cell eating" and can be compared to pinocytosis, which means "cell drinking." Certain cell types, such as macrophages and polymorphonuclear leukocytes, are specialized for incorporating and removing foreign bacteria, protozoa, fungi, damaged cells, and unneeded extracellular constituents. For example, after a bacterium becomes bound to the surface of a macrophage, cytoplasmic processes of the macrophage are extended and ultimately surround the bacterium. The edges of these processes fuse, enclosing the bacterium in an intracellular **phagocytic vacuole** (Figure 5–24).

Exocytosis is the term used to describe the fusion of a membrane-limited structure with the plasma membrane, resulting in the release of its contents into the extracellular space without compromising the integrity of the plasma membrane. A typical example is the release of stored products from secretory cells, such as those of the exocrine pancreas and the salivary glands (Figure 4–20). The fusion of membranes in exocytosis is a complex process. Because cell membranes exhibit a high density of negative charges (phosphate residues of the phospholipids), membrane-covered structures coming close to each other will not fuse but will rather repel each other, unless specific interactions facilitate the fusion process. Consequently, exocytosis is mediated by a number of specific proteins. Usually, the process is regulated by Ca^{2+}. For example, an increase in cytosolic Ca^{2+} often triggers exocytosis.

A

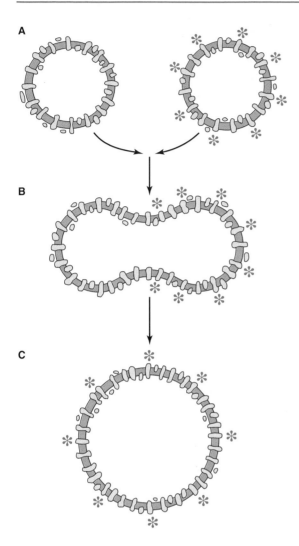

B

C

Figure 2–6. Experiment demonstrating the fluid nature of proteins within the cell membrane. The plasmalemma is shown as two parallel lines (representing the lipid portion) in which proteins are embedded. In this experiment, two types of cells derived from tissue cultures (one with a fluorescent marker [**right**] and one without) are fused (**A**→**B**) through the action of the Sendai virus. Minutes after the fusion of the membranes, the fluorescent marker of the labeled cell spreads to the entire surface of the fused cells (**C**). However, in many cells, most transmembrane proteins are stabilized in place by anchoring to elements of the cytoskeleton.

During endocytosis, portions of the cell membrane become an endocytotic vesicle; during exocytosis, the membrane is returned to the cell surface. This phenomenon is called **membrane trafficking.** In several systems, membranes are conserved and reused several times during repeated cycles of endocytosis; the significance of membrane trafficking for cell economy is self-evident.

Signal Reception

Cells in a multicellular organism need to communicate with one another to regulate their development into tissues, to control their growth and division, and to coordinate their functions. Many cells form communicating junctions that couple adjacent cells, allowing the exchange of ions and small molecules (see Chapter 4). Through these channels, also called gap junctions, signals pass directly from cell to cell without reaching the extracellular fluid. In other cases, cells display membrane-bound signaling molecules that influence other cells in direct physical contact.

Extracellular signaling molecules, or messengers, mediate three kinds of communication between cells. In **endocrine signaling,** hormones are carried in the blood to target cells throughout the body; in **paracrine signaling,** chemical mediators are rapidly metabolized so that they act on local cells only; and in **synaptic signaling,** neurotransmitters act only on adjacent nerve cells through special contact areas called **synapses** (see Chapter 9). In some cases, paracrine signals act on the same cell type that produced the messenger molecule, a phenomenon called **autocrine signaling.** Each cell type in the body contains a distinctive set of receptor proteins that enable it to respond to a complementary set of signaling molecules in a specific, programmed way.

Signaling molecules differ in their water solubility. Small **hydrophobic signaling molecules,** such as steroid and thyroid hormones, diffuse through the plasma membrane of the target cell and activate receptor proteins inside the cell. In contrast, **hydrophilic signaling molecules,** including neurotransmitters, most hormones, and local chemical mediators (paracrine signals), activate receptor proteins on the surface of target cells. These receptors, which span the cell membrane, relay information to a series of intracellular intermediaries that ultimately pass the signal to its final destination in either the cytoplasm or the nucleus. The numerous intercellular hydrophilic messengers rely on membrane proteins that direct the flow of information from the receptor to the rest of the cell. The best studied of these proteins are the **G proteins,** so named because they bind to guanine nucleotides. Once a **first messenger** (hormone, neurotransmitter, paracrine signal) binds to a receptor, conformational changes occur in the receptor; this, in turn, activates the G protein-guanine diphosphate (GDP) complex (Figure 2–8). A guanine diphosphate–guanine triphosphate (GDP-GTP) exchange releases the α subunit of the G protein, which acts on other membrane-bound intermediaries called **effectors.** Often, the effector is an enzyme that converts an inactive precursor molecule into an active **second messenger,** which can diffuse through the cytoplasm and carry the signal beyond the cell membrane. Second messengers trigger a cascade of molecular reactions that lead to changes in cell behavior.

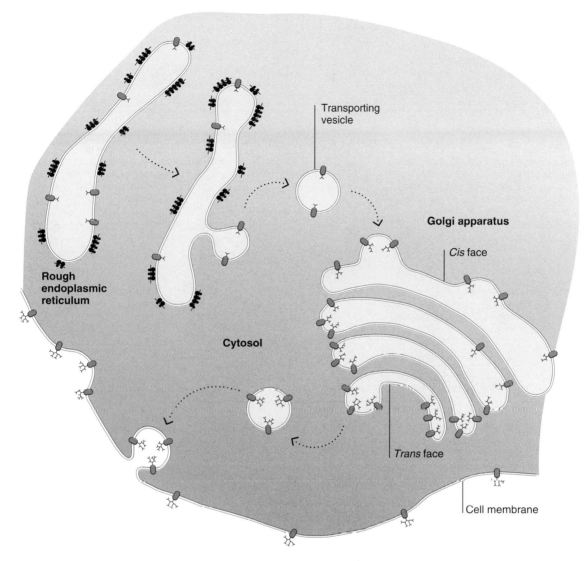

Figure 2–7. The proteins of the plasmalemma are synthesized in the rough endoplasmic reticulum and then transported in vesicles to the Golgi complex, where they may be modified and transferred to the cell membrane. This example shows the synthesis and transport of a glycoprotein, which is an integral protein of the membrane. (Redrawn and reproduced, with permission, from Junqueira LC, Carneiro J: *Biologia Celular e Molecular,* 6th ed. Editora Guanabara, 1997.)

The examples listed in Table 2–2 illustrate the diversity of G proteins present in various tissues and their roles in regulating important cell functions.

Several diseases have been shown to be due to defective receptors. For example, pseudohypoparathyroidism and a type of dwarfism are due to nonfunctioning parathyroid and growth-hormone receptors. In these two conditions the blood contains normal levels of the respective hormones, but the target cells do not respond, because they lack normal receptors.

Signaling Mediated by Intracellular Receptors

Steroid hormones are small hydrophobic (lipid-soluble) molecules derived from cholesterol; they are transported in the blood by binding reversibly to carrier proteins in the plasma. Once released from their carrier proteins, they diffuse through the plasma membrane lipids of the target cell and bind reversibly to specific steroid hormone–receptor proteins in the cytoplasm or the nucleus. The binding of hormone activates the receptor, enabling it to bind with high affinity to specific DNA sequences that act as tran-

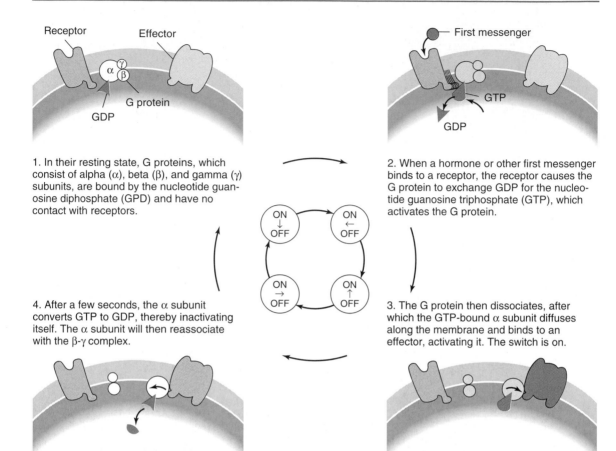

Figure 2–8. Diagram illustrating how G proteins switch effectors on and off. (Modified and reprinted, with permission, from Linder M, Gilman AG: G proteins. Sci Am, 1992:56.)

Table 2–2. A sampling of physiologic effects mediated by G proteins.

Stimulus	Affected Cell Type	G Protein	Effector	Effect
Epinephrine, glucagon	Liver cells	G_s	Adenylyl cyclase	Breakdown of glycogen
Epinephrine, glucagon	Fat cells	G_s	Adenylyl cyclase	Breakdown of fat
Luteinizing hormone	Ovarian follicles	G_s	Adenylyl cyclase	Increased synthesis of estrogen and progesterone
Antidiuretic hormone	Kidney cells	G_s	Adenylyl cyclase	Conservation of water by kidney
Acetylcholine	Heart muscle cells	G_i	Potassium channel	Slowed heart rate and decreased pumping force
Enkephalins, endorphins, opioids	Brain neurons	G_i/G_o	Calcium and potassium channels, adenylyl cyclase	Changed electrical activity of neurons
Angiotensin	Smooth muscle cells in blood vessels	G_q	Phospholipase C	Muscle contraction; elevation of blood pressure
Odorants	Neuroepithelial cells in nose	G_{olf}	Adenylyl cyclase	Detection of odorants
Light	Rod and cone cells in retina	G_t	Cyclic GMP phosphodiesterase	Detection of visual signals
Pheromone	Baker's yeast	GPA1	Unknown	Mating of cells

Reproduced, with permission, from Linder M, Gilman AG: G proteins. Sci Am 1992;267:56.

scriptional enhancers. This DNA binding increases the level of transcription from specific genes. The products of some of these activated genes may activate other genes in turn and produce a delayed secondary response, thereby extending the initial effect of the hormone. Each steroid hormone is recognized by a different member of a family of homologous receptor proteins.

Mitochondria

Mitochondria (Gr. *mitos,* thread, + *chondros,* granule) are spherical or filamentous organelles 0.5–1 μm wide that can attain a length of up to 10 μm. Their distribution in cells varies. They tend to accumulate in parts of the cytoplasm where metabolic activity is more intense, such as the apical ends of ciliated cells (Figure 17–2), in the middle piece of spermatozoa (Figure 22–5), or at the base of ion-transferring cells (Figure 4–18).

These highly efficient organelles transform the chemical energy of the metabolites present in cytoplasm into energy that is easily accessible to the cell. About 50% of this energy is stored as high-energy phosphate bonds in ATP molecules, and the remaining 50% is dissipated as heat used to maintain body temperature. Through the activity of the enzyme ATPase, ATP promptly releases energy when required by the cell to perform any type of work, whether it be osmotic, mechanical, electrical, or chemical.

Mitochondria are composed mainly of protein. Lipids are present to a lesser degree, along with small quantities of DNA and RNA. Like most cell components, mitochondrial proteins are constantly being renewed. The average half-life of mitochondrial proteins in rat liver cells, for example, is 10 days.

Mitochondria generally have a characteristic structure under the electron microscope, with small variations according to the organ and species (Figures 2–1 and 2–9). They are composed of an **outer** and an **inner mitochondrial membrane;** the latter projects folds, termed **cristae,** into the interior of the mitochondrion. These membranes enclose two compartments. The compartment located between the two membranes is termed the **intermembrane space.** The other compartment—the **intercristae,** or **matrix, space**—is enclosed by the inner membrane. Filling the matrix space is a fine granular material of variable electron density. Most mitochondria have flat, shelf-like cristae in their interiors (Figures 2–1 and 2–9), whereas cells that secrete steroids (eg, adrenal

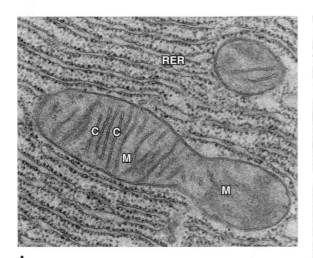

A

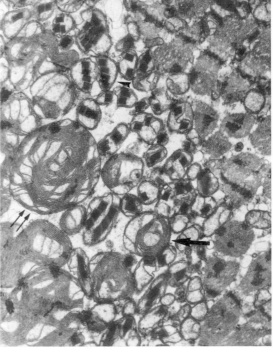

B

Figure 2–9. Structural lability of mitochondria. **A:** Electron micrograph of a section of rat pancreas. A mitochondrion with its membranes, cristae (C), and matrix (M) is seen in the center. Numerous flattened cisternae of rough endoplasmic reticulum (RER) with ribosomes on their cytoplasmic surfaces are also visible. × 50,000. **B:** Electron micrograph of striated muscle from a patient with mitochondrial myopathy. The mitochondria are profoundly modified, showing marked swelling of the matrix.

gland; see Chapter 4) frequently contain tubular cristae (Figure 4–28). The cristae increase the internal surface area of mitochondria and contain enzymes and other components of oxidative phosphorylation and electron transport systems. The adenosine diphosphate (ADP) to adenosine triphosphate (ATP) phosphorylating system is localized in globular structures connected to the inner membrane by cylindrical stalks (Figure 2–1). The globular structures are a complex of proteins with ATP synthetase activity that, in the presence of ADP plus inorganic phosphate and energy, form ATP. The chemiosmotic theory suggests that ATP synthesis occurs at the expense of a flow of protons across this globular unit (Figure 2–10).

The number of mitochondria and the number of cristae in each mitochondrion are related to the metabolic activity of the cells in which they reside. Thus, cells with a high-energy metabolism (eg, cardiac muscle, cells of some kidney tubules) have abundant mitochondria with a large number of closely packed cristae, whereas cells with a low-energy metabolism have few mitochondria with short cristae.

Between the cristae is an amorphous **matrix,** rich in protein and containing some DNA and RNA. In a great number of cell types, the mitochondrial matrix also exhibits rounded electron-dense granules rich in Ca^{2+}. Although the function of this cation in mitochondria is not completely understood, it may be important in regulating the activity of some mitochondrial enzymes; another functional role is related to the necessity of keeping the cytosolic concentration of Ca^{2+} low. Mitochondria will pump in Ca^{2+} when its concentration in the cytosol is high. Enzymes for the citric acid (Krebs) cycle and fatty acid β-oxidation are found to reside within the matrix space.

The DNA isolated from the mitochondrial matrix is double-stranded and has a circular structure, very similar to that of bacterial chromosomes. These strands are synthesized within the mitochondrion; their duplication is independent of nuclear DNA replication. Mitochondria contain the three types of RNA: ribosomal RNA (rRNA), messenger RNA (mRNA), and transfer RNA (tRNA). Mitochondrial ribosomes are smaller than cytosolic ribosomes and are comparable to bacterial ribosomes. Protein syn-

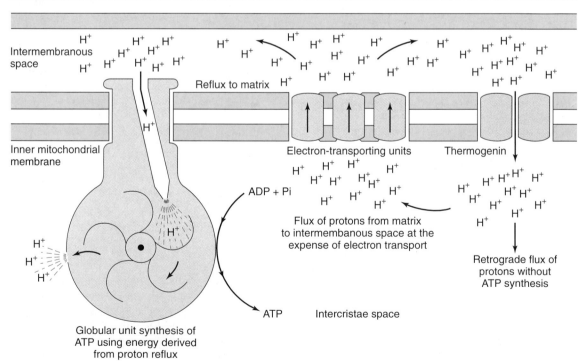

Figure 2–10. The chemiosmotic theory of mitochondrial energy transduction. Middle: The flux of protons is directed from the matrix to the intermembranous space promoted at the expense of energy derived from the electron transport system in the inner membrane. **Left:** Half the energy derived from proton reflux produces ATP; the remaining energy produces heat. **Right:** The protein thermogenin, present in multilocular adipose tissue, forms a shunt for reflux of protons. This reflux, which dissipates energy as heat, does not produce ATP (see Chapter 6).

thesis occurs in mitochondria, but because of the reduced amount of mitochondrial DNA, only a small proportion of the mitochondrial proteins are produced locally. Most are coded by nuclear DNA and synthesized in polyribosomes located in the cytosol. These proteins have a small amino acid sequence that is a signal for their mitochondrial destination, and they are transported into mitochondria by an energy-requiring mechanism.

Metabolites are degraded within mitochondria by the catalytic activity of the enzymes of the citric acid cycle, and the energy liberated in this process is partially captured through oxidative phosphorylation. The end result of these reactions is the production of CO_2, water, and heat, as well as the accumulation of energy in the high-energy compound ATP.

The initial degradation of proteins, carbohydrates, and fats is carried out in the cytoplasmic matrix. The metabolic end product of these extramitochondrial metabolic pathways is acetyl–coenzyme A (CoA), which then enters mitochondria. Within mitochondria, acetyl-CoA combines with oxaloacetate to form citric acid. Within the citric acid cycle, several reactions of decarboxylation produce CO_2, and specific reactions catalyzed by dehydrogenases result in the removal of four pairs of H^+ ions. The H^+ ions ultimately react with oxygen to form H_2O. Through the action of cytochromes *a, b,* and *c,* coenzyme Q, and cytochrome oxidase, the **electron transport system,** located in the inner mitochondrial membrane, releases energy that is captured at three points of this system through the formation of ATP from ADP and inorganic phosphate. Under aerobic conditions, the combined activity of extramitochondrial glycolysis and the citric acid cycle as well as the electron transport system gives rise to 36 molecules of ATP per molecule of glucose. This is 18 times the energy obtainable under anaerobic circumstances, when only the glycolytic pathway can be used.

In the process of mitosis, each daughter cell receives approximately half the mitochondria originally present in the parent cell. New mitochondria originate from preexisting mitochondria by accretion of material that leads to growth and subsequent division (fission) of the organelle itself.

The fact that mitochondria have some characteristics in common with bacteria has led to the hypothesis that mitochondria originated from an ancestral aerobic prokaryote that adapted to an endosymbiotic life within a eukaryotic host cell.

Several mitochondrial deficiency diseases have been described, and most of them are characterized by muscular dysfunction (Figure 2–9B). Because of their high-energy metabolism, skeletal muscle fibers are very sensitive to mitochondrial defects. These diseases usually begin with drooping of the upper eyelid and progress to difficulties in swallowing and limb weakness. They are caused by DNA mutations or defects that can occur in the mitochondria or the cell nucleus. Mitochondrial inheritance is maternal, because few, if any, mitochondria enter the ovum with the sperm nucleus. In the case of nuclear DNA defects, inheritance may be from either or both parents. In addition, mitochondrial diseases may be the result of infections and environmental toxicity and may also be associated with senility. Changes can occur in different segments of mitochondrial or nuclear DNA, affecting one or more than one gene, causing multiple symptoms and changes in mitochondrial morphology (Figure 2–9B).

RIBOSOMES

Ribosomes are small electron-dense particles, about 20×30 nm in size. They are composed of four types of ribosomal RNA (rRNA) and almost 80 different proteins.

There are two classes of ribosomes: One class is found in prokaryotes, chloroplasts, and mitochondria; the other is found in eukaryotic cells. Both classes of ribosomes are composed of two different-sized subunits.

In eukaryotic cells, most RNA molecules of both subunits are synthesized within the nucleoli. Their numerous proteins are synthesized in the cytoplasm and then enter the nucleus and associate with rRNAs. Subunits then leave the nucleus, via nuclear pores, to enter the cytoplasm and participate in protein synthesis.

Ribosomes are intensely basophilic because of the presence of numerous phosphate groups of the constituent rRNA that act as polyanions. Thus, sites in the cytoplasm that are rich in ribosomes stain intensely with basic dyes such as methylene and toluidine blue. These basophilic sites also stain with hematoxylin.

The individual ribosomes (Figure 2–11A) are held together by a strand of messenger RNA (mRNA) to form **polyribosomes (polysomes).** The message carried by mRNA is a code for the amino acid sequence of proteins being synthesized by the cell, and the ribosomes play a crucial role in decoding, or translating, this message during protein synthesis. Proteins synthesized for use within the cell and destined to remain in the cytosol (eg, hemoglobin in immature erythrocytes) are synthesized on polyribosomes existing as isolated clusters within the cytoplasm. Polyribosomes that are attached to the membranes of the endoplasmic reticulum (via their large subunits) translate mRNAs that code for proteins that are segregated into the cisternae of the reticulum (Figure 2–11B). These proteins can be secreted (eg, pancreatic and salivary enzymes) or stored in the cell (eg, enzymes of lysosomes, proteins within granules of white blood cells [leukocytes]). In addition, integral proteins of the plasma membrane are synthesized on

A. Free polyribosomes, whose proteins remain in the cytoplasm

B. Bound polyribosomes, showing protein synthesis and segregation into the rough endoplasmic reticulum

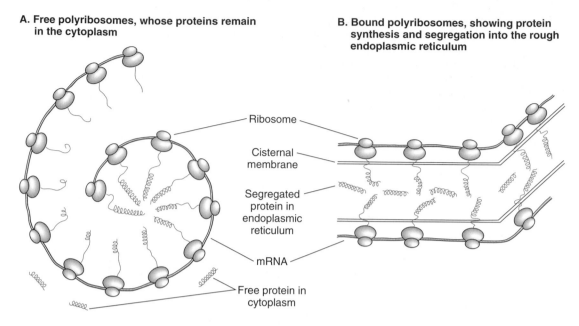

Ribosome

Cisternal membrane

Segregated protein in endoplasmic reticulum

mRNA

Free protein in cytoplasm

Figure 2–11. Diagram illustrating (**A**) the concept that cells synthesizing proteins (represented here by spirals) that are to remain within the cytoplasm possess (free) polyribosomes (ie, nonadherent to the endoplasmic reticulum). In **B,** where the proteins are segregated in the endoplasmic reticulum and may eventually be extruded from the cytoplasm (export proteins), not only do the polyribosomes adhere to the membranes of rough endoplasmic reticulum, but the proteins produced by them are injected into the interior of the organelle across its membrane. In this way, the proteins—especially enzymes such as ribonucleases and proteases, which could have undesirable effects on the cytoplasm—are separated from it.

polyribosomes attached to membranes of the endoplasmic reticulum (Figure 2–7).

Endoplasmic Reticulum

The cytoplasm of eukaryotic cells contains an anastomosing network of intercommunicating channels and sacs formed by a continuous membrane, which encloses a space called a **cisterna.** In sections, cisternae appear separated, but high-resolution microscopy of whole cells reveals that they are continuous. This membrane system is called the endoplasmic reticulum. In many places the cytosolic side of the membrane is covered by polyribosomes synthesizing protein molecules, which are injected into the cisternae. This permits the distinction between the two types of endoplasmic reticulum: **rough** and **smooth.**

A. Rough Endoplasmic Reticulum: Rough endoplasmic reticulum (RER) is prominent in cells specialized for protein secretion, such as pancreatic acinar cells (digestive enzymes), fibroblasts (collagen), and plasma cells (immunoglobulins). The RER consists of sac-like as well as parallel stacks of flattened cisternae (Figures 2–1 and 2–9), limited by membranes that are sometimes continuous with the outer membrane of the nuclear envelope. The name "rough endoplasmic reticulum" alludes to the presence of polyribosomes on the cytosolic surface of

this structure's membrane (Figures 2–1 and 2–9). The presence of polyribosomes also confers basophilic staining properties on this organelle when viewed with the light microscope.

The principal function of the RER is to segregate proteins from the cytosol that are destined for export or intracellular use. Additional functions include the initial (core) glycosylation of glycoproteins, the synthesis of phospholipids, the assembly of multichain proteins, limited proteolysis of the signal sequence of newly synthesized proteins, and certain post-translational modifications of newly formed polypeptides.

All protein synthesis begins on polyribosomes that are not attached to the endoplasmic reticulum. Messenger RNAs of proteins destined to be segregated in the endoplasmic reticulum contain an additional sequence of bases at their 5′ end that code for approximately 20–25 mainly hydrophobic amino acids called the **signal sequence.** Upon translation, the signal sequence interacts with a complex of six nonidentical polypeptides plus a 7S RNA molecule that is referred to as the **signal-recognition particle** (**SRP**). SRP inhibits further polypeptide elongation until the SRP-polyribosome complex binds to a receptor in the membrane of the RER, the **docking protein.** Upon binding to the docking protein, SRP is released from the polyribosomes, allowing the translation to continue (Figure 2–12).

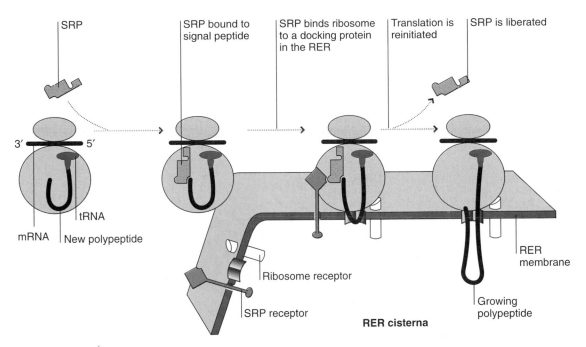

Figure 2–12. The transport of proteins across the membrane of the endoplasmic reticulum (RER). The ribosomes bind to mRNA, and the signal peptide is initially bound to a signal-recognition particle (SRP). Ribosomes bind to the RER by interacting with the SRP and a ribosomal receptor. The signal peptide is then removed by a signal peptidase (not shown). These interactions cause the opening of a pore through which the protein is extruded into the RER.

Once inside the lumen of the RER, the signal sequence is removed by a specific enzyme, **signal peptidase,** located at the inner surface of the RER. Translation of the protein continues, accompanied by intracisternal secondary and tertiary structural changes as well as certain post-translational modifications such as hydroxylation, glycosylation, sulfation, and phosphorylation.

Initial (core) glycosylation is an important post-translational modification whereby mannose oligosaccharides are added to most proteins destined for export. Proteins synthesized in the RER can have several destinations: intracellular storage (eg, in lysosomes and specific granules of leukocytes), provisional intracellular storage of proteins for export (eg, in the pancreas, some endocrine cells), and as a component of other membranes (eg, integral proteins). Proteins synthesized either in membrane-bound or free polyribosomes may remain in the cytosol or be segregated from it, according to their functions (Figure 2–13).

B. Smooth Endoplasmic Reticulum: Smooth endoplasmic reticulum (SER) also takes the form of a membranous network within the cell; however, its ultrastructure differs from that of RER in two important ways. First, SER lacks the associated polyribosomes that characterize RER. SER membranes therefore appear smooth rather than granular. Second, its cisternae are more tubular and more likely to appear

as a profusion of interconnected channels of various shapes and sizes than as stacks of flattened cisternae (Figures 2–1 and 4–28). SER is continuous with the RER; in sections, one can see continuity between membranes of the two forms.

SER not only exhibits a diversity of morphologic appearances in different cell types but is also associated with a variety of specialized functional capabilities. In cells that synthesize steroid hormones (eg, cells of the adrenal cortex), SER occupies a large portion of the cytoplasm and contains some of the enzymes required for steroid synthesis (Figure 4–28). It is abundant in liver cells, where it is responsible for the oxidation, conjugation, and methylation processes employed by the liver to degrade certain hormones and neutralize noxious substances such as alcohol and barbiturates. Another important function of SER is the synthesis of phospholipids for all cell membranes. The phospholipid molecules are transferred from the SER to other membranes (1) by vesicles that detach and are moved along cytoskeletal elements by the action of motor proteins, (2) through direct communication with the RER, or (3) by transfer proteins (Figure 2–14). SER contains the enzyme glucose-6-phosphatase, which is involved in the utilization of glucose originating from glycogen in liver cells. This enzyme is also found in RER—an example of the lack of absolute partition of functions between these organelles. SER participates in the con-

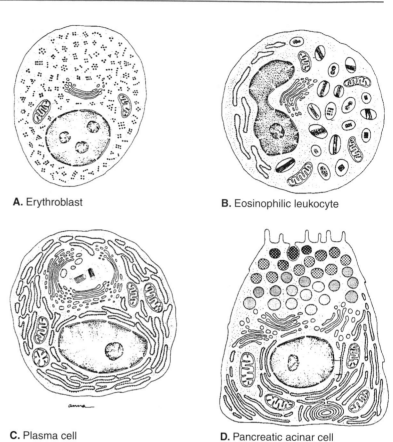

A. Erythroblast

B. Eosinophilic leukocyte

Figure 2–13. The ultrastructure of a cell that synthesizes (but does not secrete) proteins on free polyribosomes (**A**); a cell that synthesizes, segregates, and stores proteins in organelles (**B**); a cell that synthesizes, segregates, and directly exports proteins (**C**); and a cell that synthesizes, segregates, stores in supranuclear granules, and exports proteins (**D**).

C. Plasma cell

D. Pancreatic acinar cell

traction process in muscle cells, where it appears in a specialized form, called the **sarcoplasmic reticulum,** that is involved in the sequestration and release of the calcium ions that regulate muscular contraction (see Chapter 10).

Golgi Complex (Golgi Apparatus)

The Golgi complex completes post-translational modifications and packages and places an address on products that have been synthesized by the cell. This organelle is composed of three distinct smooth membrane–limited compartments (Figures 2–1, 2–15, and 2–16). The first and most obvious is a slightly curved stack of 3–10 flattened **cisternae.** The second is the numerous small **vesicles** seen around the periphery of the stack. Third, usually at one pole of the Golgi complex, are a few larger **vacuoles.** In highly polarized cells, such as mucus-secreting goblet cells (Figure 4–23), the Golgi complex occupies a characteristic position in the cytoplasm between the nucleus and the apical plasma membrane.

In most cells, there is also polarity in Golgi structure and function. Near the Golgi complex, the RER can sometimes be seen budding off small vesicles (transport vesicles) that shuttle newly synthesized proteins to the Golgi complex for further processing. The Golgi cisterna nearest this point is called the forming, convex, or *cis,* face. On the opposite side of the Golgi complex—the maturing, concave, or *trans,* face—large Golgi vacuoles accumulate (Figure 2–16). These are sometimes called **condensing vacuoles.**

These structures bud from the Golgi cisternae, generating vesicles that will transport proteins to various sites. Cytochemical methods and the electron microscope have shown that the Golgi cisternae present different enzymes at different *cis-trans* levels and that the Golgi complex is important in the glycosylation, sulfation, phosphorylation, and limited proteolysis of proteins. Furthermore, it initiates packing, concentration, and storage of secretory products. Figure 2–16 gives an overall view of the currently accepted concepts regarding transit of material through the Golgi complex.

Lysosomes

Lysosomes are sites of intracellular digestion and turnover of cellular components. Lysosomes (Gr. *lysis,* solution, + *soma,* body) are membrane-

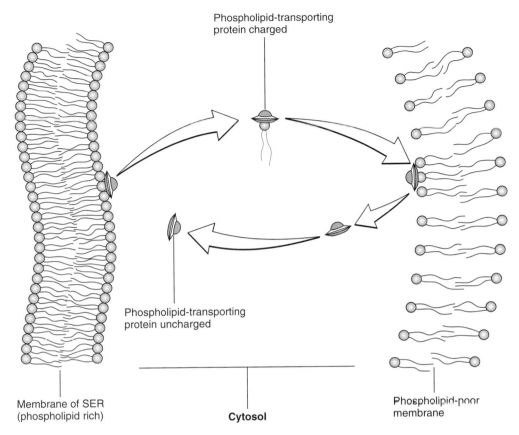

Phospholipid-transporting protein charged

Phospholipid-transporting protein uncharged

Membrane of SER (phospholipid rich)

Cytosol

Phospholipid-poor membrane

Figure 2–14. Schematic representation of a phospholipid transporting amphipathic protein. Phospholipid molecules are transported from lipid-rich (SER) to lipid-poor membranes. (Redrawn and reproduced, with permission, from Junqueira LC, Carneiro J: *Biologia Celular e Molecular,* 6th ed. Editora Guanabara, 1997.)

limited vesicles that contain a large variety of hydrolytic enzymes (more than 40) whose main function is intracytoplasmic digestion (Figures 2–17 through 2–21). Lysosomes are particularly abundant in cells exhibiting phagocytic activity (eg, macrophages, neutrophilic leukocytes). Although the nature and activity of lysosomal enzymes vary depending on the cell type, the most common enzymes are acid phosphatase, ribonuclease, deoxyribonuclease, proteases, sulfatases, lipases, and β-glucuronidase. As can be seen from this list, lysosomal enzymes are capable of breaking down most biologic macromolecules. Lysosomal enzymes have optimal activity at pH 5.

Lysosomes, which are usually spherical, range in diameter from 0.05 to 0.5 μm and present a uniformly granular, electron-dense appearance in electron micrographs. The enveloping membrane separates the lytic enzymes from the cytoplasm, an important role in that it prevents the lysosomal enzymes from attacking and digesting cytoplasmic components. The fact that the lysosomal enzymes are practically inactive at the pH of the cytosol (~7.2) is

an additional protection of the cell against leakage of lysosomal enzymes.

Lysosomal enzymes are synthesized and segregated in the RER and subsequently transferred to the Golgi complex, where the enzymes are modified and packaged as lysosomes. These enzymes have oligosaccharides attached to them but with an important modification. One or more of the mannose residues is phosphorylated at the 6' position by a phosphotransferase. There are receptors for mannose 6-phosphate-containing proteins in the RER and Golgi complex that allow these proteins to be diverted from the main secretory pathway and segregated in lysosomes. This was the first indication of how the cell manages to sort out proteins going to different destinations.

Lysosomes that have not entered into a digestive event are identified as **primary lysosomes** (Figure 2–18). They can be very small (0.05 μm in diameter) membrane-limited vesicles, and they may be impossible to identify with certainty in the absence of a histochemical test of their content. In a few cells,

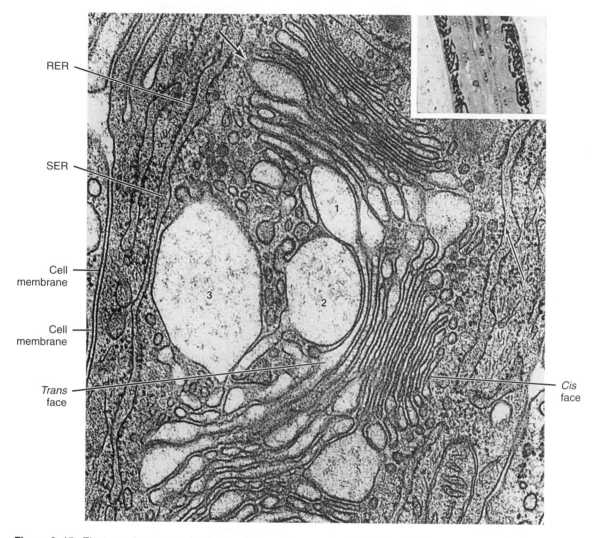

Figure 2–15. Electron micrograph of a Golgi complex of a mucous cell. To the right is a cisterna (arrow) of the rough endoplasmic reticulum containing granular material. Close to it are small vesicles containing this material. This is the *cis* face of the complex. In the center are flattened and stacked cisternae of the Golgi complex. Dilations can be observed extending from the ends of the cisternae. These dilations gradually detach themselves from the cisternae and fuse, forming the secretory granules (**1, 2,** and **3**). This is the *trans* face. Near the plasma membrane of two neighboring cells is endoplasmic reticulum with a smooth section (SER) and a rough section (RER). × 30,000. **Inset:** The Golgi complex as seen in 1-μm sections of epididymis cells impregnated with silver. × 1200.

such as macrophages and neutrophilic leukocytes, primary lysosomes are larger, up to 0.5 μm in diameter, and thus just visible with the light microscope.

Lysosomes can digest materials taken into the cell from its environment, a process called **heterophagy.** The material is taken into a phagocytic vacuole (Figure 2–21); primary lysosomes then fuse with the membrane of the phagosome and empty their hydrolytic enzymes into the vacuole. Digestion follows, and the composite structure is now termed a **secondary lysosome.**

Secondary lysosomes are generally 0.2–2 μm in diameter and present a heterogeneous appearance in electron microscopes because of the wide variety of materials they may be digesting (Figure 2–21). Again, the only sure guide to their identification is the histochemical detection of hydrolytic enzymes (eg, acid phosphatase). Secondary lysosomes resulting from the fusion of phagocytosed materials with primary lysosomes are named **phagosomes,** or **phagolysosomes.**

After digestion of the contents of the secondary lysosome, nutrients diffuse through the lysosomal limiting membrane and enter the cytosol. Indigestible compounds are retained within the vacuoles, which are now called **residual bodies** (Figures 2–20 and

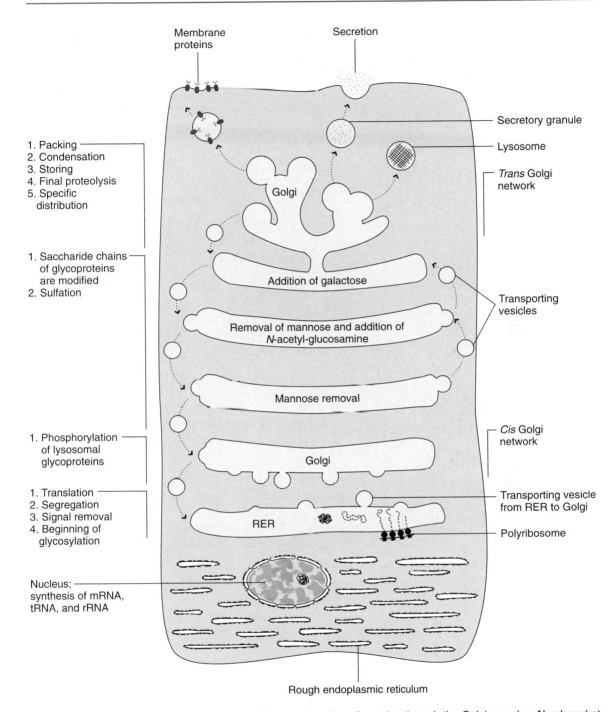

Membrane proteins

Secretion

Secretory granule

Lysosome

Trans Golgi network

Golgi

1. Packing
2. Condensation
3. Storing
4. Final proteolysis
5. Specific distribution

1. Saccharide chains of glycoproteins are modified
2. Sulfation

Addition of galactose

Transporting vesicles

Removal of mannose and addition of *N*-acetyl-glucosamine

Mannose removal

Cis Golgi network

Golgi

1. Phosphorylation of lysosomal glycoproteins

1. Translation
2. Segregation
3. Signal removal
4. Beginning of glycosylation

Transporting vesicle from RER to Golgi

RER

Polyribosome

Nucleus; synthesis of mRNA, tRNA, and rRNA

Rough endoplasmic reticulum

Figure 2–16. Main events occurring during trafficking and sorting of proteins through the Golgi complex. Numbered at the left are the main molecular processes that take place in the compartments indicated. Note that the labeling of lysosomal enzymes starts early in the *cis* Golgi network. In the *trans* Golgi network, the glycoproteins combine with specific receptors that guide them to their destination. On the left side of the drawing is the returning flux of membrane, from the Golgi to the endoplasmic reticulum. (Redrawn and reproduced, with permission, form Junqueira LC, Carneiro J: *Biologia Celular e Molecular,* 6th ed. Editora Guanabara, 1997.)

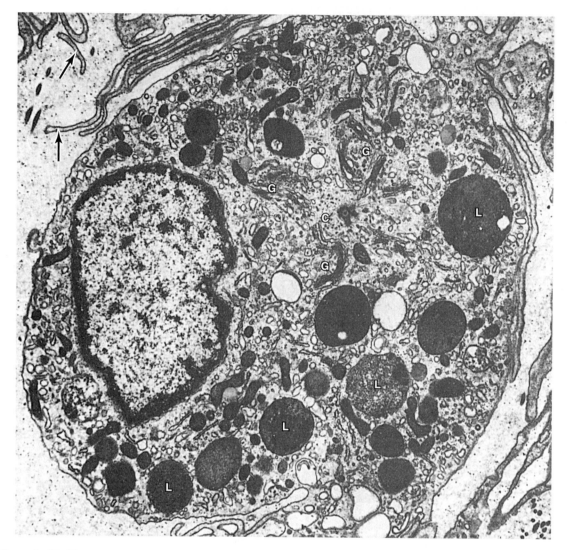

Figure 2–17. Electron micrograph of a mesenteric macrophage. Note the abundant cytoplasmic extensions (arrows). In the center is a centriole (C) surrounded by Golgi cisternae (G). Secondary lysosomes (L) are abundant. × 15,000.

2–21). In some long-lived cells (eg, neurons, heart muscle, hepatocytes), large quantities of residual bodies accumulate and are referred to as **lipofuscin, or age pigment.**

Another function of lysosomes concerns the turnover of cytoplasmic organelles. Under certain conditions, organelles or portions of cytoplasm may become enclosed by a membrane. Primary lysosomes fuse with this structure and initiate the lysis of the enclosed cytoplasm. The resulting secondary lysosomes are known as **autophagosomes** (Gr. *autos,* self, + *phagein,* to eat, + *soma*), indicating that their contents are intracellular in origin. Cytoplasmic digestion by autophagosomes is enhanced in cells undergoing atrophy (as in prostatic epithelial cells after castration) and in secretory cells that have accumu-

lated excess secretory product. The digested products of lysosomal hydrolysis are recycled by the cell to be reutilized by the cytoplasm.

In some cases, primary lysosomes release their contents extracellularly, and their enzymes act in the extracellular milieu. An example is the destruction of bone matrix by the collagenases synthesized and released by osteoclasts during normal bone tissue formation (see Chapter 8). Lysosomal enzymes acting in the extracellular milieu also play a significant role in the response to inflammation or injury. Several possible pathways relating to lysosome activities are schematically illustrated in Figure 2–21.

Lysosomes play an important role in the me-

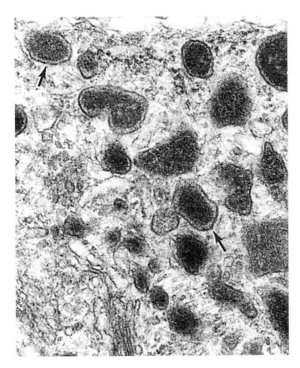

Figure 2–18. Electron micrograph of the cytoplasm of a macrophage showing primary lysosomes (arrows) characterized by uniform granular content and a limiting membrane. × 45,000.

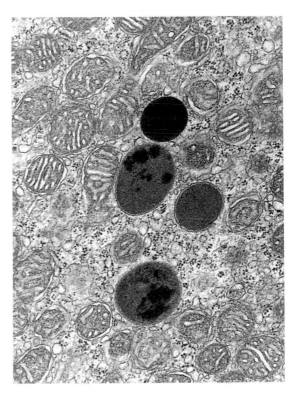

Figure 2–19. Electron micrograph showing four dark secondary lysosomes surrounded by numerous mitochondria.

tabolism of several substances in the human body, and consequently many diseases have been ascribed to deficiencies of lysosomal enzymes. In **metachromatic leukodystrophy,** there is an intracellular accumulation of sulfated cerebrosides caused by lack of lysosomal sulfatase. In most of these diseases, a specific lysosomal enzyme is absent or inactive, and certain molecules (glycogen, cerebrosides, gangliosides, sphingomyelin, glycosaminoglycans, etc) are not digested. As a result, these substances accumulate in the cells, interfering with their normal functions. This diversity of affected cell types explains the variety of clinical symptoms observed in lysosomal diseases (Table 2–3).

I-cell disease (*i*nclusion cell disease) is a rare inherited condition clinically characterized by defective physical growth and mental retardation and is due to a deficiency in a phosphorylating enzyme normally present in the Golgi complex. Lysosomal enzymes coming from the RER are not phosphorylated in the Golgi complex. Nonphosphorylated protein molecules are not separated to form lysosomes, instead following the secretory pathway. The secreted lysosomal enzymes are present in the blood of patients with I-cell disease, whereas their lysosomes are empty. Cells of these patients show large inclusion granules that interfere with normal cellular metabolism.

Peroxisomes, or Microbodies

Peroxisomes (peroxide + *soma*) are spherical membrane-limited organelles whose diameter ranges from 0.5 to 1.2 μm (see Figure 2–29). Their homogeneous matrix contains D- and L-amino oxidases and hydroxyacid oxidase. In some species, but not humans, a crystalline nucleoid is present that is composed of urate oxidase. All these enzymes oxidize their substrate and reduce O_2 and H_2O_2. Peroxisomes also contain catalase, an enzyme that decomposes hydrogen peroxide to water and oxygen (2 H_2O_2 → 2 H_2O + O_2), protecting the cell from the effects of hydrogen peroxide, which could damage many important cellular constituents.

Peroxisomes contain enzymes involved in lipid metabolism. Thus, the β-oxidation of long-chain fatty acids (18 carbons and longer) is preferentially accomplished by peroxisomal enzymes that differ from their mitochondrial counterparts. Certain hydroxylation reactions leading to the formation of bile acids also have been localized in highly purified peroxisomal fractions.

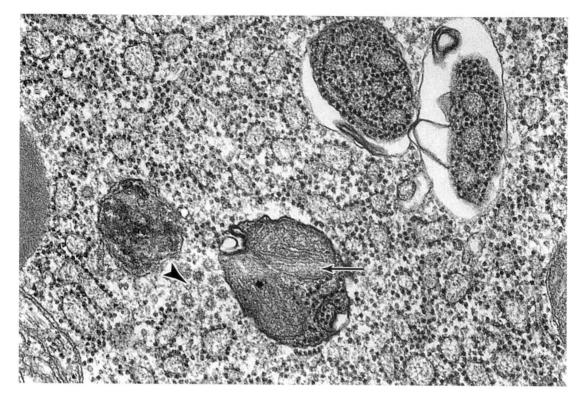

Figure 2–20. Section of a pancreatic acinar cell showing autophagosomes. **Upper right:** Two portions of the rough endoplasmic reticulum segregated by a membrane. **Center:** An autophagosome containing mitochondria (arrow) plus rough endoplasmic reticulum. **Left:** A residual body, with indigestible material. Arrowhead shows a cluster of coated vesicles.

Peroxisomal enzymes (catalase, enzymes of β-oxidation) are synthesized on free cytosolic polyribosomes, with a small sequence of amino acids located near the carboxyl terminus that functions as an import signal. Proteins with this signal are recognized by receptors located in the membrane of peroxisomes and internalized into the organelle. The peroxisome grows in size and is divided into two smaller peroxisomes, by a mechanism not completely understood.

Deficiency in peroxisomal enzymes causes the fatal Zellweger syndrome, with severe muscular impairment, liver and kidney lesions, and disorganization of the central and peripheral nervous systems. Electron microscopy reveals empty peroxisomes in liver and kidney cells of these patients.

Secretory Granules

Secretory granules are found in those cells that store a product until its release is signaled by a metabolic, hormonal, or neural message (regulated secretion). These granules are surrounded by a membrane and contain a concentrated form of the secretory product (Figure 2–22). The contents of some secretory granules may be up to 200 times more concentrated than in the cisternae of the RER. Secretory granules containing digestive enzymes are usually referred to as **zymogen granules.**

THE CYTOSKELETON

The cytoplasmic cytoskeleton is a complex network of microtubules, microfilaments, and intermediate filaments (Figure 2–23). These structural proteins provide for the shaping of cells and also play an important role in the movements of organelles and intracytoplasmic vesicles. The cytoskeleton also participates in the movement of entire cells.

Microtubules

Within the cytoplasmic matrix of eukaryotic cells are tubular structures known as microtubules (Figure 2–24). They have an outer diameter of 24 nm, consisting of a dense wall 5 nm thick and a hollow core 14 nm wide. Microtubule lengths are variable, and individual tubules can attain lengths of several micrometers. Occasionally, arms or bridges are found linking two or more tubules (Figure 2–25).

The subunit of a microtubule is a heterodimer composed of α and β **tubulin** molecules of closely

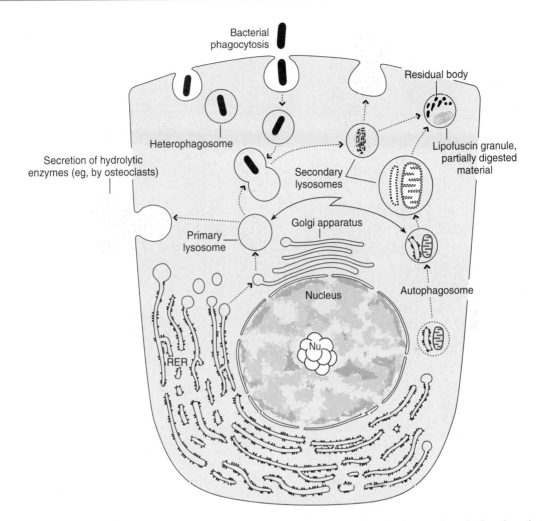

Figure 2–21. Current concepts of the functions of lysosomes. Synthesis occurs in the rough endoplasmic reticulum (RER), and the enzymes are packaged in the Golgi complex. Note the heterophagosomes, in which bacteria are being destroyed, and the autophagosomes, with RER and mitochondria in the process of digestion. Heterophagosomes and autophagosomes arc secondary lysosomes. The result of their digestion can be excreted, but sometimes the secondary lysosome creates a residual body, containing remnants of undigested molecules. In some cells, such as osteoclasts, the lysosomal enzymes are secreted to the extracellular environment.

Table 2–3. Examples of diseases caused by lysosomal enzyme failure and accumulation of undigested material in different cell types.

Disease	Faulty Enzyme	Main Cell Type Affected	Main Organs Affected
Hurler	α L-iduronidase	Fibroblasts and osteoblasts accumulate dermatan sulfate	Skeleton and nervous system
Sanfilippo Syndrome A	Heparan sulfate sulfamidase	Fibroblasts accumulate heparan sulfate	Skeleton and nervous system
Tay-Sachs	Hexosaminidase-A	Nerve cells accumulate glycolipids	Nervous system
Gaucher	β D-glycosidase	Macrophages accumulate glycolipids	Liver and spleen
I-cell disease	Phosphotransferase	Fibroblasts and osteoblasts accumulate dermatan sulfate	Skeleton and nervous system

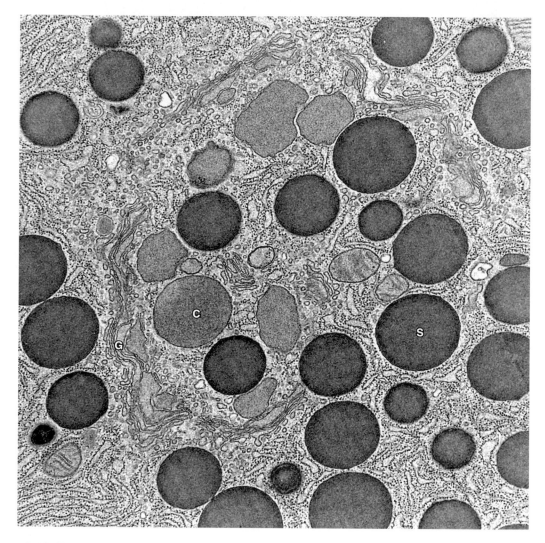

Figure 2–22. Electron micrograph of a pancreatic acinar cell from the rat. Numerous mature secretory granules (S) are seen in association with condensing vacuoles (C) and the Golgi complex (G). × 18,900.

related amino acid composition, each with a molecular mass of about 50 kDa.

Under appropriate conditions (in vivo or in vitro), tubulin subunits polymerize to form microtubules. With special staining procedures, tubulin can be seen as heterodimers organized into a spiral. A total of 13 units are present in one complete turn of the spiral (Figure 2–25).

Polymerization of tubulins to form microtubules is believed to be directed by a variety of structures collectively known as **microtubule organizing centers.** These structures include basal bodies, centrioles, and the centromeres of chromosomes. Microtubule growth, via subunit polymerization, generally occurs more rapidly at one end of existing microtubules. This end is referred to as the plus (+) end, and the other extremity is the minus (−) end. Tubulin poly-

merization is under control of the concentration of Ca^{2+} and of the *microtubule associated proteins*, or **MAPs.** Microtubule stability is variable; for example, microtubules of cilia are stable, whereas microtubules of the mitotic spindle have a short duration. The antimitotic alkaloid colchicine binds specifically to tubulin, and when the complex tubulin-colchicine binds to microtubules, it prevents the addition of more tubulin in the plus (+) extremity. Mitotic microtubules are broken down because the depolymerization continues, mainly at the minus (−) end, and the lost tubulin units are not replaced. Another alkaloid that interferes with the mitotic microtubule is taxol, which accelerates the formation of microtubules but at the same time stabilizes them. All cytosolic tubulin is used in stable microtubules, and no tubulin is left for the formation of the mitotic spindle. Another al-

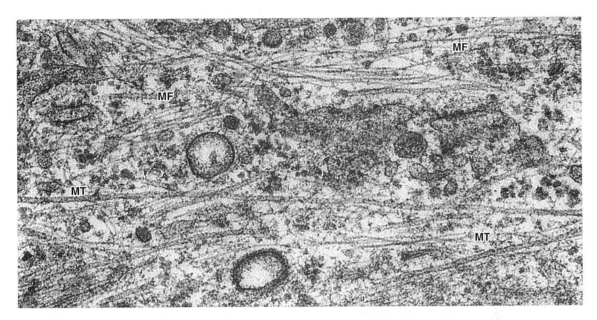

Figure 2–23. Electron micrograph of fibroblast cytoplasm. Note the microfilaments (MF) and microtubules (MT). × 60,000. (Courtesy of E Katchburian.)

kaloid, vinblastine, acts by depolymerizing formed microtubules and, in a second step, aggregating to form paracrystalline arrays of tubulin.

> The antimitotic alkaloids are useful tools in cell biology (eg, colchicine is used to arrest chromosomes in metaphase and to prepare karyotypes) and in cancer chemotherapy (eg, vinblastine, vincristine, and taxol are used to arrest cell proliferation in tumors). Because tumor cells proliferate rapidly, they are more affected by antimitotic drugs than are normal cells. However, chemotherapy has many undesirable consequences. For example, some normal blood-forming cells and the epithelial cells that cover the digestive tract also show a high rate of proliferation and are adversely affected by chemotherapy.

Microtubules are considered to play a significant role in the development and maintenance of cell form, based on the observation that they are normally quite straight and never exhibit oblique bends. These observations suggest that microtubules are rigid. Microtubules are usually present in a proper orientation, either to effect development of a given cellular asymmetry or to maintain it. Procedures that disrupt microtubules generally result in the loss of this cellular asymmetry.

Microtubules have also been implicated in the intracellular transport of organelles and vesicles, such as secretory granules. Time-lapse cinematography of living cells reveals a significant movement and redistribution of cytoplasmic components (eg, mitochondria, vesicles). Examples include axoplasmic transport in neurons, melanin transport in pigment cells, chromosome movements along the mitotic spindle, and vesicle movements between the endoplasmic reticulum and the Golgi complex and between the Golgi complex and the cell membrane. In each of these examples, movement is related to the presence of complex microtubule networks, and such activities are suspended if microtubules are disrupted. The transport guided by microtubules is under the control of special proteins called **motor proteins,** because they use energy to move molecules and vesicles inside the cell.

Microtubules provide the basis for several complex cytoplasmic components, including centrioles, basal bodies, cilia, and flagella. **Centrioles** are cylindrical structures (0.15 µm in diameter and 0.3–0.5 µm in length) composed primarily of highly organized microtubules (Figure 2–25). Each centriole is composed of nine sets of microtubule triplets arranged in the fashion of a pinwheel. The microtubules are so close together that adjacent microtubules of a triplet share a common wall. A single pair of centrioles is normally found in nondividing cells. In each pair, the long axes of the centrioles are at right angles to each other. Before cell division, more specifically during the S period of the interphase, each centriole duplicates itself. During mito-

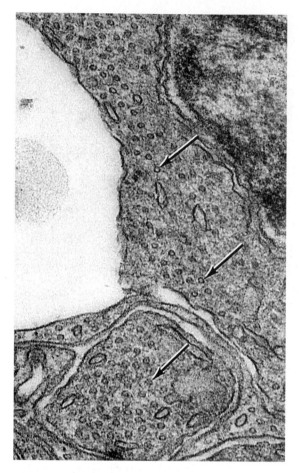

Figure 2–24. Electron micrograph of a section of a photosensitive retinal cell of a monkey. Note the accumulation of transversely sectioned microtubules (arrows). Reduced slightly from × 80,000.

sis, the resulting two pairs move to opposite poles of the cell and become organizing centers for the developing mitotic spindle.

In nondividing cells, centriole pairs are usually found in a juxtanuclear position close to the Golgi complex. Associated with the centrioles are dense **pericentriolar bodies** from which microtubules seem to arise, suggesting that these bodies represent an organizing center for microtubule formation. The pair of centrioles, in conjunction with the Golgi complex, constitutes the **cytocenter,** or cell center.

Cilia and **flagella** are motile processes with a highly organized microtubule core. Ciliated cells usually possess a large number of cilia that range from 2 to 10 μm in length. Flagellated cells normally have only one flagellum, which ranges in length from 100 to 200 μm. In humans, the spermatozoa is the only cell type with a flagellum. Both cilia and flagella have a diameter of 0.3–0.5 μm and possess the same core organization.

This core consists of nine pairs of microtubules surrounding two central tubules. This sheaf of tubules, possessing the characteristic **9 + 2 pattern,** is called an axoneme (Gr. *axon,* axis, + *nema,* thread). Each of the nine peripheral pairs (**doublets**) shares a common wall of two to three heterodimers (Figure 2–25). The tubules in the central pair are separated from each other and enclosed within a **central sheath.** Adjacent doublets are linked to each other via protein bridges called **nexins** and to the central sheath by **radial spokes.** The tubule units of each doublet are identified as subfibers A and B. Subfiber A is a complete microtubule with 13 heterodimers, whereas subfiber B has only 10 or 11 heterodimers. Extending from the surface of subfiber A are pairs of arms formed by the protein **dynein,** which has ATPase activity (Figure 2–25).

At the base of each cilium or flagellum is a **basal body.** This body is essentially identical to a centriole except at its basal end, which has a complex central organization resembling a cartwheel. The C tubule ends at the apical end of the basal body, whereas the A and B tubules are continuous with the corresponding tubules of the ciliary or flagellar axoneme. In developing cilia or flagella, the basal bodies act as a template to control the assembly of the axoneme subunits.

The undulating motion exhibited by cilia and flagella is propagated by sliding of adjacent doublets within the axoneme. This sliding mechanism is mediated by two protein extensions from the A microtubule, formed mainly by the protein dynein (dynein arms). These arms exhibit ATPase activity (Figure 2–25B). The dynein arms on microtubule A of one doublet are believed to bind to and walk along the surface of microtubule B of the adjacent doublet.

The sliding process occurring between adjacent pairs of microtubules does not occur freely and is constrained by the presence of nexin and the radial spokes. Thus, forces developed during the sliding process bend the cilia or flagella and account for their movements.

> Several mutations have been described in the proteins of the cilia and flagella. One of these is termed the **immotile cilia syndrome of Kartagener** and is characterized by the absence of dynein arms in cilia and flagella, leading to immotile spermatozoa, male infertility, and chronic respiratory infections caused by the lack of the cleansing action of cilia in the respiratory tract.

Microfilaments

Contractile activity in muscle cells results primarily from an interaction between two proteins: **actin** and **myosin.** Actin is present in muscle as a thin (5–7 nm in diameter) filament composed of globular subunits organized into a double-stranded helix (Figure 2–26). Structural and biochemical studies reveal that

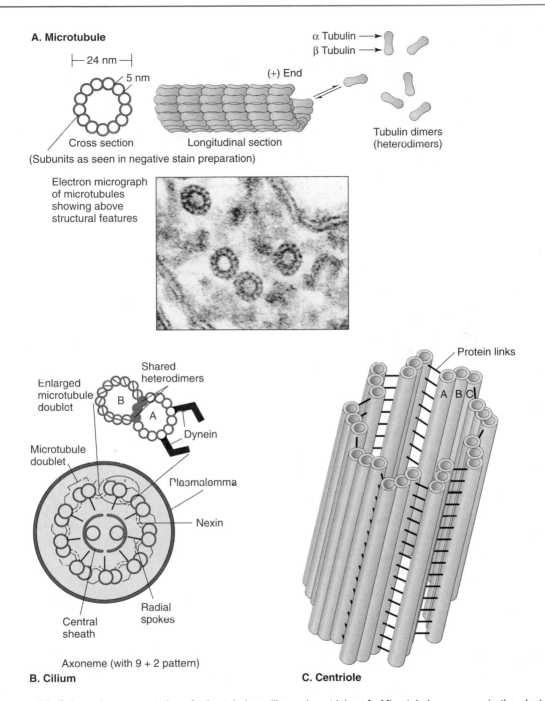

Figure 2–25. Schematic representation of microtubules, cilia, and centrioles. **A:** Microtubules as seen in the electron microscope after fixation with tannic acid in glutaraldehyde. The unstained tubulin subunits are delineated by the dense tannic acid. Cross sections of tubules reveal a ring of 13 subunits of dimers arranged in a spiral. Changes in microtubule length are due to the addition or loss of individual tubulin subunits. **B:** A cross section through a cilium reveals a core of microtubules called an axoneme. The axoneme consists of two central microtubules surrounded by 9 microtubule doublets. In the doublets, microtubule A is complete and consists of 13 subunits, whereas microtubule B shares 2 or 3 heterodimers with A. When activated by ATP, the dynein arms link adjacent tubules and provide for the sliding of doublets against each other. **C:** Centrioles consist of 9 microtubule triplets linked together in a pinwheel-like arrangement. In the triplets, microtubule A is complete and consists of 13 subunits, whereas tubules B and C share tubulin subunits. Under normal circumstances, these organelles are found in pairs with the centrioles disposed at right angles to one another.

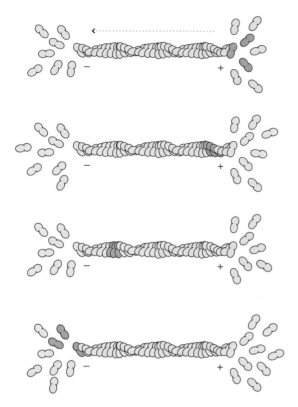

Figure 2–26. The cytosolic actin filament. Actin dimers are added to the plus (+) end and removed at the minus (–) end, dynamically lengthening or shortening the filament, as required by the cell. (Redrawn and reproduced, with permission, from Junqueira LC, Carneiro J: *Biologia Celular e Molecular,* 6th ed. Editora Guanabara, 1997.)

unorganized fashion within the cytoplasm (Figure 2–23).

Although actin filaments in muscle cells are structurally stable, microfilaments in nonmuscle cells readily dissociate and reassemble. Microfilament polymerization appears to be under the direct control of minute changes in Ca^{2+} and cAMP levels. A large number of actin-binding proteins have been demonstrated in a wide variety of cells, and much current research is focused on how these proteins regulate the state of polymerization and lateral aggregation of microfilaments. Their importance can be deduced from the fact that only about half the cell's actin is in the form of microfilaments.

Presumably, most microfilament-related activities depend upon the interaction of **myosin** with actin. (The structure and activity of the thick myosin filaments are described in the section on muscle tissues.) Myosin is present in unpolymerized form in most motile nonmuscle cells, polymerizing to form filaments only when participating in cell movement. Myosin-actin interactions are described in detail in the discussion of muscle tissue (see Chapter 10).

Intermediate Filaments

Ultrastructural and immunocytochemical investigations reveal that a third major filamentous structure is present in almost all eukaryotic cells. In addition to the thin (actin) and thick (myosin) filaments, cells contain a class of intermediate-sized filaments with an average diameter of 10–12 nm (Figure 2–27 and Table 2–4). Several proteins that form intermediate

there are several types of actin and that this protein is present in all cells.

The differences in amino acid composition are related to specific functional roles of the various actins found in the cytoplasm. Within cells, microfilaments can be organized in many forms. (1) In skeletal muscle, they assume a paracrystalline array integrated with thick (16-nm) myosin filaments. (2) In most cells, microfilaments form a thin sheath just beneath the plasmalemma, called the **cell cortex.** These filaments appear to be associated with membrane activities such as endocytosis, exocytosis, and cell migratory activity. (3) Microfilaments are intimately associated with several cytoplasmic organelles, vesicles, and granules. The filaments are believed to play a role in moving and shifting cytoplasmic components (cytoplasmic streaming). (4) Microfilaments are associated with myosin and form a "purse-string" ring of filaments whose constriction results in the cleavage of mitotic cells. (5) In most cells, microfilaments are found scattered in what appears to be an

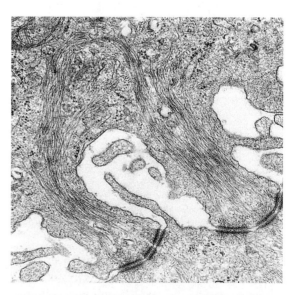

Figure 2–27. Electron micrograph of a skin epithelial cell showing cytokeratin (intermediate) filaments associated with desmosomes.

Table 2–4. Examples of intermediate filaments found in eukaryotic cells

Filament Type	Cell Type	Examples
Cytokeratins	Epithelium	Both keratinizing and nonkeratinizing epithelia
Vimentin	Mesenchymal cells	Fibroblasts, chondroblasts, macrophages, endothelial cells, vascular smooth muscle
Desmin	Muscle	Striated and smooth muscle (except vascular smooth muscle)
Gilial fibrillary acidic proteins	Glial cells	Astrocytes
Neurofilaments	Neurons	Most, but probably not all, neurons

filaments have been isolated and localized by immunocytochemical means.

Keratins (Gr. *keras,* horn) are found in most epithelia and constitute a family of approximately 20 proteins (molecular mass 40–68 kDa). They are coded by a family of genes and have different chemical and immunologic properties. This diversity of keratin is not surprising and is probably related to the various roles these proteins play in the epidermis, nails, hooves, horns, feathers, scales, and the like that provide animals with defense against abrasion and loss of water and heat and supply them with camouflage, decoration, and physical protection.

Vimentin filaments are characteristic of cells of mesenchymal origin. (Mesenchyme is an embryonic tissue.) Vimentin is a single protein (56–58 kDa) and may copolymerize with desmin or glial fibrillary acidic protein.

Desmin (skeletin) is found in smooth muscle and in the Z disks of skeletal and cardiac muscle (53–55 kDa).

Glial filaments (glial fibrillary acidic [GFA] protein) are characteristic of astrocytes but are not found in neurons, muscle, mesenchymal cells, or epithelia (51 kDa).

Neurofilaments consist of at least three high-molecular-weight polypeptides (68, 140, and 210 kDa). Intermediate filament proteins have different chemical structures and different roles in cellular function.

The presence of a specific type of intermediate filament in tumors can reveal which cell origi-

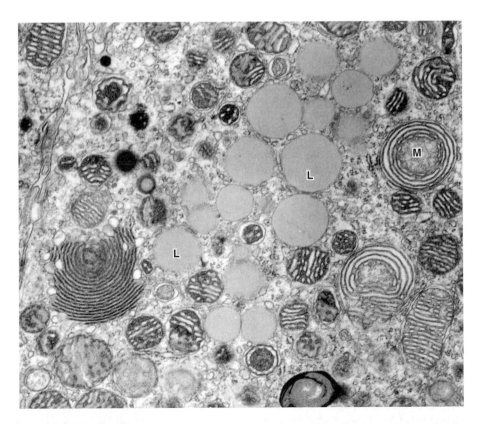

Figure 2–28. Section of adrenal gland showing lipid droplets (L) and abundant anomalous mitochondria (M). × 19,000.

nated the tumor, information important for diagnosis and treatment (see Table 1–3). Identification of intermediate filament proteins by means of immunocytochemical methods is a routine procedure.

Cytoplasmic Deposits

Cytoplasmic deposits are usually transitory components of the cytoplasm, composed mainly of accumulated metabolites or other substances. The accumulated molecules occur in several forms, one of them being lipid droplets in adipose tissue, adrenal cortex cells, and liver cells (Figure 2–28). Carbohydrate accumulations are also visible in several cells in the form of glycogen. After impregnation with lead salts, glycogen appears as collections of electron-dense particles (Figure 2–29). Proteins are stored in glandular cells as **secretory granules** or **secretory vesicles** (Figure 2–22); these are periodically released into the extracellular medium.

Deposits of colored substances—**pigments**—are often found in cells. They may be synthesized by the cell (eg, in the skin melanocytes) or come from outside the body (eg, carotene). One of the most common pigments is **lipofuscin,** a yellowish-brown substance present mainly in permanent cells (eg, neurons, cardiac muscle) that increases in quantity with age. Its chemical constitution is complex. It is believed that granules of lipofuscin derive from secondary lysosomes and represent deposits of indigestible substances. A widely distributed pigment, **melanin,** is abundant in the epidermis and in the pigment layer of the retina in the form of dense intracellular membrane-limited granules.

Cytosol

At one time, it was believed that the cytoplasm intervening between the discrete organelles and deposits was unstructured. This belief was reinforced by the use of homogenization and centrifugation of

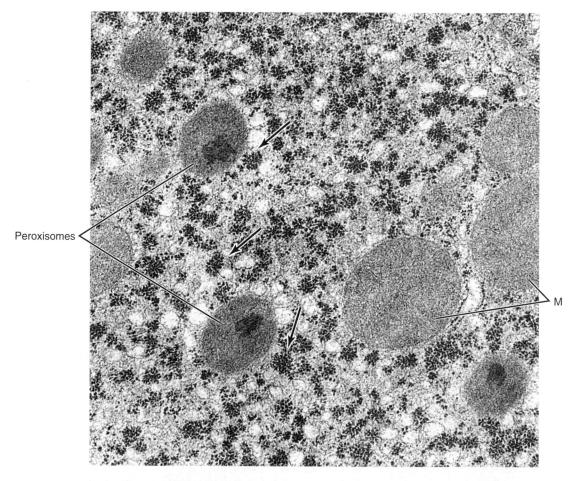

Peroxisomes

M

Figure 2–29. Electron micrograph of a section of a liver cell showing glycogen inclusions as accumulations of electron-dense particles (arrows). The dark structures with a dense core are peroxisomes. Mitochondria (M) are also shown. × 30,000.

Table 2–5. Some human and animal diseases related to altered cellular components.

Cell Component Involved	Disease	Molecular Defect	Morphologic Change	Clinical Consequence
Mitochondrion	Mitochondrial cytopathy	Defect of oxidative phosphorylation	Increase in size and number of muscle mitochondria	High basal metabolism without hyperthyroidism
Microtubule	Kartagener's syndrome	Lack of dynein in cilia and flagella	Lack of arms of the doublet microtubules	Immotile cilia and flagella with male sterility and chronic respiratory infection
	Mouse (*Acomys*) diabetes	Reduction of tubulin in pancreatic β cells	Reduction of microtubules in β cells	High blood sugar content (diabetes)
Lysosome	Metachromatic leukodystrophy	Lack of lysosomal sulfatase	Accumulation of lipid (cerebroside) in tissues	Motor and mental impairment
	Hurler disease	Lack of lysosomal α-L-iduronidase	Accumulation of dermatan sulfate in tissues	Growth and mental retardation
Secretory granule	Proinsulin diabetes	Defect of proinsulin-cleaving enzyme	None	High blood proinsulin content (diabetes)
Golgi complex	I-cell disease	Phosphotransferase deficiency	Inclusion-particle storage in fibroblasts	Psychomotor retardation, bone abnormalities

the homogenates to yield fractions consisting of recognizable organelles. The final supernatant produced by this process, after the separation of organelles, is called the **cytosol,** or soluble ground substance. The cytosol constitutes about half the total volume of the cell. Homogenization of cells disrupts a delicate **microtrabecular lattice** that incorporates microfilaments of actin, microtubules, enzymes, and other soluble constituents into a structured cytosol, or cytomatrix (*kytos* + L. *matrix,* mold). This matrix coordinates the intracellular movements of organelles and provides an explanation for the viscosity of the cytoplasm. Soluble (not membrane-bound) enzymes, such as those of the glycolytic pathway, for example, function more efficiently when organized in a sequence instead of having to rely on random collisions with their substrates. The cytosol may provide a framework for this organization. It contains thousands of enzymes that produce building blocks for larger molecules and break down small molecules to liberate energy. All machinery to synthesize proteins (rRNA, mRNA, tRNA, enzymes, and other factors) is contained in the cytosol. The role of the RER is to segregate some of the newly formed protein molecules into its cisternae.

Cell Components & Diseases

Many diseases are related to molecular alterations in specific cell components. In several of these diseases, structural changes can be detected by light or electron microscopy or by cytochemical techniques. Table 2–5 lists some of these diseases and emphasizes the importance of understanding the many cell components in pathobiology.

REFERENCES

Afzelius BA, Eliasson R: Flagellar mutants in man: on the heterogeneity of the immotile-cilia syndrome. J Ultrastruct Res 1979;69:43.

Alberts B et al: *Molecular Biology of the Cell,* 3rd ed. Garland, 1994.

Barrit GJ: *Communication Within Animal Cells.* Oxford Univ Press, 1992.

Bittar EW (editor): *Membrane Structure and Function.* 4 vols. Wiley, 1980–1981.

Bretscher MS: The molecules of the cell membrane. Sci Am 1985;253:100.

Brinkley BR: Microtubule organizing centers. Annu Rev Cell Biol 1985;1:145.

Brown MS et al: Recycling receptors: the round-trip itinerary of migrant membrane proteins. Cell 1983;32:663.

Cooper, GM: *The Cell: A Molecular Approach.* ASM Press/Sinauer Associates, Inc., 1997.

Darnell J et al: *Molecular Cell Biology,* 2nd ed. Scientific American Books, 1990.

DeDuve C: *A Guided Tour of the Living Cell.* Freeman, 1984.

DeDuve C: Microbodies in the living cell. Sci Am 1983; 248:74.

Dingle JT (editor): *Lysosomes in Biology and Pathology,* 6 vols. Elsevier/North-Holland, 1969–1979.

Dustin P: *Microtubules,* 2nd ed. Springer-Verlag, 1984.

Farquhar MG: Progress in unraveling pathways of Golgi traffic. Annu Rev Cell Biol 1985;1:447.

Fawcett D: *The Cell,* 2nd ed. Saunders, 1981.

Krstić RV: *Ultrastructure of the Mammalian Cell.* Springer-Verlag, 1979.

Osborn M, Weber K: Intermediate filaments: cell-type-specific markers in differentiation and pathology. Cell 1982;31:303.

Palade GE: Intracellular aspects of the process of protein synthesis. Science 1975;189:347.

Pfeffer SR, Rothman JE: Biosynthetic protein transport and sorting in the endoplasmic reticulum. Annu Rev Biochem 1987;56:829.

Rothman J: The compartmental organization of the Golgi apparatus. Sci Am 1985;253:74.

Singer SJ, Nicholson GL: The fluid mosaic model of the structure of cell membranes. Science 1972;175:720.

Trent RJ: *Molecular Medicine. An Introductory Text for Students.* Churchill Livingstone, 1993.

Tzagoloff A: *Mitochondria.* Plenum, 1982.

Weber K, Osborn M: The molecules of the cell matrix. Sci Am 1985;253:110.

Wolfe SL: *Molecular and Cellular Biology.* Wadsworth, 1993.

The Cell Nucleus

3

In the nucleus, the DNA of the cell is so well organized that it can be partially or totally duplicated with few, if any, mistakes.

The nucleus of the cell appears as a rounded or elongated structure, usually in the center of the cell. In mammalian tissues, its diameter usually varies between 5 and 10 µm. The nucleus comprises the **nuclear envelope, chromatin, nucleolus,** and **nuclear matrix** (Figure 3–1). The size and morphologic features of nuclei in a specific tissue tend to be uniform, with rare exceptions.

In a tumor, the presence of nuclei with irregular features (eg, variable size, atypical chromatin patterns) and the capacity to invade neighboring tissues are the main morphologic characteristics used by pathologists to estimate the degree of malignancy.

Nuclear Envelope

In the light microscope, a nuclear membrane—a thin line surrounding the nucleus—can be observed. This nuclear membrane is mainly a thin layer of heterochromatin that lines and binds to the internal surface of the nuclear envelope (Figures 3–2 and 3–3). Electron microscopy, however, shows that the nucleus is actually surrounded by two parallel unit membranes separated by a narrow space (40–70 nm) called the **perinuclear cisterna.** Together, the paired membranes and the intervening space make up the nuclear envelope. Closely associated with the internal membrane of the nuclear envelope is a protein structure called the **fibrous lamina,** which varies in thickness from 80 to 300 nm, depending on the cell examined. This structure does not block nuclear pores. The fibrous lamina is composed of three main polypeptides, called **lamins,** that form part of the nuclear matrix. During interphase, the chromatin adjacent to the centromeres of chromosomes is associated with the fibrous lamina. The pattern of association is very regular from cell to cell within a tissue. This finding has given rise to the idea that chromatin has a definite organization within the nucleus. Polyribosomes are frequently attached to the outer membrane, and this portion of the nuclear envelope is sometimes continuous with the rough endoplasmic reticulum (Figure 3–1). When covered with polyribosomes, the nuclear envelope functions as rough endoplasmic reticulum, synthesizing polypeptide chains and segregating them in the perinuclear cistern between its two membranes. Around the nuclear envelope, at sites where the inner and outer membranes fuse, there are circular gaps, the **nuclear pores** (Figures 3–3 and 3–4), that provide pathways between the nucleus and the cytoplasm. Nuclear pores have an average diameter of 70 nm. The pores are not open but show a **pure complex** made of several proteins. Although the permeability of the nucleus to molecules is variable, all pores are permeable to some macromolecules (eg, messenger RNA, cytoplasmic proteins), and molecular complexes such as ribosome subunits.

Chromatin

Two types of chromatin can be distinguished with both the light and electron microscopes (Figures 3–1 and 3–2). **Heterochromatin** (Gr. *heteros*, other, + *chroma*, color), which is electron-dense and appears as coarse granules in the electron microscope, is visible in the light microscope (after appropriate staining) as basophilic clumps of nucleoprotein. **Euchromatin** is visible as an organized structure only in the electron microscope. When viewed with the light microscope, however, lightly stained areas in the nucleus correspond to the euchromatin recognized using electron microscopy. The proportion of heterochromatin to euchromatin accounts for the light-to-dark appearance of nuclei in tissue sections as seen in light and electron microscopes. The intensity of nuclear staining of the chromatin is frequently used to distinguish and identify different tissues and cell types in the light microscope. The morphologic characteristics of chromatin are therefore used throughout this book to aid in the study and identification of cells and tissues.

Chromatin is composed mainly of coiled strands of DNA bound to basic proteins (histones); its structure is schematically presented in Figure 3–5. The

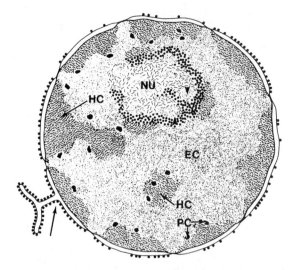

Figure 3–1. Structure of a nucleus. The nuclear envelope merges with the endoplasmic reticulum (arrow). Heterochromatin (HC) and euchromatin (EC) are shown. The large dark dots (PC) are perichromatin granules. Fibrillar and granular portions can be distinguished in the nucleolus (NU). The heterochromatin surrounding the nucleolus forms the **nucleolus-associated chromatin.** Portions of euchromatin are interspersed with nucleolar material (arrowhead). This chromatin contains the genes that specify ribosomal RNAs.

basic structural unit of chromatin is the nucleosome, which consists of a core of four types of histones: two copies each of histones H2A, H2B, H3, and H4, around which are wrapped 166 DNA base pairs. An additional 48–base pair segment forms a link between adjacent nucleosomes, and another type of histone (H1 or H5) is bound to this DNA. This organization of chromatin has been referred to as "beads-on-a-string." Nonhistone proteins are also associated with chromatin, but their arrangement is less well understood.

The next higher order of organization of chromatin is the 30-nm fiber commonly referred to as a **solenoid.** In this structure, nucleosomes become coiled around an axis, with six nucleosomes per turn, to form the 30-nm chromatin fiber. One assumes that there must be higher orders of coiling, especially in the condensation of chromatin into chromosomes during mitosis and meiosis.

Chromatin DNA is the major form of DNA in the cell and consequently carries most of the genetic information. Within the chromatin, the precursors of the messenger, ribosomal, and transfer ribonucleic acids (mRNA, rRNA, and tRNA) are synthesized.

The nucleoprotein of chromatin is coiled, and the degree of coiling varies during cell activity. The chromatin pattern of a nucleus has been considered a guide to the cells' activity. In general, cells with light nuclei are more active than those with condensed,

dark nuclei. In light-stained nuclei (with few heterochromatin clumps), more DNA surface is available for the transcription of genetic information. In dark-stained nuclei, the coiling of DNA makes less surface available.

Careful study of the chromatin of mammalian cell nuclei reveals a heterochromatin mass that is frequently observed in female cells but not in male cells. This chromatin clump is the **sex chromatin** and is one of the two X chromosomes present in female cells during interphase. The X chromosome that constitutes the sex chromatin remains tightly coiled and visible, whereas the other X chromosome is uncoiled and not visible. Evidence suggests that the sex chromatin is genetically inactive. The male has one X chromosome and one Y chromosome as sex determinants; the X chromosome is uncoiled, and therefore no sex chromatin is visible. In human epithelial cells, sex chromatin appears as a small granule attached to the nuclear envelope. The cells lining the internal surface of the cheek are frequently used to study sex chromatin. Blood smears are also often used, in which case the sex chromatin appears as a drumstick-like appendage to the nuclei of the neutrophilic leukocytes (Figure 3–6).

The study of sex chromatin has wide applicability in medicine, because it permits determination of genetic sex in patients whose external sex organs do not permit assignment of gender, as in hermaphroditism and pseudohermaphroditism. Sex chromatin is essential for the study of other anomalies involving the sex chromosomes—eg, Klinefelter syndrome, in which testicular abnormalities, azoospermia, and other symptoms are associated with the presence of XXY chromosomes in the cell.

The study of chromosomes of animals, and particularly of humans, made considerable progress after the development of methods that induce cells to divide, arrest mitotic cells during metaphase, and cause cell rupture. Mitosis can be induced by phytohemagglutinin and can be arrested in metaphase by colchicine. Cells are immersed in a hypotonic solution, which causes swelling, after which cells are flattened and broken between a glass slide and a coverslip.

The pattern of chromosomes obtained in a human cell after staining is illustrated in Figure 3–7. In addition to the X and Y sex chromosomes, the remaining chromosomes are customarily grouped according to their morphologic characteristics, in 22 successively numbered pairs.

The number and characteristics of chromosomes encountered in an individual are known as the **karyotype** (Figure 3–7). The study of karyotypes has revealed chromosomal alterations as-

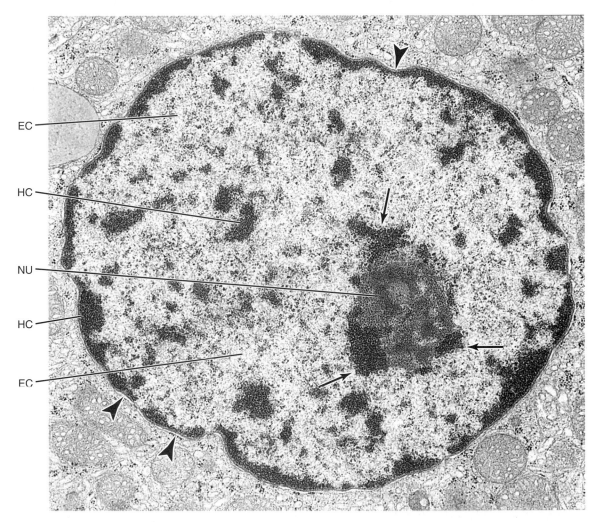

Figure 3–2. Electron micrograph of a nucleus, showing the heterochromatin (HC) and euchromatin (EC). Unlabeled arrows indicate the nucleolus-associated chromatin around the nucleolus (NU). Arrowheads indicate the perinuclear cisterna. Underneath the cisterna is a layer of heterochromatin designated a **nuclear membrane** by optical microscopists. × 26,000.

sociated with tumors, leukemias, and several types of genetic diseases.

Until recently, recognition of individual chromosomes was difficult, because different chromosomes of the same karyotype often had the same general morphologic characteristics. The development of techniques that reveal segmentation of chromosomes in transverse, differentially stained bands permitted not only the identification of individual chromosomes but also the detailed study of genetic deletion and translocation. These techniques are based mainly on the appearance of transverse bands in chromosomes previously treated with saline or enzyme solution and stained with fluorescent dyes or Giemsa's blood-staining technique. In situ hybridization is also a valuable technique for localizing DNA sequences (genes) in chromosomes. All these procedures have revolutionized the field of cytogenetics and have made possible many important observations in human cytogenetics, including the chromosomal localization of several genes.

Nucleolus

The nucleolus is a spherical structure, up to 1 mm in diameter, that is rich in rRNA and protein. It is usually basophilic when stained with hematoxylin and eosin. As seen with the electron microscope, the nucleolus consists of three distinct components: (1) From one to several pale-staining regions are composed of **nucleolar organizer DNA**—sequences of bases that code for rRNA (Figure 3–8). In the human

Nucleus

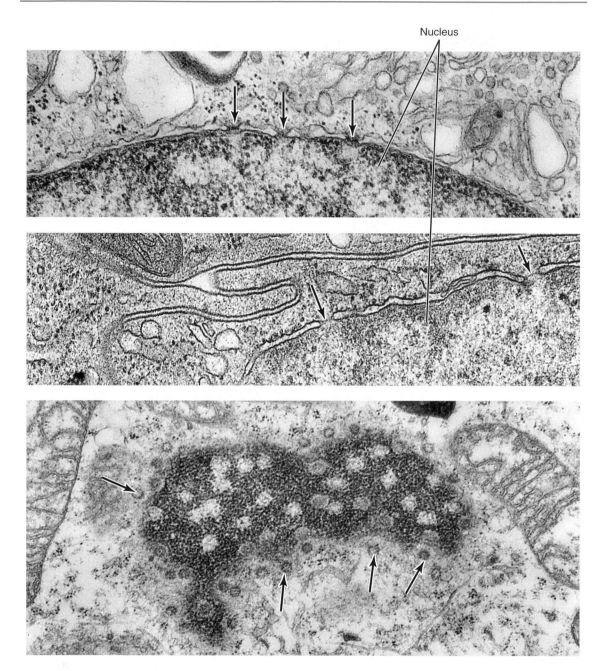

Figure 3–3. Electron micrographs of nuclei showing their envelopes, composed of two membranes and the nuclear pores (arrows). The two upper pictures are of transverse sections; the bottom is of a tangential section. Chromatin, frequently condensed below the nuclear envelope, is not usually seen in the pore regions. × 80,000.

genome, five pairs of chromosomes contain nucleolar organizers. (2) Closely associated with the nucleolar organizers are densely packed 5- to 10-nm ribonucleoprotein fibers composing the **pars fibrosa,** which consists of primary transcripts of rRNA genes. (3) The **pars granulosa** consists of 15- to 20-nm granules (maturing ribosomes; see Figure 3–8). Proteins, synthesized in the cytoplasm, become associated with rRNAs in the nucleolus; ribosome subunits then

migrate into the cytoplasm. Heterochromatin is often attached to the nucleolus (**nucleolus-associated chromatin**), but the functional significance of the association is not known (see Figures 3–1 and 3–2).

Large nucleoli are encountered in embryonic cells during their proliferation, in cells that are actively synthesizing proteins, and in rapidly growing malignant tumors. The nucleolus dis-

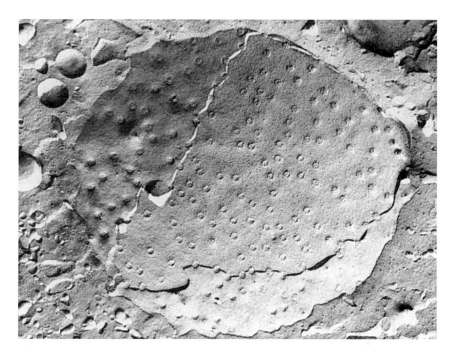

Figure 3–4. Electron micrograph of a rat intestine preparation obtained by cryofracture, showing the two components of the nuclear envelope and the nuclear pores. (Courtesy of P Pinto da Silva.)

perses during cell division but reappears in the telophase stage of mitosis.

Nuclear Matrix

The nuclear matrix is the component that fills the space between the chromatin and the nucleoli in the nucleus. It is composed mainly of proteins (some of which have enzymatic activity), metabolites, and ions. When its nucleic acids and other soluble components are removed, a continuous fibrillar structure remains, forming the **nucleoskeleton.** The fibrous lamina of the nuclear envelope is part of the nuclear matrix. The nucleoskeleton probably contributes to the formation of a protein base to which DNA loops are bound.

CELL DIVISION

Cell division, or mitosis (Gr. *mitos,* a thread), can be observed with the light microscope. During this process, the parent cell divides, and each of the daughter cells receives a chromosomal karyotype identical to that of the parent cell. Essentially, a longitudinal duplication of the chromosomes takes place, and these chromosomes are distributed to the daughter cells. The phase during which the cell does not undergo division is called **interphase,** during which the nucleus appears as it is normally observed in microscope preparations. The process of mitosis is

dynamic and continuous but is subdivided into phases to facilitate its study (Figures 3–9 and 3–10).

The **prophase** of mitosis is characterized by the gradual coiling of nuclear chromatin, giving rise to several individual rod- or hairpin-shaped bodies (chromosomes) that stain intensely. The nuclear envelope remains unaltered, and the chromosomes appear to be coiled in the nucleus. The centrioles separate, and a pair of centrioles migrates to each pole of the cell. Simultaneously, the microtubules of the mitotic spindle appear between the two pairs of centrioles (Figure 3–9).

During **metaphase,** the nuclear envelope and the nucleolus disappear. The chromosomes migrate to the equatorial plane of the cell, where each divides longitudinally to form two chromatids. The chromatids attach to the microtubules of the mitotic spindle (Figures 3–11 and 3–12) at a plaque-like, electron-dense region, the **centromere** (Gr. *kentron,* center, + *meros,* part), or **kinetochore** (Gr. *kinetos,* moving, + *chora,* central region).

In **anaphase,** the sister chromatids separate from each other and migrate toward the opposite poles of the cell, following the direction of the spindle microtubules. Throughout this process, the centromeres move away from the center, pulling along the remainder of the chromosome. Immunofluorescence shows microtubular protein (tubulin), actin, and myosin in the spindle region. These proteins may participate with microtubules in the process of chro-

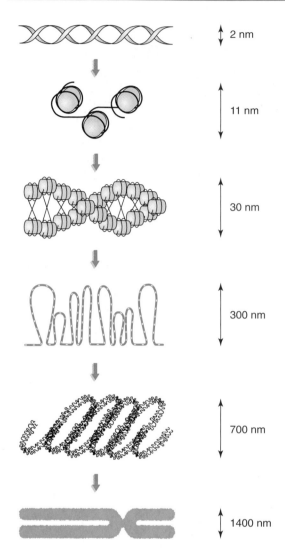

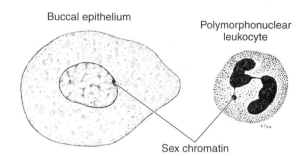

Figure 3–6. Morphologic features of sex chromatin in human female oral (buccal) epithelium and in a polymorphonuclear leukocyte. In the epithelium, sex chromatin appears as a small, dense granule adhering to the nuclear envelope. In the leukocyte, it has a drumstick shape.

Figure 3–5. The orders of chromatin packing believed to exist in the metaphase chromosome. Starting at the top, the 2-nm DNA double helix is shown; next is the association of DNA with histones to form filaments of nucleosomes of 11 nm and 30 nm. Through further condensation, filaments with diameters of 300 nm and 700 nm are formed. Finally, the bottom drawing shows a metaphase chromosome, which exhibits the maximum packing of DNA.

mosome migration to the cell poles, but the mechanism of this process is still a subject for discussion.

Telophase is characterized by the reappearance of nuclei in the daughter cells. The chromosomes revert to their semidispersed state, and the nucleoli, chromatin, and nuclear envelope reappear. While these nuclear alterations are taking place, a constriction develops at the equatorial plane of the parent cell and progresses until the cytoplasm and its organelles are divided in two. Microfilaments containing both actin

and myosin accumulate in a belt-like shape beneath the cell membrane in the region of mitotic constriction.

Most tissues undergo constant turnover because of continuous cell division and the ongoing death of cells. Nerve tissue and cardiac muscle cells are exceptions, since they do not multiply postnatally and therefore cannot regenerate. The turnover rate of cells varies greatly from one tissue to another—rapid in the epithelium of the alimentary canal and the epidermis, slow in the pancreas and the thyroid.

THE CELL CYCLE

Mitosis is the visible manifestation of cell division, but other processes, not so easily observed with the light microscope, play a fundamental role in cell multiplication. Principal among these is the phase in which DNA, the main chromosomal component, replicates. This process can be analyzed by introducing labeled radioactive DNA precursors (eg, ^{3}H-thymidine) into the cell and tracing them by means of biochemical and autoradiographic methods. DNA replication has been shown to occur during **interphase,** when no visible phenomena of cell division can be seen with the microscope. This alternation between mitosis and interphase, known as the **cell cycle,** occurs in all tissues with cell turnover. A careful study of the cell cycle reveals that it can be divided into two stages: mitosis, consisting of the four phases already described (prophase, metaphase, anaphase, and telophase), and interphase (Figure 3–13).

Interphase is itself divided into three phases: G_1 (presynthesis), S (DNA synthesis), and G_2 (post–DNA duplication). Synthesis and replication of DNA and centrioles take place in the S phase. The sequence of these phases and the times involved are illustrated in Figure 3–13. During the G_1 (for gap) phase, RNA and protein synthesis take place, and the

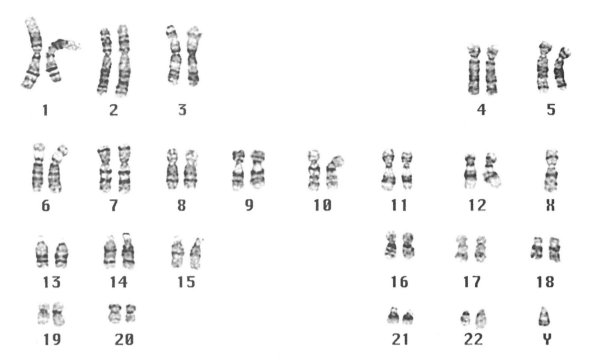

Figure 3–7. Human karyotype preparation made by means of a banding technique. Each chromosome has a particular pattern of banding that facilitates its identification and also the relationship of the banding pattern to genetic anomalies. The chromosomes are grouped in numbered pairs according to their morphologic characteristics

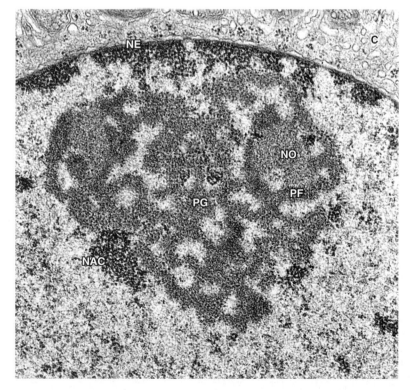

Figure 3–8. Nucleolus in a human adrenocortical cell. The nucleolar organizer DNA (NO), pars fibrosa (PF), pars granulosa (PG), nucleolus-associated chromatin (NAC), nuclear envelope (NE), and cytoplasm (C) are shown.

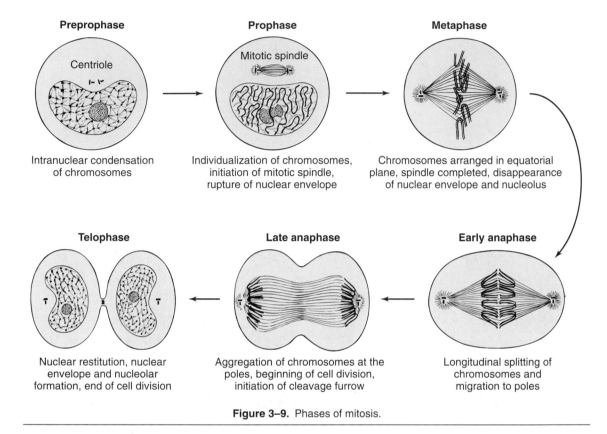

Preprophase

Centriole

Intranuclear condensation
of chromosomes

Prophase

Mitotic spindle

Individualization of chromosomes,
initiation of mitotic spindle,
rupture of nuclear envelope

Metaphase

Chromosomes arranged in equatorial
plane, spindle completed, disappearance
of nuclear envelope and nucleolus

Telophase

Nuclear restitution, nuclear
envelope and nucleolar
formation, end of cell division

Late anaphase

Aggregation of chromosomes at the
poles, beginning of cell division,
initiation of cleavage furrow

Early anaphase

Longitudinal splitting of
chromosomes and
migration to poles

Figure 3–9. Phases of mitosis.

cell volume, previously reduced to one-half by mitosis, is restored to its normal size. In cells that are not
continuously dividing, the cell cycle activities may
be temporarily or permanently suspended. Cells in
such a developmental state (eg, muscle, nerve) are
referred to as being in a G_0 phase.

Regulation of the mammalian cell cycle is complex and currently under intense investigation. It is

known that cultured cells deprived of serum stop proliferating and arrest in G_0. The essential components
provided by serum are highly specific proteins called
growth factors, which are required only in very low
concentrations. In animals, proliferation of most cell
types depends on specific combinations of growth
factors rather than a single factor. Thus, a relatively
small number of growth factors may be used in vari-

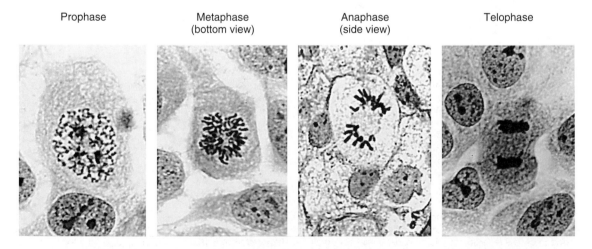

Prophase

Metaphase
(bottom view)

Anaphase
(side view)

Telophase

Figure 3–10. Photomicrograph showing the four main phases of mitosis in animal cells.

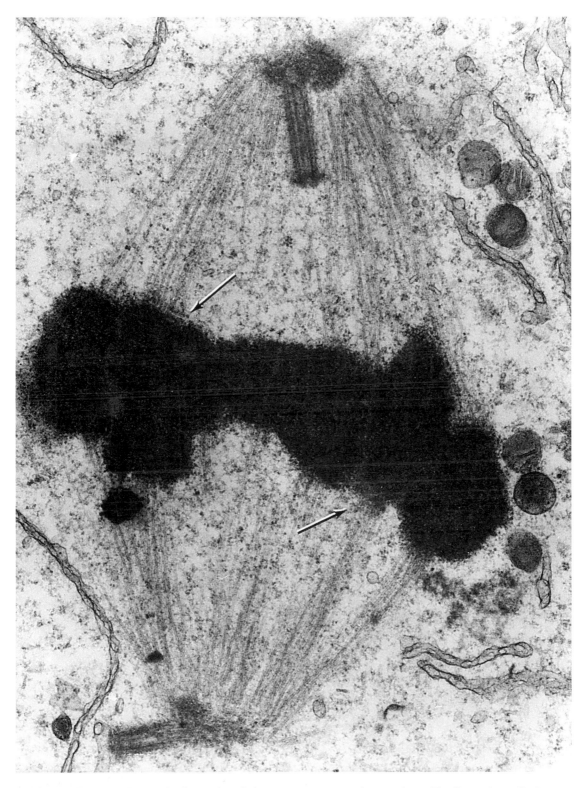

Figure 3–11. Electron micrograph of a section of a rooster spermatocyte in metaphase. The figure shows the two centrioles in each pole, the mitotic spindle formed by microtubules, and the chromosomes in the equatorial plate. The arrows show the insertion of microtubules in the centromeres. Reduced from × 19,000. (Courtesy of R McIntosh.)

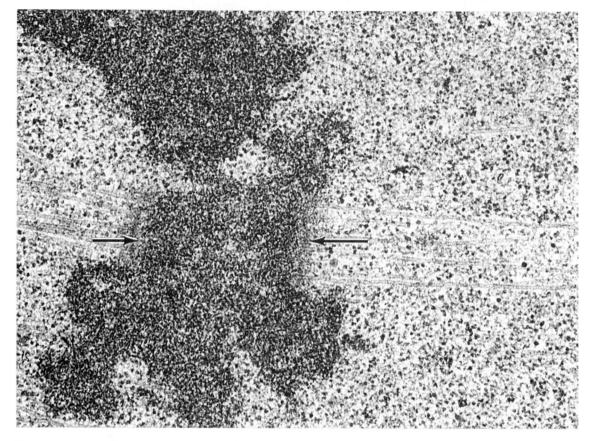

Figure 3–12. Electron micrograph of the metaphase of a human lung cell in tissue culture. Note the insertion of microtubules in the centromeres (arrows) of the densely stained chromosomes. Reduced from × 50,000. (Courtesy of R McIntosh.)

ous combinations to selectively regulate the proliferation of each of the many types of cells present in the animal. Some growth factors are being used in medicine. One example is erythropoietin, which stimulates proliferation, differentiation, and survival of red blood cell (erythrocyte) precursors in the bone marrow.

The cell cycle is also regulated by a variety of signals that inhibit progression through the cycle. DNA damage arrests the cell cycle not only in G_2, but also at a checkpoint in G_1. G_1 arrest may permit repair of the damage to take place before the cell enters S phase, where the damaged DNA would be replicated. In mammalian cells, arrest at the G_1 checkpoint is mediated by the action of a protein known as p53. The gene encoding p53 is often mutated in human cancers, thus reducing the cell's ability to repair damaged DNA. Inheritance of damaged DNA by daughter cells results in an increased frequency of mutations and general instability of the genome, which may contribute to the development of cancer.

Processes that occur during the G_2 phase are the accumulation of energy to be used during mitosis and

the synthesis of tubulin to be assembled in microtubules during mitosis.

Rapidly growing tissues (eg, intestinal epithelium) frequently contain cells in mitosis, whereas slowly growing tissues do not. The increased number of mitotic figures and abnormal mitoses in tumors is an important characteristic that distinguishes malignant from benign tumors. The organism has elaborate regulatory systems that control cell reproduction by either stimulating or inhibiting mitosis. Normal cell proliferation and differentiation are controlled by a group of genes called **proto-oncogenes;** altering the structure or expression of these genes promotes the production of tumors. Altered proto-oncogenes are present in tumor-producing viruses and are probably derived from cells. Altered oncogene activity can be induced by a change in the DNA sequence (mutation), an increase in the number of genes (gene amplification), or gene rearrangement, in which genes are relocated near an active promoter site. Altered

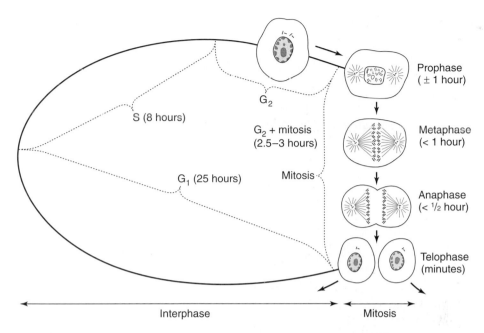

Figure 3–13. Phases of the cell cycle in bone tissue. The G_1 phase (presynthesis) varies in duration, which depends on many factors, including the rate of cell division in the tissue. In bone tissue, G_1 lasts 25 hours. The S phase (DNA synthesis) lasts about 8 hours. The G_2-plus-mitosis phase lasts 2.5–3 hours. The times indicated are courtesy of RW Young.

oncogenes have been associated with several tumors and hematologic neoplasia. Proteins that stimulate mitotic activity in various cell types include nerve growth factor, epithelial growth factor, fibroblast growth factor, and precursors of erythrocyte growth factor (erythropoietin); there is an extensive and rapidly growing list of these proteins (see Chapter 13). Several factors that inhibit cell reproduction are collectively called **chalones.** Cell proliferation is usually regulated by precise mechanisms that can, when necessary, stimulate or retard mitosis according to the needs of the organism. Several factors (eg, chemical substances, certain types of radiation, viral infections) can induce abnormal cell proliferation that bypasses normal regulation mechanisms for controlled growth and results in the formation of tumors.

The term **tumor,** initially used to denote any localized swelling in the body caused by inflammation or abnormal cell proliferation, is now usually used as a synonym for **neoplasm** (Gr. *neos,* new, + *plasma,* thing formed). Neoplasm can be defined as an abnormal mass of tissue formed by uncoordinated cell proliferation. Neoplasms are either benign or malignant according to their characteristics of slow growth and no invasiveness (benign) or rapid growth and great capacity to invade other tissues and organs (malignant) (Figure 3–14). Between these extremes are many tumors with intermediate properties. **Cancer** is the common term for all malignant tumors. Cancers are of great importance in medicine and are responsible for 20–30% of all deaths.

APOPTOSIS, OR PROGRAMMED CELL DEATH

Cell proliferation for renewal and growth is a process of self-evident physiologic significance. Less evident, but no less important for body functions and health, is the process of programmed cell death called **apoptosis.** A few examples of apoptosis will illustrate its significance.

Most T lymphocytes originating in the thymus have the ability to attack and destroy body components and would cause serious damage if they entered the blood circulation. Inside the thymus, T lymphocytes receive signals that activate the apoptotic program encoded in their chromosomes. T lymphocytes are destroyed by apoptosis before leaving the thymus, just as are T lymphocytes that display activated surface receptors to foreign molecules (see Chapter 14).

Most cells of the body can activate their apoptotic program when major changes occur in their DNA,

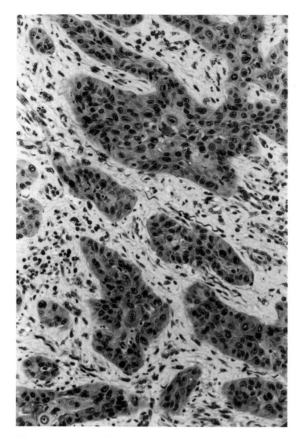

Figure 3–14. Photomicrograph of a malignant neoplasm (cancer) invading the neighboring connective tissue, which appears light-stained. The neoplasm shows compact masses of dark-stained cells.

eg, just before a tumor appears. In this way, apoptosis prevents the proliferation of malignant cells that develop as a result of accumulated mutations in the DNA. To form a clone and develop into a tumor, the malignant cell needs to deactivate the genes that control the apoptotic process.

Apoptosis was first discovered in developing embryos, where programmed cell death is an essential process for shaping the embryo (morphogenesis). Later investigators observed that apoptosis is also a common event in the tissues of normal adults.

In apoptosis, the cell and its nucleus become compact, decreasing in size. At this stage the apoptotic cell shows a dark-stained nucleus (pyknotic nucleus), easily identified with the light microscope. Next, the chromatin is cut into pieces by DNA endonucleases. During apoptosis the cell shows cytoplasmic large vesicles (blebs) that detach from the cell surface. These detached fragments are contained within the plasma membrane, which is changed in such a way that all cell remnants are readily engulfed, or phagocytosed, by macrophages. However, the apoptotic fragments do not elicit in macrophages the synthesis of the molecules that trigger the inflammatory process (see below).

The accidental death of cells, a pathologic process, is called **necrosis.** Necrosis can be caused by microorganisms, viruses, chemicals, and other harmful agents. Necrotic cells swell; their organelles increase in volume; and finally they burst, releasing their contents into the extracellular space. Macrophages engulf the debris of necrotic cells by phagocytosis and then secrete molecules that activate other immunodefensive cells to promote inflammation.

REFERENCES

Alberts B et al: *Molecular Biology of the Cell,* 3rd ed. Garland, 1994.

Barrit GJ: *Communication Within Animal Cells.* Oxford Univ Press, 1992.

Bostock CJ, Sumner AT: *The Eukaryotic Chromosome.* North-Holland, 1978.

Cooper, GM. *The Cell: A Molecular Approach.* ASM Press/Sinauer Associates, Inc., 1997

Darnell J et al: *Molecular Cell Biology,* 2nd ed. Scientific American Books, 1990.

DeDuve C: *A Guided Tour of the Living Cell.* Freeman, 1984.

Duke RC et al: Cell suicide in health and disease. Sci Am 1996;275(6):48.

Fawcett D: *The Cell,* 2nd ed. Saunders, 1981.

Goodman, SR. *Medical Cell Biology.* Lippincott, 1994.

Jordan EG, Cullis CA (editors): *The Nucleolus.* Cambridge Univ Press, 1982.

Kornberg RD, Klug A: The nucleosome. Sci Am 1981;244:52.

Krstić RV: *Ultrastructure of the Mammalian Cell.* Springer-Verlag, 1979.

Lloyd D et al: *The Cell Division Cycle.* Academic Press, 1982.

Trent RJ: *Molecular Medicine. An Introductory Text for Students.* Churchill Livingstone, 1993.

Watson JD et al: *Recombinant DNA,* 2nd ed. Scientific American Books, 1992.

Wolfe SL: *Molecular and Cellular Biology.* Wadsworth, 1993.

Epithelial Tissue

4

Despite its complexity, the human body is composed of only **four basic types of tissue:** epithelial, connective, muscular, and nervous. These tissues, which are formed by cells and molecules generically called **extracellular matrix,** do not exist as isolated units but rather in association with one another and in variable proportions, forming different organs and systems of the body. The main characteristics of these basic types of tissue are shown in Table 4–1.

Each tissue is composed of several cell types. Approximately 200 types of cells are recognized in the human body. Almost all cell types can undergo abnormal changes in their growth that can generate tumors (neoplasms). Tumors can be derived from virtually every stage of differentiation for each cell type, and each type of tumor has its own biologic characteristics. The enormous diversity of recognized tumors (several hundred types) helps explain the difficulty of diagnosis and clinical and surgical treatment.

An interesting observation regarding the tissue origin of cancer is worth noting. In children up to age 10, most tumors develop (in decreasing order) from hematopoietic organs, nerve tissues, connective tissues, and epithelial tissues. This proportion gradually changes, and after age 45, more than 90% of all tumors are of epithelial origin.

Connective tissue is characterized by the abundance of extracellular material produced by its cells; muscle tissue is composed of elongated cells that have the specialized function of contraction; and nerve tissue is composed of cells with elongated processes extending from the cell body that have the specialized functions of receiving, generating, and transmitting nerve impulses. Organs can be divided into **parenchyma,** which is composed of the cells responsible for the main functions typical of the organ, and **stroma,** which is the supporting tissue. Except in the brain and spinal cord, the stroma is made of connective tissue.

Epithelial tissues are composed of closely aggregated polyhedral cells with very little extracellular substance. These cells have strong adhesion and form cellular sheets that cover the surface of the body and line its cavities.

The principal functions of epithelial (Gr. *epi,* upon, + *thele,* nipple) tissues are the covering and lining of surfaces (eg, skin), absorption (eg, the intestines), secretion (eg, the epithelial cells of glands), sensation (eg, neuroepithelium), and contractility (eg, myoepithelial cells). Because all external and internal surfaces of the body are lined by epithelial cells, everything that enters or leaves the body must cross an epithelial sheet.

Epithelia are derived from all three embryonic germ layers. Most of the epithelium that lines the skin, mouth, nose, and anus has an ectodermal origin. The lining of the respiratory system, the digestive tract, and the glands of the digestive tract (eg, the pancreas and the liver) is derived from the endoderm. Other epithelia (eg, the endothelial lining of blood vessels) originate from mesoderm.

THE FORMS & CHARACTERISTICS OF EPITHELIAL CELLS

The forms and dimensions of epithelial cells are varied, ranging from high **columnar** to **cuboidal** to low **squamous** cells and including all intermediate forms (Figure 4–1). Their common polyhedral form results from their juxtaposition in cellular layers or masses. A similar phenomenon might be observed if a large number of inflated rubber balloons were compressed into a limited space. Epithelial cell nuclei have a distinctive shape, varying from spherical to elongated or elliptic. The nuclear form often corresponds roughly to the cell shape; thus, cuboidal cells have spherical nuclei, and squamous cells have flattened nuclei. The long axis of the nucleus is always parallel to the main axis of the cell.

Since the boundaries between cells are frequently indistinguishable with the light microscope, the form of the cell nucleus is a clue to the shape and number of cells. Nuclear form is also of value in determining whether the cells are arranged in layers, a primary morphologic criterion for classifying epithelia (Figures 4–1 and 4–2).

Table 4–1. Main characteristics of the four basic types of tissues.

Tissue	Cells	Extracellular Matrix	Main Functions
Nervous	Intertwining elongated processes	None	Transmission of nervous impulses
Epithelial	Aggregated polyhedral cells	Only small amount	Lining of surface or body cavities, glandular secretion
Muscle	Elongated contractile cells	Moderate amount	Movement
Connective	Several types of fixed and wandering cells	Abundant amount	Support and protection

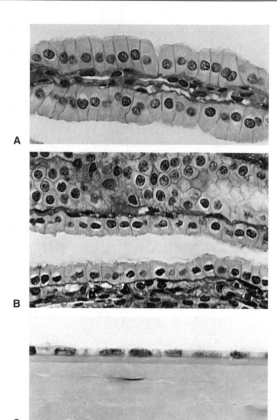

Figure 4–1. Examples of simple epithelia. **A:** Simple columnar type from the intestine. **B:** Simple cuboidal epithelium from the kidney. **C:** Simple squamous epithelium from the cornea. × 300.

Basal Laminae & Basement Membranes

All epithelial cells in contact with subjacent connective tissue have, at their basal surfaces, a sheet-like extracellular structure called the **basal lamina.** This structure is visible only with the electron microscope, where it appears as a dense layer, 20–100 nm thick, consisting of a delicate network of fine fibrils (**lamina densa**). In addition, basal laminae may have electron-lucent layers on one or both sides of the lamina densa, called **laminae rarae** or **laminae lucidae.** The main components of basal laminae are **type IV collagen,** the glycoproteins **laminin** and **entactin,** and **proteoglycan** (eg, the heparan sulfate proteoglycan called perlecan). The precise molecular composition of these components varies between and within tissues. Basal laminae are attached to the underlying connective tissues by anchoring fibrils formed by a special type of collagen (type VII) and by bundles of microfibrils that are part of the elastic system of the superficial dermis (Figures 4–3 and 4–4).

Basal laminae are found not only in epithelial tissues but also where other cell types come into contact with connective tissue (Figure 4–3B). Around muscle, adipose, and Schwann cells, basal laminae provide a barrier that limits or regulates exchanges of macromolecules between connective tissue and other tissues. Basal laminae are also found between adjacent epithelial layers, such as in lung alveoli and in the renal glomerulus (Figure 4–3A). In these cases, the basal lamina is thicker as a result of fusion of the basal laminae of each epithelial cell layer.

The components of basal laminae are secreted by epithelial, muscle, adipose, and Schwann cells. In some instances, reticular fibers are closely associated with the basal lamina, forming the **reticular lamina** (Figures 4–3B and 4–4B). The reticular fibers are produced by connective tissue cells.

Basal laminae have many functions. In addition to simple structural and filtering functions, they are also able to influence cell polarity; regulate cell proliferation and differentiation by binding with growth factors; influence cell metabolism; organize the proteins in adjacent plasma membrane (affecting signal transduction); and serve as pathways for cell migration. The basal lamina seems to contain the information necessary for certain cell-to-cell interactions, such as the reinnervation of denervated muscle cells. The presence of the basal lamina around a muscle cell is necessary for the establishment of new neuromuscular junctions.

The passage of tumor cells across a basal lamina attests to the invasive quality of these cells and is an important clue to the pathologist in evaluating the degree of malignancy of certain tumors.

The term **basement membrane** is used to specify a periodic acid–Schiff (PAS)-positive layer, visible with the light microscope, beneath epithelia (Figure 4–5) and in the kidney glomerulus and lung alveoli. The basement membrane is usually formed by the fusion of either two basal laminae (Figure 4–3A) or a basal lamina and a reticular lamina (Figure 4–3B) and is therefore thicker. The use of the terms base-

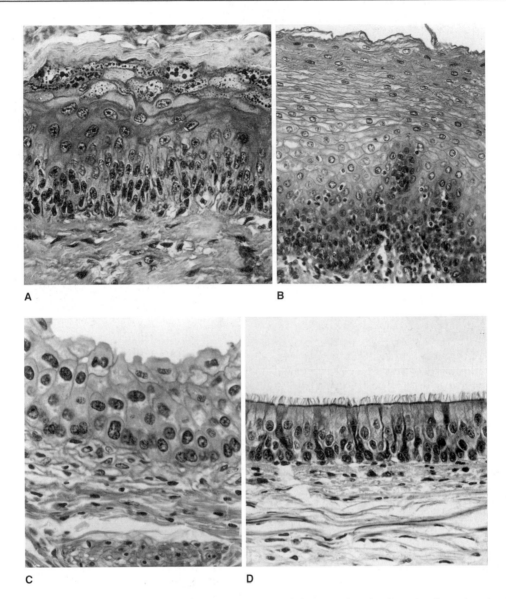

Figure 4–2. Photomicrographs of more complex types of epithelial tissue made using hematoxylin-and-eosin stain. **A:** Stratified squamous keratinized epithelium. **B:** Stratified squamous nonkeratinized epithelium. **C:** Transitional epithelium. **D:** Ciliated pseudostratified columnar epithelium. × 500.

ment membrane and basal lamina is not agreed upon by all investigators; the two terms are often used indiscriminately, causing confusion. In this book, "basal lamina" is used to denote the lamina densa and the variable presence of laminae rarae, which are structures seen with the electron microscope. "Basement membrane" is used to denote the thicker structures seen with the light microscope (Figure 4–5).

Intercellular Junctions

Several membrane-associated structures promote cell aggregation and contribute to cohesion and communication between cells. Epithelial cells are extremely cohesive, and relatively strong mechanical forces are necessary to separate them. Intercellular adhesion is especially marked in epithelial tissues that are subjected to traction and pressure (eg, the skin). Adhesion is due in part to the binding action of the glycoproteins, which are integral membrane proteins of the plasma membrane, and of a small amount of intercellular proteoglycan. Some glycoproteins lose their adhesiveness in the absence of calcium.

In addition to the cohesive effects of intercellular macromolecules and ions, the lateral membranes of epithelial cells exhibit several specializations that

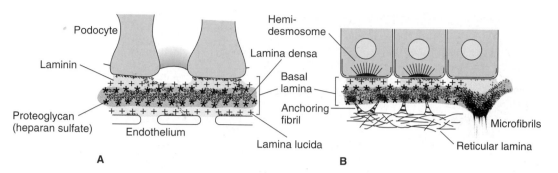

Figure 4–3. Two types of basement membranes. **A:** The thickness of this type of membrane results from fusion of two basal laminae produced by an epithelial and an endothelial cell layer, as found in the kidney glomerulus (shown here) and in the alveoli of the lung. It consists of a thick central **lamina densa** (darker colored zone) with a **lamina lucida** (**lamina rara;** lighter colored zone) on either side. **B:** The more common type of basement membrane that separates and binds epithelia to connective tissue is formed by association of the **basal** and **reticular laminae.** Note the presence of the anchoring fibrils formed by type VII collagen, which binds the basal lamina to the subjacent collagen. Note also the microfibrils grouped in a bundle that perforate the basal lamina, binding this structure to the elastic fiber system (see Figure 4–4).

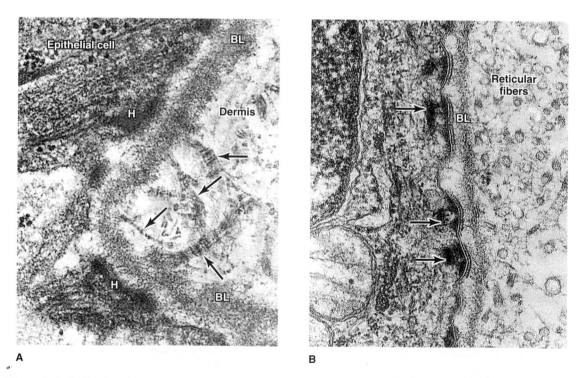

Figure 4–4. A: Section of human skin showing hemidesmosomes (H) at the epithelial–connective tissue junction. Note the anchoring fibrils (arrows) that apparently insert into the basal lamina (BL). The characteristically irregular spacing of these fibrils distinguishes them from collagen fibrils. × 54,000. (Courtesy of FM Guerra Rodrigo.) **B:** Section of skin showing the basal lamina (BL) and hemidesmosomes (arrows). This is a typical example of a basement membrane formed by a basal lamina and a reticular lamina (to the right of the basal lamina in this micrograph). × 80,000.

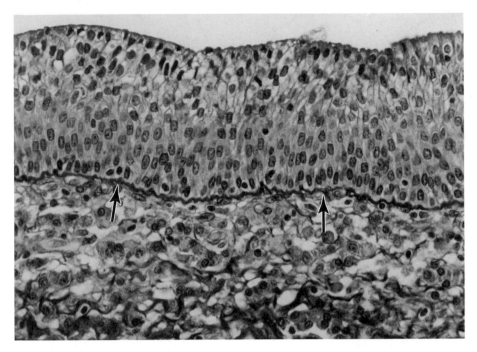

Figure 4–5. Photomicrograph of a section of the male urethra showing stratified columnar epithelium separated from the underlying connective tissue by a basement membrane (arrows). Picrosirius-hematoxylin stain.

form **intercellular junctions.** These junctions serve not only as sites of **adhesion** but also as **seals** to prevent the flow of materials through the intercellular space (the **paracellular pathway**) and to provide a mechanism for communication between adjacent cells. In some epithelia the various junctions are present in a definite order from the apex toward the base of the cell.

Tight junctions, or **zonulae occludentes** (singular, **zonula occludens**), are the most apical of the junctions. The Latin terminology gives important information about the geometry of the junction. "Zonula" refers to the fact that the junction forms a band completely encircling the cell, and "occludens" refers to the membrane fusions that close off the intercellular space. In properly stained thin sections viewed in the electron microscope, the outer leaflets of adjacent membranes are seen to fuse, giving rise to a local pentalaminar appearance. One to several of these fusion sites may be observed, depending on the epithelium (Figures 4–6 and 4–7). After cryofracture (Figure 4–8), the replicas show anastomosing ridges and grooves that form a net-like structure corresponding to the fusion sites observed in conventional thin sections. The number of ridges and grooves, or fusion sites, has a high correlation with the leakiness of the epithelium. Epithelia with one or very few fusion sites (eg, proximal renal tubule) are more per-

meable to water and solutes than are epithelia with numerous fusion sites (eg, urinary bladder). Thus, the principal function of the tight junction is to form a more or less tight seal that prevents the flow of materials between epithelial cells (paracellular pathway) in either direction (from apex to base or from base to apex; see Figure 4–19).

In many epithelia, the next type of junction encountered is the **zonula adherens** (Figures 4–6 and 4–7). This junction encircles the cell and is believed to provide for the adhesion of one cell to its neighbor. A noteworthy feature of this junction is the insertion of numerous actin microfilaments into dense plaques of material on the cytoplasmic surfaces of the junctional membranes. The plaques contain myosin, tropomyosin, α-actinin, and vinculin. The microfilaments arise from the **terminal web,** a web of several types of filaments in the apical cytoplasm. In this region, most cytoplasmic organelles are excluded, and the terminal web is believed to provide a certain rigidity to the apex of the cell (see Figure 4–10). Both junctions are responsible for a structure known as the **terminal bar** (see Figures 4–13 and 4–14).

A **gap junction,** or nexus, can occur almost anywhere along the lateral membranes of most epithelial cells. Gap junctions are found in nearly all mammalian tissues; skeletal muscle is a major exception.

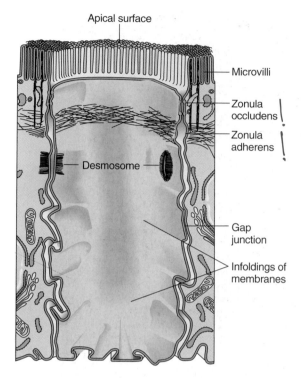

Figure 4–6. The main structures that participate in cohesion among epithelial cells. The drawing shows three cells from the intestinal epithelium. The cell in the middle was emptied of its contents to show the inner surface of its membrane. The zonula occludens and zonula adherens form a continuous ribbon around the cell apex, whereas the desmosomes and gap junctions make spotlike plaques. The zonula occludens is formed by multiple ridges where the outer laminae of apposed membranes fuse. (Redrawn and reproduced, with permission, from Krstić RV: *Ultrastructure of the Mammalian Cell*. Springer-Verlag, 1979.)

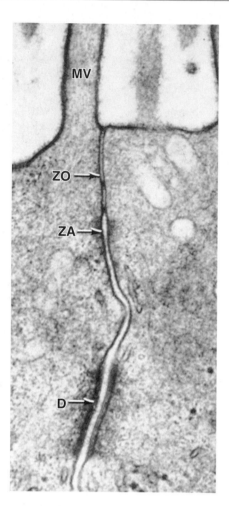

Figure 4–7. Electron micrograph of a section of epithelial cells in the large intestine showing a junctional complex with its zonula occludens (ZO), zonula adherens (ZA), and desmosome (D). Also shown is a microvillus (MV). × 80,000.

They are characterized, in conventional electron micrographs, by the close (2-nm) apposition of adjacent cell membranes (Figure 4–9A and C). After cryofracture, aggregates of intramembrane particles are found in circular patches in the plasma membrane (Figure 4–9B).

Gap junction protein units, called **connexins,** form hexamers with a hydrophilic pore about 1.5 nm in diameter in the center. This individual unit of the gap junction is called a **connexon,** and connexons in adjacent cell membranes are aligned to form a hydrophilic channel between the two cells (Figure 4–9A). Molecular cloning studies have demonstrated that connexins are a family of related proteins that are distributed differently and form channels with differing physiologic properties. Gap junctions permit the exchange between cells of molecules with molecular mass < 1500 Da. In addition, signaling molecules such as some hormones, cyclic AMP and GMP, and ions can move through gap junctions, causing the cells in many tissues to act in a coordinated manner rather than as independent units. A typical example is heart muscle cells, where gap junctions are greatly responsible for the heart's coordinated beat.

Gap junctions between previously isolated cells can be formed rapidly. Metabolic inhibitors—especially those that block oxidative phosphorylation—can inhibit the formation of junctions or can undo junctions already present between cells. New junctions can be formed in the absence of protein synthesis, however, in which case, connexons may form from subunits diffusely scattered in the plasma membrane.

The final type of junction is the **desmosome** (Gr.

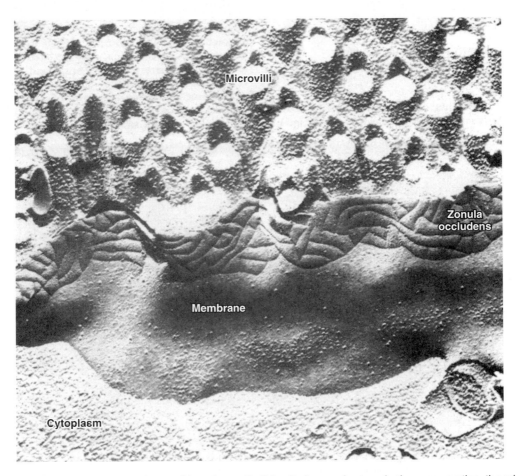

Figure 4–8. Electron micrograph of a small-intestine epithelial cell after cryofracture. In the upper portion, the microvilli are fractured transversely; in the lower portion, the fracture crosses through the cytoplasm of the intestinal epithelial cell. The grooves, which actually lie in the lipid (middle) layer of each plasmalemma, reveal that the membranes of adjoining cells were fused in the zonula occludens. × 100,000. (Courtesy of P Pinto da Silva.)

desmos, band, + *soma,* body), or **macula adherens** (see Figures 4–6 and 4–7). The desmosome is a complex disk-shaped structure at the surface of one cell that is matched with an identical structure at the surface of the adjacent cell. The cell membranes in this region are very straight and are usually somewhat farther apart (> 30 nm) than the usual 20 nm. In addition, some desmosomes possess a line of dense material in the intercellular space. Inside the membrane of each cell and separated from it by a short distance is a circular plaque of material called an **attachment plaque,** made up of at least 12 proteins. Groups of intermediate keratin filaments are inserted into the attachment plaque or make hairpin turns and return to the cytoplasm. Desmosomes are distributed in patches along the lateral membranes of most epithelial cells and are the only type of junction present in the stratified squamous epithelium of the skin. The

only function of desmosomes appears to be that of providing an especially firm adhesion of one cell to the next. The description here applies to the more complex desmosomes, many cells have a simpler structure with a similar function.

In the contact zone between certain epithelial cells and the basal lamina, **hemidesmosomes** (Gr. *hemi,* half, + *desmos* + *soma*) can often be observed. These structures take the form of half a desmosome on the epithelial cell plasmalemma and probably serve to bind the epithelial cell to the subjacent basal lamina (Figure 4–4B).

From the functional point of view, junctions between cells can be classified as **adhering junctions** (zonulae adherentes, hemidesmosomes, and desmosomes), **impermeable junctions** (zonulae occludentes), and **communicating junctions** (gap junctions).

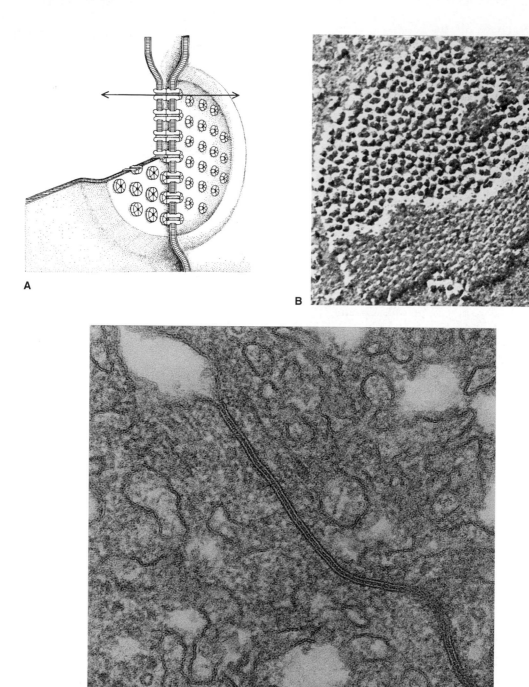

Figure 4–9. A: Model of a gap junction (oblique view) depicting the structural elements that allow the exchange of nutrients and signal molecules between cells without loss of material into the intercellular space. The communicating pipes are formed by pairs of abutting particles, which are in turn composed of six dumbbell-shaped protein subunits that span the lipid bilayer of each cell membrane. The channel passing through the cylindrical bridges (arrow in A) is about 1.5 nm in diameter, limiting the size of the molecules that can pass through it. Fluids and tracers in the intercellular space can permeate the gap junction by flowing around the protein bridges. (Reproduced, with permission, from Staehelin LA, Hull BE: Junctions between living cells. Sci Am 1978;238:41. Copyright © 1978 by Scientific American, Inc. All rights reserved.) **B:** Gap junction between living cells as seen on a cryofracture preparation. The junction appears as a plaque-like agglomeration of intramembrane protein particles. × 45,000. (Courtesy of P Pinto da Silva). **C:** Gap junction between two rat liver cells. At the junction, two apposed membranes are separated by a 2-nm-wide electron-dense space, or gap. × 193,000. (Courtesy of MC Williams.)

SPECIALIZATIONS OF THE CELL SURFACE

Structural specializations reflect specific activities at the various cell surfaces and are an important part of cell polarity.

Microvilli

When viewed in the electron microscope, most cells are seen to have projections rising from the surface. These projections may be short or long finger-like extensions or folds that pursue a sinuous course, and they range in number from a few to many. In absorptive cells, such as the lining epithelium of the small intestine and the cells of the proximal renal tubule, orderly arrays of many hundreds of microvilli (Gr. *mikros,* small, + L. *villus,* tuft of hair) are encountered (Figures 4–10 and 4–11). Each microvillus is about 1 μm high and 0.08 μm wide. Covering the microvillus is a filamentous coat of variable thickness, the **glycocalyx,** which contains glycoproteins and is thus PAS-positive. The complex of microvilli and glycocalyx is easily seen in the light microscope and is called the **brush,** or **striated, border** (see Figure 15–21).

Each microvillus is an extension of the cytoplasm of the cell and is covered by plasma membrane, thereby greatly increasing the surface area of the apex of the cell with a consequent increase in its absorptive efficiency. Within the microvilli are clusters of 20–30 actin microfilaments (Figure 4–11) that are cross-linked to each other and to the surrounding plasma membrane by several other proteins. The basal ends of these microfilaments intermingle with microfilaments of the terminal web just beneath the microvilli.

Stereocilia

Stereocilia are long, nonmotile processes of cells of the epididymis that are actually longer branched microvilli and should not be confused with true cilia. In the epididymis, stereocilia increase the cell surface area, facilitating the movement of molecules into and out of the cell.

Cilia & Flagella

Cilia are elongated, motile structures on the surface of epithelial cells, 5–10 μm long and 0.2 μm in diameter—much longer than the microvilli and different in structure. They are surrounded by the cell membrane and contain a central pair of microtubules. At the periphery inside the membrane, arranged in a circle, are nine more pairs of microtubules, all of

Terminal web   Microvilli   Cell coat

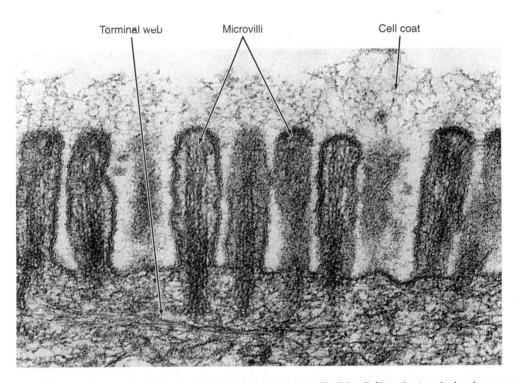

Figure 4–10. Electron micrograph of the apical region of an intestinal epithelial cell. Note the terminal web composed of a horizontal network that contains mainly actin microfilaments. The vertical microfilaments that constitute the core of the microvilli are clearly seen. An extracellular cell coat (glycocalyx) is bound to the plasmalemma of the microvilli. × 45,000.

Microvilli   Microfilaments

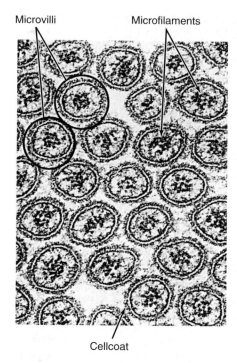

Cellcoat

Figure 4–11. Electron micrograph of a section from the apical region of a cell from the intestinal lining showing cross-sectioned microvilli. In their interiors, note the microfilaments in a cross section. The surrounding unit membrane can be clearly discerned and is covered by a layer of glycocalyx, or cell coat. × 100,000.

which run in the direction of the long axis (Figures 2–25 and 4–12).

Cilia are inserted into **basal bodies,** which are electron-dense structures at the apical pole just below the cell membrane (Figure 4–12). Basal bodies have a structure analogous to that of the centrioles (see Chapter 2).

In living organisms, cilia have a rapid back-and-forth movement. Ciliary movement is frequently coordinated to permit a current of fluid or particulate matter to be propelled in one direction over the ciliated epithelium. ATP is the source of energy for ciliary motion. A ciliated cell of the trachea is estimated to have about 250 cilia.

Flagella, present in the human body only in spermatozoa, are similar in structure to cilia but are much longer and are mostly limited to one flagella per cell.

TYPES OF EPITHELIA

Epithelia are divided into two main groups according to their structure and function: **covering epithelia** and **glandular epithelia.** This is an arbitrary division, for there are covering epithelia in which all cells secrete (eg, the surface epithelium of the stomach) or in which glandular cells are sparse among covering cells (eg, mucous cells in the small intestine or trachea).

Covering Epithelia

Covering epithelia are tissues in which the cells are organized in layers that cover the external surface or line the cavities of the body. They can be classified according to the number of cell layers and the morphologic features of the cells in the surface layer (Table 4–2). **Simple epithelium** contains only one layer of cells, and **stratified epithelium** contains more than one layer (Figures 4–1, 4–2, 4–13, and 4–14).

Simple epithelium can, according to cell shape, be **squamous, cuboidal,** or **columnar.** The endothelium that lines blood vessels and the mesothelium that lines certain body cavities are examples of simple squamous epithelium (Figure 4–13A).

> Because endothelial and mesothelial cells are both derived from mesenchyme (an embryonic tissue) rather than from ectodermal or endodermal cells, they have characteristic mesenchymal features, such as cytoskeletal intermediate filaments composed of vimentin rather than of keratin, which is found in the intermediate filaments of other epithelia. However, they differ in their ultrastructure, physiology, and response to several types of insults. They even produce different types of tumors.

An example of cuboidal epithelium is the surface epithelium of the ovary (Figure 4–13B), and an example of columnar epithelium is the lining of the small intestine (Figures 15–21 and 15–24).

Stratified epithelium is classified according to the cell shape of its superficial layer: **squamous, cuboidal, columnar,** and **transitional.** Pseudostratified epithelium forms a separate group, discussed below.

Stratified squamous keratinized epithelium is found mainly in the skin. Its cells form many layers, and the cells closer to the underlying connective tissue are usually cuboidal or columnar. The cells become irregular in shape and flatten as they get progressively closer to the surface, where they are thin and squamous (Figure 4–14A; see Chapter 18 for more detailed information).

Stratified squamous nonkeratinized epithelium lines wet cavities (eg, mouth, esophagus, vagina), in contrast to the skin, whose surface is dry. Stratified squamous nonkeratinized epithelium is characterized by a surface layer of flattened living cells that retain their nuclei. This is not the case with the keratinized variety of this epithelium, in which the surface cells are dead and their nuclei are not discernible (compare Figures 4–2A and 4–2B).

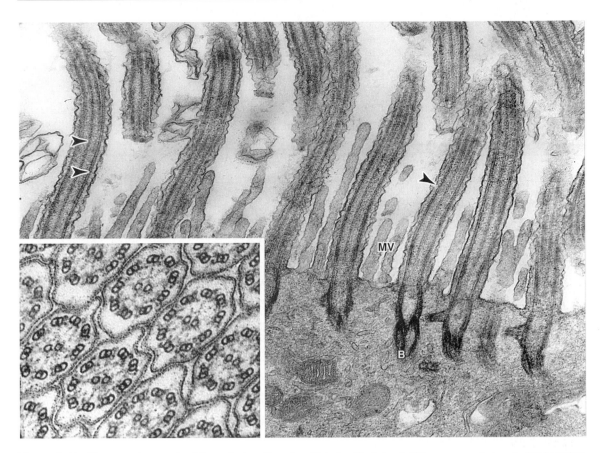

Figure 4–12. Electron micrograph of the apical portion of a ciliated epithelial cell. Cilia are seen in longitudinal section. At the left, arrowheads point to the central and peripheral microtubules of the axoneme. The arrowhead at right indicates the plasma membrane surrounding the cilium. Each cilium has a basal body (B) from which it grows. Microvilli (MV) are shown. × 59,000. **Inset:** Cilia in cross section. The 9 + 2 array of microtubules in each cilium is evident. × 80,000. (Reproduced, with permission, from Junqueira LCU, Salles LMM: Ultra-Estrutura e Função Celular. Edgard Blücher, 1975.)

Stratified columnar epithelium is rare; it is present in the human body only in small areas, such as the ocular conjunctiva and the large ducts of salivary glands.

Transitional epithelium, which lines the urinary bladder, the ureter, and the upper part of the urethra, is characterized by a surface layer of dome-like facet cells that are neither squamous nor columnar (Figures 4–2C and 4–14B). The form of these cells changes according to the degree of distention of the bladder. It is not unusual for these cells to be binucleate. This type of epithelium is discussed in detail in Chapter 19.

Pseudostratified epithelium is so called because the nuclei appear to lie in various layers. Although all cells are attached to the basal lamina, some do not reach the surface. The best-known example of this tissue is the ciliated pseudostratified columnar epithelium in the respiratory passages (Figures 4–2D and 4–14C).

Two other types of epithelium warrant brief mention. **Neuroepithelial cells** are cells of epithelial origin with specialized sensory functions (eg, cells of taste buds). **Myoepithelial cells** are branched cells that contain myosin and a large number of actin microfilaments. They are specialized for contraction, mainly of the acini of the mammary, sweat, and salivary glands.

Glandular Epithelia

Glandular epithelia are tissues formed by cells specialized to produce a fluid secretion that differs in composition from blood or extracellular fluid. This secretion is usually accompanied by the intracellular synthesis of macromolecules. These macromolecules are generally stored in the cells in small membrane-bound vesicles called **secretory granules.**

The chemical nature of these macromolecules is variable. Glandular epithelial cells may synthesize, store, and secrete proteins (eg, pancreas), lipids (eg,

Table 4–2. Common types of covering epithelia in the human body.

Number of Cell Layers	Cell Form	Examples of Distribution	Main Function
Simple (one layer)	Squamous	Lining of vessels (endothelium). Serous lining of cavities; pericardium, pleura, peritoneum (mesothelium).	Facilitates the movement of the viscera (mesothelium), active transport by pinocytosis (mesothelium and endothelium), secretion of biologically active molecules (mesothelium)
	Cuboidal	Covering the ovary, thyroid.	Covering, secretion.
	Columnar	Lining of intestine, gallbladder.	Protection, lubrication, absorption, secretion.
Pseudostratified (layers of cells with nuclei at different levels; not all cells reach surface but all adhere to basal lamina)		Lining of trachea, bronchi, nasal cavity.	Protection, secretion; cilia-mediated transport of particles trapped in mucus out of the air passages.
Stratified (two or more layers)	Squamous keratinized (dry)	Epidermis.	Protection; prevents water loss.
	Squamous nonkeratinized (moist)	Mouth, esophagus, larynx, vagina, anal canal.	Protection, secretion; prevents water loss.
	Cuboidal	Sweat glands, developing ovarian follicles.	Protection, secretion.
	Transitional	Bladder, ureters, renal calyces.	Protection, distensibility.
	Columnar	Conjunctiva.	Protection.

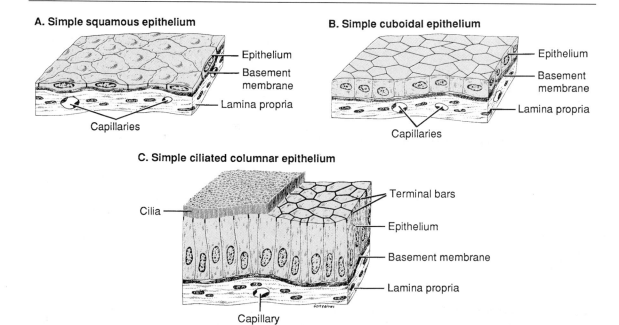

Figure 4–13. Diagrams of simple epithelial tissue. **A:** Simple squamous epithelium. **B:** Simple cuboidal epithelium. **C:** Simple ciliated columnar epithelium. All are separated from the subjacent connective tissue by a basement membrane. In C, note the terminal bars that correspond in light microscopy to the zonula occludens and the zonula adherens of the junctional complex.

A. Stratified squamous epithelium

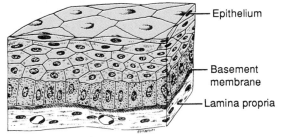

- Epithelium
- Basement membrane
- Lamina propria

B. Transitional epithelium

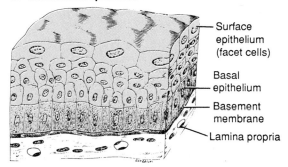

- Surface epithelium (facet cells)
- Basal epithelium
- Basement membrane
- Lamina propria

C. Ciliated pseudostratified epithelium

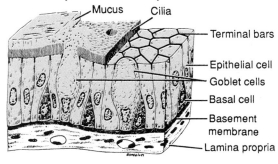

- Mucus
- Cilia
- Terminal bars
- Epithelial cell
- Goblet cells
- Basal cell
- Basement membrane
- Lamina propria

Figure 4–14. Diagrams of stratified epithelial tissue. **A:** Stratified squamous epithelium. **B:** Transitional epithelium. **C:** Ciliated pseudostratified epithelium. The goblet cells secrete mucus, which forms a continuous mucous layer over the ciliary layer.

adrenal, sebaceous glands), or complexes of carbohydrates and proteins (eg, salivary glands). The mammary glands secrete all three substances. Less common are the cells of glands that have low synthesizing activity (eg, sweat glands) and that secrete mostly substances transferred from the blood to the lumen of the gland.

A gland may contain active synthesizing cells in association with cells specializing in ion transport. This occurs in most major mammalian salivary glands, in which secretory acini coexist with ion-transporting structures called **striated ducts** (see Chapter 16).

Types of Glandular Epithelia

The epithelia that form the glands of the body can be classified according to various criteria. Unicellular glands consist of isolated glandular cells, and multicellular glands are composed of clusters of cells. An example of a unicellular gland is the **goblet cell** of the lining of the small intestine or of the respiratory tract (Figure 4–14C). The term "gland," however, is usually used to designate large, complex aggregates of glandular epithelial cells, such as in the salivary glands and the pancreas.

Glands always arise from covering epithelia by means of cell proliferation and invasion of subjacent connective tissue, followed by further differentiation (Figure 4–15). **Exocrine** (Gr. *exo*, outside, + *krinein*, to separate) glands retain their connection with the surface epithelium from which they originated. This connection takes the form of tubular ducts lined with epithelial cells through which the glandular secretions pass to reach the surface. **Endocrine** (Gr. *endon*, within, + *krinein*) glands are those whose connection with the surface from which they originated was obliterated during development. These glands are therefore ductless, and their secretions are picked up and transported to their site of action by the bloodstream rather than by a duct system.

Two types of endocrine glands can be differentiated according to cell grouping. In the first type, the agglomerated cells form anastomosing cords interspersed between dilated blood capillaries (eg, adrenal gland, parathyroid, anterior lobe of the pituitary; see Figure 4–15). In the second type, the cells line a vesicle or follicle filled with noncellular material (eg, the thyroid gland; Figure 4–15).

Exocrine glands have a **secretory portion,** which contains the cells responsible for the secretory process, and **ducts,** which transport the secretion to the exterior of the gland (Figure 4–15). **Simple**

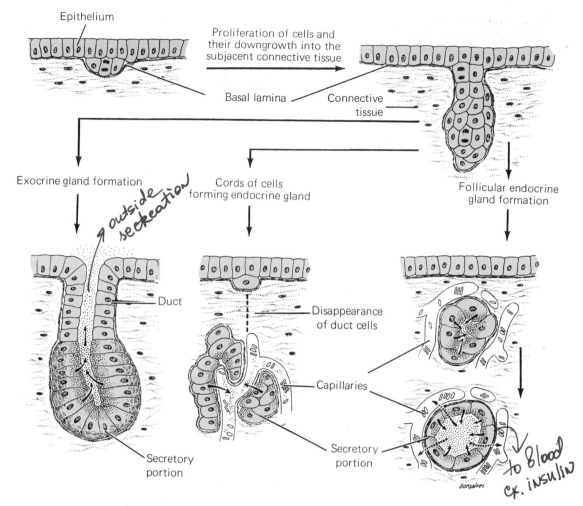

Figure 4–15. Formation of glands from covering epithelia. Epithelial cells proliferate and penetrate connective tissue. They may—or may not—maintain contact with the surface. When contact is maintained, exocrine glands are formed; without contact, endocrine glands are formed. The cells of these glands can be arranged in cords or follicles. The lumens of the follicles accumulate large quantities of secretion; cells of the cords store only small quantities in their cytoplasm. (Redrawn and reproduced, with permission, from Ham AW: *Histology,* 6th ed. Lippincott, 1969.)

glands have only one unbranched duct, whereas **compound glands** have ducts that branch repeatedly. The cellular organization within the secretory portion differentiates the glands further. Simple glands can be tubular, coiled tubular, branched tubular, or acinar. Compound glands can be tubular, acinar, or tubuloacinar (Figure 4–16). Some organs have both endocrine and exocrine functions, and one cell type may function both ways—eg, in the liver, where cells that secrete bile into the duct system also secrete some of their products into the bloodstream. In other organs, some cells are specialized in exocrine secretion and others are specialized in endocrine secretion; in the pancreas, for example, the acinar cells secrete digestive enzymes into the intestinal lumen, whereas the islet cells secrete insulin and glucagon into the blood.

According to the way in which the secretory products leave the cell, glands can be classified as **merocrine** (Gr. *meros,* part, + *krinein*) or **holocrine** (Gr. *holos,* whole, + *krinein*). In merocrine glands (eg, the pancreas), the secretory granules leave the cell by exocytosis with no loss of other cellular material. In holocrine glands (eg, sebaceous glands), the product of secretion is shed with the whole cell—a process that involves destruction of the secretion-filled cells. In an intermediate type—the **apocrine** (Gr. *apo,* away from, + *krinein*) gland—the secretory product is discharged together with parts of the apical cytoplasm.

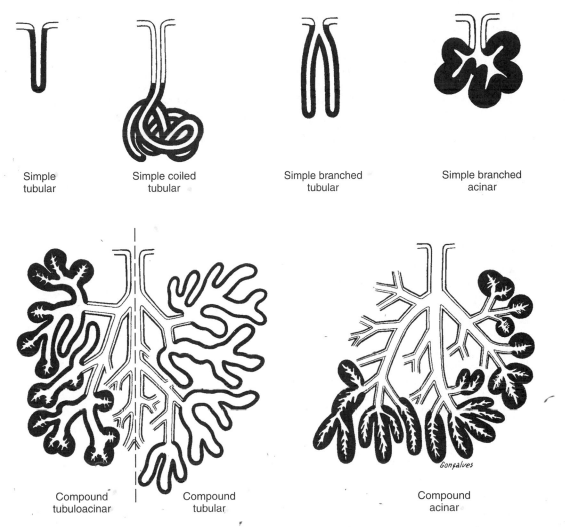

Simple
tubular

Simple coiled
tubular

Simple branched
tubular

Simple branched
acinar

Compound
tubuloacinar

Compound
tubular

Compound
acinar

Gonçalves

Figure 4–16. Principal types of exocrine glands. The part of the gland formed by secretory cells is shown in black; the remainder shows the ducts. The compound glands have branching ducts.

Multicellular glands usually have a surrounding capsule of connective tissue and septa that divides the gland into lobules. These lobules then subdivide, and in this way the connective tissue separates and binds together the glandular components. Blood vessels and nerves also penetrate and subdivide in the gland.

GENERAL BIOLOGY OF EPITHELIAL TISSUES

Underlying the covering epithelial tissues that line the body cavities is a layer of connective tissue, the **lamina propria,** which is bound to the epithelium by the basal lamina. The lamina propria not only serves to support the epithelium but also binds it to neigh-

boring structures. The area of contact between epithelium and lamina propria is increased by irregularities in the connective tissue surface in the form of evaginations called **papillae** (L.. diminutive of *papula,* nipple; singular, **papilla**). Papillae occur most frequently in epithelial tissues subject to stress, such as the skin and the tongue.

Polarity

An important feature of epithelia is their polarity; ie, they have a free, or apical, surface and a basal surface that rests on a basal lamina. Since blood vessels do not normally penetrate an epithelium, all nutrients must pass out of the capillaries in the underlying lamina propria. These nutrients and precursors of products of the epithelial cells then diffuse across the basal lamina and are taken up through the basolateral surface of the epithelial cell, usually by an energy-dependent process. Receptors for chemical messengers (eg, hormones, neurotransmitters) that influence the activity of epithelial cells are localized in the basolateral membranes. In absorptive epithelial cells, the apical cell membrane contains, as integral membrane proteins, enzymes such as disaccharidases and peptidases, which complete the digestion of molecules to be absorbed. Tight junctions help to prevent the integral membrane proteins of the various cell membrane regions from intermingling.

Nutrition

Because blood vessels do not penetrate the epithelium, there is no direct contact between epithelial cells and blood vessels. Epithelial nutrition depends, therefore, on the diffusion of metabolites through the basal lamina and often through parts of the lamina propria as well. The diffusion process is probably enhanced by the papillae, which increase the area of contact between epithelium and lamina propria. Reduced diffusion probably limits the thickness of the epithelium.

Innervation

Most epithelial tissues receive a rich supply of sensory nerve endings from nerve plexuses in the lamina propria. Everyone is aware of the exquisite sensitivity of the cornea, the epithelium covering the anterior surface of the eye. This sensitivity is due to the great number of sensory nerve fibers that ramify between corneal epithelial cells.

Renewal of Epithelial Cells

Epithelial tissues are labile structures whose cells are renewed continuously by means of mitotic activity. The renewal rate is variable; it can be fast in such tissues as the intestinal epithelium, which is replaced every week, or slow, as in the pancreas, where cell renewal takes about 2 months. In stratified and pseudostratified epithelial tissues, mitosis takes place within the germinal layer, the cells closest to the basal lamina.

Metaplasia

Under certain abnormal conditions, one type of epithelial tissue may undergo transformation into another type. This process is called **metaplasia** (Gr. *metaplasis*, transformation). The following examples illustrate this process.

In heavy cigarette smokers, the ciliated pseudostratified epithelium lining the bronchi can be transformed into stratified squamous epithelium.

In individuals with chronic vitamin A deficiency, epithelial tissues of the type found in the bronchi and urinary bladder are gradually replaced by stratified squamous epithelium.

Metaplasia is not restricted to epithelial tissue; it may also occur in connective tissue. Metaplasia is reversible.

Control of Glandular Activity

Usually, glands are sensitive to both neural and endocrine control. However, one form of control frequently dominates the other. For example, exocrine secretion in the pancreas depends mainly on stimulation by the hormones secretin and cholecystokinin (Gr. *chole*, bile, + *kystis*, bladder, + *kinein*, to move). In contrast, the salivary glands are principally under neural control.

The neural and endocrine control of glands occurs through the action of chemical substances called **chemical messengers.** Neurotransmitters are the messengers produced by nerve cells, and hormones are the messengers produced by endocrine glands.

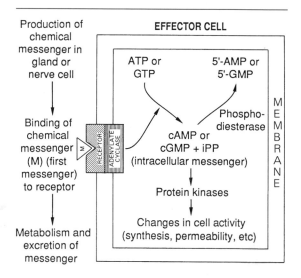

Figure 4–17. The activation of adenylate cyclase by the first messenger causes the production of cyclic AMP (cAMP) or cGMP from ATP or GTP, respectively. Adenylate cyclase is located in the cell membrane, and a specific first-messenger (M) receptor binds with this enzyme. The resulting intracellular (second) messengers are produced inside the cell, while the first messenger remains outside. The actions of many neurotransmitters and hormones are mediated by cAMP or cGMP. The action of the first messengers on different cell types depends on the presence of specific receptors associated with adenylate cyclase. Although cGMP is usually found in lower concentrations than is cAMP, it mediates a variety of cellular activities. In some cells, both cAMP and cGMP are known to interact, one stimulating a specific cellular activity and the other inhibiting it. (Based on Sutherland EW: Studies on the mechanism of hormone action. Science 1972;177:401. Copyright © 1972 by the American Association for the Advancement of Science.)

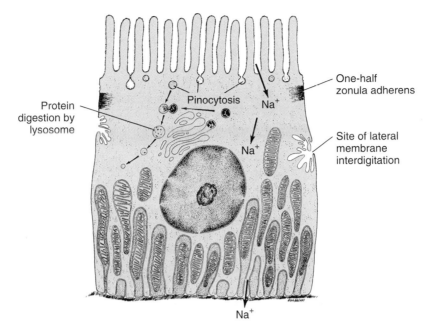

Figure 4–18. Ultrastructure of a proximal convoluted tubule cell of the kidney. Invaginations of the basal cell membrane outline regions filled with elongated mitochondria. This typical disposition is present in ion-transporting cells. Interdigitations from neighboring cells interlock with those of this cell. Protein being absorbed by pinocytosis and digested by lysosomes is shown in the upper left portion of the diagram. Sodium ions diffuse passively through the apical membranes of renal epithelial cells. These ions are then actively transported out of the cells by Na+/K+-ATPase located in the basolateral membranes of the cells. Energy for this sodium pump is supplied by nearby mitochondria. This is an example of a cell with more than one function; it transports ions in addition to providing for protein digestion.

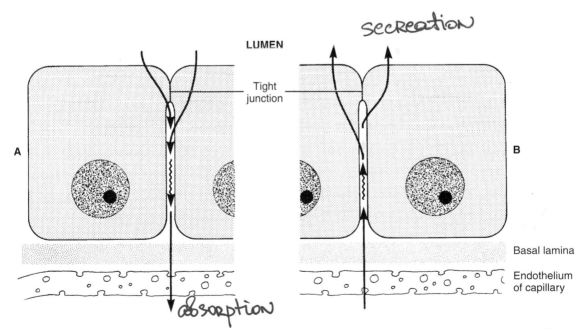

Figure 4–19. Ion and fluid transport can occur in different directions, depending on which tissue is involved. **A:** The direction of transport is from the lumen to the blood vessel, as in the gallbladder and intestine. This process is called **absorption. B:** Transport is in the opposite direction, as in the choroid plexus, ciliary body, and sweat gland. This process is called **secretion.** Note the use of the intercellular space in the transport process. Also note that the presence of occluding junctions is necessary to maintain compartmentalization and consequent control over ion distribution.

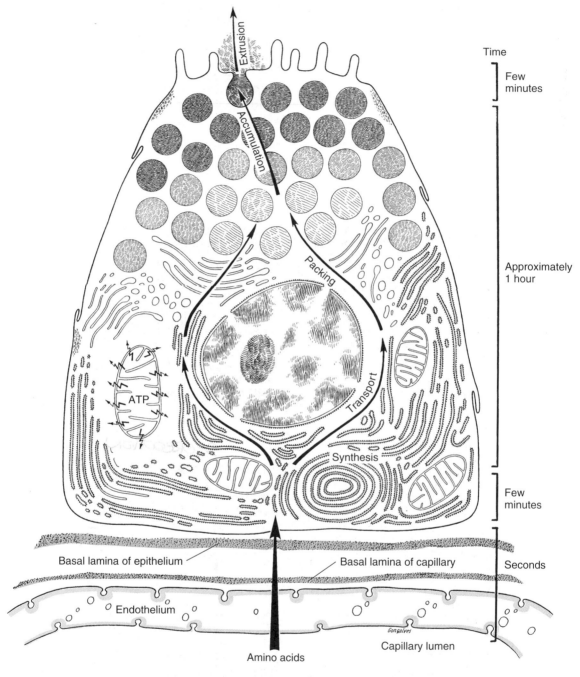

Figure 4–20. Diagram of a serous (pancreatic acinar) cell. Note its evident polarity, with abundant basal rough endoplasmic reticulum. The Golgi complex and zymogen granules are in the supranuclear region. The secretory process is described in the text. To the right is a scale indicating the approximate time necessary for each step. The darker color marks the epithelial and endothelial basal laminae; the lighter color highlights the endothelial cell membrane.

Chemical messengers act by one of two mechanisms. In the first mechanism, the messenger enters the cell, reacts with intracellular receptors, and activates one or more genes, initiating the production of specific proteins. Steroid hormones, which are capable of easily crossing the cell membrane, exhibit this type of action.

The second mechanism is related to the interaction of a chemical messenger with a receptor located in the outer surface of the cell membrane. This chemical substance, referred to as the **first messenger,** acts by inducing the synthesis of additional messengers, the **intracellular (second) messengers,** which initi-

ate a series of events that ultimately promote a specific cell activity (Figure 4–17). Protein or polypeptide hormones and neurotransmitters do not readily cross the cell membrane and act via second messengers.

Cells That Transport Ions

All cells have the ability to transport certain ions against a concentration and electrical-potential gradient, using ATP as an energy source. This is called **active transport,** to distinguish it from passive diffusion down a concentration gradient. In mammals, the sodium ion (Na^+) concentration in the extracellular

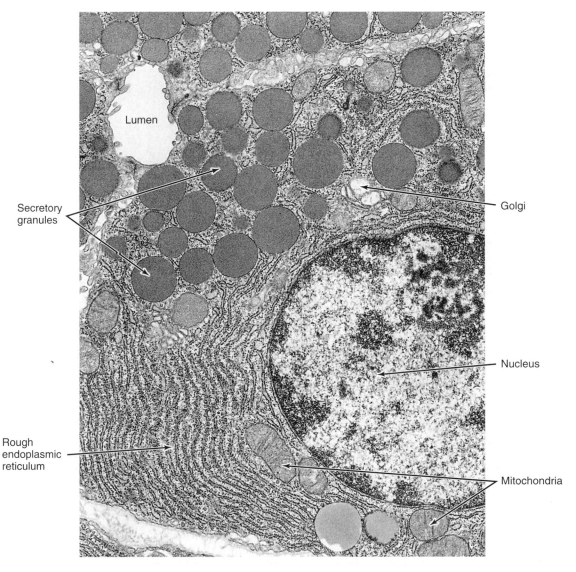

Figure 4–21. Electron micrograph of a frog pancreatic cell. Note the nucleus, mitochondria, Golgi complex, secretory (zymogen) granules in various stages of condensation, and rough endoplasmic reticulum. × 13,000. (Courtesy of KR Porter.)

fluid is 140 mmol/L, whereas the intracellular concentration is 5–15 mmol/L. In addition, the interior of the cells is electrically negative with respect to the extracellular environment. Under these conditions, Na^+ would tend to diffuse down both an electrical gradient and a concentration gradient. The cell uses the energy stored in ATP to actively extrude Na^+ by means of Mg^{2+}-activated Na^+/K^+-ATPase (**sodium pump**), thereby maintaining the required low intracellular sodium concentration.

Some epithelial cells (eg, proximal and distal renal tubules, striated ducts of salivary glands) use the sodium pump to transfer sodium across the epithelium, from its apex to its base; this is known as **transcellular transport.** The apical surface of the proximal renal tubule cell is freely permeable to Na^+. To maintain electrical and osmotic balance, equimolar amounts of chloride and water follow the Na^+ ion into the cell. The basal surfaces of these cells are elaborately folded; many long invaginations of the basal plasma membrane are seen in electron micrographs (Figures 4–18 and 19–14). In addition, there is elaborate interdigitation of basal processes between adjacent cells. It has been shown that Mg^{2+}-activated Na^+/K^+-ATPase is localized in these invaginations of the basal plasma membrane but is also present in the lateral membranes. Located between the invaginations are vertically oriented mitochondria that supply the energy (ATP) for the active extrusion of Na^+ from the base of the cell. Chloride and water again follow passively. In this way, sodium is returned to the circulation and not lost in massive amounts in the urine.

Tight junctions play an important role in the trans-

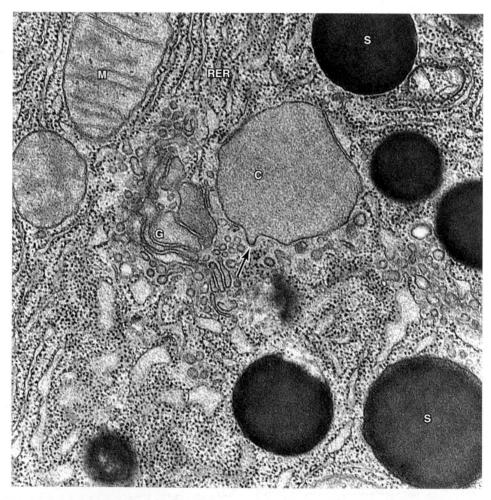

Figure 4–22. Electron micrograph of part of a rat pancreatic acinar cell showing a condensing vacuole (C), which is presumed to be receiving a small quantity of secretory product (arrow) from the Golgi complex (G). M, mitochondrion; RER, rough endoplasmic reticulum; S, mature condensed secretory (zymogen) granule. × 40,000.

port process. Because of their relative impermeability to ions, water, and larger molecules, they prevent back-diffusion of materials already transported across the epithelium. Otherwise, a great deal of energy would be wasted.

Ion transport and the consequent flow of fluid may occur in opposite directions (ie, apical → basal, basal → apical) in different epithelial tissues. In the intestine, proximal convoluted tubules of the kidney, striated ducts of the salivary glands, gallbladder, etc, the flow is from the apex of the cell to its basal region. Flow is in the opposite direction in other epithelial sheets, such as the choroid plexus and ciliary body. In both cases, the tight junctions seal the apical portions of the cells and provide for inner and outer tissue compartments (Figure 4–19).

Cells That Transport by Pinocytosis

In various cells of the body, pinocytotic vesicles, which form abundantly on plasmalemma surfaces, permit the transport of macromolecules across the plasma membrane. This activity is clearly observed in the simple squamous epithelia that line the blood vessels (endothelia) or the body cavities (mesothelia). These cells have few organelles other than the abundant pinocytotic vesicles found on the cell surfaces and in the cytoplasm. These observations, in conjunction with results obtained by injection of electron-dense colloidal particles (eg, ferritin, colloidal gold, thorium) followed by observation with the electron microscope, indicate that the vesicles transporting the injected materials flow in both directions through the cells (Figures 11–4 and 11–6).

Calculations based on these studies suggest that a pinocytotic vesicle can cross these cells in 2 or 3 minutes.

Serous Cells

The acinar cells of the pancreas and parotid glands are typical examples of the serous cell type. They are polyhedral or pyramidal, with central, rounded nuclei and well-defined polarity. In the basal infranuclear region, serous cells exhibit an intense basophilia, which results from local accumulation of rough endoplasmic reticulum in the form of parallel arrays of cisternae studded with abundant polyribosomes (Figure 4–20). In the apical region just above the nucleus lies a well-developed Golgi complex and many rounded, protein-rich, membrane-bound **secretory granules.** In cells that produce digestive enzymes (eg, pancreatic acinar cells), structures containing enzymes are called **zymogen granules** (Figures 4–20, 4–21, and 4–22). From the Golgi cisternae pinch off large membrane-bound **condensing vacuoles** or **immature secretory granules** (Figure 4–22). They become more dense as water is removed, forming the **mature secretory granules,** which accumulate until

the cell is stimulated to secrete. When the cells release their secretory products, the membranes of secretory granules fuse to the cell membrane, and the granule contents spill out of the cell in a process called **exocytosis.** Because their surfaces have the same electrical charge, membrane lipid bilayers repel each other. Therefore, fusion of cell membranes is a rather complex process assisted and controlled by proteins. The movements of secretory granules, as

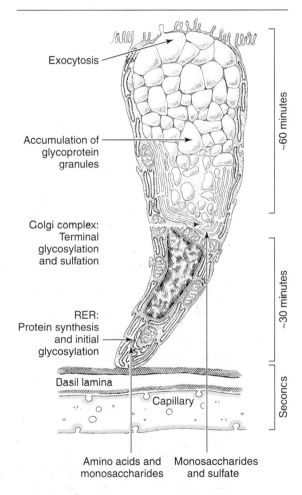

Figure 4–23. Diagram of a mucus-secreting intestinal goblet cell showing a typically constricted base, where the mitochondria and rough endoplasmic reticulum (RER) are located. The protein part of the glycoprotein complex is synthesized in the endoplasmic reticulum. A well-developed Golgi complex is present in the supranuclear region. In cells that secrete sulfated polysaccharides, the process of sulfation occurs in the Golgi complex. Darker color highlights the epithelial and endothelial basal laminae. (Redrawn after Gordon and reproduced, with permission, from Ham AW: *Histology,* 6th ed. Lippincott, 1969.)

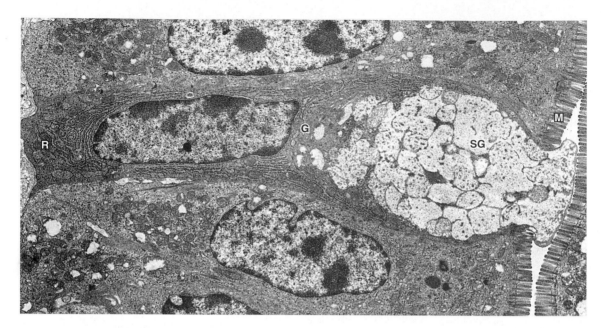

Figure 4–24. Electron micrograph of a typical goblet cell from the small intestine. The rough endoplasmic reticulum is present mainly in the basal portion of the cell (R), while the cell apex is filled with light secretory granules (SG). The Golgi complex (G) lies just above the nucleus. Typical columnar absorptive cells with microvillar borders (M) lie adjacent to the goblet cell. × 7000. (Reproduced, with permission, from Junqueira LCU, Salles LMM. Ultra-Estrutura e Função Celular, Edgard Blücher, 1975.)

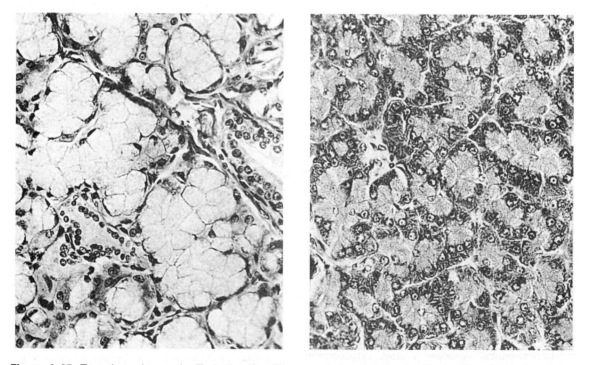

Figure 4–25. Two photomicrographs illustrating the differences between mucous cells (sublingual gland), **left,** and serous cells (pancreas), **right.** × 300.

well as all other cytoplasmic structures, are under the influence of cytoskeletal and motor proteins of the cytosol.

Mucus-Secreting Cells

The most thoroughly studied mucus-secreting cell is the **goblet cell** of the intestines. This cell is characterized by the presence of numerous large, lightly staining granules containing strongly hydrophilic glycoproteins called **mucins.** Secretory granules fill the extensive apical pole of the cell, and the nucleus is usually located in the cell base. This region is rich in rough endoplasmic reticulum (Figures 4–23 and 4–24). The Golgi complex, located just above the nucleus, is exceptionally well developed, indicative of its important function in this cell. Data obtained by autoradiography suggest that, in this cell, proteins are synthesized in the cell base where most rough endoplasmic reticulum is located. Monosaccharides are added to the core protein by enzymes—**glycosyltransferases**—located in the endoplasmic reticulum and in the Golgi apparatus. When mucins are released from the cell, they become highly hydrated and form mucus, a viscous, elastic, protective lubricating gel.

The goblet cell of the intestines is only one of several types of cells that synthesize mucin glycoproteins. Other types are found in the stomach, salivary glands, respiratory tract, and genital tract. These mucous cells show great variability in their morphologic features and in the chemical nature of their secretions. Figure 4–25 illustrates the structural differences between mucous and serous cells.

The Diffuse Neuroendocrine System (DNES)

Studies initially performed in the digestive system revealed the presence of endocrine cells interspersed among nonendocrine cells. The cytoplasm of the endocrine cells contains either polypeptide hormones or the biogenic amines epinephrine, norepinephrine, or 5-hydroxytryptamine (serotonin). In some cases, more than one of these compounds is present in the same cell. Many, but not all, of these cells are able to take up amine precursors and exhibit amino acid decarboxylase activity. These characteristics explain the acronym APUD (*a*mine *p*recursor *u*ptake and *de*carboxylation) by which they are known. Because some of these cells stain with silver salts, they are also called **argentaffin** and **argyrophil** cells.

Because not all endocrine cells concentrate amine precursors, the APUD designation has largely been replaced by DNES (*d*iffuse *n*euroendocrine *s*ystem). DNES cells are derived from the embryonic nervous system and can be identified and localized by immunocytochemical methods or other cytochemical techniques for specific amines. These cells are widespread throughout the organism and include about 35 types of cells in the respiratory, urinary, and gastrointestinal systems; thyroid; and hypophysis. Some DNES cells are known as **paracrine cells** because they produce chemical signals that diffuse into the surrounding extracellular fluid to regulate the function of neighboring cells without passing through the vascular system. Many of the polypeptide hormones and amines produced by DNES cells also act as chemical mediators in the nervous system. DNES polypeptide-secreting cells generally have distinctive, dense granules about 100–400 nm in diameter (Figure 4–26). Table 4–3 presents some of the best-characterized polypeptide hormone–producing cells.

Apudomas are tumors derived from polypeptide-secreting cells of the DNES. Clinical symptoms result from hypersecretion of the specific chemical messenger involved. The diagnosis is usually confirmed by using immunocytochemical methods on sections of the tumor biopsies.

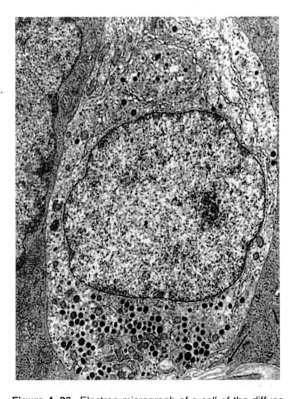

Figure 4–26. Electron micrograph of a cell of the diffuse neuroendocrine system. Note the accumulation of secretory granules in the basal region of the cell. The Golgi complex seen in the upper part of the micrograph shows some secretory granules; it is here that these granules first appear. The arrow indicates the basal lamina.

Table 4–3. Some of the best-characterized polypeptide-producing cells present in humans.

Hormone Produced	Major Action	Mechanism of Action			Location
		Neurocrine	Endocrine	Paracrine	
Gastrin	Activates secretion of gastic acid and pepsin		+		Gastric antrum, duodenum (G cell)
Cholecystokinin (CCK)	Activates secretion of pancreatic enzymes	+	+		Duodenum, jejunum (I cell)
Secretin	Activates secretion of pancreatic bicarbonate		+		Duodenum, jejunum (S cell)
Gastric inhibitory polypeptide (GIP)	Enhances insulin release, inhibits gastric-acid secretion		+		Small intestine
Vasoactive intestinal polypeptide (VIP)	Causes smooth-muscle relaxation; stimulates pancreatic-bicarbonate secretion	+			Pancreas (D1 cell)
Motilin	Causes intestinal motility		+		Small intestine (EC2 cell)
Somatostatin	Has numerous inhibitory effects	+		+	Stomach, duodenum, pancreas (D cell)
Calcitonin	Regulates calcium metabolism		+		Thyroid gland (C cell)
Insulin	Regulates glucose metabolism		+		Pancreas (B cell)

Myoepithelial Cells

Several exocrine glands (eg, sweat, lacrimal, salivary, mammary) contain stellate or spindle-shaped myoepithelial cells (Figure 4–27). These cells embrace gland acini as an octopus might embrace a rounded boulder. They are more longitudinally arranged along ducts. Myoepithelial cells are located between the basal lamina and the basal pole of secretory or ductal cells. They are connected to each other and to the epithelial cells by gap junctions and desmosomes. The cytoplasm contains numerous actin microfilaments, as well as tropomyosin and myosin. Myoepithelial cells also contain intermediate (10–12 nm in diameter) filaments that belong to the keratin family, which confirms their epithelial origin. The function of myoepithelial cells is to contract around the secretory or conducting portion of the gland and thus to help propel secretory products toward the exterior.

Steroid-Secreting Cells

Cells that secrete steroids are found in various organs of the body (eg, testes, ovaries, adrenals). They are endocrine cells specialized for synthesizing and secreting steroids with hormonal activity and have the following characteristics (Figure 4–28):

1. They are polyhedral or rounded acidophilic cells with a central nucleus and a cytoplasm that is usually—but not invariably—rich in lipid droplets.

2. The cytoplasm of steroid-secreting cells contains an exceptionally rich smooth endoplasmic reticulum, which takes the form of anastomosing tubules. Smooth endoplasmic reticulum contains the enzymes necessary to synthesize cholesterol from acetate and other substrates and to transform the pregnenolone produced in the mitochondria into androgens, estrogens, and progestogens.

3. The spherical or elongated mitochondria that are present usually contain tubular cristae rather than the shelf-like cristae that are common in mitochondria of other epithelial cells. In addition to being the main site of energy production for cell function, these organelles have the necessary enzymatic equipment not only to cleave the cholesterol side chain and produce pregnenolone but also to participate in subsequent reactions that result in steroid hormones. The process of steroid synthesis results, therefore, from close collaboration between smooth endoplasmic reticulum and mitochondria, a striking example of cooperation between cell organelles (Figure 21–4). This

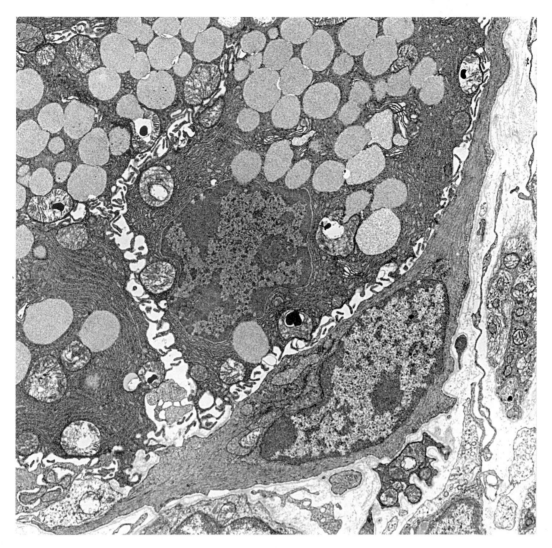

Figure 4–27. Electron micrograph of salivary gland showing secretory cells in the upper left; in the lower right of the image is a myoepithelial cell that embraces the secretory acinus. Contraction of the myoepithelial cell compresses the acinus and aids in the expulsion of secretory products.

process also explains the close proximity observed between these two organelles in steroid-secreting cells.

Epithelial Cell–Derived Tumors

Both benign and malignant tumors can arise from most types of epithelial cells. A **carcinoma** (Gr. *karkinos,* cancer, + *oma,* tumor) is a malignant tumor of epithelial cell origin. Malignant tumors derived from glandular epithelial tissue are usually called **adenocarcinomas** (Gr. *adenos,* gland, + *karkinos*); these are by far the most common tumors in adults.

Carcinomas composed of differentiated cells reflect cell-specific morphologic features and behaviors (eg, the production of keratins, mucins, and hormones). Undifferentiated carcinomas are often difficult to diagnose by morphologic analysis alone. Since these carcinomas usually contain keratins, the detection of keratins by immunocytochemistry often helps to determine the diagnosis and treatment of these tumors (see Table 1–3).

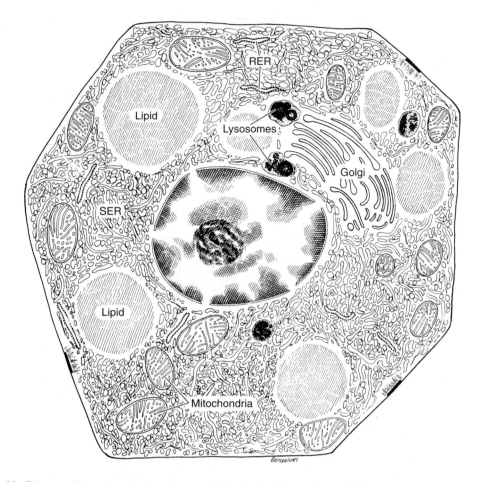

Figure 4–28. Diagram of the ultrastructure of a hypothetical steroid-secreting cell. Note the abundance of the smooth endoplasmic reticulum (SER), lipid droplets, Golgi complex, and lysosomes. The numerous mitochondria have tubular cristae. They not only produce the energy necessary for the activity of the cell but are also involved in steroid hormone synthesis. Rough endoplasmic reticulum (RER) is also shown.

REFERENCES

Alberts B et al: *Molecular Biology of the Cell,* 3rd ed. Garland, 1994.

Berridge MJ, Oschman JL: *Transporting Epithelia.* Academic Press, 1972.

Darnell J et al: *Molecular Cell Biology,* 2nd ed. Scientific American Books, 1990.

Farquhar MG, Palade GE: Junctional complexes in various epithelia. J Cell Biol 1963;17:375.

Fawcett D: *The Cell,* 2nd ed. Saunders, 1981.

Hall PF: Cellular organization for steroidogenesis. Int Rev Cytol 1984;86:53.

Hertzberg EL et al: Gap junctional communication. Annu Rev Physiol 1981;43:479.

Hull BE, Staehelin LA: The terminal web: a reevaluation of its structure and function. J Cell Biol 1979;81:67.

Jamieson JD, Palade, GE: Intracellular transport of secre-

tory protein in the pancreatic exocrine cell. 4. Metabolic requirements. J Cell Biol 1968;39:589.

Kefalides NA: *Biology and Chemistry of Basement Membranes.* Academic Press, 1978.

Krstić RV: *Illustrated Encyclopedia of Human Histology.* Springer-Verlag, 1984.

Krstić RV: *Ultrastructure of the Mammalian Cell.* Springer-Verlag, 1979.

Mooseker MS: Organization, chemistry, and assembly of the cytoskeletal apparatus of the intestinal brush border. Annu Rev Cell Biol 1985;1:209.

Simons K, Fuller SD: Cell surface polarity in epithelia. Annu Rev Cell Biol 1985;1:243.

Staehelin LA, Hull BE: Junctions between living cells. Sci Am 1978;238:41.

Connective Tissue

5

The connective tissues are responsible for providing and maintaining form in the body. Functioning in a mechanical role, they provide a matrix that connects and binds the cells and organs and ultimately gives support to the body. Unlike the other tissue types (epithelium, muscle, and nerve), which are formed mainly by cells, the major constituent of connective tissue is its **extracellular matrix,** composed of **protein fibers, ground substance,** and **tissue fluid.** Tissue fluid consists primarily of bound water of solvation. Embedded within the extracellular matrix are the **connective tissue cells.**

Structurally, connective tissue can be divided into three classes of components: **cells, fibers,** and **ground substance.** The wide variety of connective tissue types in the body reflects variations in the composition and amount of these three components, which are responsible for the remarkable structural, functional, and pathologic diversity of connective tissue.

Connective tissue serves a variety of functions, the most conspicuous being structural. The capsules that surround the organs of the body and the internal architecture that supports their cells are composed of connective tissue. This tissue also makes up tendons, ligaments, and the areolar tissue that fills the spaces between organs. Bone, cartilage, and adipose tissue are specialized types of connective tissue that support the soft tissues of the body and store fat.

The role of connective tissue in defending the organism is related to its phagocytic and immunocompetent cells as well as to the cells that produce pharmacologically active substances that are important in modulating inflammation. Phagocytic cells engulf inert particles and microorganisms that enter the body. Specific proteins called **antibodies** are produced by plasma cells in the connective tissue. The antibodies combine with foreign proteins of bacteria and viruses—or with the toxins produced by bacteria—and combat the biologic activity of these harmful agents. In addition, components of connective tissue matrix provide a physical barrier, preventing the dispersion of microorganisms that pass through the epithelia.

Because of its close association with blood vessels, connective tissue plays an important role in cell nutrition. The connective tissue matrix serves as the medium through which nutrients and metabolic wastes are exchanged between cells and their blood supply.

Most connective tissues develop from the middle layer of the embryo, the **mesoderm.** Some of the connective tissues of the head, however, derive from the neural crest, a derivative of the ectoderm. Mesodermal cells migrate from their site of origin, surrounding and penetrating developing organs. These are the **mesenchymal cells,** and the tissue they form is called **mesenchyme.** Mesenchymal cells are characterized by an oval nucleus with prominent nucleoli and fine chromatin. Their relatively small amount of cytoplasm extends as multiple thin processes away from the nucleus. The space between mesenchymal cells is occupied by a viscous ground substance containing few fibers. In addition to being the point of origin of all types of connective tissue cells, mesenchyme develops into other types of structures, such as blood cells and blood vessels.

GROUND SUBSTANCE

The intercellular ground substance, a complex mixture of glycoproteins and proteoglycans (see Chapter 7) that participate in binding cells to the fibers of connective tissues, is colorless and transparent. It fills the space between cells and fibers of the connective tissue; it is viscous and acts as both a lubricant and a barrier to the penetration of invaders. When fixed for histologic analysis, its components aggregate and appear as granular material in the electron microscope (Figure 5–1). The ground substance is formed mainly of two classes of components: **glycosaminoglycans** and **structural glycoproteins.**

Glycosaminoglycans (originally called **acid mucopolysaccharides**) are linear polysaccharides formed by repeating disaccharide units usually composed of a uronic acid and a hexosamine. The hexosamine can be **glucosamine** or **galactosamine,** and

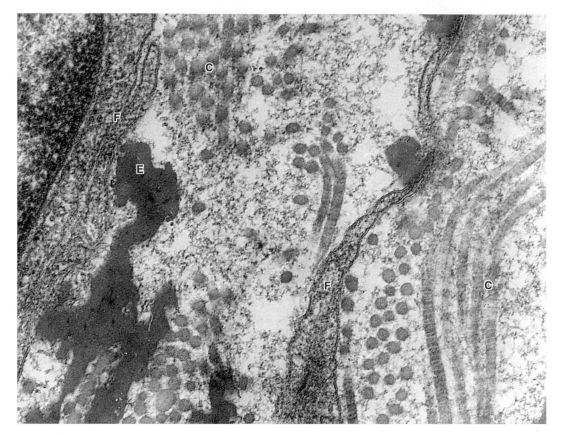

Figure 5–1. Electron micrograph showing the structural organization of the connective tissue matrix. The ground substance is a fine granular material that fills the spaces between the collagen (C) and elastic (E) fibers and surrounds fibroblast cells and processes (F). The granularity of ground substance is an artifact of the glutaraldehyde–tannic acid fixation procedure. × 100,000.

the uronic acid can be **glucuronic** or **iduronic acid.** With the exception of hyaluronic acid, these linear chains are bound covalently to a protein core (Figure 5–2), forming a **proteoglycan molecule.** This molecule is a three-dimensional structure that can be pictured as a test tube brush, with the wire stem representing the protein core and the bristles representing the glycosaminoglycans. In cartilage, the proteoglycan molecules have been shown to be bound to a hyaluronic acid chain, forming larger molecules— proteoglycan aggregates. Because of the abundance of hydroxyl, carboxyl, and sulfate groups in the carbohydrate moiety of most proteoglycans, the proteoglycans are intensely hydrophilic and act as polyanions. With the exception of hyaluronic acid, all other glycosaminoglycans are sulfated to some degree in the adult state. The carbohydrate portion of proteoglycans constitutes 80–90% of the weight of this macromolecule. Because of these characteristics, proteoglycans can bind to a great number of cations (usually sodium) by electrostatic (ionic) bonds. Pro-

teoglycans are intensely hydrated structures with a thick layer of solvation water surrounding the molecule. When fully hydrated, proteoglycans fill a much larger volume (domain) than they do in their anhydrous state.

The main proteoglycans are composed of a core protein associated with the four main glycosaminoglycans: **dermatan sulfate, chondroitin sulfate, keratan sulfate,** and **heparan sulfate.** Table 5–1 shows the chemical composition and tissue distribution of the glycosaminoglycans.

Dermatan sulfate is found mainly in dermis, tendons, ligaments, and fibrous cartilage, all structures that contain **collagen** (Gr. *kolla,* glue, + *genin,* to produce) fibers (collagen type I). Chondroitin sulfate predominates in hyaline and elastic cartilages, which are rich in collagen type II. Keratan sulfate is found in the cornea. Heparan sulfate seems to be associated mainly with **reticular fibers,** which contain collagen type III, and with basal laminae. The various collagen types are discussed below. The electrostatic in-

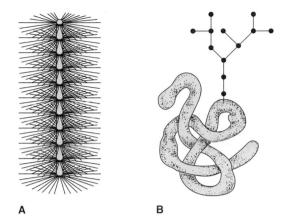

A   **B**

Figure 5–2. The molecular structure of proteoglycans and glycoproteins. **A:** Proteoglycans contain a core of protein (vertical rod in drawing) to which molecules of glycosaminoglycans (GAGs) are covalently bound. A GAG is an unbranched polysaccharide made up of repeating disaccharides; one component is an amino sugar, and the other is uronic acid. Proteoglycans contain a greater amount of carbohydrate than do glycoproteins. **B:** Glycoproteins are globular protein molecules to which branched chains of monosaccharides are covalently attached. (Reproduced, with permission, from Junqueira LA, Carneiro J: *Biologia Celular e Molecular,* 5th ed. Editora Guanabara Koogan. Rio de Janeiro, 1991.)

teraction between their acidic groups and the basic amino acid residues of collagen causes proteoglycans to bind to collagen (Figure 7–3).

The synthesis of proteoglycans begins in the rough endoplasmic reticulum with the synthesis of the protein moiety of the molecule. Glycosylation is initiated in the rough endoplasmic reticulum and com-

pleted in the Golgi complex, where sulfation also occurs (see Chapter 2).

The degradation of proteoglycans is carried out by several cell types and depends on the presence of several lysosomal enzymes. The turnover of proteoglycans is rapid—2–4 days for hyaluronic acid and 7–10 days for sulfated proteoglycans. Several disorders have been described in which a deficiency in lysosomal enzymes causes glycosaminoglycan degradation to be blocked, with the consequent accumulation of these compounds in tissues. The lack of specific hydrolases in the lysosomes has been found to be the cause of several disorders in humans, including Hurler syndrome, Hunter syndrome, Sanfilippo syndrome, and Morquio syndrome.

Because of their high viscosity, intercellular substances act as a barrier to the penetration of bacteria and other microorganisms. Bacteria that produce **hyaluronidase,** an enzyme that hydrolyzes hyaluronic acid and other glycosaminoglycans, have great invasive power since they reduce the viscosity of the connective tissue ground substance.

Structural glycoproteins are compounds that contain a protein moiety to which carbohydrates are attached. In contrast to proteoglycans, the protein moiety usually predominates, and these molecules do not contain the linear polysaccharides formed by repeating disaccharides containing hexosamines. Instead, the carbohydrate moiety of glycoproteins is frequently a branched structure.

Several glycoproteins have been isolated from connective tissue, and they play an important role not

Table 5–1. Composition and distribution of glycosaminoglycans in connective tissue and their interactions with collagen fibers.

Glycosaminoglycan	Repeating Disaccharides		Distribution	Electrostatic Interaction with Collagen
	Hexuronic Acid	**Hexosamine**		
Hyaluronic acid	D-glucuronic acid	D-glucosamine	Umbilical cord, synovial fluid, vitreous humor, cartilage	. . .
Chondroitin 4-sulfate	D-glucuronic acid	D-galactosamine	Cartilage, bone, cornea, skin, notochord, aorta	High levels of interaction, mainly with collagen type II
Chondroitin 6-sulfate	D-glucuronic acid	D-galactosamine	Cartilage, umbilical cord, skin, aorta (media)	High levels of interaction, mainly with collagen type II
Dermatan sulfate	L-iduronic acid or D-glucoronic acid	D-galactosamine	Skin, tendon, aorta (adventitia)	Low levels of interaction, mainly with collagen type I
Heparan sulfate	D-glucuronic acid or L-iduronic acid	D-galactosamine	Aorta, lung, liver, basal laminae	Intermediate levels of interaction, mainly with collagen types III and IV
Keratan sulfate (cornea)	D-galactose	D-galactosamine	Cornea	None
Keratan sulfate (skeleton)	D-galactose	D-glucosamine	Cartilage, nucleus pulposus, annulus fibrosus	None

only in the interaction between neighboring adult and embryonic cells but also in the adhesion of cells to their substrate. **Fibronectin** (L. *fibra,* fiber, + *nexus,* interconnection) is a glycoprotein synthesized by fibroblasts and some epithelial cells. This molecule, with a molecular mass of 222–240 kDa, has binding sites for cells, collagen, and glycosaminoglycans. Interactions at these sites help to mediate normal cell adhesion and migration. **Laminin** is a large glycoprotein that participates in the adhesion of epithelial cells to the basal lamina, a structure rich in laminin.

Cells interact with extracellular matrix components by using cell-surface molecules (**matrix receptors**) that bind to collagen, fibronectin, and laminin. These receptors are the **integrins,** a family of transmembrane linker proteins (Figure 5–3). Integrins bind their ligands in the extracellular matrix with relatively low affinity, allowing cells to explore their environment without losing attachment to it or becoming glued to it. Clearly, integrins must interact with the cytoskeleton, usually the actin microfilaments. (The integrin found in hemidesmosomes is an exception and binds to keratin intermediate filaments.) The interactions that integrins mediate between the extracellular matrix and the cytoskeleton operate in both directions and play an important role in orienting both the cells and the matrix in a tissue (Figure 5–4).

Participation of fibronectin and laminin has been postulated in both embryonic development and the increased ability of cancer cells to invade other tissues. The importance of fibronectin is shown by the fact that mice whose fibronectin has been inactivated die during early embryogenesis. Further information on the structure and function of laminin and fibronectin is presented in Figure 5–5. **Chondronectin** is present in cartilage, where it mediates the adhesion of chondrocytes to type II collagen.

In connective tissue, in addition to the ground substance, there is a very small quantity of fluid—called **tissue fluid**—that is similar to blood plasma in its content of ions and diffusible substances. Tissue fluid contains a small percentage of plasma proteins of low molecular weight that pass through the capillary walls as a result of the hydrostatic pressure of the blood.

Edema

Water in the intercellular substance of connective tissue comes from the blood, passing through the capillary walls into the intercellular regions of the tissue. The capillary wall is only slightly permeable to macromolecules but permits the passage of water and small molecules, including low-molecular-weight proteins.

Blood brings to connective tissue the various nutrients required by the cells and carries metabolic waste products away to the detoxifying and excretory organs, such as liver and kidneys.

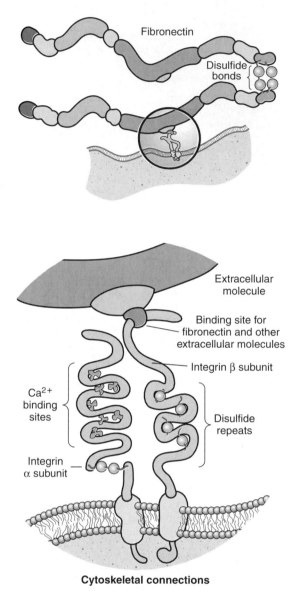

Cytoskeletal connections

Figure 5–3. Integrin cell-surface matrix receptor. By binding to a matrix protein and to the actin cytoskeleton (via α-actinin) inside the cell, the integrin serves as a transmembrane link. The molecule is a heterodimer, with α and β chains. The head portion may protrude some 20 nm from the surface of the cell membrane into the extracellular matrix.

Two forces act on the water contained in the capillaries: the hydrostatic pressure of the blood, a consequence of the pumping action of the heart, which forces water to pass through the capillary walls; and the colloid osmotic pressure of the blood plasma, which draws water back into the capillaries (Figure 5–6). Osmotic pressure is due mainly to plasma proteins. Because

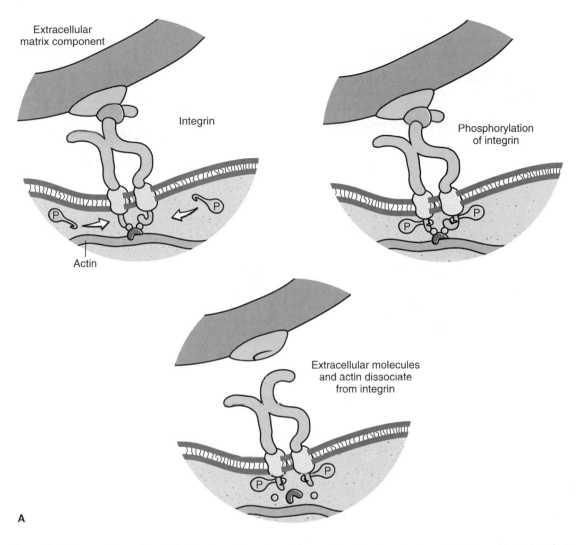

A

Figure 5–4. How cells regulate their attachment to extracellular matrix molecules via phosphorylation of integrins. **A:** Intracellular signaling activates integrins to attach to matrix ligands and to the actin cytoskeleton, whereas phosphorylation dissociates these links, thus relaxing the cells' grip on the matrix. (*Continued*)

the ions and low-molecular-weight compounds that pass easily through the capillary walls have approximately the same concentration inside and outside these blood vessels, the osmotic pressures they exert are approximately equal on either side of the capillaries and cancel each other. The colloid osmotic pressure exerted by the blood protein macromolecules—which are unable to pass through the capillary walls—is not counterbalanced by outside pressure and tends to bring water back into the blood vessel.

Normally, water passes through capillary walls to the surrounding tissues at the arterial end of a capillary, because the hydrostatic pres-

sure there is greater than the colloid osmotic pressure; the hydrostatic pressure, however, decreases along the length of the capillary toward the venous end. As the hydrostatic pressure falls, osmotic pressure rises because of the progressive increase in the concentration of proteins, which is caused by the passage of water from the capillaries. As a result of this increase in protein concentration and decrease in hydrostatic pressure, osmotic pressure becomes greater than hydrostatic pressure at the venous end of the capillary, and water is drawn back into the capillary (Figure 5–6).

The quantity of water drawn back is less than

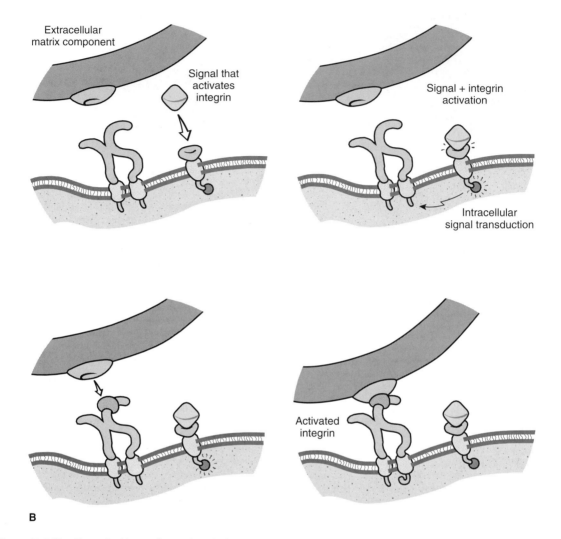

B

Figure 5–4 (Continued). How cells regulate their attachment to extracellular matrix molecules via phosphorylation of integrins. **B:** Extracellular signals also control the link between extracellular molecules and the cytoskeleton.

that which passes out through the capillaries. The water that remains in the connective tissue returns to the blood through the lymphatic vessels. The smallest lymphatic vessels are the lymphatic capillaries, which originate in connective tissue with closed ends. Lymphatic vessels drain into veins at the base of the neck (see Chapter 11 and Figure 14–1).

Because of the equilibrium that exists between the water entering and the water leaving the intercellular substance of connective tissue, there is little free water in the tissue.

In several pathologic conditions, the quantity of tissue fluid may increase considerably, causing **edema.** In tissue sections, this condition is characterized by enlarged spaces, caused by the increase in liquid, between the components of the connective tissue. Macroscopically, edema is characterized by an increase in volume that yields easily to localized pressure, causing a depression that slowly disappears (pitting edema).

Edema may result from venous obstruction or from a decrease in venous blood flow (eg, congestive heart failure). It may also be caused by chronic starvation; protein deficiency results in a lack of plasma proteins and a decrease in colloid osmotic pressure. Water therefore accumulates in the connective tissue and is not drawn back into the capillaries.

Another possible cause of edema is increased permeability of the blood capillary endothelium resulting from chemical or mechanical injury or

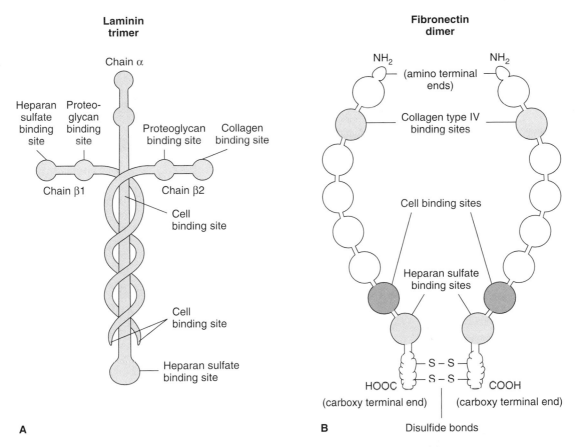

Laminin trimer

Chain α

Heparan sulfate binding site

Proteoglycan binding site

Proteoglycan binding site

Collagen binding site

Chain β1

Chain β2

Cell binding site

Cell binding site

Heparan sulfate binding site

A

Fibronectin dimer

NH₂

NH₂

(amino terminal ends)

Collagen type IV binding sites

Cell binding sites

Heparan sulfate binding sites

S – S
S – S

HOOC

COOH

(carboxy terminal end)

(carboxy terminal end)

B

Disulfide bonds

Figure 5–5. A: The structure of laminin, which is formed by three intertwined polypeptides in the shape of a cross. The figure shows sites on the molecule with a high affinity for cell membrane receptors and type IV collagen and heparan sulfate, which are components of basal laminae. Laminin thus promotes adhesion of cells to basal laminae. **B:** The structure of fibronectin. This is a dimer bound by S—S groups, formed by serially disposed coiled sites, that bind to type I collagen, heparan sulfate, other proteoglycans, and cell membrane receptors. (Reproduced, with permission, from Junqueira LA, Carneiro J: *Biologia Celular e Molecular,* 5th ed. Editora Guanabara Koogan. Rio de Janeiro, 1991.)

the release of certain substances produced in the body (eg, histamine). Edema may also be caused by the obstruction of lymphatic vessels, eg, by plugs of parasites or tumor cells.

FIBERS

Connective tissue fibers are long, slender protein polymers that are present in variable proportions in the different types of connective tissue.

The three main types of connective tissue fibers are **collagen, reticular,** and **elastic.** Collagen and reticular fibers are formed by the protein **collagen,** and elastic fibers are composed mainly of the protein **elastin.** These fibers are distributed unequally among the types of connective tissue. In many cases, the predominant fiber type is responsible for conferring specific properties on the tissue.

Evolution & Types of Collagen

During the process of evolution, a group of structural proteins that were modified by environmental influences and the functional requirements of the animal organism developed to varying degrees of rigidity, elasticity, and strength. These proteins are known collectively as **collagen,** and the chief examples among its various types are from the skin, bone, cartilage, smooth muscle, and basal lamina.

Collagen is the most abundant protein in the human body, representing 30% of its dry weight. The collagens of vertebrates are a family of proteins, produced by several cell types, that are distinguishable by their differing chemical compositions, morphologic characteristics, distribution, functions, and pathologies (Table 5–2). According to their structure and functions, they can be classified in the following groups.

Fibril-forming collagens. The molecules of fib-

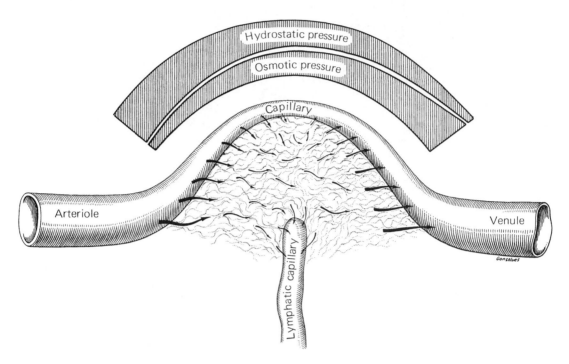

Figure 5–6. Movement of fluid through connective tissue. There is a decrease in hydrostatic pressure and an increase in osmotic pressure from the arterial to the venous ends of blood capillaries (upper part of drawing). Fluid leaves the capillary through its arterial end and repenetrates the blood at the venous end. Some fluid is drained by the lymphatic capillaries.

ril-forming collagens aggregate to form fibrils clearly visible under the electron microscope (Figure 5–7). These are collagens type I, II, III, V, and XI. Collagen type I is the most abundant and has a widespread distribution. It occurs in tissues as structures that are classically designated as **collagen fibers** and that form bones, dentin, tendons, organ capsules, dermis, etc.

Fibril-associated collagens. Fibril-associated collagens are short structures that bind collagen fibrils to one another and to other components of the extracellular matrix. They are collagens type IX and XII.

Network-forming collagen. Network-forming collagen is type IV collagen, whose molecules assemble in a meshwork that constitutes the structural component of the basal lamina.

Anchoring collagen. Anchoring collagen is type VII collagen, present in the anchoring fibrils that bind collagen fibers to the basal lamina (see Figure 4–4).

Collagen synthesis, an activity originally believed to be restricted to fibroblasts, chondroblasts, osteoblasts, and odontoblasts, has now been shown to be widespread, with many cell types producing this protein (Table 5–2). The principal amino acids that

make up collagen are glycine (33.5%), proline (12%), and hydroxyproline (10%). Collagen contains two amino acids that are characteristic of this protein: **hydroxyproline** and **hydroxylysine.**

The protein unit that polymerizes to form collagen fibrils is the elongated molecule called **tropocollagen,** which measures 280 nm in length and 1.5 nm in width. Tropocollagen consists of three subunit polypeptide chains intertwined in a triple helix (Figure 5–8). Differences in the chemical structure of these polypeptide chains are responsible for the various types of collagen.

In collagen types I, II, and III, tropocollagen molecules aggregate into microfibrillar subunits that are packed together to form **fibrils.** Hydrogen bonds and hydrophobic interactions are important in the aggregation and packing of these units. In a subsequent step, this structure is reinforced by the formation of covalent cross-links, a process catalyzed by the activity of the enzyme lysyl oxidase.

Collagen fibrils are thin, elongated structures with a variable diameter (ranging from 20 to 90 nm); they have transverse striation with a characteristic periodicity of 64 nm (Figure 5–7). The transverse striations of the collagen fibrils are determined by the overlapping arrangement of the tropocollagen molecules (Figure

Table 5-2. Main characteristics of the different collagen types.

Collagen Type	Tissue Distribution	Optical Microscopy	Ultrastructure	Site of Synthesis	Interaction with Glycosaminoglycans	Main Function	Molecular Organization
I	Dermis, tendon, bone, fibrocartilage	Thick, highly birefringent, nonargyrophilic fibers	Densely packed thick fibrils; marked variation in diameter	Fibroblasts, odontoblasts, osteoblasts, chondroblasts	Weak; mainly with dermatan sulfate	Resistance to tension	Fibril-forming collagen
II	Hyaline cartilage, intervertebral disk	Loose bundles of fibrils, visible with polarization microscopy	No fibers, th n fibrils embedded in abundant ground substance	Chondroblasts	High interaction with chondroitin sulfates	Resistance to pressure.	Fibril-forming collagen
III	Smooth muscle, reticular connective tissue	Thin, weakly birefringent, argyrophilic fibers	Loosely packed thin fibrils of uniform diameter	Smooth muscle cells, reticular cells, Schwann cells	Intermediate interaction with heparan sulfate	Structural maintenance in expansible organs	Fibril-forming collagen
IV	Basal laminae	Thin, PAS-positive, and argyrophilic	No fibrils present	Endothelial, epithelial, muscle, and Schwann cells.	Intermediate level of interaction with heparan sulfate	Support of delicate structures, filtration	Network-forming collagen
V	Dermis, tendon, bone, fibrocartilage	Forms fibrils with type I	Fibrils	Fibroblasts		Participates in type I function	Fibril-forming collagen
VII	Dermis	Not visible	Clearly visible (Fig. 4-4A)			Binding cells to subjacent connective tissue	Anchoring collagen
IX	Hyaline cartilage			Chondroblasts		Fibril lateral association	Fibril-associated collagen
XI	Hyaline cartilage, intervertebral disk	Forms fibrils with type II	Fibrils	Chondroblasts		Participates in type II function	Fibril-forming collagen
XII	Tendon, ligaments			Fibroblasts		Fibril lateral association	Fibril-associated collagen

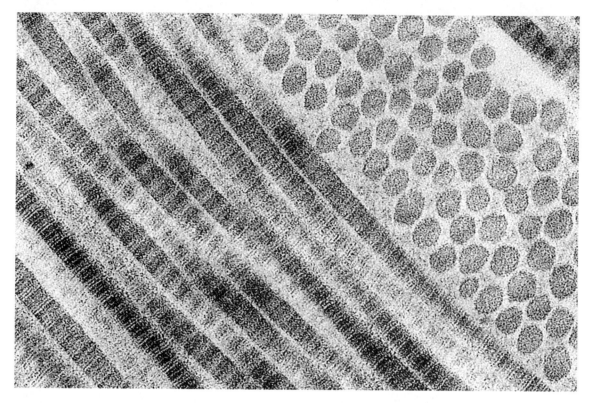

Figure 5–7. Electron micrograph of human collagen fibrils in cross and longitudinal sections. Each fibril consists of regular alternating dark and light bands that are further divided by cross-striations. Ground substance completely surrounds the fibrils. × 100,000.

5–9). The dark bands retain more of the lead-based stain used in electron-microscope studies, because their more numerous free chemical groups react more intensely with the lead solution than do the light bands. In collagen types I and III, these fibrils associate to form fibers. In collagen type I, the fibers can associate to form bundles (Figure 5–9). Collagen type II (present in cartilage) occurs as fibrils but does not form fibers (Figure 5–10). Collagen type IV, present in basal laminae, does not form either fibrils or fibers and probably occurs as unpolymerized or scarcely polymerized procollagen molecules.

Biosynthesis of Collagen Type I

Because collagen type I is widely distributed in the body, its synthesis has been thoroughly studied. This synthesis proceeds through the following steps, which are summarized in Figure 5–11:

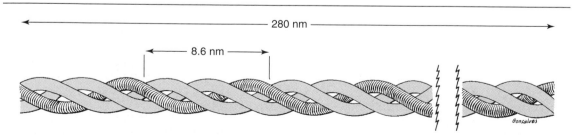

Figure 5–8. In the most abundant form of collagen, type I, each molecule (tropocollagen) is composed of two $\alpha 1$ (shown in color) and one $\alpha 2$ (shaded) peptide chains, each with a molecular mass of approximately 100 kDa, intertwined in a right-handed helix and held together by hydrogen bonds and hydrophobic interactions. Each complete turn of the helix spans a distance of 8.6 nm. The length of each tropocollagen molecule is 280 nm, and its width is 1.5 nm.

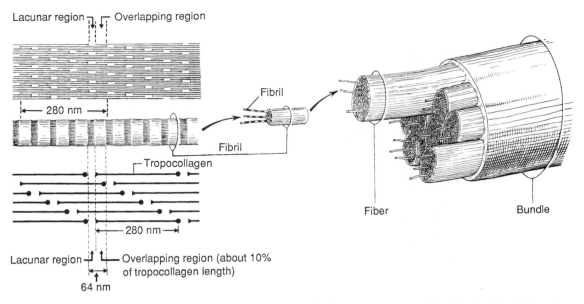

Figure 5–9. Schematic drawing of collagen molecules (tropocollagen), fibrils, fibers, and bundles. In the electron microscope, the fibrils show a 64-nm periodicity of dark and light bands. This periodicity is explained by the stepwise overlapping arrangement of rod-like tropocollagen subunits, each measuring 280 nm. This arrangement results in the production of alternating lacunar and overlapping regions that cause the cross-striations characteristic of collagen fibrils.

1. Polypeptide α chains are assembled on polyribosomes bound to rough endoplasmic reticulum membranes and injected into the cisternae as **preprocollagen** molecules. The signal peptide is clipped off, forming **procollagen.**

2. Hydroxylation of proline and lysine occurs after these amino acids are incorporated into polypeptide chains. Hydroxylation begins after the peptide chain has reached a certain minimum length and is still bound to the ribosomes. The two enzymes involved are **peptidyl proline hydroxylase** and **peptidyl lysine hydroxylase.**

3. Glycosylation of hydroxylysine occurs after its hydroxylation. Different collagen types have different amounts of carbohydrate in the form of galactose or glycosylgalactose linked to hydroxylysine.

4. Each α chain is synthesized with an extra length of peptides called **registration peptides** on both amino- and carboxyl-terminal ends. Registration peptides probably ensure that the appropriate α chains (α1, α2) assemble in the correct position as a triple helix. In addition, the extra peptides make the resulting **procollagen molecule** soluble and prevent its premature intracellular assembly and precipitation as collagen fibrils. Procollagen is transported as such out of the cell to the extracellular environment.

5. Outside the cell, specific proteases called **procollagen peptidases** remove the registration peptides. The altered protein, known as **tropocollagen,** is capable of assembling into polymeric collagen fibrils. The hydroxyproline residues contribute to the stability of the tropocollagen triple helix, forming hydrogen bonds between its polypeptide chains.

6. Collagen fibrils aggregate spontaneously to form fibers. Proteoglycans and structural glycoproteins play an important role in the aggregation of tropocollagen to form fibrils and in the formation of fibers from fibrils.

7. Fibrillar structure is reinforced by the formation of covalent cross-links between tropocollagen molecules. This process is catalyzed by the action of the enzyme **lysyl oxidase,** which also acts in the extracellular space.

The other fibrillar collagens are probably formed according to the same pattern described for collagen type I, with only minor differences.

The synthesis of collagen involves a cascade of unique post-translational biochemical modifications of the original procollagen polypeptide. All these modifications are critical to the structure and function of normal mature collagen. Because there are so many steps in collagen biosynthesis, there are many points at which the process can be interrupted or changed by faulty enzymes or by disease processes.

It should not be surprising, therefore, that a large number of pathologic conditions are directly attributable to insufficient or abnormal collagen synthesis. Table 5–3 lists examples of the many disorders caused by collagen biosyn-

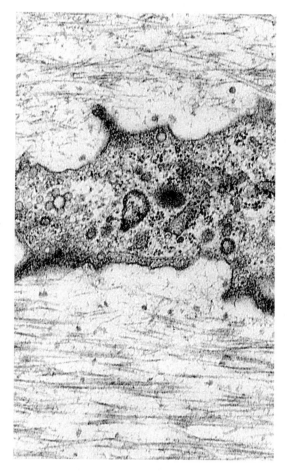

Figure 5–10. Electron micrograph of hyaline cartilage matrix showing the fine collagen fibrils of collagen type II interspersed with abundant ground substance. Transverse striations of the fibrils are barely visible because of the interaction of collagen with chondroitin sulfate. In the center is a portion of a chondrocyte. Compare the appearance of these fibrils with those of fibrocartilage. (See Figure 7–8.) × 14,000.

The degradation of collagen is initiated by specific enzymes called **collagenases.** These enzymes cut the collagen molecule into two parts that are susceptible to further degradation by nonspecific proteases.

Collagen Fibers

Collagen fibers (made of collagen type I) are the most numerous fibers in connective tissue. Although fresh collagen fibers are colorless strands, when they are present in great numbers the tissues in which they lie (eg, tendons, aponeuroses) are white.

The orientation of the elongated tropocollagen molecules in collagen fibers makes them birefringent. When fibers containing collagen are stained with an acidic dye composed of elongated molecules (eg, Sirius red) that bind to collagen in an array parallel to its molecules, the collagen's normal birefringence increases considerably. Because this increase in birefringence occurs only in oriented collagen structures, it is used as a specific method for their detection (Figure 5–12).

Collagen fibers are inelastic and, because of their molecular configuration, have a tensile strength greater than that of steel. Consequently, collagen imparts a unique combination of flexibility and strength to the tissues in which it lies.

Collagen fibers consist of closely packed thick fibrils with an average diameter of 75 nm in mammals. The diameter of the fibers depends on the number of fibrils they contain. In many parts of the body, collagen fibers lie parallel to each other, forming **collagen bundles** (Figure 5–9).

Because of the long and tortuous course of collagen fibers, their morphologic characteristics are better studied in spread preparations (Figure 5–13) than in histologic sections. Mesentery is frequently used for this purpose; when spread on a slide, this tissue is sufficiently thin to be stained and examined under the microscope. Mesentery consists of a central portion of connective tissue lined on both surfaces by a simple squamous epithelium, the mesothelium. The collagen fibers in a spread preparation appear as elongated and tortuous cylindrical structures of indefinite length, with a diameter that varies from 1 to 20 μm.

In the light microscope, collagen fibers are acidophilic; they stain pink with eosin, blue with Mallory's trichrome stain, green with Masson's trichrome stain, and red with Sirius red.

Reticular Fibers

Reticular fibers are extremely thin, with a diameter between 0.5 and 2 μm, and they form an extensive network in certain organs. They are not visible in hematoxylin-and-eosin (H&E) preparations but can be easily stained black by impregnation with silver salts. Because of their affinity for silver salts, these fibers are called **argyrophilic** (Gr. *argyros,* silver, + *philein,* to love) (Figure 5–14).

thesis failure. In addition to these disorders, several diseases result from an overaccumulation of collagen. In **progressive systemic sclerosis,** almost all organs may present an excessive accumulation of collagen (**fibrosis**). This occurs mainly in the skin, digestive tract, muscles, and kidneys, causing hardening and functional impairment of the involved organs. **Keloid** is a local swelling caused by abnormal amounts of collagen that form in scars of the skin. Keloids, which occur most often in individuals of black African descent, can be a troublesome clinical problem to manage; not only can they be disfiguring, but excision is almost always followed by recurrence.

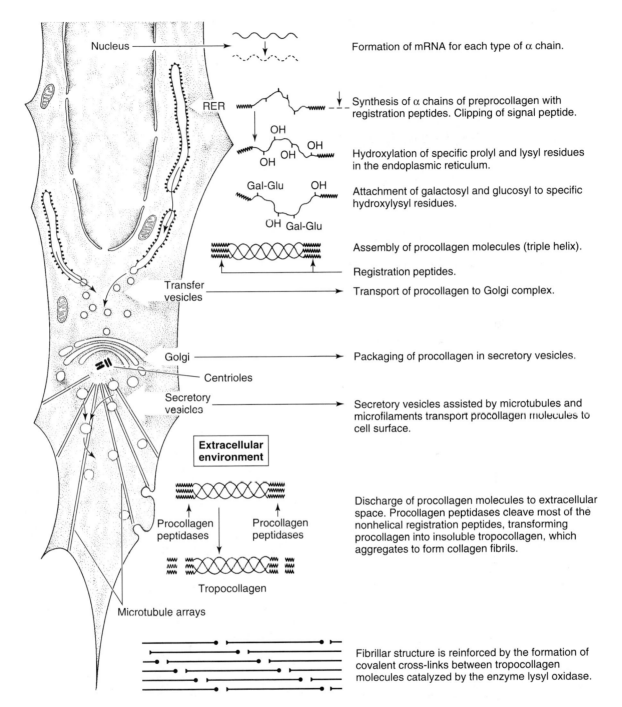

Nucleus — Formation of mRNA for each type of α chain.

RER — Synthesis of α chains of preprocollagen with registration peptides. Clipping of signal peptide.

OH — Hydroxylation of specific prolyl and lysyl residues in the endoplasmic reticulum.

Gal-Glu   OH — Attachment of galactosyl and glucosyl to specific hydroxylysyl residues.

Assembly of procollagen molecules (triple helix).

Registration peptides.

Transfer vesicles — Transport of procollagen to Golgi complex.

Golgi — Packaging of procollagen in secretory vesicles.

Centrioles

Secretory vesicles — Secretory vesicles assisted by microtubules and microfilaments transport procollagen molecules to cell surface.

Extracellular environment

Procollagen peptidases   Procollagen peptidases — Discharge of procollagen molecules to extracellular space. Procollagen peptidases cleave most of the nonhelical registration peptides, transforming procollagen into insoluble tropocollagen, which aggregates to form collagen fibrils.

Tropocollagen

Microtubule arrays

Fibrillar structure is reinforced by the formation of covalent cross-links between tropocollagen molecules catalyzed by the enzyme lysyl oxidase.

Figure 5–11. Collagen synthesis. The assembly of the triple helix and the hydroxylation and glycosylation of procollagen molecules are simultaneous processes that begin as soon as the three chains cross the membrane of the rough endoplasmic reticulum (RER).

Table 5–3. Examples of clinical disorders resulting from defects in collagen synthesis.

Disorder	Defect	Symptoms
Ehlers-Danlos type IV	Faulty transcription or translation of type III	Aortic and/or intestinal rupture
Ehlers-Danlos type VI	Faulty lysine hydroxylation	Augmented skin elasticity, rupture of eyeball
Ehlers-Danlos type VII	Decrease in procollagen peptidase activity	Increased articular mobility, frequent luxation
Scurvy	Lack of vitamin C (cofactor for proline hydroxylase)	Ulceration of gums, hemorrhages
Osteogenesis imperfecta	Change of one nucleotide in genes for collagen type I	Spontaneous fractures, cardiac insufficiency

Reticular fibers are also PAS-positive. Both PAS-positivity and argyrophilia are considered to be due to the high content of glycoproteins associated with these fibers. Reticular fibers contain 6–12% hexoses as opposed to 1% in collagen fibers. Immunocytochemical and histochemical evidence reveals that reticular fibers (in contrast to collagen fibers, which consist of collagen type I) are composed mainly of collagen type III in association with other types of collagen, glycoproteins, and proteoglycans. They are formed by loosely packed, thin (average 35-nm) fibrils (Figure 5–15) bound together by abundant small interfibrillar bridges probably composed of proteoglycans and glycoproteins. Because of their small diameter, reticular fibers are weakly birefringent when stained with Sirius red and observed by means of polarizing microscopy.

Reticular fibers are particularly abundant in smooth muscle, endoneurium, and the framework of hematopoietic (or hemopoietic) organs (eg, spleen, lymph nodes, red bone marrow) and constitute a net-

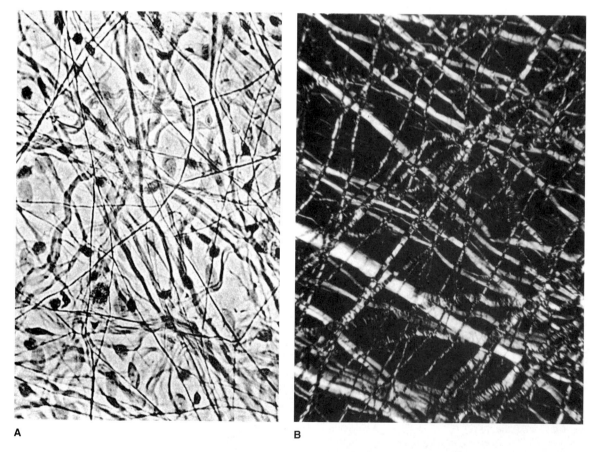

A   B

Figure 5–12. A: Whole mesentery spread on a microscope slide. The preparation was stained by the Weigert method for elastic fibers and photographed under the phase contrast microscope. The thin, taut filaments are elastic fibers that branch and form a woven network. Collagen fibers are the thick and wavy structures. × 200. **B:** A similar preparation stained with Sirius red and observed by means of polarization microscopy. Collagen fibers are the only structures revealed. The birefringence of collagen is due to the tight packing and paracrystalline assembly of its tropocollagen subunits. × 300.

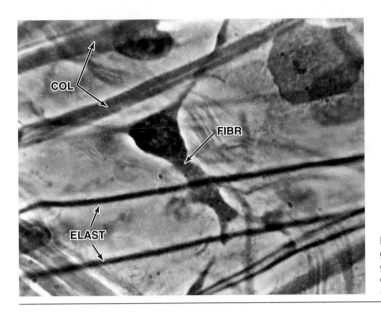

Figure 5–13. Phase contrast photomicrograph of a piece of mesentery spread on a glass slide. Shown are a fibroblast (FIBR), collagen fibers (COL), and elastic fibers (ELAST). H&E stain. × 800.

work around the cells of parenchymal organs (eg, liver, endocrine glands). The small diameter and the loose disposition of reticular fibers create a flexible network in organs that are subjected to changes in form or volume, such as the arteries, spleen, liver, uterus, and intestinal muscle layers.

> Ehlers-Danlos type IV disease, a deficiency of collagen type III, is characterized by ruptures in arteries and the intestine (Table 5–3). Both structures are rich in reticular fibers.

The Elastic Fiber System

The elastic fiber system is composed of three types of fibers—oxytalan, elaunin, and elastic. The structures of the elastic fiber system develop through three successive stages (Figure 5–16). In the first stage, the fiber consists of a bundle of 10-nm microfibrils composed of various glycoproteins, including one with a large molecule called **fibrillin**. These **oxytalan** (Gr. *oxys,* thin) fibers can be found in the zonule fibers of the eye (Figure 24–13) and in the dermis (Figure 18–7) where the dermis connects the elastic system to the basal lamina. In the second stage of development, an irregular deposition of the protein **elastin** appears between the oxytalan fibers, forming the **elaunin** (Gr. *elaunem,* to drive) fibers. These structures are found around sweat glands and in the dermis. During the

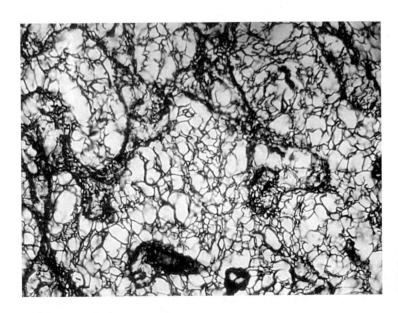

Figure 5–14. Section from a lymph node stained with silver. Note the thin black lines, which are the argyrophilic reticular fibers. × 200.

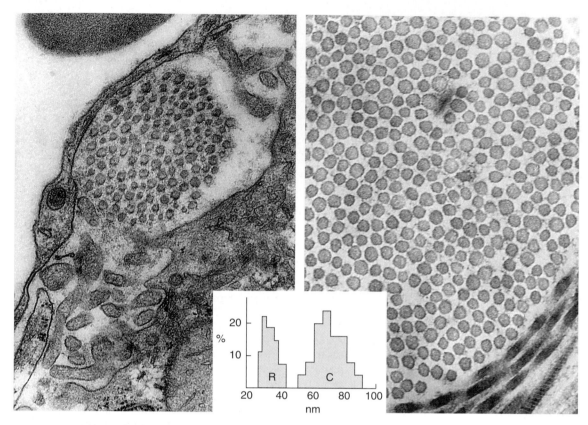

Figure 5–15. Electron micrograph of cross sections of reticular (**left**) and collagen (**right**) fibers. Note that each fiber type is composed of numerous smaller collagen fibrils. Reticular fibers (R) are significantly narrower in diameter than collagen fibrils (C; see histogram **inset**); in addition, the constituent fibrils reveal an abundant surface-associated granularity not present on regular collagen fibrils (**right**). × 70,000.

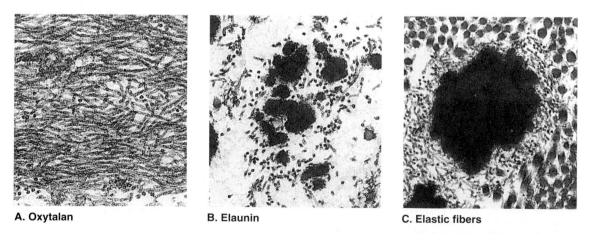

A. Oxytalan **B. Elaunin** **C. Elastic fibers**

Figure 5–16. Electron micrographs of developing elastic fibers. **A:** In early stages of formation, developing fibers consist of numerous small glycoprotein microfibrils. **B:** With further development, amorphous aggregates of elastin are found among the microfibrils. **C:** The amorphous elastin accumulates, ultimately occupying the center of an elastic fiber delineated by microfibrils. Note the collagen fibrils, seen in cross section. (Courtesy of GS Montes.)

third stage, elastin gradually accumulates until it occupies the center of the fiber bundles, which are further surrounded by a thin sheath of microfibrils. These are the **elastic fibers,** the most numerous component of the elastic fiber system.

Oxytalan fibers are highly resistant to pulling forces, but the elastic fibers, which are rich in the protein elastin, stretch easily in response to tension. The elastic fiber system, by using different proportions of microfibrils and elastin, constitutes a family of fibers whose variable functional characteristics are adapted to local tissue requirements.

Proelastin is a globular molecule (molecular mass 70 kDa) produced by fibroblasts in connective tissue and by smooth muscle cells in blood vessels. Proelastin polymerizes, producing elastin, the amorphous rubber-like glycoprotein that predominates in mature fibers. Elastin is resistant to boiling, acid and alkali extraction, and digestion by the usual proteases. It is easily hydrolyzed by pancreatic **elastase.**

The amino acid composition of elastin resembles that of collagen, because both are rich in glycine and proline. Elastin contains two unusual amino acids, **desmosine** and **isodesmosine,** formed by covalent reactions among four lysine residues. These reactions effectively cross-link elastin and are thought to account for the rubber-like qualities of this protein, which forms fibers at least five times more extensible than rubber. Figure 5–17 presents a model that illustrates the elasticity of elastin.

Elastin also occurs in a nonfibrillar form as **fenestrated membranes** (elastic laminae) present in the walls of some blood vessels.

Mutations in the fibrillin gene result in Marfan syndrome, a disease characterized by a lack of resistance in the tissues rich in elastic fibers. Because the large arteries are rich in components of the elastic system and because the blood pressure is high in the aorta, patients with this disease often experience aortic ruptures, a life-threatening condition.

CELLS

Some cells of connective tissue, such as fibroblasts and adipose cells, are produced locally and remain in the connective tissue; others, such as leukocytes, come from other territories and can be transient inhabitants of connective tissue (Figure 5–18). The various functions of these cells are summarized in Table 5–4.

Cells of the connective tissue interact, creating complex mechanisms that help to defend the organism from invasion. Thus, macrophages can influence antibody production by lymphocyte-derived plasma cells. Lymphocytes and mast cells can also produce substances that participate in the inflammatory process.

Fibroblasts

Fibroblasts are the most common cells in connective tissue (Figure 5–19) and are responsible for the synthesis of fibers and intercellular ground substance. Two stages of activity—active and quiescent—are observed in these cells. Cells with intense synthetic activity are morphologically distinct from the quiescent fibroblasts that are scattered within the matrix they have already synthesized. Some histologists reserve the term **fibroblast** to denote the active cell and **fibrocyte** to denote the quiescent cell.

The active fibroblast has an abundant and irregularly branched cytoplasm. Its nucleus is ovoid, large, and pale-staining, with fine chromatin and a prominent nucleolus. The cytoplasm is rich in rough endoplasmic reticulum, and the Golgi complex is well developed (Figures 5–20 and 5–21).

The fibrocyte (Figure 5–20), a smaller cell than the fibroblast, tends to be spindle-shaped. It has fewer processes than the fibroblast; a smaller, darker, elongated nucleus; an acidophilic cytoplasm; and a small amount of rough endoplasmic reticulum. When it is adequately stimulated, such as during wound healing, the fibrocyte reverts to the fibroblast state and its synthetic activities are reactivated. In such instances the cell reassumes the form and appearance of a fibroblast. The **myofibroblast,** a cell with features of both fibroblasts and smooth muscle, is also observed during wound healing. These cells have the morphologic characteristics of fibroblasts but contain increased amounts of actin microfilaments and myosin. Their activity is responsible for wound clo-

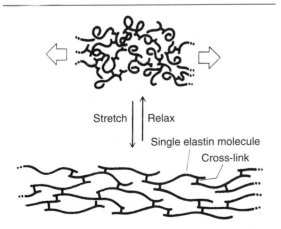

Figure 5–17. Elastin molecules are joined by covalent bonds to generate an extensive cross-linked network. Because each elastin molecule in the network can expand and contract like a random coil, the entire network can stretch and recoil like a rubber band. (Reproduced, with permission, from Alberts B et al: *Molecular Biology of the Cell.* Garland, 1983.)

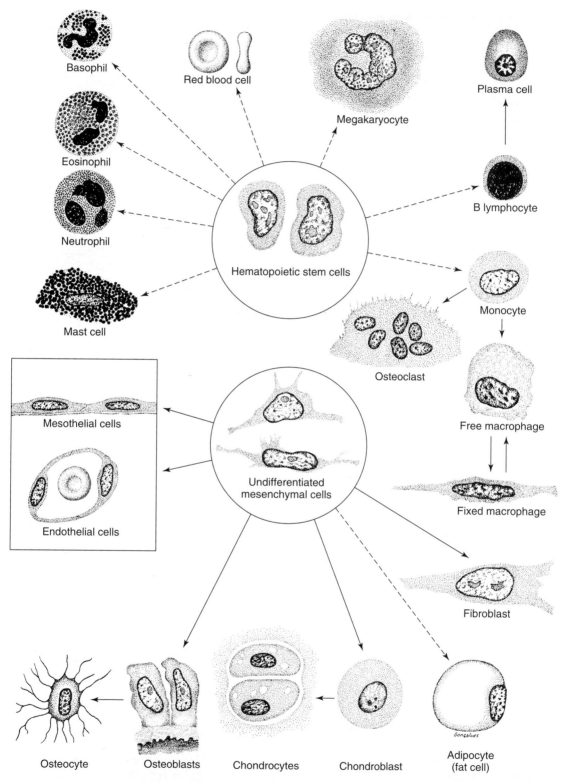

Figure 5–18. Simplified representation of the connective tissue cell lineages derived from the multipotential embryonic mesenchyme cell. Dotted arrows indicate that intermediate cell types exist between the examples illustrated. The two cells in the rectangle are epithelial cells that still maintain some mesenchymal characteristics. Note that the cells are not drawn in proportion to actual sizes, eg, adipocyte, megakaryocyte, and osteoclast cells are significantly larger than other illustrated cells.

Table 5–4. Functions of connective tissue cells.

Cell Type	Main Product or Activity	Main Function
Fibroblast, chondroblast, osteoblast, odontoblast	Production of fibers and ground substance	Structural
Plasma cell	Production of antibodies	Immunologic
Lymphocyte	Production of immunocompetent cells	Immunologic
Eosinophilic leukocyte	Phagocytosis of antigen-antibody complex	Immunologic
Macrophage, neutrophilic leukocyte	Phagocytosis of foreign substances, bacteria	Defense
Mast cell basophilic leukocyte	Liberation of pharmacologically active substances (eg, histamine)	Defense
Adipose cell	Storage of neutral fats, heat production	Energy reservoir; heat production

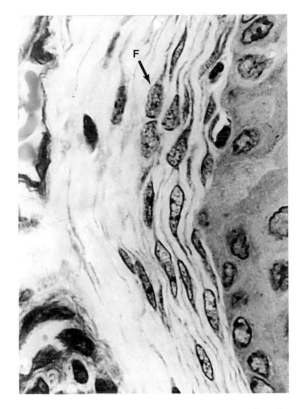

Figure 5–19. Photomicrograph of loose connective tissue showing several fibroblasts (F), which are the elongated cells in the center of the illustration. A few collagen fibers are near the fibroblasts.

sure after tissue injury, a process called **wound contraction.**

Fibroblasts synthesize collagen, reticular and elastic fibers, and the glycosaminoglycans and glycoproteins of the intercellular ground substance. In adults, fibroblasts in connective tissue rarely undergo division. Mitoses are observed only when the organism requires additional fibroblasts, eg, when connective tissue is damaged.

Macrophages: The Mononuclear Phagocyte System

Macrophages were discovered and initially characterized by their phagocytic capacity. When a vital dye such as trypan blue or India ink is injected into an animal, macrophages engulf and accumulate the dye in their cytoplasm in the form of granules or vacuoles visible in the light microscope. Macrophages derive mainly from bone marrow precursor cells that divide, producing **monocytes** (Gr. *monos,* single, + *kytos,* cell) that circulate in the blood. In a second step, these cells migrate into the connective tissue, where they mature and are called **macrophages** (Gr. *macro,* large, + *phagein,* to eat). Tissue macrophages can proliferate locally, producing more such cells.

Macrophages, which are distributed throughout the body, are present in most organs and constitute the **mononuclear phagocyte system** (Table 5–5). In certain regions, macrophages have special names, eg, Kupffer cells in the liver, microglial cells in the central nervous system, and osteoclasts in bone tissue. At one time, most of the body's macrophages were

considered to be constituents of what was referred to as the **reticuloendothelial system.** Certain components of this system, notably the reticular cells of lymphoid organs, are excluded from the mononuclear phagocyte system. Conversely, a few cell types not originally considered components of the reticuloendothelial system (eg, alveolar macrophages of the lung, microglia, Langerhans cells of the skin) are included in the mononuclear phagocyte system.

Although mononuclear phagocytes have a wide spectrum of morphologic features that correspond to their state of functional activity and to the tissue they inhabit, they are characterized by an irregular surface with pleats, protrusions, and indentations—a morphologic expression of their active pinocytotic and phagocytic activities. They generally have a well-developed Golgi complex, many lysosomes, and a prominent rough endoplasmic reticulum (Figure 5–22). The process of monocyte-to-macrophage transformation results in an increase in protein synthesis and cell size. Increases in the Golgi complex and in the number of lysosomes, microtubules, and microfilaments are also apparent. Macrophages measure between 10 and 30 μm and usually have an oval or kidney-shaped nucleus located eccentrically.

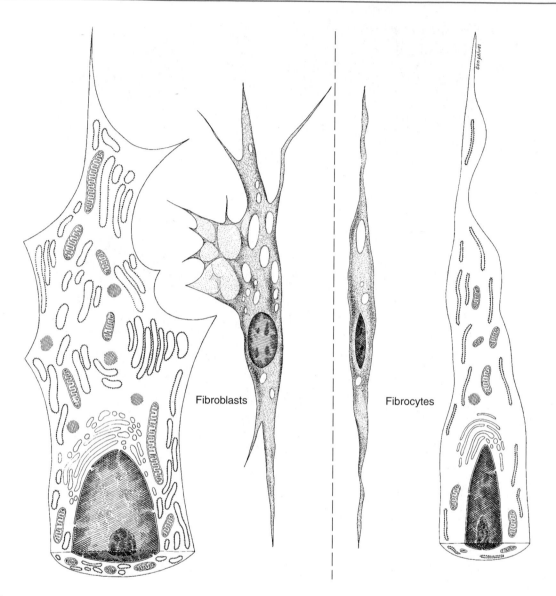

Figure 5–20. Active (**left**) and quiescent (**right**) fibroblasts. External morphologic characteristics and ultrastructure of each cell are shown. Fibroblasts that are actively engaged in synthesis are richer in mitochondria, lipid droplets, Golgi complex, and rough endoplasmic reticulum than are quiescent fibroblasts, often called fibrocytes.

Macrophages are long-living cells and may survive for months in the tissues. When adequately stimulated, these cells may increase in size, forming **epithelioid** (Gr. *epi,* upper, + *thele,* nipple, + *eidos,* resemblance) cells, or several may fuse to form **multinuclear giant cells** (Figure 5–23)—cell types that are usually found only in pathologic conditions.

The major functions of macrophages are the ingestion of particles, digestion of these particles by lysosomes, and secretion of an impressive array of substances that participate in defensive and reparative functions. Macrophages ingest a particle by surrounding it with thin extensions of the cell surface that ultimately fuse, isolating the particle within a phagocytic vacuole. Next, lysosomes fuse with the phagocytic vacuole and digest the contents. The currently accepted hypothesis regarding the mechanism of phagocytosis is summarized in Figure 5–24. Macrophages are antigen-presenting cells (see Chapter 14) and also participate in cell-mediated resistance to infection by bacteria, viruses, protozoa, fungi, and metazoa (eg, parasitic worms); in cell-

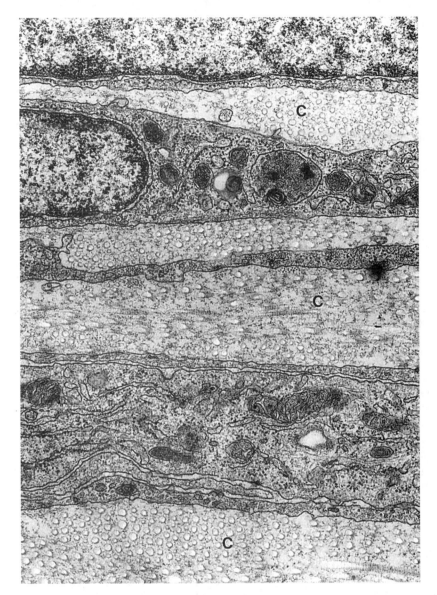

Figure 5–21. Electron micrograph revealing portions of several flattened fibroblasts in dense connective tissue. Abundant mitochondria, rough endoplasmic reticulum, and vesicles distinguish these cells from the less active fibrocytes. Multiple strata of collagen fibrils (C) lie among the fibroblasts. × 30,000.

mediated resistance to tumors; and in extrahepatic bile production, iron and fat metabolism, and the destruction of aged erythrocytes.

The diversity of the macrophage's morphologic characteristics extends to its metabolism, which also varies according to this cell's functional activity and environment. Thus, lung macrophages exhibit a high level of aerobic glycolysis (probably related to the high oxygen tension available locally), whereas peritoneal macrophages have a high level of anaerobic glycolysis.

When macrophages are stimulated (by injection of foreign substances or by infection), they change their morphologic characteristics and metabolism. They are then called **activated macrophages** and acquire characteristics not present in their nonactivated state. These activated macrophages, in addition to showing an increase in their capacity for phagocytosis and intracellular digestion, exhibit enhanced metabolic and lysosomal enzyme activity. They can also secrete several substances that participate

Table 5–5. Distribution and main functions of the cells of the mononuclear phagocyte system.

Cell Type	Location	Main Function
Monocyte	Blood	Precursor of macrophages
Macrophage	Connective tissue, lymphoid organs, lungs	Production of cytokines, chemotactic factors, and several other molecules that participate in inflammation (defense); antigen presentation
Kupffer cell	Liver	Same as macrophages
Microglia cell	Nerve tissue of the central nervous system	Same as macrophages
Langerhans cell	Skin	Antigen presentation
Osteoclast	Bone (fusion of several macrophages)	Digestion of bone
Multinuclear giant cell	Connective tissue (fusion of several macrophages)	Digestion or segregation of foreign bodies

in inflammation and repair (eg, collagenase) and exhibit increased tumor cell–killing capacity (Figure 5–25).

Mast Cells

Mast cells are oval to round connective tissue cells, 20–30 μm in diameter, whose cytoplasm is filled with basophilic granules. The rather small and spherical nucleus is centrally situated; it is frequently obscured by the cytoplasmic granules (Figure 5–26).

The secretory granules are 0.3–2.0 μm in diameter. Their interior is heterogeneous in appearance, with a prominent scroll-like substructure (Figure 5–27). The principal function of mast cells is the storage of chemical mediators of the inflammatory response.

Mast cell granules are metachromatic because of their content of glycosaminoglycans. **Metachromasia** is a property of certain basic aniline dyes (eg, toluidine blue) in which the stained material takes on a different color (purple-red) from that of the applied dye (blue). Other constituents of mast cell granules are histamine, neutral proteases, and eosinophil

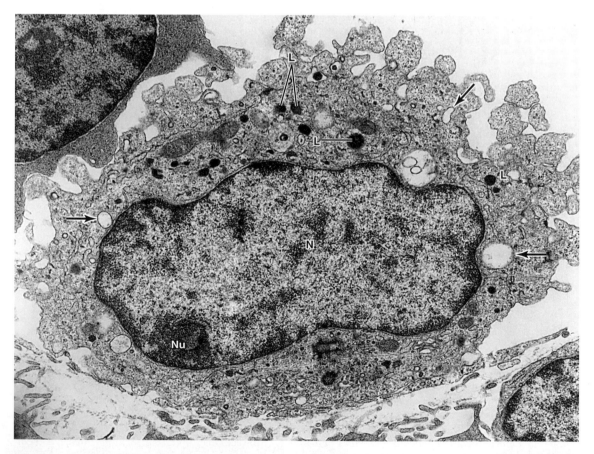

Figure 5–22. Electron micrograph of a macrophage. Note the secondary lysosomes (L), the nucleus (N), and the nucleolus (Nu). The arrows indicate phagocytic vacuoles.

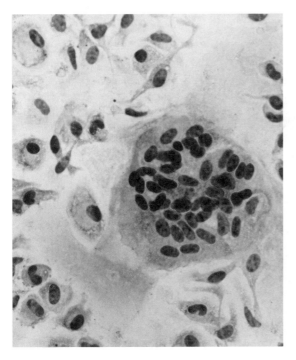

Figure 5–23. Photomicrograph of a multinuclear giant cell, surrounded by macrophages.

chemotactic factor of anaphylaxis (ECF-A). Mast cells also release leukotrienes, but these substances are not stored in the cell. Rather, they are synthesized from membrane phospholipids and immediately released upon appropriate stimulation.

There are at least two populations of mast cells in connective tissues. One type is called the **connective tissue mast cell,** in which the proteoglycan in the granules is mainly heparin, a substance with anticoagulant activity. In the second type, the **mucosal mast cell,** the granules contain chondroitin sulfate instead of heparin. The two types also react differently to pharmacologic agents.

Mast cells originate from stem cells in the bone marrow. Although they are, in many respects, similar to basophilic leukocytes, they have a separate stem cell.

The surface of mast cells contains specific receptors for IgE, a type of immunoglobulin produced by plasma cells. Most IgE molecules are bound to the surface of mast cells and blood basophils; very few remain in the plasma.

Release of the chemical mediators stored in mast cells promotes the allergic reactions known as **immediate hypersensitivity reactions,** because they occur within a few minutes after penetration by an antigen of an individual previously sensitized to the same or a very simi-

1. Coating

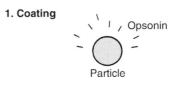

2. Opsonization

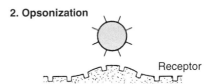

3. Recognition and binding

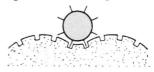

4. Ingestion

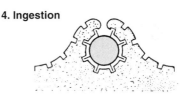

5. Fusion with lysosomes

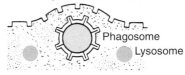

6. Killing

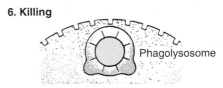

7. Killing and digestion

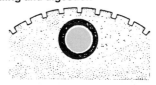

Figure 5–24. Phagocytosis of foreign particles. **1:** Coating of a foreign particle by substances such as immunoglobulins (opsonins) for which the phagocyte has receptors. **2:** Binding of opsonized particle to phagocyte. **3** and **4:** Uptake of the opsonized particle involving sequential interaction of phagocyte membrane receptors with the particle ("zippering"). Subsequent events include fusion of the phagocytic vacuole with lysosomes and killing and digestion of the foreign particle (**5, 6,** and **7**). (Redrawn and reproduced, with permission, from Stites DP et al [editors]: *Basic & Clinical Immunology,* 6th ed. Appleton & Lange, 1987.)

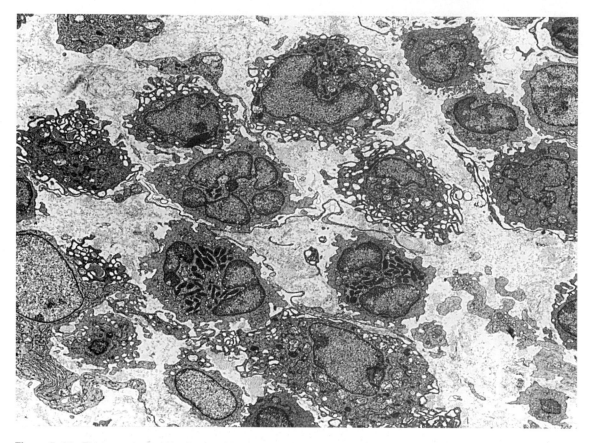

Figure 5–25. Electron micrograph of several macrophages and two eosinophils in a region adjacent to a tumor. This figure illustrates the participation of macrophages in tissue reaction to tumor invasion.

lar antigen. There are many examples of immediate hypersensitivity reaction; a dramatic one is **anaphylactic shock,** a potentially fatal condition. The process of anaphylaxis consists of the following sequential events: The first exposure to an antigen (allergen), such as bee venom, results in production of the IgE class of immunoglobulins (antibodies) by plasma cells. IgE is avidly bound to the surface of mast cells. A second exposure to the antigen results in binding of the antigen to IgE on the mast cells. This event triggers release of the mast cell granules, liberating histamine, leukotrienes, ECF-A, and heparin (Figure 5–28).

Histamine causes contraction of smooth muscle (mainly of the bronchioles) and dilates and increases the permeability of blood capillaries. Any liberated histamine is inactivated immediately after release. Leukotrienes produce slow contractions in smooth muscle, and ECF-A attracts blood eosinophils. Heparin is a blood anticoagulant, but blood clotting remains normal in humans during anaphylactic shock.

Mast cells are widespread in the human body but are particularly abundant in the dermis and in the digestive and respiratory tracts.

Plasma Cells

There are few plasma cells in most connective tissues. They are numerous in sites subject to penetration by bacteria and foreign proteins (eg, intestinal mucosa) and in areas where there is chronic inflammation.

Plasma cells are large, ovoid cells that have a basophilic cytoplasm owing to their richness in rough endoplasmic reticulum (Figures 5–29, 5–30, and 5–31). The juxtanuclear Golgi complex and the centrioles occupy a region that appears pale in regular histologic preparations.

The nucleus of the plasma cell is spherical and eccentrically placed, containing compact, coarse hete-

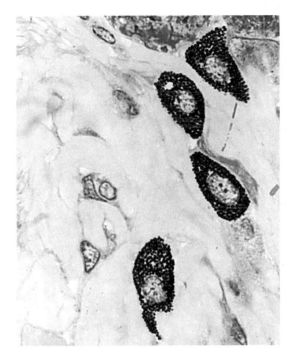

Figure 5–26. Thin section of connective tissue. Four mast cells appear with their conspicuous granules, stained by toluidine blue × 800.

rochromatin alternating with lighter areas of approximately equal size. This configuration resembles the face of a clock, with the heterochromatin clumps corresponding to the numerals. Thus, the nucleus of a plasma cell is commonly described as having a clock-face appearance.

Plasma cells are derived from B lymphocytes and are responsible for the synthesis of the antibodies. Antibodies are immunoglobulins produced in response to penetration by antigens. Each antibody is specific for the one antigen that gave rise to its production and reacts specifically with molecules possessing similar epitopes (see Chapter 14). The results of the antibody-antigen reaction are variable. The capacity of the reaction to neutralize harmful effects caused by antigens is important. An antigen that is a toxin (eg, tetanus, diphtheria) may lose its capacity to do harm when it combines with its respective antibody. Plasma cells seldom divide; their average life is 10–20 days.

Adipose Cells

Adipose cells (adipocytes; L. *adeps,* fat, + Gr. *kytos*) are connective tissue cells that have become specialized for storage of neutral fats or for the production of heat. Often called **fat cells,** they are discussed in detail in Chapter 6.

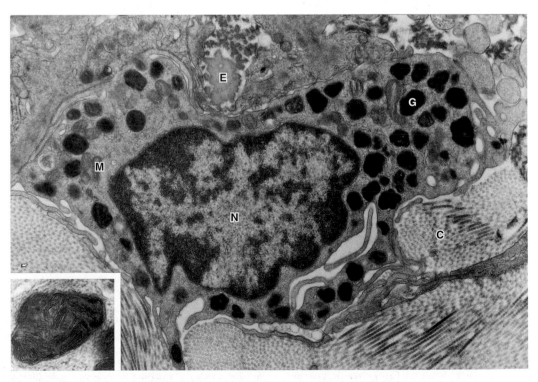

Figure 5–27. Electron micrograph of a human mast cell. The granules (G) contain heparin and histamine. Note the characteristic scroll-like structures within the granules. M, mitochondrion: C, collagen fibrils: E, elastic fibril; N, nucleus. × 14,700. **Inset:** Higher magnification view of a mast cell granule. × 44,600 (Courtesy of MC Williams.)

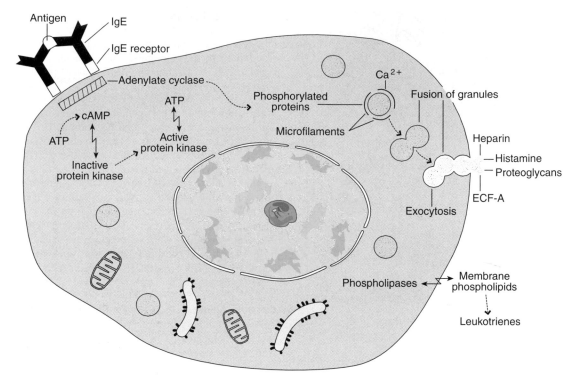

Figure 5–28. Mast-cell secretion. After a second exposure to an antigen (eg, bee venom), IgE molecules bound to surface receptors are cross-linked by the antigen. This activates adenylate cyclase and results in the phosphorylation of certain proteins. At the same time, Ca^{2+} enters the cell. These events lead to intracellular fusion of specific granules and exocytosis of their contents. In addition, phospholipases act on membrane phospholipids to produce leukotrienes. The process of extrusion does not damage the cell, which remains viable and synthesizes new granules. ECF-A, eosinophil chemotactic factor of anaphylaxis.

Leukocytes

Leukocytes (Gr. *leukos,* white, + *kytos*), or white blood corpuscles, are frequently found in connective tissue. They migrate through the walls of capillaries and venules from the blood to connective tissues, by a process called diapedesis. This process increases greatly during inflammation. Leukocytes do not return to the blood after having resided in connective tissue, except for the lymphocytes that circulate continuously in various compartments of the body (blood, lymph, connective tissues, lymphatic organs). A detailed analysis of the structure and functions of leukocytes is presented in Chapter 12.

TYPES OF CONNECTIVE TISSUE

There are several types of connective tissue that consist of the basic components already described—fibers, cells, and ground substance. The names given to the various types denote either the component that predominates in the tissue or a structural characteris-

tic of the tissue. Figure 5–32 illustrates the main types of connective tissue.

Connective Tissue Proper

There are two classes of connective tissue proper: loose and dense.

A. Loose Connective Tissue: Loose connective tissue, also called **areolar** tissue, is the more abundant of the two types. It fills spaces between groups of muscle cells, supports epithelial tissue, and forms a layer that sheathes the lymphatic and blood vessels. Loose connective tissue is also found in the papillary layer of the dermis, in the hypodermis, in the serosal linings of peritoneal and pleural cavities, and in glands and the mucous membranes (wet membranes that line the hollow organs) supporting the epithelial cells.

Loose connective tissue (Figure 5–33A) comprises all the main components of connective tissue proper. The most numerous cells are fibroblasts and macrophages, but all the other types of connective tissue cells are also present. Collagen, elastic, and

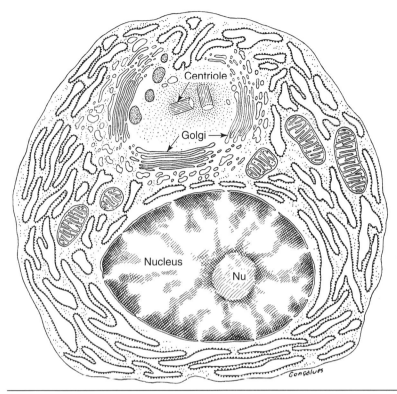

Figure 5–29. Ultrastructure of a plasma cell. The cell contains a well-developed rough endoplasmic reticulum, with dilated cisternae containing immunoglobulins (antibodies). In plasma cells, the secreted proteins do not aggregate into secretory granules. Nu, nucleolus. (Redrawn and reproduced, with permission, from Ham AW: *Histology,* 6th ed. Lippincott, 1969.)

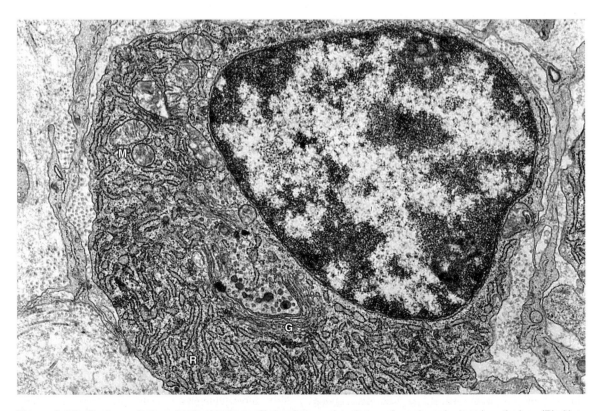

Figure 5–30. Electron micrograph of a plasma cell showing an abundance of rough endoplasmic reticulum (R). Note that many cisternae are dilated. M, mitochondria: G, Golgi complex. × 18,000.

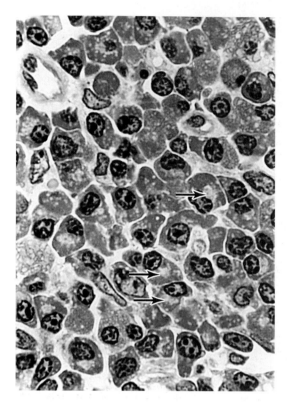

Figure 5–31. Photomicrograph of plasma cells. Note the coarse chromatin and light juxtanuclear area corresponding to the region of the Golgi complex and centriole (arrows). Compare with Figures 5–27 and 5–28. × 600.

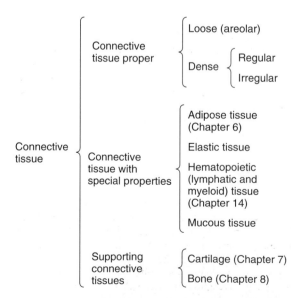

Figure 5–32. Simplified scheme classifying the principal types of connective tissue, which are discussed in the chapters indicated.

reticular fibers appear in this tissue, although the proportion of reticular fibers is small. Loose connective tissue has a delicate consistency; it is flexible, well vascularized, and not very resistant to stress.

B. Dense Connective Tissue: Dense connective tissue consists of the same components found in loose connective tissue, but there are fewer cells and a clear predominance of collagen fibers (Figure 5–33B). Dense connective tissue is less flexible and far more resistant to stress than is loose connective tissue. It is known as **dense irregular** connective tissue when the collagen fibers are arranged in bundles without a definite orientation. The collagen fibers form a three-dimensional network in dense irregular tissue and provide resistance to stress from all directions. This type of tissue is encountered in such areas as the dermis.

The collagen bundles of **dense regular** connective tissue are arranged according to a definite pattern. The collagen fibers of this tissue are aligned with the linear orientation of fibroblasts in response to prolonged stresses exerted in the same direction; they consequently offer great resistance to traction forces.

Tendons are the most common example of dense regular connective tissue. These elongated cylindrical structures attach striated muscle to bone; by virtue of their richness in collagen fibers, they are white and inextensible. They have parallel, closely packed bundles of collagen separated by a small quantity of intercellular ground substance. Their fibrocytes contain elongated nuclei parallel to the fibers and sparse cytoplasmic folds that envelop portions of the collagen bundles. The cytoplasm of these fibrocytes is rarely revealed in H&E stains—not only because it is sparse but also because it stains the same color as the fibers (Figures 5–34 and 5–35).

The collagen bundles of the tendons (primary bundles) aggregate into larger bundles (secondary bundles) that are enveloped by loose connective tissue containing blood vessels and nerves. Externally, the tendon is surrounded by a sheath of dense connective tissue. In some tendons, this sheath is made up of two layers, both lined by squamous cells of mesenchymal origin. One layer is attached to the tendon, and the other lines the neighboring structures. A cavity containing a viscous fluid (similar to the fluid of synovial joints) is formed between the two layers. This fluid, which contains water, proteins, glycosaminoglycans, glycoproteins, and ions, is a lubricant that permits an easy sliding movement of the tendon within its sheath.

Elastic Tissue

Elastic tissue is composed of bundles of thick, parallel elastic fibers. The space between these fibers is occupied by thin collagen fibers and flattened fibroblasts. The abundance of elastic fibers in this tissue confers on it a typical yellow color and great elasticity. Elastic tissue, which occurs infrequently, is pre-

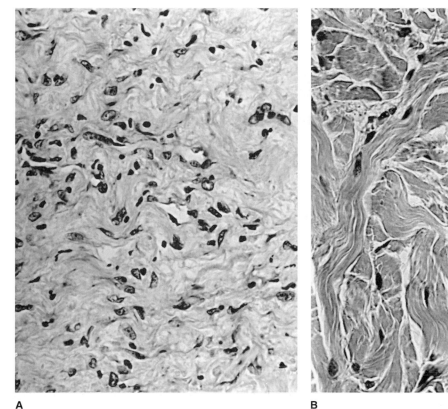

A   B

Figure 5–33. Photomicrographs of sections showing two varieties of connective tissue frequently found in several organs. **A:** Loose connective tissue. Note the abundance of cells, most of which are fibroblasts. × 400. **B:** Dense irregular connective tissue, which contains many randomly oriented collagen fibers, sparse ground substance, and few cells. × 320.

sent in the yellow ligaments of the vertebral column and in the suspensory ligament of the penis.

Reticular Tissue

Reticular tissue is a specialized loose connective tissue that provides the architectural framework of the myeloid (bone marrow) and lymphoid (lymph nodules and nodes, spleen) hematopoietic organs. In this form of connective tissue, **reticular cells** elaborate a fine matrix of branched reticular fibers. Reticular cells are fibroblasts specialized for secreting the constituents of reticular fibers. The reticular cells are dispersed along this matrix and sheathe the reticular fibers and ground substance with cytoplasmic processes. The resulting cell-lined trabecular system creates a sponge-like structure (Figure 5–36) within which cells and fluids are freely mobile.

In addition to the reticular cells, cells of the mononuclear phagocyte system are strategically dispersed along the trabeculae. These cells monitor the slow flow of materials through the sinus-like spaces and remove invaders by phagocytosis.

Mucous Tissue

Mucous tissue has an abundance of ground substance composed chiefly of hyaluronic acid. It is a jelly-like tissue containing very few fibers. The cells in this tissue are mainly fibroblasts. Mucous tissue is the principal component of the umbilical cord, where it is referred to as **Wharton's jelly.** It is also found in the pulp of young teeth.

HISTOPHYSIOLOGY

Connective tissues have the functions of support, packing, storage, defense, repair, and transport. The functions of support and packing are obvious—epithelial, muscular, and nerve tissues are associated with connective tissue that supports and fills the tissue spaces between their cells. The support function is carried out mainly by connective tissue fibers.

Fibers, predominantly composed of collagen, constitute tendons, aponeuroses, capsules of organs, and membranes that envelop the central nervous system

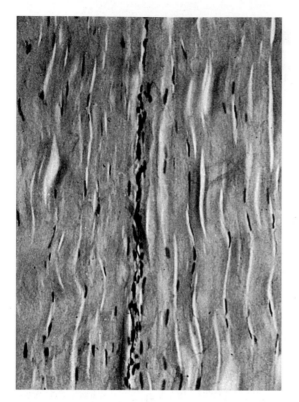

Figure 5–34. Dense regular connective tissue (longitudinal section through a tendon). Numerous collagen bundles are in parallel array, and fibrocyte nuclei are seen between the collagen bundles. H&E stain. × 320.

(**meninges**). They also make up the trabeculae and walls inside several organs, forming the most resistant component of the **stroma** (support tissue) of these organs.

Storage

Lipids, which are important nutritional reserves, are stored in adipose tissue (see Chapter 6). In addition, because of its richness in glycosaminoglycans, loose connective tissue stores water and electrolytes. The most abundant electrolyte is sodium. Although only a small proportion of connective tissue consists of plasma proteins, it is estimated that because of its wide distribution, as much as one third of the plasma proteins of the body are stored in the intercellular connective tissue matrix.

Defense

Several defense mechanisms depend upon the cells and intercellular components of connective tissue. This tissue contains a number of cell types, each with several functions (summarized in Table 5–4), creating a complex network of activities that can initiate and regulate defense mechanisms in the body.

One of these important mechanisms has been extensively studied; it is called **inflammation.**

Inflammation is a vascular and cellular defensive reaction against foreign substances, in most cases pathogenic bacteria or irritating chemical substances. The classic signs of inflammation were first described by Celsus (first century A.D.) as redness and swelling with heat and pain (*rubor et tumor cum calore et dolore*). Much later, disturbed function (*functio laesa*) was added as the fifth cardinal sign.

Inflammation begins with the local release of **chemical mediators of inflammation,** substances of various origin (mainly from cells and blood plasma proteins) that induce some of the events characteristic of inflammation, eg, **increase of blood flow** and **vascular permeability, chemotaxis,** and **phagocytosis.**

Increased vascular permeability is caused by the action of vasoactive substances; an example is histamine, which is liberated from mast cells and basophilic leukocytes. Histamine promotes the permeability of endothelial cells, mainly in capillaries and venules (see Chapter 11). Increases in blood flow and vascular permeability are responsible for local swelling (edema), redness, and heat. Pain is due mainly to the action of chemical mediators on nerve endings. **Chemotaxis** (Gr. *chemeia,* alchemy, + *taxis,* orderly arrangement), the phenomenon by which specific cell types are attracted by some molecules, is responsible for the migration of large quantities of specific cell types to regions of inflammation.

As a consequence of chemotaxis, leukocytes cross the walls of venules and capillaries by the process of **diapedesis,** invading the inflamed area.

During the initial or **acute phase** of inflammation, the neutrophils predominate; when inflammation enters the **chronic phase,** the cell population changes. The main types of cells in the chronic phase are lymphocytes and macrophages, which come from the blood, and plasma cells, which originate from B lymphocytes. Macrophages in the area of inflammation are wandering connective tissue cells that have migrated to that site, or they may differentiate from monocytes that arrive via the circulation.

The cells in the inflamed area engulf (phagocytose) the remains of the cells and fibers altered by inflammation and participate in producing antibodies against invading microorganisms. Surrounding connective tissue frequently forms a fibrous retaining wall, or capsule, around the inflamed area. Some bacteria of the genus *Clostridium* that cause gas gangrene produce collagenase, which greatly increases the invasive power of these microorganisms.

Repair

Connective tissue has great regenerative capacity, and the areas destroyed by inflammation or traumatic injury are easily repaired. The spaces

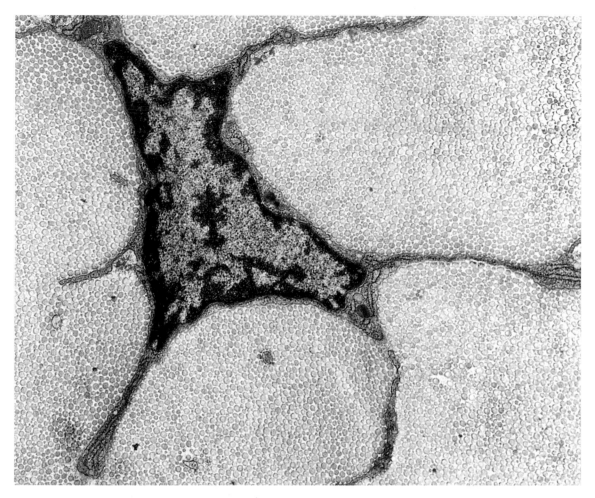

Figure 5–35. Electron micrograph of the rarely seen cytoplasm of fibrocytes in dense regular connective tissue. The sparse cytoplasm of the fibrocyte is divided into numerous thin cytoplasmic processes that interdigitate among the coarse collagen fibers. Note that the thick collagen fibers are composed of smaller parallel collagen fibrils of various diameters. × 25,000.

left after injury to tissues whose cells do not divide (eg, cardiac muscle) are filled by connective tissue, which forms a scar. The healing of surgical incisions depends on the reparative capacity of connective tissue. The main cell type involved in repair is the fibroblast.

Transport

There is a close association between connective tissue and blood and lymphatic capillaries. These vessels, except in nerve tissue, are always sheathed by connective tissue. Consequently, the connective tissue carries nutrients from the blood to various cells in the body and moves metabolic wastes from the cells to the blood.

Hormonal Effects

Various hormones influence the metabolism of connective tissue. An example is the hormone cortisol (hydrocortisone), which is produced by the cortical layer of the adrenal gland and inhibits the synthesis of fibers by connective tissue cells. Adrenocorticotropic hormone (ACTH), released by the pituitary, which stimulates the production of cortisol, has the same effect. Injection of either cortisol or ACTH has a detrimental effect on wound healing. These hormones suppress or attenuate the inflammatory process; their action is also directed against the cells of the connective tissue (lymphocytes, plasma cells, etc).

Hypothyroidism causes an accumulation of glycosaminoglycans in connective tissues. Adult hypothyroidism causes myxedema (mucous edema) and is associated with an excess of glycosaminoglycans in skin connective tissue.

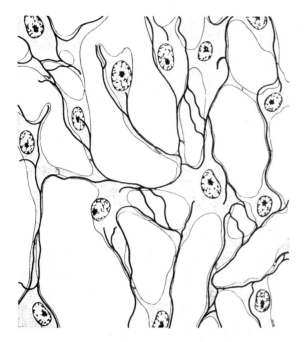

Figure 5–36. Reticular connective tissue showing only the attached cells and the fibers (free cells are not represented). Reticular fibers are enveloped by the cytoplasm of reticular cells; the fibers, however, are extracellular, being separated from the cytoplasm by the cell membrane. Within the sinus-like spaces, cells and tissue fluids of the organ are freely mobile.

Nutritional Factors

Vitamin C (ascorbic acid) deficiency leads to scurvy, a disease characterized by the degeneration of connective tissue. Without this vitamin, fibroblasts synthesize defective collagen, and the defective fibers are not replaced. This process leads to a general degeneration of connective tissue that becomes more pronounced in areas where collagen renewal takes place at a faster rate. The periodontal ligament that holds teeth in their sockets exhibits a relatively high collagen turnover; consequently, this ligament is markedly affected by scurvy, which leads to a loss of teeth. Ascorbic acid is a cofactor for proline hydroxylase, which is essential for the normal synthesis of collagen.

Renewal of Collagen

Collagen is a stable protein, and its renewal is very slow, with a **turnover rate** that differs in various anatomic structures. The collagen of tendons is renewed very slowly or not at all, whereas the collagen of loose connective tissue is renewed more rapidly.

REFERENCES

Deyl Z, Adam M: *Connective Tissue Research: Chemistry, Biology and Physiology.* Liss, 1981.

Gay S, Miller EJ: *Collagen in the Physiology and Pathology of Connective Tissue.* Gustav Fischer, 1978.

Hay ED (editor): *Cell Biology of Extracellular Matrix,* 2nd ed. Plenum, 1991.

Junqueira LCU et al: Picrosirius staining plus polarization microscopy, a specific method for collagen detection in tissue sections. Histochem J. 1979;11:447.

Junqueira LCU, Montes GS: Biology of collagen proteoglycan interaction. Arch Histol Jpn 1983;6:589.

Kefalides NA et al: Biochemistry and metabolism of basement membranes. Int Rev Cytol 1979;1:167.

Krstić RV: *Illustrated Encyclopedia of Human Histology.* Springer-Verlag, 1984.

Mathews MB: *Connective Tissue, Macromolecular Structure and Evolution.* Springer-Verlag, 1975.

Montes GS et al: Collagen distribution in tissues. In: *Ultrastructure of the Connective Tissue Matrix.* Ruggieri A, Motta PM (editors). Martinus Nijhoff, 1984.

Montes GS, Junqueira LCU: The use of the picrosirius-polarization method for the study of biopathology of collagen. Mem Inst Oswaldo Cruz. 1991;86(suppl):1.

Prockop DJ et al: The biosynthesis of collagen and its disorders. N Engl J Med 1979;01:13.

Sandberg LB et al: Elastin structure, biosynthesis, and relation to disease state. N Engl J Med 1981;04:556.

Van Furth R (editor): *Mononuclear Phagocytes: Functional Aspects.* 2 vols. Martinus Nijhoff, 1980

Adipose Tissue

6

Adipose tissue is a special type of connective tissue in which adipose (L. *adeps,* fat) cells (**adipocytes**) predominate. These cells can be found isolated or in small groups within the connective tissue itself; most are found in large aggregates, making up the adipose tissues that are spread throughout the body. Adipose tissue is, in a sense, one of the largest organs in the body. In men of normal weight, adipose tissue represents 15–20% of the body weight; in women of normal weight, 20–25% of body weight.

Adipose tissue is the largest repository of energy (in the form of triglycerides) in the body. The other organs that store energy (in the form of glycogen) are the liver and skeletal muscle. Since eating is a periodic activity and the supply of glycogen is limited, there must be a large store of calories that can be mobilized between meals. Because triglycerides are of lower density than glycogen and have a higher caloric value (9.3 kcal/g for triglycerides versus 4.1 kcal/g for carbohydrates), adipose tissue is a very efficient storage tissue. It is in a state of continuous turnover and is sensitive to both nervous and hormonal stimuli. Subcutaneous layers of adipose tissue help to shape the surface of the body, whereas deposits in the form of pads act as shock absorbers, chiefly in the soles and palms. Since fat is a poor heat conductor, it contributes to the thermal insulation of the body. Adipose tissue also fills up spaces between other tissues and helps to keep some organs in position. There are two known types of adipose tissue that have different locations, structures, colors, and pathologic characteristics. **Unilocular** (**common,** or **yellow**) **adipose tissue** is composed of cells that, when completely developed, contain one large central droplet of yellow fat in their cytoplasm. **Multilocular** (or **brown**) adipose tissue is composed of cells that contain numerous lipid droplets and abundant brown mitochondria. Both types of adipose tissue have a rich blood supply.

UNILOCULAR ADIPOSE TISSUE

Cells of unilocular adipose tissue have only one large fat vacuole; they are the main energy depot for the organism.

The color of unilocular adipose tissue varies from white to dark yellow, depending on the diet; it is due mainly to the presence of carotenoids dissolved in fat droplets of the cells. Almost all adipose tissue in adults is of this type. It is found throughout the human body except for the eyelids, the penis, the scrotum, and all of the auricle of the external ear but the lobule. The distribution and density of adipose deposits are determined by age and sex.

In the newborn, unilocular adipose tissue has a uniform thickness throughout the body. As the baby matures, the tissue tends to disappear from some parts of the body and increase in others. Its distribution is partly regulated by sex hormones and adrenocortical hormones, which control the accumulation of fat and are largely responsible for male or female body contour.

Histologic Structure

Unilocular adipose cells are spherical when isolated but are polyhedral in adipose tissue, where they are closely packed. Each cell is between 50 and 150 μm in diameter. Since lipid droplets are removed by the alcohol and xylol used in routine histologic techniques, each cell appears in standard microscope preparations as a thin ring of cytoplasm surrounding the vacuole left by the dissolved lipid droplet—the **signet ring cell.** Consequently, these cells have eccentric and flattened nuclei (Figure 6–1). The rim of cytoplasm that remains after removal of the stored triglycerides (neutral fats) may rupture and collapse, distorting the tissue structure.

The thickest portion of the cytoplasm surrounds the nucleus of these cells and contains a Golgi complex, filamentous and ovoid mitochondria, poorly developed cisternae of the rough endoplasmic reticulum, and free polyribosomes. The rim of cytoplasm surrounding the lipid droplet contains vesicles of smooth endoplasmic reticulum, occasional microtubules, and numerous pinocytotic vesicles. Electron-microscope studies reveal that each adipose cell usually possesses minute lipid droplets in addition to the single large droplet seen with the light microscope; the droplets are not surrounded by a membrane. Each adipose cell is surrounded by a basal lamina.

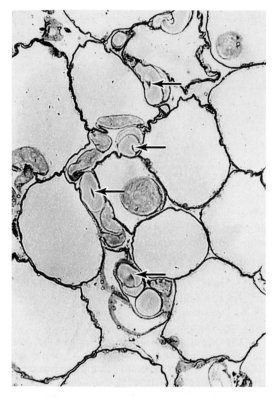

Figure 6–1. Photomicrograph of unilocular adipose tissue. The arrows show blood capillaries. Hematoxylin-and-eosin stain.

Unilocular adipose tissue is subdivided into incomplete lobules by a partition of connective tissue containing a rich vascular bed and network of nerves. Reticular fibers form a fine interwoven network that supports individual fat cells and binds them together.

Although blood vessels are not always apparent, adipose tissue is richly vascularized. If the amount of cytoplasm in fat cells is taken into consideration, the ratio of blood volume to cytoplasm volume is greater in adipose tissue than in striated muscle.

Histophysiology

The lipids stored in adipose cells are chiefly triglycerides, ie, esters of fatty acids and glycerol. Fatty acids stored by these cells have their origin in dietary fats that are brought to adipose tissue cells in the form of chylomicron triglycerides, in triglycerides synthesized in the liver and transported to adipose tissue in the form of **very low-density lipoproteins** (**VLDL**), and by the synthesis of free fatty acids and glycerol from glucose to form triglycerides in adipose cells.

Chylomicrons (Gr. *chylos,* juice, + *micros,* small) are particles up to 3 μm in diameter, formed in in-

testinal epithelial cells and transported in blood plasma and mesenteric lymph. They consist of a central core, composed mainly of triglycerides and a small quantity of cholesterol esters, surrounded by a stabilizing monolayer consisting of apolipoproteins, cholesterol, and phospholipids. VLDL have proportionately more lipid in their surface layer because they are smaller (providing a greater surface-to-volume ratio), have different apolipoproteins at the surface, and contain a higher proportion of cholesterol esters to triglycerides than do chylomicrons. Chylomicrons and VLDL are hydrolyzed at the luminal surfaces of blood capillaries of adipose tissue by lipoprotein lipase, an enzyme synthesized by the adipocyte and transferred to the capillary cell membrane. Free fatty acids enter the adipocyte by mechanisms that are not completely understood. Both an active transport system and free diffusion seem to be involved. The numerous pinocytotic vesicles seen at the surfaces of adipocytes are probably not involved. The fatty acids cross the following layers (in order) in passing from the endothelium into the adipose cell: (1) capillary endothelium, (2) capillary basal lamina, (3) connective tissue ground substance, (4) adipocyte basal lamina, and (5) adipocyte plasma membrane. The movement of fatty acids across the cytoplasm into the lipid droplet is incompletely understood but may utilize specific carrier proteins (Figure 6–2). Within the adipocyte, the fatty acids combine with glycerol phosphate, an intermediate product of glucose metabolism, to form triglyceride molecules. These are then deposited in the triglyceride droplets. Mitochondria and smooth endoplasmic reticulum are organelles that participate actively in the process of lipid uptake and storage.

Adipose cells can synthesize fatty acids from glucose, a process accelerated by insulin. Insulin also stimulates the uptake of glucose into the adipose cells and increases the synthesis of lipoprotein lipase.

Stored lipids are mobilized by humoral and neurogenic mechanisms, resulting in the liberation of fatty acids and glycerol into the blood. Triglyceride lipase, an enzyme known as **hormone-sensitive lipase,** is activated by adenylate cyclase when the tissue is stimulated by norepinephrine. Norepinephrine is liberated at the endings of the postganglionic sympathetic nerves present in adipose tissue. The activated enzyme breaks down triglyceride molecules, which are located mainly at the surface of the lipid droplets. The relatively insoluble fatty acids are transported in association with serum albumin to other tissues of the body, whereas the more soluble glycerol remains free and is taken up by the liver.

Growth hormone, glucocorticoids, prolactin, corticotropin, insulin, and thyroid hormone also have roles at various stages in the metabolism of adipose tissue.

Both unilocular and multilocular adipose tissues

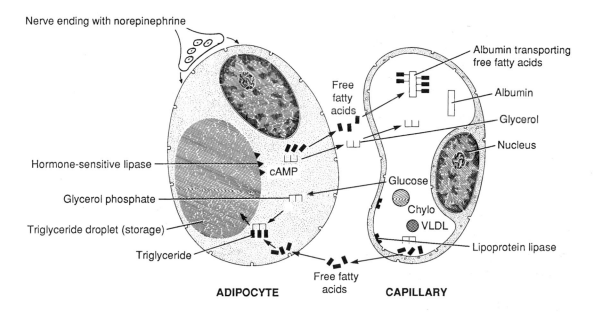

Figure 6–2. The process of lipid storage and release by the adipocyte. Triglycerides are transported in blood from the intestine and liver by lipoproteins known as chylomicrons (Chylo) and very low-density lipoproteins (VLDL). In adipose tissue capillaries, these lipoproteins are partly broken down by lipoprotein lipase, releasing free fatty acids and glycerol. The free fatty acids diffuse from the capillary into the adipocyte, where they are re-esterified to glycerol phosphate, forming triglycerides. These resulting triglycerides are stored in droplets until needed. Norepinephrine from nerve endings stimulates the cyclic AMP (cAMP) system (see Figure 4–17), which activates hormone-sensitive lipase. Hormone-sensitive lipase hydrolyzes stored triglycerides to free fatty acids and glycerol. These substances diffuse into the capillary, where free fatty acids are bound to the hydrophobic moiety of albumin for transport to distant sites for use as an energy source.

are richly innervated by the sympathetic division of the autonomic nervous system. In unilocular adipose tissue, nerve endings are found only in the walls of blood vessels; the adipocytes are not directly innervated. Multilocular fat cells do receive direct sympathetic innervation: Release of the neurotransmitter norepinephrine activates the hormone-sensitive lipase described above. This innervation plays an important role in the mobilization of fats when the body is subjected to long periods of fasting or severe cold.

In response to body needs, lipids are not mobilized uniformly in all parts of the body. Subcutaneous, mesenteric, and retroperitoneal deposits are the first to be mobilized, whereas adipose tissue in the hands, feet, and retro-orbital fat pads resists long periods of starvation. After such periods of starvation, unilocular adipose tissue loses nearly all its fat and contains polyhedral or spindle-shaped cells with very few lipid droplets. These cells remain as quiescent adipocytes and do not modulate into fibroblasts or other types of connective tissue cells.

Obesity in adults may result from an excessive accumulation of fat in unilocular tissue cells that become larger than usual (**hypertrophic obesity**). An increase in the number of adipocytes causes **hyperplastic obesity.**

Histogenesis

Adipose cells develop from mesenchymally derived lipoblasts. These cells have the appearance of fibroblasts but are able to accumulate fat in their cytoplasm. Lipid accumulations are isolated from one another at first but soon fuse to form the single larger droplet that is characteristic of unilocular tissue cells (Figure 6–3). Lipoblasts or immature adipose cells that contain more than one lipid droplet are considered to be in the multilocular stage.

The human being is one of the few mammals born with fat stores, which begin to accumulate at the 30th week of gestation. After birth, the development of new adipose cells is common around small blood vessels, where undifferentiated mesenchymal cells are usually found.

It is believed that during a finite postnatal period, nutritional and other influences can result in an increase in the number of adipocytes, but the cells do not increase in number after that period. They accumulate more lipid only under conditions of excess

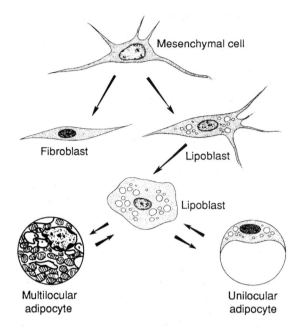

Figure 6–3. Development of fat cells. Undifferentiated mesenchymal cells are transformed into lipoblasts that accumulate fat and thus give rise to mature fat cells. When a large amount of lipid is mobilized by the body, mature unilocular fat cells return to the lipoblast stage. Undifferentiated mesenchymal cells also give rise to a variety of other cell types, including fibroblasts. The mature fat cell is larger than that shown here in relation to the other cell types.

caloric intake (overfeeding). This early increase in the number of adipocytes may predispose an individual to hyperplastic obesity in later life.

MULTILOCULAR ADIPOSE TISSUE

Cells of multilocular adipose tissue have several fat vacuoles and many mitochondria. When stimulated, they transform stored chemical energy to heat.

Multilocular adipose tissue is also called **brown fat** because of its color, which is due to both the large number of blood capillaries in this tissue and the numerous mitochondria (containing colored cytochromes) in the cells. Compared to unilocular tissue, which is present throughout the body, brown adipose tissue has a more limited distribution. (Because it is more abundant in hibernating animals, it was at one time called the **hibernating gland.**)

In rats and several other mammals, multilocular adipose tissue is found mainly around the shoulder girdle. In the human embryo and newborn, this tissue is encountered in several areas and remains restricted to these locations after birth (Figure 6–4). In humans, this tissue appears to be important mainly in the first months of postnatal life, when it produces heat and thus protects the newborn against cold. It is greatly reduced in adulthood.

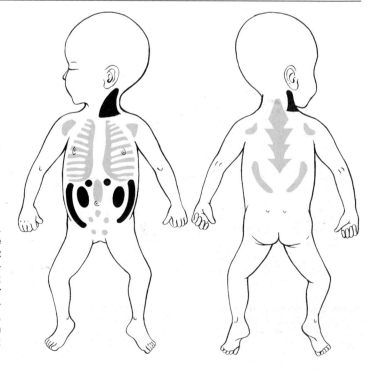

Figure 6–4. Distribution of adipose tissue. In a human newborn, multilocular adipose tissue constitutes 2–5% of the body weight and is distributed as shown. The black areas indicate multilocular adipose tissue; shaded areas are a mixture of multilocular and unilocular adipose tissue. (Modified, redrawn, and reproduced, with permission, from Merklin RJ: Growth and distribution of human fetal brown fat. Anat Rec 1974; 178:637.)

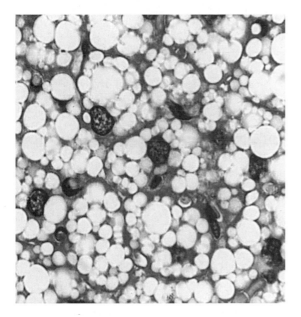

Figure 6–5. Photomicrograph of multilocular adipose tissue with its characteristic cells containing central spherical nuclei and multiple lipid droplets. × 1000.

Histologic Structure

Multilocular tissue cells are polygonal and smaller than cells of unilocular adipose tissue. Their cytoplasm contains a great number of lipid droplets of various sizes (Figures 6–5 and 6–6), a spherical and central nucleus, and numerous mitochondria with abundant long cristae.

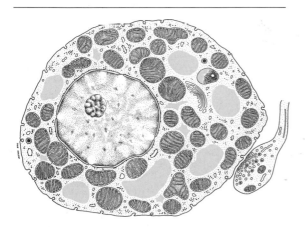

Figure 6–6. Multilocular adipose tissue. Note the central nucleus, multiple fat droplets, and abundant mitochondria. A sympathetic nerve ending is shown at the lower right.

Multilocular adipose tissue resembles an endocrine gland in that its cells assume an almost epithelial arrangement of closely packed masses associated with blood capillaries. This tissue is subdivided by partitions of connective tissue into lobules that are better delineated than are unilocular adipose tissue lobules. Cells of this tissue receive direct sympathetic innervation.

Histophysiology

The physiology of multilocular adipose tissue is best understood in the study of hibernating species.

In animals ending their hibernation period, or in newborn mammals (including humans) who are exposed to a cold environment, nerve impulses liberate norepinephrine into the tissue. This neurotransmitter activates the hormone-sensitive lipase present in adipose cells, promoting hydrolysis of triglycerides to fatty acids and glycerol. Liberated fatty acids are metabolized, with a consequent increase in oxygen consumption and heat production, elevating the temperature of the tissue and warming the blood passing through it. Heat production is increased, because the mitochondria in cells of this tissue have a transmembrane protein called **thermogenin** in their inner membrane. Thermogenin permits the backflow of protons previously transported to the intermembranous space without passing through the ATP-synthetase system in the mitochondrial globular units. Consequently, the energy generated by proton flow is not used to synthesize ATP but is dissipated as heat (Figure 2–10). Warmed blood circulates throughout the body, heating the body and carrying fatty acids not metabolized in the adipose tissue. These fatty acids are used by other organs.

Thermogenin is reduced in quantity in obese animals and increased in animals subjected to low temperatures. Its increase may explain the ability of some individuals to overeat without becoming obese; conversely, its reduction may be related to obesity.

Histogenesis

Multilocular adipose tissue develops differently from unilocular tissue. The mesenchymal cells that constitute this tissue resemble epithelium (thus suggesting an endocrine gland) before they accumulate fat. Apparently, there is no formation of multilocular adipose tissue after birth, and one type of adipose tissue is not transformed into another.

Tumors of Adipose Tissues

Unilocular adipocytes can generate very common benign tumors called **lipomas.** Malignant adipocyte-derived tumors (**liposarcomas**) are among the more common tumors of connective tissue. Tumors of the multilocular adipose cells (**hibernomas**) are relatively rare.

REFERENCES

Angel A et al (editors): *The Adipocyte and Obesity: Cellular and Molecular Mechanisms.* Raven Press, 1983.

Forbes, GB: The companionship of lean and fat. Basic Life Sci 1993;60:1.

Napolitano L: The differentiation of white adipose cells: an electron microscope study. J Cell Biol 1963;8:663.

Nedergaard J, Lindberg O: The brown fat cell. Int Rev Cytol 1982;4:310.

Renold AE, Cahill GF Jr (editors): *Handbook of Physiology.* Section 5: *Adipose Tissue.* American Physiological Society, 1965.

Slavin BG: The cytophysiology of mammalian adipose cells. Int Rev Cytol 1972;3:297.

Cartilage

7

Cartilage is characterized by an extracellular matrix enriched with glycosaminoglycans and proteoglycans, macromolecules that interact with collagen and elastic fibers. Variations in the composition of these matrix components produce three types of cartilage.

Cartilage is a specialized form of connective tissue in which the firm consistency of the extracellular matrix allows the tissue to bear mechanical stresses without permanent distortion. Another function of cartilage is to support soft tissues. Because it is smooth-surfaced and resilient, cartilage is a shock-absorbing and sliding area for joints and facilitates bone movements. Cartilage is also essential for the development and growth of long bones both before and after birth (see Chapter 8).

Cartilage consists of cells (**chondrocytes;** Gr. *chondros,* cartilage, + *kytos,* cell) and an extensive **extracellular matrix** composed of fibers and ground substance. Chondrocytes synthesize and secrete the extracellular matrix, and the cells themselves are located in matrix cavities called **lacunae.** Collagen, hyaluronic acid, proteoglycans, and small amounts of several glycoproteins are the principal macromolecules present in all types of cartilage matrix. Elastic cartilage, characterized by its great pliability, contains significant amounts of the protein elastin in the matrix.

Since collagen and elastin are flexible, the firm gel-like consistency of cartilage depends on electrostatic bonds between collagen fibers and the glycosaminoglycan side chains of matrix proteoglycans. It also depends on the binding of water (solvation water) to the negatively charged glycosaminoglycan chains that extend from the proteoglycan core proteins. The importance of matrix proteoglycans can be observed after intravenous injection of papain in rabbits. Within hours after injection, the cartilages supporting the ears of the rabbits lose their turgidity and the ears droop (Figure 7–1, inset). The loss of turgidity is due to digestion of proteoglycan core proteins and the consequent dissolution of glycosaminoglycan side chains (Figure 7–1).

As a consequence of various functional requirements, three forms of cartilage have evolved, each exhibiting variations in matrix composition. In the matrix of **hyaline cartilage,** the most common form, type II collagen is the principal collagen type. The more pliable and distensible **elastic cartilage** possesses, in addition to collagen type II, an abundance of elastic fibers within its matrix. **Fibrocartilage,** present in regions of the body subjected to pulling forces or the demands of weight bearing, is characterized by a matrix containing a dense network of coarse type I collagen fibers.

In all three forms, cartilage is avascular and is nourished by the diffusion of nutrients from capillaries in adjacent connective tissue (perichondrium) or by synovial fluid from joint cavities. In some instances, blood vessels traverse cartilage to nourish other tissues, but these vessels do not supply nutrients to the cartilage. As might be expected of cells in an avascular tissue, chondrocytes exhibit low metabolic activity. Cartilage has no lymphatic vessels or nerves.

The **perichondrium** (Figures 7–2 and 7–4) is a sheath of dense connective tissue that surrounds cartilage in most places, forming an interface between the cartilage and the tissue supported by the cartilage. The perichondrium harbors the vascular supply for the avascular cartilage and also contains nerves and lymphatic vessels. Articular cartilage, which covers the surfaces of the bones of movable joints, is devoid of perichondrium and is sustained by the diffusion of oxygen and nutrients from the synovial fluid.

HYALINE CARTILAGE

Hyaline cartilage (Figure 7–2) is the most common and best studied of the three forms. Fresh hyaline cartilage is bluish-white and translucent. In the embryo, it serves as a temporary skeleton until it is gradually replaced by bone.

In adult mammals, hyaline cartilage is located in the articular surfaces of the movable joints, in the walls of larger respiratory passages (nose, larynx, trachea, bronchi), in the ventral ends of ribs, where they

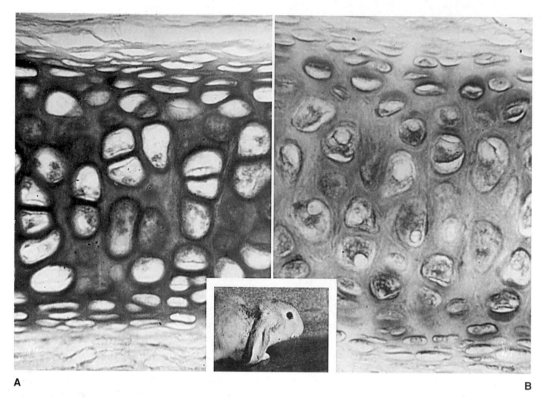

Figure 7–1. Sections of rabbit ear cartilage with its proteoglycan stained by alcian blue. **A:** A control (uninjected) animal. **B:** An animal previously injected intravenously with papain, an enzyme that hydrolyzes the proteoglycan moiety of the cartilage matrix. Note the decrease of proteoglycan content in the cartilage of the injected animal (less intense staining by alcian blue). **Inset:** The collapsed ear of the papain-injected animal. This experiment dramatically illustrates the functional role of proteoglycans in cartilage matrix. × 600.

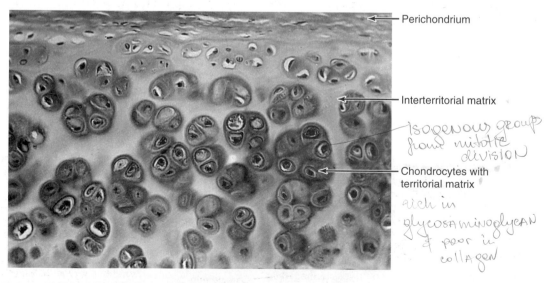

Perichondrium

Interterritorial matrix

isogenous groups from mitotic division

Chondrocytes with territorial matrix

rich in glycosaminoglycan & poor in collagen

Figure 7–2. Photomicrograph of hyaline cartilage. Most chondrocytes are organized in isogenous groups. An enriched concentration of glycosaminoglycans in the matrix—the territorial, or capsular, matrix—is present around the chondrocytes. The upper part of the figure shows the perichondrium. Hematoxylin-and-eosin stain. × 300.

articulate with the sternum, and in the **epiphyseal plate,** where it is responsible for the longitudinal growth of bone (see Chapter 8).

Matrix

Forty percent of the dry weight of hyaline cartilage consists of collagen embedded in a firm, hydrated gel of proteoglycans and structural glycoproteins. In routine histologic preparations, the collagen is indiscernible for two reasons: the collagen is in the form of fibrils, which have submicroscopic dimensions; and the refractive index of the fibrils is almost the same as that of the ground substance in which they are embedded. Although the collagen fibrils in hyaline cartilage have a 64-nm periodicity, the striations are not clearly seen in the electron microscope, because they are masked by the interaction of collagen with the proteoglycans (see Figure 5–10). Hyaline cartilage contains primarily type II collagen.

Cartilage proteoglycans contain chondroitin 4-sulfate, chondroitin 6-sulfate, and keratan sulfate, covalently linked to core proteins. Up to 200 of these proteoglycans are noncovalently associated with long molecules of hyaluronic acid, forming **proteoglycan aggregates** that interact with collagen (Figure 7–3). The aggregates can be up to 4 μm in length. Structurally, proteoglycans resemble bottle brushes, the protein core being the stem and the radiating glycosaminoglycan chains the bristles.

The high content of solvation water bound to the negative charges of glycosaminoglycans acts as a shock absorber or biomechanical spring; this is of great functional importance, especially in articular cartilages (see Chapter 8).

In addition to type II collagen and proteoglycan, an important component of cartilage matrix is the structural glycoprotein **chondronectin,** a macromolecule that binds specifically to glycosaminoglycans

and collagen type II, mediating the adherence of chondrocytes to the extracellular matrix. The cartilage matrix surrounding each chondrocyte is rich in glycosaminoglycan and poor in collagen. This peripheral zone, called the **territorial,** or **capsular,** matrix, histochemically exhibits an intense basophilia, metachromasia, and greater PAS-positivity than does the matrix located between the capsules, the **interterritorial matrix** (Figures 7–2 and 7–4).

Perichondrium →chondroblasts→ chondrocytes

Except in the articular cartilage of joints, all hyaline cartilage is covered by a layer of dense connective tissue, the perichondrium, which is essential for the growth and maintenance of cartilage (Figures 7–2 and 7–4). It is rich in collagen type I fibers and contains numerous fibroblasts. Although cells in the inner layer of the perichondrium resemble fibroblasts, they are chondroblasts and easily differentiate into chondrocytes.

Chondrocytes

At the periphery of hyaline cartilage, young chondrocytes have an elliptic shape, with the long axis parallel to the surface. Farther in, they are round and may appear in groups of up to eight cells originating from mitotic divisions of a single chondrocyte (Figure 7–2). These groups are called **isogenous** (Gr. *isos,* equal, + *genos,* family).

Cartilage cells and the matrix shrink during routine histologic preparation, resulting in both the irregular shape of the chondrocytes and their retraction from the capsule. In living tissue, and in properly prepared sections, the chondrocytes fill the lacunae completely (Figure 7–5).

Chondrocytes synthesize collagen (mainly type II), proteoglycans, hyaluronic acid, and chondronectin. *function of chondrocytes*

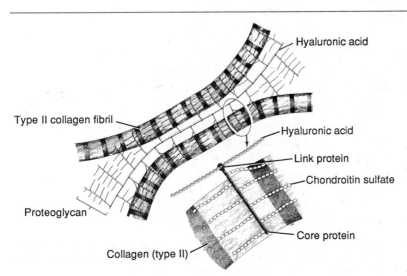

Hyaluronic acid
Type II collagen fibril
Hyaluronic acid
Link protein
Chondroitin sulfate
Proteoglycan
Core protein
Collagen (type II)

Figure 7–3. Schematic representation of molecular organization in cartilage matrix. Link proteins noncovalently bind the protein core (lighter color) of proteoglycans to the linear hyaluronic acid molecules (darker color). The chondroitin sulfate side chains of the proteoglycan electrostatically bind to the collagen fibrils, forming a cross-linked matrix. The oval outlines the area shown larger in the lower part of the figure.

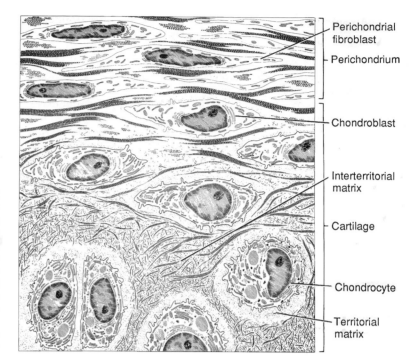

Perichondrial fibroblast

Perichondrium

Chondroblast

Interterritorial matrix

Cartilage

Chondrocyte

Territorial matrix

Figure 7–4. Diagram of the area of transition between the perichondrium and the hyaline cartilage. As perichondrial cells differentiate into chondrocytes, they become round, with an irregular surface. Cartilage (interterritorial) matrix contains numerous fine collagen fibrils except around the periphery of the chondrocytes, where the matrix consists primarily of glycosaminoglycans; this peripheral region is called the territorial, or capsular, matrix.

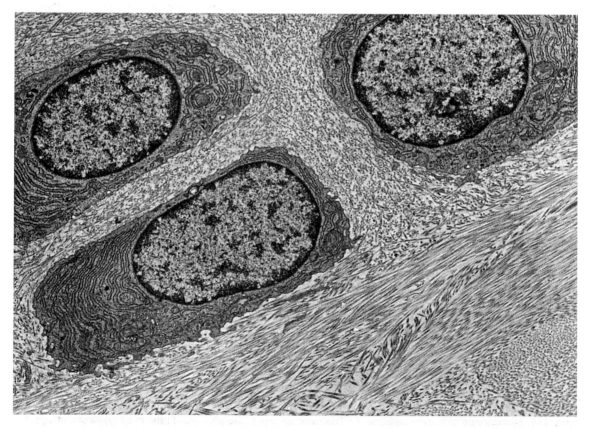

Figure 7–5. Electron micrograph of fibrocartilage, showing three chondrocytes in their lacunae. Note the abundance of rough endoplasmic reticulum. Chondrocytes synthesize the cartilage matrix. Fine collagen fibers, sectioned in several places, are prominent around the chondrocytes. × 3750.

Histophysiology

Because cartilage is devoid of blood capillaries, chondrocytes respire under low oxygen tension. Hyaline cartilage cells metabolize glucose mainly by anaerobic glycolysis to produce lactic acid as the end product. Nutrients from the blood cross the perichondrium to reach more deeply placed cartilage cells. Mechanisms include diffusion and transport of water and solute promoted by the pumping action of intermittent cartilage compression and decompression. Because of this, the maximum width of the cartilage is limited. The nutrients diffuse through the solvation water of the matrix.

Chondrocyte function depends on a proper hormonal balance. The synthesis of sulfated glycosaminoglycans is accelerated by growth hormone, thyroxine, and testosterone and is slowed by cortisone, hydrocortisone, and estradiol. Cartilage growth depends mainly on the hypophyseal growth hormone **somatotropin.** This hormone does not act directly on cartilage cells but promotes the synthesis of **somatomedin C** in the liver. Somatomedin C acts directly on cartilage cells, promoting their growth.

Cartilage cells can give rise to benign (**chondroma**) or malignant (**chondrosarcoma**) tumors.

Histogenesis

Cartilage derives from the mesenchyme (Figure 7–6). The first modification observed is the rounding up of the mesenchymal cells, which retract their extensions, multiply rapidly, and form mesenchymal condensations. The cells formed by this direct differentiation of mesenchymal cells, now called **chondroblasts,** have a ribosome-rich basophilic cytoplasm. Synthesis and deposition of the matrix then begin to separate the chondroblasts from one another. The differentiation of cartilage takes place from the center outward; therefore, the more central cells have the characteristics of chondrocytes, whereas the peripheral cells are typical chondroblasts. The superficial mesenchyme develops into chondroblasts and fibroblasts of the perichondrium.

Growth

The growth of cartilage is attributable to two processes: **interstitial growth,** resulting from the mitotic division of preexisting chondrocytes; and **appositional growth,** resulting from the differentiation of perichondrial cells. In both cases, newly formed chondrocytes synthesize collagen fibrils and ground substance. Real growth is thus much greater than that from the simple increase in the number of cells. Interstitial growth is the less important of the two

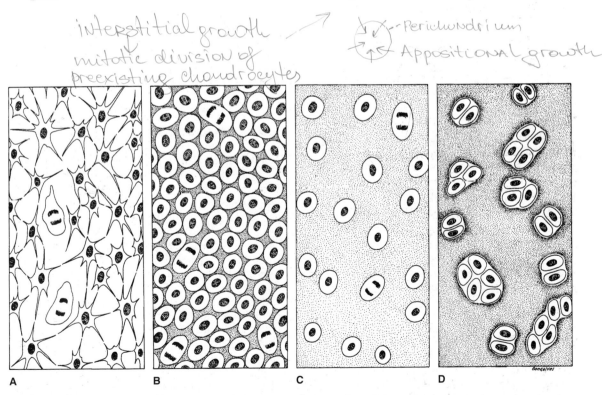

Figure 7–6. Histogenesis of hyaline cartilage. **A:** The mesenchyme is the precursor tissue of all types of cartilage. **B:** Mitotic proliferation of mesenchymal cells gives rise to a highly cellular tissue. **C:** Chondroblasts are separated from one another by the formation of a great amount of matrix. **D:** Multiplication of cartilage cells gives rise to isogenous groups, each surrounded by a condensation of territorial (capsular) matrix.

processes. It occurs only during the early phases of cartilage formation, when it increases tissue mass by expanding the cartilage matrix from within. Interstitial growth also occurs in the epiphyseal plates of long bones and within articular cartilage. In the epiphyseal plates, interstitial growth is important in increasing the length of long bones and in providing a cartilage model for endochondral bone formation (see Chapter 8). In articular cartilage, as the cells and matrix near the articulating surface are gradually worn away, the cartilage must be replaced from within, since there is no perichondrium there to add cells by apposition. In cartilage found elsewhere in the body, interstitial growth becomes less pronounced as the matrix becomes increasingly rigid from the cross-linking of matrix molecules. Cartilage then grows in girth only by apposition. Chondroblasts of the perichondrium proliferate and become chondrocytes once they have surrounded themselves with cartilaginous matrix and are incorporated into the existing cartilage (Figures 7–2 and 7–4).

Degenerative Changes

In contrast to other tissues, hyaline cartilage is more susceptible to degenerative aging processes. Calcification of the matrix, preceded by an increase in the size and volume of the chondrocytes and followed by their death, is a common process in some cartilage, providing a model for bone development (see Endochondral Ossification, Chapter 8). Asbestiform degeneration, frequent in aged cartilage, is due to the formation of localized aggregates of thick, abnormal collagen fibrils.

Regeneration

Except in young children, damaged cartilage regenerates with difficulty and often incompletely, by activity of the perichondrium, which invades the injured area and generates new cartilage. In extensively damaged areas—and occasionally in small areas—the perichondrium produces a scar of dense connective tissue instead of forming new cartilage.

ELASTIC CARTILAGE

Elastic cartilage is found in the auricle of the ear, the walls of the external auditory canals, the auditory (eustachian) tubes, the epiglottis, and the cuneiform cartilage in the larynx.

Elastic cartilage is essentially identical to hyaline cartilage except that it contains an abundant network of fine elastic fibers in addition to collagen type II fibrils. Fresh elastic cartilage has a yellowish color due to the presence of elastin in the elastic fibers, which can be demonstrated by standard elastin stains, eg, orcein (Figure 7–7).

The chondrocytes of elastic and hyaline cartilage tissues are similar, and elastic cartilage is frequently

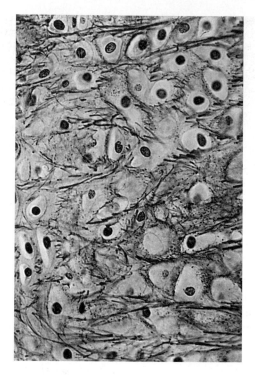

Figure 7–7. Photomicrograph of elastic cartilage, stained for elastic fibers. × 350.

found to be gradually continuous with hyaline cartilage. Like hyaline cartilage, elastic cartilage possesses a perichondrium.

FIBROCARTILAGE

Fibrocartilage is a tissue intermediate between dense connective tissue and hyaline cartilage. It is found in intervertebral disks, in attachments of certain ligaments to the cartilaginous surface of bones, and in the symphysis pubis. Fibrocartilage is always associated with dense connective tissue, and the border areas between these two tissues are not clear-cut, showing a gradual transition.

Fibrocartilage contains chondrocytes similar to those of hyaline cartilage, either singly or in isogenous groups. The chondrocytes are very often arranged in long rows (Figure 7–8). The fibrocartilage matrix is acidophilic, because it contains a great number of coarse type I collagen fibers, which are easily seen under the microscope.

In fibrocartilage, the numerous collagen fibers either form irregular bundles between the groups of chondrocytes or are aligned in a parallel arrangement along the columns of chondrocytes (Figure 7–8). This orientation depends on the stresses acting on fibrocartilage, since the collagen bundles take up a di-

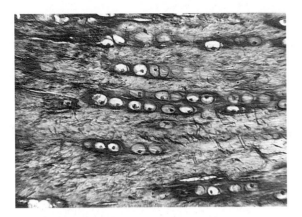

Figure 7–8. Photomicrograph of fibrocartilage. Note the rows of chondrocytes separated by collagen fibers. Picrosirius-hematoxylin stain. × 500.

rection parallel to those stresses. There is no identifiable perichondrium in fibrocartilage.

INTERVERTEBRAL DISKS

Each intervertebral disk is situated between two vertebrae and held to them by means of ligaments. The disks have two components: the cartilaginous annulus fibrosus and the liquid nucleus pulposus. The intervertebral disk acts as a lubricated cushion that prevents adjacent vertebrae from being eroded by abrasive forces during movement of the spinal column. The nucleus pulposus serves as a shock absorber to cushion the impact between vertebrae.

The **annulus fibrosus** has an external layer of dense connective tissue, but it is mainly composed of overlapping laminae of fibrocartilage in which collagen bundles are orthogonally arranged in adjacent layers. The multiple lamellae, with the 90-degree registration of type I collagen fibers in adjacent layers, provide the disk with unusual resilience that enables it to withstand the pressures generated by impinging vertebrae. In tangential section, the disk presents a characteristic herringbone pattern as a result of the orthogonal alignment of collagen in alternating lamellae.

The **nucleus pulposus** is situated in the center of the annulus fibrosus. It is derived from the notochord and consists of a few rounded cells embedded in a viscous matrix rich in hyaluronic acid and type II collagen fibrils. In children, the nucleus pulposus is large, but it gradually becomes smaller with age and is partially replaced by fibrocartilage.

Herniation of the Intervertebral Disk

Rupture of the annulus fibrosus, which most frequently occurs in the posterior region where there are fewer collagen bundles, results in expulsion of the liquid nucleus pulposus and a concomitant flattening of the disk. As a consequence, the disk frequently dislocates or slips from its position between the vertebrae. If it moves toward the spinal cord, it can compress the nerves and result in severe pain and neurologic disturbances. The pain accompanying a slipped disk may be perceived in areas innervated by the compressed nerve fibers—usually the lower lumbar region.

REFERENCES

Anderson DR: The ultrastructure of elastic and hyaline cartilage in the rat. Am J Anat 1964;14:403.

Chakrabarti B, Park JW: Glycosaminoglycans: structure and interaction. CRC Crit Rev Biochem 1980;8:225.

Eyre DR, Muir H: The distribution of different molecular species of collagen in fibrous, elastic and hyaline cartilages of the pig. Biochem J 1975;51:595.

Hall BK (editor): *Cartilage,* Vol 1: *Structure, Function, and Biochemistry.* Academic Press, 1983.

Jasin, HE: Structure and function of the articular cartilage surface. Scand J Rheumatol 1995;101:51.

Junqueira LCU et al: Quantitation of collagen-proteoglycan interaction in tissue sections. Connect Tissue Res 1980;7:91.

Reddy AH (editor): *Extracellular Matrix Structure and Functions.* Liss, 1985.

Stockwell RA: *Biology of Cartilage Cells.* Cambridge Univ Press, 1979.

Thomas L: Reversible collapse of rabbit ears after intravenous papain, and prevention of recovery by cortisone. J Exp Med 1956;104:245.

Zambrano NZ et al: Collagen arrangement in cartilages. Acta Anat 1982;113:26.

Bone

As the main constituent of the adult skeleton, bone tissue supports fleshy structures, protects such vital organs as those in the cranial and thoracic cavities, and harbors the bone marrow, where blood cells are formed. Bone also serves as a reservoir of calcium, phosphate, and other ions that can be released or stored in a controlled fashion to maintain constant concentrations of these important ions in body fluids.

In addition to these functions, bones form a system of levers that multiply the forces generated during skeletal muscle contraction and transform them into bodily movements.

Bone is a specialized connective tissue composed of intercellular calcified material, the **bone matrix,** and three cell types: **osteocytes** (Gr. *osteon,* bone, + *kytos,* cell), which are found in cavities (**lacunae**) within the matrix (Figure 8–1); **osteoblasts** (*osteon* + Gr. *blastos,* germ), which synthesize the organic components of the matrix; and **osteoclasts** (*osteon* + Gr. *klastos,* broken), which are multinucleated giant cells involved in the resorption and remodeling of bone tissue.

Since metabolites are unable to diffuse through the calcified matrix of bone, the exchanges between osteocytes and blood capillaries depend on communication through the **canaliculi** (L. *canalis,* canal), thin, cylindrical spaces that perforate the matrix (Figure 8–2).

All bones are lined on both internal and external surfaces by layers of tissue containing osteogenic cells—**endosteum** on the internal surface and **periosteum** on the external surface.

Because of its hardness, bone is difficult to section with the microtome, and special techniques must be used for its study. A common technique that permits the observation of the cells and organic matrix is based on the decalcification of bone preserved by standard fixatives. The mineral is removed by immersion in a solution containing a calcium-chelating substance (eg, ethylenediaminetetraacetic acid [EDTA]). The decalcified tissue is then embedded, sectioned, and stained.

BONE CELLS

Osteoblasts

Osteoblasts are responsible for the synthesis of the organic components of bone matrix (type I collagen, proteoglycans, and glycoproteins). Deposition of the inorganic components of bone also depends on the presence of viable osteoblasts. Osteoblasts are exclusively located at the surfaces of bone tissue, side by side, in a way that resembles simple epithelium (Figure 8–3). When they are actively engaged in matrix synthesis, osteoblasts have a cuboidal to columnar shape and basophilic cytoplasm. When their synthesizing activity declines, they flatten, and cytoplasmic basophilia declines.

Some osteoblasts are gradually surrounded by newly formed matrix and become **osteocytes.** During this process a space called a **lacuna** is formed. Lacunae are occupied by osteocytes and their extensions, along with a small amount of extracellular noncalcified matrix.

During matrix synthesis, osteoblasts have the ultrastructure of cells actively synthesizing proteins for export. Osteoblasts are polarized cells. Matrix components are secreted at the cell surface, which is in contact with older bone matrix, producing a layer of new (but not yet calcified) matrix, called **osteoid,** between the osteoblast layer and the previously formed bone. This process, **bone apposition,** is completed by subsequent deposition of calcium salts into the newly formed matrix.

The fluorescent antibiotic tetracycline interacts with great affinity with recently deposited mineralized bone matrix. Based on this interaction, a method was developed to measure the rate of bone apposition—an important parameter in the study of bone growth and the diagnosis of bone growth diseases. Tetracycline is administered twice to patients, with an interval of 5 days between injections. A bone biopsy is then performed, and the sections are studied by means

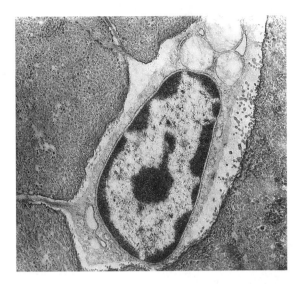

Figure 8–1. Section of the bone showing an osteocyte with its cytoplasmic processes surrounded by matrix. Ultrastructure compatible with a low level of synthetic activity is apparent in both nucleus and cytoplasm.

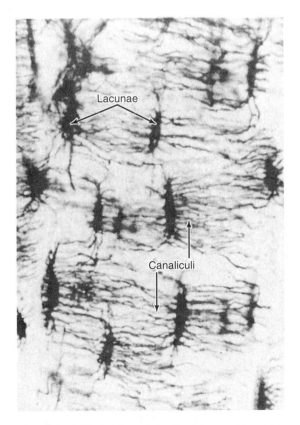

Figure 8–2. Photomicrograph of a bone section. Lacunae and canaliculi appear black. × 900.

of fluorescence microscopy. The distance between the two fluorescent layers is proportional to the rate of bone apposition. This procedure is of diagnostic importance in such diseases as **osteomalacia,** in which mineralization is impaired, and **osteitis fibrosa cystica,** in which increased osteoclast activity results in removal of bone matrix and fibrous degeneration.

Osteocytes

Osteocytes, which derive from osteoblasts, lie in the lacunae situated between lamellae (L. diminutive of *lamina,* leaf) of matrix. Only one osteocyte is found in each lacuna. The thin, cylindrical matrix canaliculi house cytoplasmic processes of osteocytes. Processes of adjacent cells make contact via gap junctions, and molecules are passed via these structures from cell to cell. Some molecular exchange between osteocytes and blood vessels also takes place through the small amount of extracellular substance located between osteocytes (and their processes) and the bone matrix. This exchange can provide nourishment for a chain of about 15 cells.

When compared with osteoblasts, the flat, almond-shaped osteocytes exhibit a significantly reduced rough endoplasmic reticulum (see Figure 8–1) and Golgi complex and more condensed nuclear chromatin. These cells are actively involved in the maintenance of the bony matrix, and their death is followed by resorption of this matrix.

Osteoclasts

Osteoclasts are very large, branched motile cells. Dilated portions of the cell body (Figure 8–4) contain from 5 to 50 (or more) nuclei. In areas of bone undergoing resorption, osteoclasts lie within enzymatically etched depressions in the matrix known as **Howship's lacunae.** Osteoclasts are derived from the fusion of bone marrow-derived cells, and belong to the mononuclear phagocyte system (see Chapter 5).

In active osteoclasts, the surface-facing bone matrix is folded into irregular, often subdivided projections, forming a **ruffled border.** Surrounding the ruffled border is a cytoplasmic zone—the **clear zone**—that is devoid of organelles, yet rich in actin microfilaments. This zone is a site of adhesion of the osteoclast to the bone matrix and creates a microenvironment in which bone resorption occurs (Figure 8–5).

The osteoclast secretes collagenase and other enzymes and pumps protons into a subcellular pocket (the microenvironment referred to above), promoting the localized digestion of collagen and dissolving calcium salt crystals. Osteoclast activity is controlled by cytokines (small signaling proteins that act as local mediators) and hormones. Osteoclasts have receptors for calcitonin, a thyroid hormone, but not for parathyroid hormone. However, osteoblasts have receptors for parathyroid hormone and, when activated

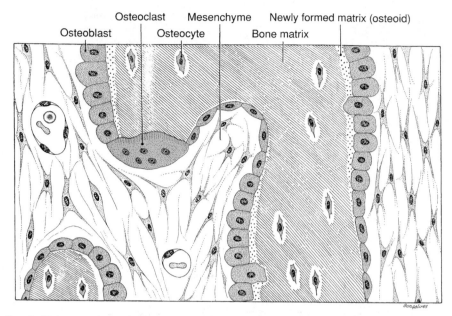

Figure 8–3. Events that occur during intramembranous ossification. Osteoblasts (lighter color) are synthesizing collagen, which forms a strand of matrix that traps cells. As this occurs, the osteoblasts gradually differentiate to become osteocytes. The lower part of the drawing shows an osteoblast being trapped in newly formed bone matrix.

by this hormone, produce a cytokine called osteoclast stimulating factor.

> Ruffled borders are related to the activity of osteoclasts. In the genetic disease **osteopetrosis,** which is characterized by dense, heavy bones ("marble bones"), the osteoclasts lack ruffled borders, and bone resorption is defective.

BONE MATRIX

Inorganic matter represents about 50% of the dry weight of bone matrix. Calcium and phosphorus are especially abundant, but bicarbonate, citrate, magnesium, potassium, and sodium are also found. X-ray diffraction studies have shown that calcium and phosphorus form hydroxyapatite crystals with the

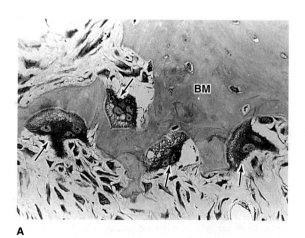

A

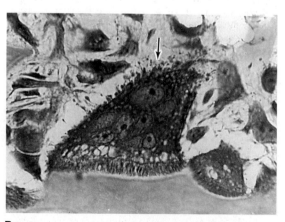

B

Figure 8–4. **A:** Photomicrograph of a bone section showing four osteoclasts (arrows). Note the ruffled borders close to the bone matrix (BM). × 600. **B:** Higher magnification of osteoclast (arrow) showing in detail the ruffled border and the erosion of bone matrix closed to it. Note the size of the osteoclast and the presence of several nuclei. × 1200.

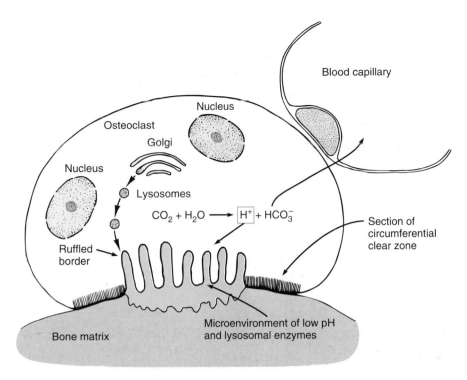

Blood capillary

Osteoclast

Nucleus

Golgi

Nucleus

Lysosomes

$CO_2 + H_2O \longrightarrow \boxed{H^+} + HCO_3^-$

Ruffled
border

Section of
circumferential
clear zone

Microenvironment of low pH
and lysosomal enzymes

Bone matrix

Figure 8–5. Bone resorption. Lysosomal enzymes packaged in the Golgi complex and hydrogen ions produced are released into the confined microenvironment created by the attachment between bone matrix and the osteoclast's peripheral clear zone. The acidification of this confined space facilitates the dissolution of calcium phosphate from bone and is the optimal pH for the activity of lysosomal hydrolases. Bone matrix is thus removed and the products of bone resorption are taken up by the osteoclast's cytoplasm, probably digested further, and transferred to blood capillaries.

composition $Ca_{10}(PO_4)_6(OH)_2$. Significant quantities of amorphous (noncrystalline) calcium phosphate are also present. In electron micrographs, hydroxyapatite crystals of bone appear as plates that lie alongside the collagen fibrils but are surrounded by ground substance. The surface ions of hydroxyapatite are hydrated, and a layer of water and ions forms around the crystal. This layer, the **hydration shell,** facilitates the exchange of ions between the crystal and the body fluids.

The organic matter in bone matrix is type I collagen and ground substance, which contains proteoglycan aggregates and several specific structural glycoproteins. Some of the glycoproteins are produced by osteoblasts and demonstrate affinity for both hydroxyapatite and the cell membrane; they might be involved in binding osteoblasts or osteoclasts to bone matrix. Bone glycoproteins may also be responsible for promoting calcification of bone matrix. Other tissues containing type I collagen are not normally calcified and do not contain these glycoproteins. Because of its high collagen content, decalcified bone matrix intensely binds stains for collagen fibers.

The association of hydroxyapatite with collagen fibers is responsible for the hardness and resistance of bone tissue. After a bone is decalcified, its shape

is preserved, but it becomes as flexible as a tendon. Removal of the organic part of the matrix—which is mainly collagenous—also leaves the bone with its original shape; however, it becomes fragile, breaking and crumbling easily when handled.

PERIOSTEUM & ENDOSTEUM

External and internal surfaces of bone are covered by layers of bone-forming cells and connective tissue called periosteum and endosteum.

The **periosteum** consists of an outer layer of collagen fibers and fibroblasts (Figure 8–6). Bundles of periosteal collagen fibers, called **Sharpey's fibers,** penetrate the bone matrix, binding the periosteum to bone. The inner, more cellular layer of the periosteum is composed of fibroblast-like cells called **osteoprogenitor cells,** with the potential to divide by mitosis and differentiate into osteoblasts. Autoradiographic studies demonstrate that these cells take up ^{3}H-thymidine, which is subsequently encountered in osteoblasts. Osteoprogenitor cells play a prominent role in bone growth and repair.

The **endosteum** (Figure 8–6) lines all internal cavities within the bone and is composed of a single

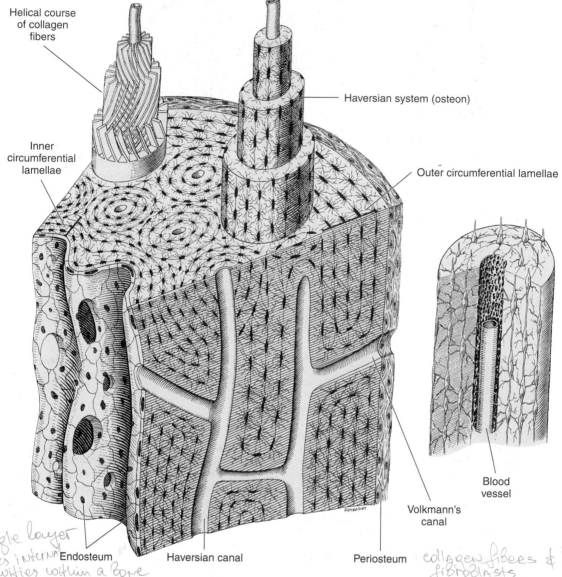

Helical course
of collagen
fibers

Inner
circumferential
lamellae

Haversian system (osteon)

Outer circumferential lamellae

Blood
vessel

Volkmann's
canal

single layer
lines internal
cavities within a bone
Endosteum   Haversian canal   Periosteum
collagen fibres &
fibroblasts

Figure 8–6. Schematic drawing of the wall of a long-bone diaphysis showing three types of lamellar bone: haversian system and outer and inner circumferential lamellae. (For interstitial lamellae, see Figure 8–10.) The protruding haversian system on the left shows the orientation of collagen fibers in each lamella. At the right is a haversian system showing lamellae, a central blood capillary, and many osteocytes with their processes.

layer of flattened osteoprogenitor cells and a very small amount of connective tissue. The endosteum is therefore considerably thinner than the periosteum.

The principal functions of periosteum and endosteum are nutrition of osseous tissue and provision of a continuous supply of new osteoblasts for repair or growth of bone.

TYPES OF BONE

Gross observation of bone in cross section shows dense areas without cavities—corresponding to **compact bone**—and areas with numerous interconnecting cavities—corresponding to **cancellous (spongy) bone** (Figure 8–7). Under the microscope, however,

periosteum > provide nutrition of
endosteum > osseous tissue and
provision of a continuous supply of new osteoblasts
for repair & growth of bone

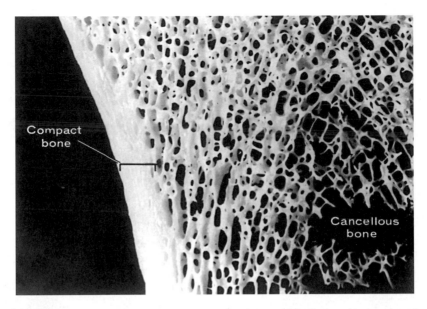

Figure 8–7. Thick section of bone illustrating the cortical compact bone and the lattice of trabeculae of cancellous bone. (Courtesy of DW Fawcett.)

both compact bone and the trabeculae separating the cavities of cancellous bone have the same basic histologic structure.

In long bones, the bulbous ends—called **epiphyses** (Gr. *epiphysis,* an excrescence)—are composed of spongy bone covered by a thin layer of compact bone. The cylindrical part—**diaphysis** (Gr. *diaphysis,* a growing between)—is almost totally composed of compact bone, with a small component of spongy bone on its inner surface around the bone marrow cavity (see Figure 8–13). Short bones usually have a core of spongy bone completely surrounded by compact bone. The flat bones that form the calvaria have two layers of compact bone called **plates** (tables), separated by a layer of spongy bone called the **diploë.**

Microscopic examination of bone shows two varieties: **primary, immature,** or **woven bone** and **secondary, mature,** or **lamellar bone.** Primary bone is the first bone tissue to appear in embryonic development and in fracture repair and other repair processes. It is characterized by random disposition of fine collagen fibers, in contrast to the organized lamellar disposition of collagen in secondary bone.

Primary Bone Tissue

Primary bone tissue is usually temporary and is replaced in adults by secondary bone tissue except in a very few places in the body, eg, near the sutures of the flat bones of the skull, in tooth sockets, and in the insertions of some tendons.

In addition to the irregular array of collagen fibers,

other characteristics of primary bone tissue are a lower mineral content (it is more easily penetrated by x-rays) and a higher proportion of osteocytes than that in secondary bone tissue.

Secondary Bone Tissue

Secondary bone tissue is the variety usually found in adults. It characteristically shows collagen fibers arranged in lamellae (3–7 μm thick) that are parallel to each other or concentrically organized around a vascular canal. The whole complex of concentric lamellae of bone surrounding a canal containing blood vessels, nerves, and loose connective tissue is called a **haversian system,** or **osteon** (Figures 8–6 and 8–8). Lacunae containing osteocytes are found between and occasionally within the lamellae. In each lamella, collagen fibers are parallel to each other. Surrounding each haversian system is a deposit of amorphous material called the **cementing substance** that consists of mineralized matrix with few collagen fibers.

In compact bone (eg, the diaphysis of long bones), the lamellae exhibit a typical organization consisting of **haversian systems, outer circumferential lamellae, inner circumferential lamellae,** and **interstitial lamellae** (Figures 8–6 and 8–9).

Inner circumferential lamellae are located around the marrow cavity, and outer circumferential lamellae are located immediately beneath the periosteum. There are more outer than inner lamellae.

Between the two circumferential systems are numerous haversian systems, including triangular or ir-

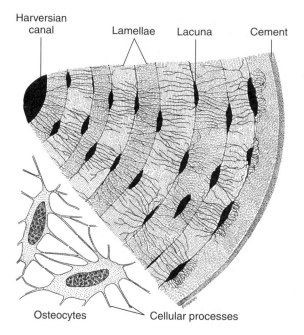

Harversian canal   Lamellae   Lacuna   Cement

Osteocytes   Cellular processes

Figure 8–8. Schematic drawing of two osteocytes and part of a haversian system. Collagen fibers of contiguous lamellae are sectioned at different angles. Note the numerous canaliculi that permit communication between lacunae and with the haversian canals. Although it is not apparent in this simplified diagram, each lamella consists of multiple lamellae in which the parallel arrays of collagen fibers in adjacent lamellae are oriented in different directions. The presence of large numbers of lamellae with differing fiber orientations provides the bone with great strength, despite its light weight. (Redrawn and reproduced, with permission, from Leeson TS, Leeson CR: *Histology,* 2nd ed. Saunders, 1970.)

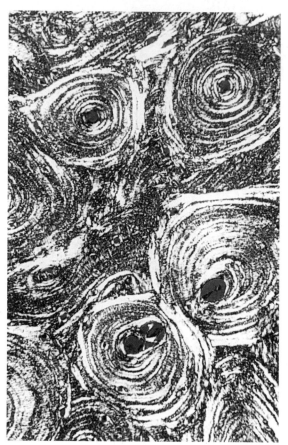

Figure 8–9. Transverse section of decalcified diaphysis; polarized light micrograph showing the alternating light and dark bands of the haversian system. This alternating birefringence is due to the presence of collagen fibers disposed in different orientations in contiguous lamellae. Note the interstitial lamellae and haversian systems. × 50.

regularly shaped groups of parallel lamellae called **interstitial** (or **intermediate**) **lamellae.** These structures are lamellae left by haversian systems destroyed during growth and remodeling of bone (Figure 8–10).

Each haversian system is a long, often bifurcated cylinder parallel to the long axis of the diaphysis. It consists of a central canal surrounded by 4–20 concentric lamellae. Each endosteum-lined canal contains blood vessels, nerves, and loose connective tissue. The haversian canals communicate with the marrow cavity, the periosteum, and one another through transverse or oblique Volkmann's canals (Figure 8–6). Volkmann's canals do not have concentric lamellae; instead, they perforate the lamellae. All vascular canals found in bone tissue come into existence when matrix is laid down around preexisting blood vessels.

Examination of haversian systems with polarized light shows bright anisotropic layers alternating with dark isotropic layers (Figure 8–9). When observed under polarized light at right angles to their length, collagen fibers are birefringent (anisotropic). The alternating bright and dark layers are due to the changing orientation of collagen fibers in the lamellae. In each lamella, fibers are parallel to each other and follow a helical course. The pitch of the helix is, however, different for different lamellae, so that at any given point, fibers from adjacent lamellae intersect at approximately right angles (Figure 8–6).

There is great variability in the diameter of haversian canals. Each system is formed by successive deposits of lamellae, starting inward from the periphery, so that younger systems have larger canals. In mature haversian systems, the most recently formed lamella is the one closest to the central canal.

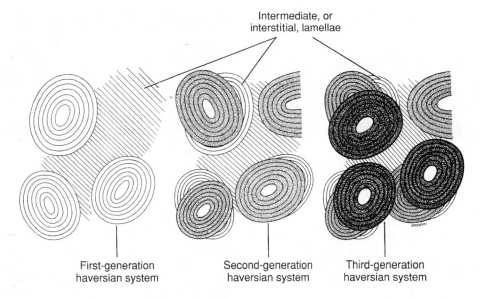

Figure 8–10. Schematic drawing of diaphyseal bone remodeling showing three generations of haversian systems and their successive contributions to the formation of intermediate, or interstitial, lamellae. Remodeling is a continuous process responsible for bone adaptations, especially during growth.

HISTOGENESIS

Bone can be formed in two ways: by direct mineralization of matrix secreted by osteoblasts (*intramembranous ossification*) or by deposition of bone matrix on a preexisting cartilage matrix (*endochondral ossification*).

In both processes, the bone tissue that appears first is primary, or woven. Primary bone is a temporary tissue and is soon replaced by the definitive lamellar, or secondary, bone. During bone growth, areas of primary bone, areas of resorption, and areas of secondary bone appear side by side. This combination of bone synthesis and removal (**remodeling**) occurs not only in growing bones but also throughout adult life, although its rate of change in adults is considerably slower.

Intramembranous Ossification

Intramembranous ossification, the source of most of the flat bones, is so called because it takes place within condensations of mesenchymal tissue. The frontal and parietal bones of the skull—as well as parts of the occipital and temporal bones and the mandible and maxilla—are formed by intramembranous ossification. This process also contributes to the growth of short bones and the thickening of long bones.

In the mesenchymal condensation layer, the starting point for ossification is called a **primary ossification center.** The process begins when groups of cells differentiate into osteoblasts. Osteoblasts pro-

duce bone matrix and calcification follows, resulting in the encapsulation of some osteoblasts, which then become osteocytes (Figures 8–11 and 8–12). These islands of developing bone form walls that delineate elongated cavities containing capillaries, bone marrow cells, and undifferentiated cells. Several such groups arise almost simultaneously at the ossification center, so that the fusion of the walls gives the bone a spongy structure. The connective tissue that remains among the bone walls is penetrated by growing blood vessels and additional undifferentiated mesenchymal cells, giving rise to the bone marrow cells.

The ossification centers of a bone grow radially and finally fuse together, replacing the original connective tissue. The fontanelles of newborn infants, for example, are soft areas in the skull that correspond to parts of the connective tissue that are not yet ossified.

In cranial flat bones there is a marked predominance of bone formation over bone resorption at both the internal and external surfaces. Thus, two layers of compact bone (internal and external plates) arise, whereas the central portion (diploë) maintains its spongy nature.

The portion of the connective tissue layer that does not undergo ossification gives rise to the endosteum and the periosteum of intramembranous bone.

Endochondral Ossification

Endochondral (Gr. *endon,* within, + *chondros,* cartilage) ossification takes place within a piece of hyaline cartilage whose shape resembles a small version,

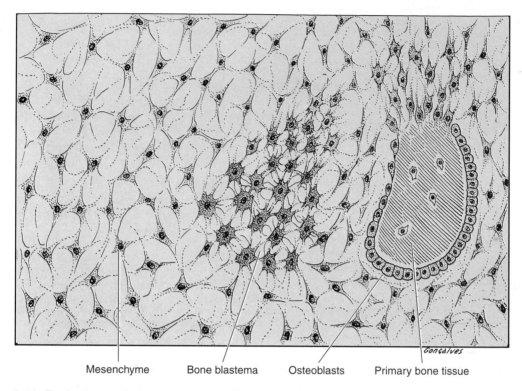

Mesenchyme   Bone blastema   Osteoblasts   Primary bone tissue

Figure 8–11. The beginning of intramembranous ossification. Mesenchymal cells round up and form a blastema, from which osteoblasts differentiate, producing primary bone tissue.

or model, of the bone to be formed. This type of ossification is principally responsible for the formation of short and long bones (Figures 8–13 and 8–14).

Endochondral ossification of a long bone consists of the following sequence of events. Initially, the first bone tissue appears as a hollow bone cylinder that surrounds the mid portion of the cartilage model. This structure, the **bone collar,** is produced by intramembranous ossification within the local perichondrium. In the next step, the local cartilage undergoes a degenerative process characterized by cell enlargement (hypertrophy), matrix calcification, and cell death, resulting in a three-dimensional structure formed by the remnants of the calcified cartilage matrix (Figure 8–15). This process begins at the central portion of the cartilage model (diaphysis), where blood vessels penetrate through the bone collar previously perforated by osteoclasts, bringing osteoprogenitor cells to this region. Next, osteoblasts adhere to the calcified cartilage matrix and produce continuous layers of primary bone that surround the cartilaginous matrix remnants. At this stage, the calcified cartilage appears basophilic, and the primary bone is eosinophilic. In this way the **primary ossification center** is produced (Figure 8–13). Then, **secondary ossification centers** appear at the swellings in the extremities of the cartilage model (epiphyses). During their expansion and remodeling, the primary and

secondary ossification centers produce cavities that are gradually filled with bone marrow.

In the secondary ossification centers, cartilage remains in two regions: the **articular cartilage,** which persists throughout adult life and does not contribute to bone growth in length, and the **epiphyseal cartilage,** also called **epiphyseal plate,** which connects the two epiphyses to the diaphysis (Figures 8–15 and 8–16). The epiphyseal cartilage is responsible for the growth in length of the bone, and it disappears in adults, which is why bone growth ceases in adulthood.

The closure of the epiphyses follows a chronologic order according to each bone and is complete at about 20 years of age. Through x-ray examination of the growing skeleton, it is possible to determine the "bone age" of a young person, noting which epiphyses are open and which are closed. Once the epiphyses have closed, growth in length of bones becomes impossible, although widening may still occur.

Epiphyseal cartilage is divided into five zones (Figure 8–16), starting from the epiphyseal side of cartilage: (1) The **resting zone** consists of hyaline cartilage without morphologic changes in the cells. (2) In the **proliferative zone,** chondrocytes divide rapidly and form columns of stacked cells parallel to the long axis of the bone. (3) The **hypertrophic cartilage zone** contains large chondrocytes whose cyto-

Layer of osteoblasts   Bone tissue   Layer of osteoblasts   Blood vessel

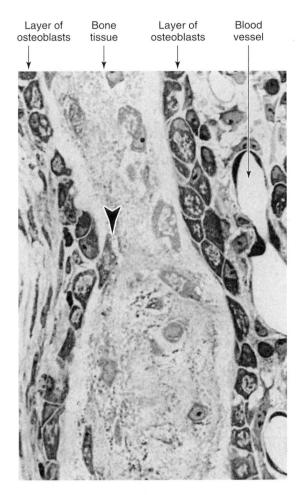

Figure 8–12. Photomicrograph of intramembranous ossification from the head of a young rat. The newly formed, growing bone is enclosed by a layer of darkly stained (basophilic) osteoblasts. The bone, which appears more lightly colored, shows young osteocytes recently enclosed by the forming matrix. The arrowhead shows one osteoblast trapped by the matrix synthesized by these cells.

plasm has accumulated glycogen. The resorbed matrix is reduced to thin septa between the chondrocytes. (4) Simultaneous with the death of chondrocytes in the **calcified cartilage zone,** the thin septa of cartilage matrix become calcified by the deposit of hydroxyapatite (Figures 8–15 and 8–16). (5) In the **ossification zone,** endochondral bone tissue appears. Blood capillaries and osteoprogenitor cells formed by mitosis of cells originating from the periosteum invade the cavities left by the chondrocytes. The osteoprogenitor cells form osteoblasts, which are distributed in a discontinuous layer over the septa of calcified cartilage matrix. Ultimately, the osteoblasts deposit bone matrix over the three-dimensional calcified cartilage matrix (Figures 8–14 and 8–15).

In summary, growth in length of a long bone oc-

curs by proliferation of chondrocytes in the epiphyseal plate adjacent to the epiphysis. At the same time, chondrocytes of the diaphyseal side of the plate hypertrophy; their matrix becomes calcified, and the cells die. Osteoblasts lay down a layer of primary bone on the calcified cartilage matrix. Because the rates of these two opposing events (proliferation and destruction) are approximately equal, the epiphyseal plate does not change thickness. Instead, it is displaced away from the middle of the diaphysis, resulting in growth in length of the bone.

Mechanisms of Calcification

No hypothesis to explain the events occurring during calcium phosphate deposition on bone matrix is yet generally accepted.

It is known that calcification begins by the deposition of calcium salts on collagen fibrils, a process induced by proteoglycans and high-affinity calcium-binding glycoproteins. The deposition of calcium salts is probably accelerated by the ability of osteoblasts to concentrate them in intracytoplasmic vesicles and to release, when necessary, their contents to the extracellular medium.

Calcification is aided, in some unknown way, by alkaline phosphatase, which is produced by osteoblasts and is present at ossification sites.

BONE GROWTH & REMODELING

Bone growth is generally associated with partial resorption of preformed tissue and the simultaneous laying down of new bone (exceeding the rate of bone loss). This process permits the shape of the bone to be maintained while it grows. The rate of bone remodeling (**bone turnover**) is very active in young children, where it can be 200 times faster than that in adults. Bone remodeling is related to several factors: strain and stress imposed by muscular contraction and body movements; pregnancy; hormones; and growth factors.

Cranial bones grow mainly because of the formation of bone tissue by the periosteum between the sutures and on the external bone surface. At the same time, resorption takes place on the internal surface. Since bone is an extremely plastic tissue, it responds to the growth of the brain and forms a skull of adequate size. The skull will be small if the brain does not develop completely and will be larger than normal in a person suffering from hydrocephalus, a disorder characterized by abnormal accumulation of spinal fluid and dilatation of the cerebral ventricles.

Fracture Repair

When a bone is fractured, bone matrix is destroyed and bone cells adjoining the fracture die. The damaged blood vessels produce a localized hemorrhage and form a blood clot.

During repair, the blood clot, cells, and dam-

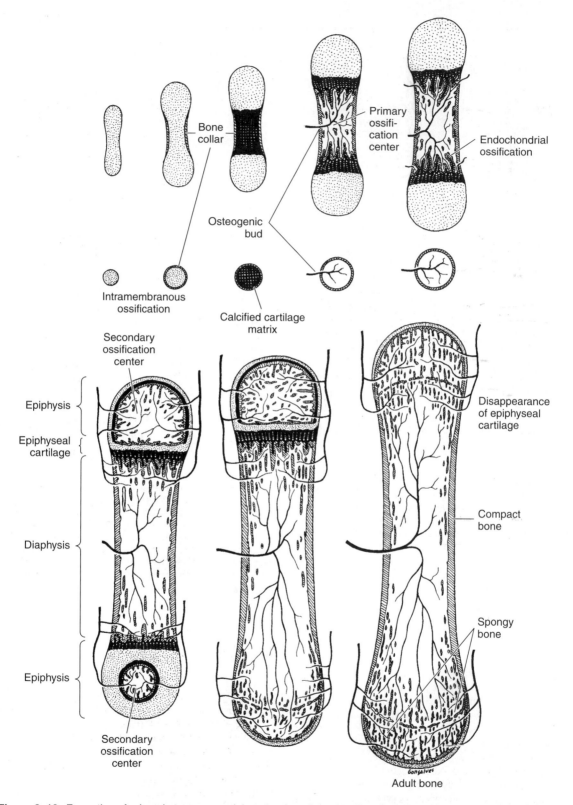

Figure 8–13. Formation of a long bone on a model made of cartilage. Hyaline cartilage is stippled; calcified cartilage is black, and bone tissue is indicated by oblique lines. The five small drawings in the middle row represent cross sections through the middle regions of the figures shown in the upper row. Note the formation of the bone collar and primary and secondary ossification centers. Epiphyseal fusion with diaphysis, with disappearance of the epiphyseal cartilage, occurs at different times in the same bone. (Redrawn and reproduced, with permission, from Bloom W, Fawcett DW: *A Text-book of Histology,* 9th ed. Saunders, 1968.)

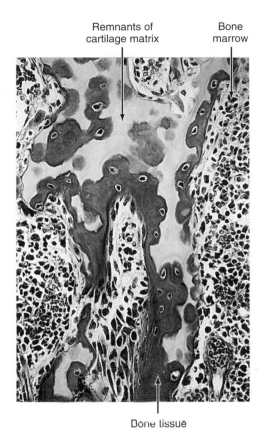

Figure 8–14. Photomicrograph of endochondral ossification from the finger of a human fetus. Remnants of calcified cartilage matrix appear covered by dark primary bone tissue. Calcified cartilage matrix has no cells, whereas bone matrix contains many osteocytes. × 238.

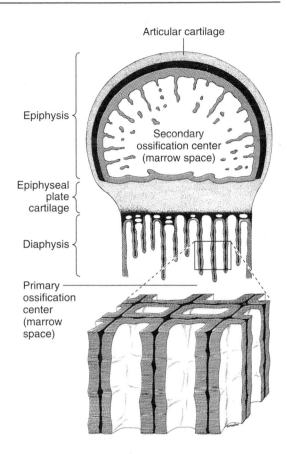

Figure 8–15. Schematic drawings showing the three-dimensional shape of bone in the epiphyseal plate area. Hyaline cartilage is stippled, calcified cartilage is black, and bone tissue is shown in color. The upper drawing shows the region represented three-dimensionally in the lower drawing. (Redrawn and reproduced, with permission, from Ham AW: *Histology,* 6th ed. Lippincott, 1969.)

aged bone matrix are removed by macrophages. The periosteum and the endosteum around the fracture respond with intense proliferation of osteoprogenitor cells, producing a connective tissue that surrounds the fracture and penetrates between the extremities of the fractured bone (Figure 8–17).

Primary bone is then formed by endochondral and intramembranous ossification, both processes contributing simultaneously to the healing of fractures. Repair progresses in such a way that irregularly formed trabeculae of primary bone temporarily unite the extremities of the fractured bone, forming a **bone callus** (Figure 8–17).

Stresses imposed on the bone during repair and during the patient's gradual return to activity serve to remodel the bone callus. If these stresses are identical to those that occurred during the growth of the bone—and therefore influence its structure—the primary bone tissue of the callus is gradually resorbed and replaced by secondary tissue, remodeling the bone and restoring its original structure (Figure 8–17).

HISTOPHYSIOLOGY

Plasticity

Despite its hardness, bone is capable of remodeling its internal structure according to the various stresses to which it is subjected. For example, the positions of the teeth in the jawbone can be modified by lateral pressures produced by orthodontic appliances. Bone is formed on the side where traction is applied and is resorbed where pressure is exerted (on the opposite side). In this way, teeth move within the jawbone while the alveolar bone is being remodeled.

Calcium Reserve

The skeleton contains 99% of the total calcium of the body and acts as a calcium reservoir. The concentration of calcium in the blood and tissues is quite

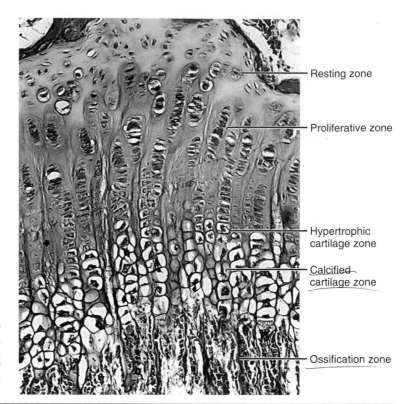

Figure 8–16. Photomicrograph of the epiphyseal plate, showing its five zones, the changes that take place in the cartilage, and the formation of bone. Hematoxylin-and-eosin stain. × 110.

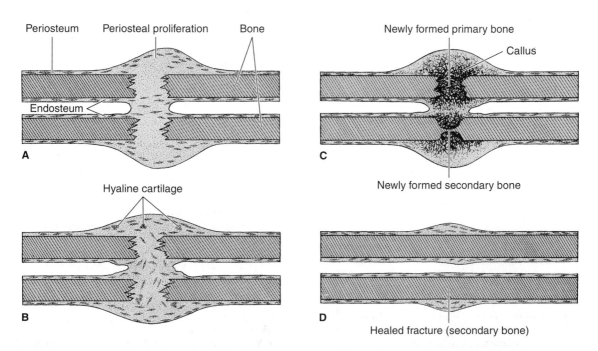

Figure 8–17. Repair of a fractured bone by formation of new bone tissue through periosteal and endosteal cell proliferation.

stable because of a continuous interchange between blood calcium and bone calcium.

Bone calcium is mobilized by two mechanisms, one rapid and the other slow. The first is the simple transfer of ions from hydroxyapatite crystals to interstitial fluid—from which, in turn, calcium passes into the blood. This purely physical mechanism, which takes place mainly in spongy bone, is aided by the large surface area of the hydroxyapatite crystals. The younger, slightly calcified lamellae that exist even in adult bone (because of continuous remodeling) receive and lose calcium more readily. These lamellae are more important for the maintenance of calcium concentration in the blood than are the older, greatly calcified lamellae, whose role is mainly that of support and protection.

The second mechanism for controlling blood calcium level depends on the action of hormones on bone. **Parathyroid hormone** activates and increases the number of cells (osteoclasts), promoting resorption of the bone matrix with the consequent liberation of calcium.

Another hormone, **calcitonin,** which is synthesized mainly by the parafollicular cells of the thyroid gland, inhibits matrix resorption. Calcitonin has an inhibitory effect on osteoclast activity.

Since the concentration of calcium in tissues and blood must be kept constant, nutritional deficiency of calcium results in decalcification of bones; decalcified bones are more likely to fracture and are more transparent to x-rays. Decalcification of bone may also be caused by excessive production of parathyroid hormone (hyperparathyroidism), which results in increased osteoclastic activity, intense resorption of bone, elevation of blood Ca^{2+} and $(PO_4)^{3-}$ levels, and abnormal deposits of calcium in several organs, mainly the kidneys and arterial walls.

The opposite occurs in **osteopetrosis** (L. *petra,* stone), a disease caused by a defect in osteoclast function that results in overgrowth, thickening, and hardening of bones. This process produces obliteration of the bone marrow cavities, depressing blood cell formation with consequent anemia and frequent infections that may be fatal.

Nutrition

Especially during growth, bone is sensitive to nutritional factors. Insufficient dietary protein causes a deficiency of amino acids and leads to reduced synthesis of collagen by osteoblasts. Deficiency of calcium leads to incomplete calcification of the organic bone matrix, owing either to the lack of calcium in the diet or to the lack of the steroid prohormone vitamin D, which is important for the absorption of Ca^{2+} and $(PO_4)^{3-}$ by the small intestine.

Another vitamin that acts directly on bone is vitamin C, which is essential for collagen synthesis. Vitamin C deficiency interferes with bone growth and hinders repair of fractures by altering collagen deposition.

Calcium deficiency in children causes **rickets,** a disease in which the bone matrix does not calcify normally and the epiphyseal plate becomes distorted by the normal strains of body weight and muscular activity. Ossification processes at this level are consequently hindered, and the bones not only grow more slowly but also become deformed.

Calcium deficiency in adults gives rise to **osteomalacia** (*osteon* + Gr. *malakia,* softness), which is characterized by deficient calcification of recently formed bone and partial decalcification of already calcified matrix. Osteomalacia should not be confused with **osteoporosis.** In osteomalacia, there is a decrease in the amount of calcium per unit of bone matrix. Osteoporosis, frequently found in immobilized patients and in postmenopausal women, is a decrease in bone mass caused by decreased bone formation, increased bone resorption, or both. In osteoporosis, the ratio of mineral to organic matrix is unchanged in the otherwise morphologically normal bone.

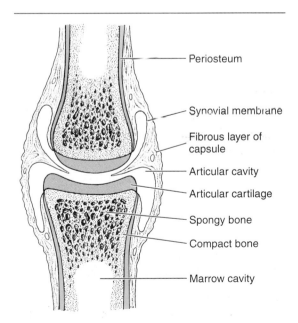

Figure 8–18. Schematic drawing of a diarthrosis. The capsule is formed by two parts: the external fibrous layer and the synovial layer (synovial membrane) that lines the articular cavity except for the cartilaginous areas (in blue).

Hormonal Factors

In addition to parathyroid hormone and calcitonin, several other hormones act on bone. The anterior lobe of the pituitary synthesizes growth hormone, which stimulates overall growth—especially that of epiphyseal cartilage. Consequently, lack of growth hormone during the growing years causes **pituitary dwarfism;** an excess of growth hormone causes excessive growth of the long bones, resulting in **gigantism.** Adult bones cannot increase in length when stimulated by an excess of growth hormone because of the lack of epiphyseal cartilage, but they do increase in width by periosteal growth. In adults, an increase in growth hormone causes **acromegaly,** a disease in which the bones—mainly the long ones—become very thick.

The sex hormones, both male (androgens) and female (estrogens), have a complex effect on bones and are, in a general way, stimulators of bone formation. They influence the time of appearance and development of ossification centers and accelerate the closure of epiphyses.

Precocious sexual maturity caused by sex hormone–producing tumors retards bodily growth, since the epiphyseal cartilage is quickly replaced by bone (closure of epiphysis). In hormone deficiencies caused by castration or by abnormal development of the gonads, epiphyseal cartilage remains functional for a longer period of time, resulting in tall stature. Thyroid hormone deficiency in children, as in **cretinism,** is associated with **dwarfism.**

Interrelationships Between Bone Cells

Autoradiographic studies performed after the administration of ^{3}H-thymidine to young animals—whose bone cells proliferate rapidly—reveal that osteoblasts and osteocytes do not divide after having been formed from the **osteoprogenitor cell.** These studies also show that osteoblasts usually give rise to osteocytes, which can remain as such for long periods (in secondary bone) or short periods (in primary bone). Both osteoblasts and osteocytes can revert to osteoprogenitor cells. The ability of the cells related to bone production both to turn over rapidly and to modulate back to osteoprogenitor cells confers a high plasticity that permits the cells to adapt quickly to changing conditions.

Although bone tumors are uncommon (0.5% of all cancer deaths), bone cells may escape the normal controls of proliferation to become benign (eg, **osteoblastoma, osteoclastoma**) or malignant (eg, **osteosarcoma**) tumors. Os-

teosarcomas show pleomorphic (Gr. *pleion,* more, + *morphe,* form) and mitotically active osteoblasts associated with osteoid. Most cases of this aggressive malignant tumor occur in adolescents and young adults. The lower end of the femur, the upper tibia, and the upper humerus are the most common locations. In addition to the tumors originating from bone cells, the skeleton is often the site of metastases from malignant tumors originating in other organs. The most frequent bone metastases are from breast, lung, prostate, kidney, and thyroid tumors.

JOINTS

Joints are regions where bones are capped and surrounded by connective tissues that hold the

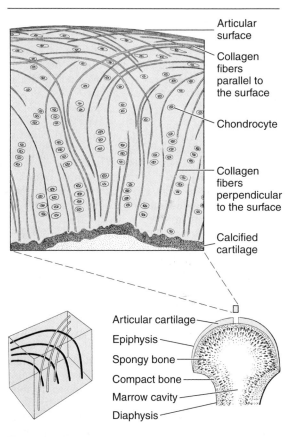

Figure 8–19. Articular surfaces of diarthrosis are covered by hyaline cartilage that is devoid of perichondrium. The upper drawing shows that in this cartilage, collagen fibers are first perpendicular and then bend gradually, becoming parallel to the cartilage surface. Deeply located chondrocytes are globular and are arranged in vertical rows. Superficially placed chondrocytes are flattened; they are not organized in groups. The lower left drawing shows the organization of collagen fibers in articular cartilage in three dimensions.

bones together and determine the type and degree of movement between them. Joints may be classified as **diarthroses,** which permit free bone movement, and **synarthroses** (Gr. *syn,* together, + *arthrosis,* articulation), in which very limited or no movement occurs. There are three types of synarthroses, based on the type of tissue uniting the bone surfaces: **synostosis, synchondrosis,** and **syndesmosis.**

Synostosis

In synostosis (*syn + osteon* + Gr. *osis,* condition), bones are united by bone tissue and no movement takes place. In older adults, this type of synarthrosis unites the skull bones, which, in children and young adults, are united by dense connective tissue.

Synchondrosis

Synchondroses (*syn + chondros*) are articulations in which the bones are joined by hyaline cartilage.

The epiphyseal plates of growing bones are one example, and in the adult human, synchondrosis unites the first rib to the sternum.

Syndesmosis

As with synchondrosis, a syndesmosis permits a certain amount of movement. The bones are joined by an interosseous ligament of dense connective tissue (eg, the pubic symphysis).

Diarthrosis

Diarthroses (Figure 8–18) are joints that generally unite long bones and have great mobility, such as the elbow and knee joints. In a diarthrosis, ligaments and a capsule of connective tissue maintain the contact at the ends of the bone. The capsule encloses a sealed **articular cavity** that contains **synovial fluid,** a colorless, transparent, viscous fluid. Synovial fluid is a blood plasma dialysate with a high concentration of

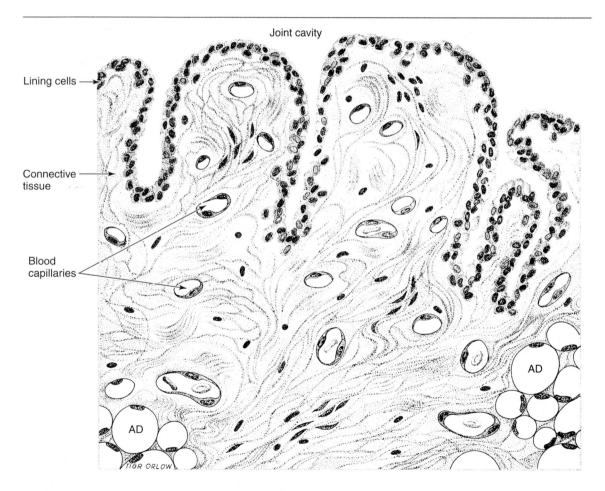

Figure 8–20. Histologic structure of the synovial membrane, with its lining cells in epithelioid arrangement. There is no basal lamina between the lining cells and the underlying connective tissue. This tissue is rich in blood capillaries and contains a variable number of adipose cells (AD). (Reproduced, with permission, from Cossermelli W: *Reumatologia Basica,* Sarvier, 1971.)

hyaluronic acid produced by cells of the synovial layer. The sliding of articular surfaces covered by hyaline cartilage (Figure 8–18) and having no perichondrium is facilitated by the lubricating synovial fluid, which also supplies nutrients and oxygen to the avascular articular cartilage.

The collagen fibers of the articular surface cartilage are disposed as gothic arches, a convenient arrangement to distribute the forces generated by pressure in this tissue (Figure 8–19).

The resilient articular cartilage is also a very efficient absorber of the intermittent mechanical pressures to which many joints are subjected. Proteoglycan molecules, found isolated or aggregated in a network, contain a large amount of water. These matrix components, rich in highly branched hydrophilic

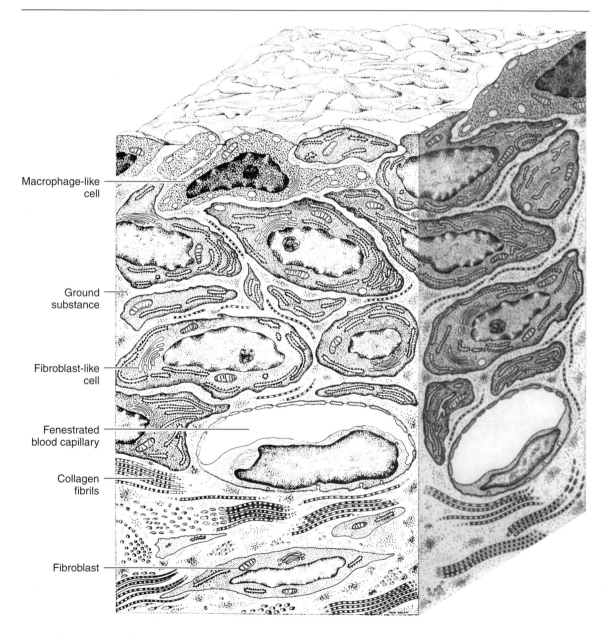

Figure 8–21. Schematic representation of the ultrastructure of synovial membrane. The two covering cell types are separated by a small amount of connective tissue ground substance. No basal lamina is seen separating the lining cells from the connective tissue. Blood capillaries are of the fenestrated type, which facilitates exchange of substances between blood and synovial fluid.

glycosaminoglycans, function as a biomechanical spring. When pressure is applied, water is forced out of the cartilage matrix into the synovial fluid. When water is expelled, another mechanism that contributes to cartilage resilience enters into play. This is the reciprocal electrostatic repulsion of the negatively charged carboxyl and sulfate groups in the glycosaminoglycan molecules. These charges are also responsible for separating the glycosaminoglycan branches and thus creating spaces to be occupied by water. When the pressure is released, water is attracted back into the interstices of the glycosaminoglycan branches. These water movements are brought about by the use of the joint. They are essential for nutrition of the cartilage and for facilitating the interchange of O_2, CO_2, and other molecules between the synovial fluid and the articular cartilage.

The capsules of diarthroses (Figure 8–18) vary in structure according to the joint. Generally, however, this capsule is composed of two layers, the external **fibrous layer** and the internal **synovial layer** (Figure 8–20).

The synovial layer is formed by two types of cells. One resembles fibroblasts and the other has the aspect and behavior of macrophages (Figure 8–21). The fibrous layer is made of dense connective tissue that is better developed in parts subject to great strain. This layer envelops the ligaments of the joint and some of the tendons inserted into the bone near the joint.

REFERENCES

Bourne GH (editor): *The Biochemistry and Physiology of Bone,* 2nd ed. 4 vols. Academic Press, 1971–1976.

Ghadially FN: *Fine Structure of Synovial Joints.* Butterworth, 1983.

Gothlin G, Ericsson JLE: The osteoclast: review of ultrastructure, origin and structure-function relationship. Clin Orthop 1976;120:201.

Gunness M, Hock JM: Anabolic effect of parathyroid hormone on cancellous and cortical bone histology. Bone 1993;14:277.

Hancox NM: *Biology of Bone.* Cambridge Univ Press, 1972.

Holtrop ME: The ultrastructure of bone. Ann Clin Lab Sci 1975;5:264.

Jotereau FV, LeDouarin NM: The developmental relationship between osteocytes and osteoclasts: a study using the quail-chick nuclear marker in endochondral ossification. Dev Biol 1978;63:253.

Levick JR: Synovial fluid hydraulics. Sci & Med 1996;3(5):52.

Marks SC Jr, Popoff SN: Bone cell biology: the regulation of development, structure, and function in the skeleton. Amer J Anat 1988;183:1.

Mundy GR et al: The effects of cytokines and growth factors on osteoblastic cells. Bone 1995;17:71S.

Ross PD et al: Bone mass and beyond. risk factors for fractures. Calcified Tissue International 1993;53:S134.

Termine JD et al: Osteonectin, a bone-specific protein linking mineral to collagen. Cell 1981;26:99.

Urist MR: *Fundamental and Clinical Bone Physiology.* Lippincott, 1980.

Nerve Tissue & the Nervous System

The human nervous system is by far the most complex system in the human body and is formed by a network of more than 100 million nerve cells (**neurons**), assisted by many more glial cells. Each neuron has, on average, at least a thousand interconnections with other neurons, forming a very complex system for communication.

Neurons provide rapid communication between groups of serially disposed cells, permitting rapid transmission of information over long distances.

Neurons are grouped as **circuits.** Like electronic circuits, neural circuits are highly specific combinations of elements that make up systems of various sizes and complexities. Although a neural system may be a single circuit, in most cases it is a combination of two or more circuits that interact to generate a function. A neural function is a set of coordinated processes intended to produce a definite result. A number of elementary circuits may be combined to form higher-order systems; higher-order systems may combine to create systems of even higher orders.

Nerve tissue is distributed throughout the body as an integrated communications network. Anatomically, the nervous system is divided into the **central nervous system,** consisting of the brain and the spinal cord; and the **peripheral nervous system,** composed of nerve fibers and small aggregates of nerve cells called **nerve ganglia** (Figure 9–1).

Structurally, nerve tissue consists of two cell types: **nerve cells,** or **neurons,** which usually show numerous long processes; and several types of **glial cells** (Gr. *glia,* glue), which have short processes, support and protect neurons, and participate in neural activity, neural nutrition, and the defense processes of the central nervous system.

The study of nerve tissue has recently progressed rapidly owing to the use of markers that identify neurons and glia cells and the use of molecules that flow in a retrograde direction, permitting a more precise study of neuronal circuits.

Neurons respond to environmental changes (**stimuli**) by altering electrical potentials that exist between the inner and outer surfaces of their membranes. Cells with this property (eg, neurons, muscle cells, some gland cells) are called **excitable,** or **irritable.** Neurons react promptly to stimuli with a modification of electrical potential that may be restricted to the place that received the stimulus or may be spread (propagated) throughout the neuron by the plasma membrane. This propagation, called the **action potential,** or **nerve impulse,** is capable of traveling long distances; it transmits information to other neurons, muscles, and glands.

By creating, analyzing, identifying, and integrating information, the nervous system generates two great classes of functions: stabilization of the intrinsic conditions (eg, blood pressure, O_2 and CO_2 content, pH, blood glucose levels, and hormone levels) of the organism within normal ranges; and behavioral patterns (eg, feeding, reproduction, defense, interaction with other living creatures).

DEVELOPMENT OF NERVE TISSUE

Nerve tissues develop from embryonic ectoderm that is induced to differentiate by the underlying notochord. First, a neural plate forms; then the edges of the plate thicken, forming the neural groove. The edges of the groove grow toward each other and ultimately fuse, forming the neural tube. This structure gives rise to the entire central nervous system, including neurons, glial cells, ependymal cells, and the epithelial cells of the choroid plexus.

Cells lateral to the neural groove form the **neural crest.** These cells undergo extensive migrations and contribute to the formation of the peripheral nervous system, as well as a number of other structures. Neural crest derivatives include (1) chromaffin cells of the adrenal medulla (see Chapter 21); (2) melanocytes of skin and subcutaneous tissues (see Chapter 18); (3) odontoblasts (see Chapter 15); (4) cells of the pia mater and the arachnoid; (5) sensory neurons of cranial and spinal sensory ganglia; (6) postganglionic neurons of sympathetic and parasympathetic ganglia; (7) Schwann cells of peripheral axons; and (8) satellite cells of peripheral ganglia.

NERVOUS SYSTEM

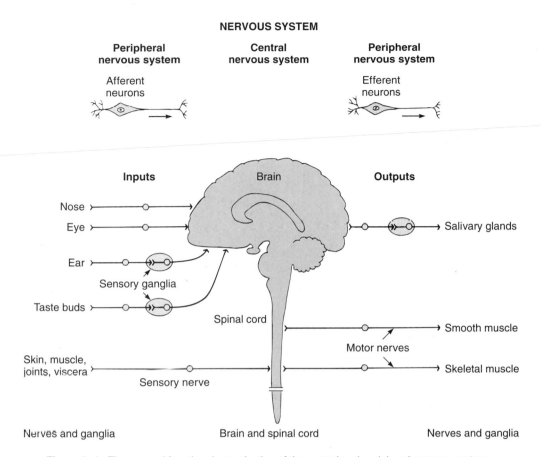

Figure 9–1. The general functional organization of the central and peripheral nervous systems.

NEURONS

Nerve cells, or neurons, are independent anatomic and functional units with complex morphologic characteristics. They are responsible for the reception, transmission, and processing of stimuli; the triggering of certain cell activities; and the release of neurotransmitters and other informational molecules.

Most neurons consist of three parts (Figure 9–2): the **dendrites,** which are multiple elongated processes specialized in receiving stimuli from the environment, sensory epithelial cells, or other neurons; the **cell body,** or **perikaryon** (Gr. *peri,* around, + *karyon,* nucleus), which represents the trophic center for the whole nerve cell and is also receptive to stimuli; and the **axon** (from Greek, meaning axis), which is a single process specialized in generating or conducting nerve impulses to other cells (nerve, muscle, and gland cells). Axons may also receive information from other neurons; this information mainly modifies the transmission of action potentials to other neurons. The distal portion of the axon is usually branched and constitutes the **terminal arborization.** Each branch of this arborization termi-

nates on the next cell in dilatations called **end bulbs** (**boutons**), which interact with other neurons or nonnerve cells, forming structures called **synapses.** Synapses transmit information to the next cell in the circuit.

Neurons and their processes are extremely variable in size and shape (Figure 9–3). Cell bodies can be spherical, ovoid, or angular; some are very large, measuring up to 150 μm in diameter—large enough to be visible to the naked eye. Other nerve cells are among the smallest cells in the body; for example, the cell bodies of granule cells of the cerebellum are only 4–5 μm in diameter.

According to the size and shape of their processes, most neurons can be placed in one of the following categories (Figures 9–3 and 9–4): **multipolar neurons,** which have more than two cell processes, one process being the axon and the others dendrites; **bipolar neurons,** with one dendrite and one axon; and **pseudounipolar neurons,** which have a single process that is close to the perikaryon and divides into two branches. The process then forms a T shape, with one branch extending to a peripheral ending and the other toward the central nervous system (Figure 9–4). In pseudounipolar neurons, stimuli that are

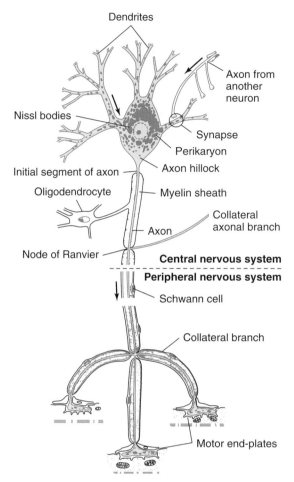

Dendrites

Axon from
another
neuron

Nissl bodies

Synapse

Perikaryon

Initial segment of axon

Axon hillock

Oligodendrocyte

Myelin sheath

Collateral
axonal branch

Axon

Node of Ranvier

Central nervous system

Peripheral nervous system

Schwann cell

Collateral branch

Motor end-plates

Figure 9–2. Motor neuron. The myelin sheath is produced by oligodendrocytes in the central nervous system
and by Schwann cells in the peripheral nervous system.
The neuronal cell body has an unusually large, euchromatic nucleus with a well-developed nucleolus. The
perikaryon contains Nissl bodies, which are also found in
large dendrites. An axon from another neuron is shown at
upper right. It has three end bulbs, one of which forms a
synapse with the neuron. Note also the three motor end-
plates, which transmit the nerve impulse to striated skeletal muscle fibers. Arrows show the direction of the nerve
impulse.

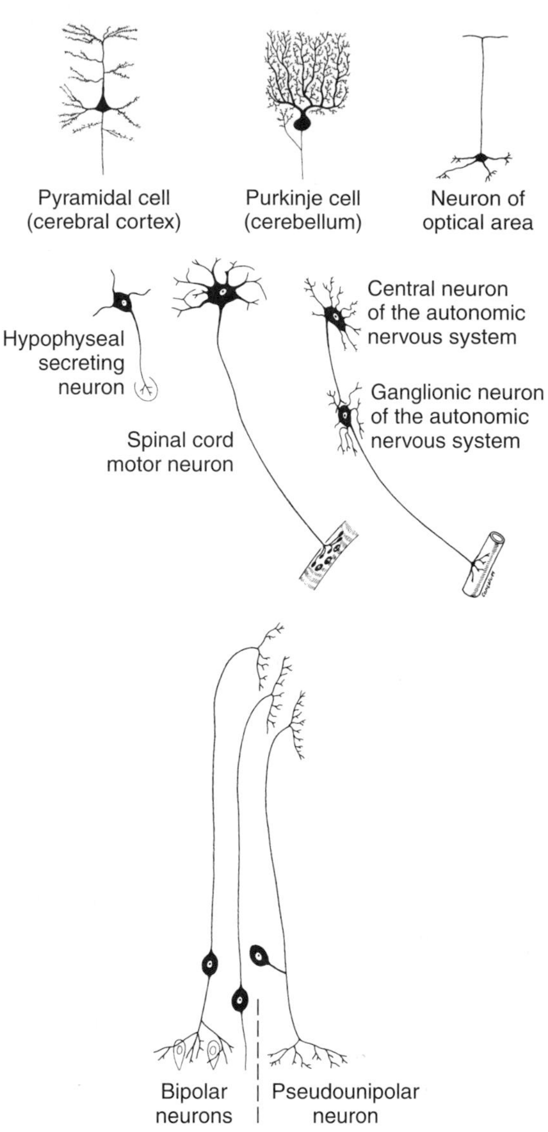

Pyramidal cell
(cerebral cortex)

Purkinje cell
(cerebellum)

Neuron of
optical area

Central neuron
of the autonomic
nervous system

Hypophyseal
secreting
neuron

Ganglionic neuron
of the autonomic
nervous system

Spinal cord
motor neuron

Bipolar
neurons

Pseudounipolar
neuron

Figure 9–3. Diagrams of several types of neurons. The
morphologic characteristics of neurons are very complex.
All neurons shown here, except for the bipolar and
pseudounipolar neurons, which are not very numerous in
nerve tissue, are of the common multipolar variety.

picked up by the dendrites travel directly to the axon
terminal without passing through the perikaryon.

During the maturation process of pseudounipolar
neurons, the central (axon) and the peripheral (dendrite) fibers fuse, becoming one single fiber. In these
neurons, the cell body does not seem to be involved
in the conduction of impulses, although it does synthesize many molecules, including neurotransmitters,
that migrate to the peripheral fibers.

Most neurons of the body are multipolar. Bipolar
neurons are found in the cochlear and vestibular gan-

glia as well as in the retina and the olfactory mucosa.
Pseudounipolar neurons are found in the spinal ganglia (the sensory ganglia located in the dorsal roots of
the spinal nerves). They are also found in most cranial ganglia.

Neurons can also be classified according to their
functional roles. **Motor (efferent) neurons** control
effector organs such as muscle fibers and exocrine
and endocrine glands. **Sensory (afferent) neurons**
are involved in the reception of sensory stimuli from
the environment and from within the body. **In-**

Main types of neurons

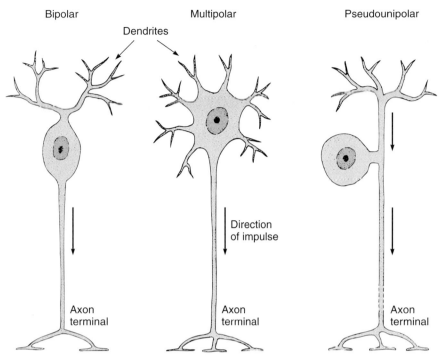

Figure 9–4. Simplified view of the three main types of neurons, according to their morphologic characteristics.

terneurons establish relationships among other neurons, forming complex functional networks or circuits (as in the retina).

During mammalian evolution there has been a great increase in the number and complexity of interneurons. Highly developed functions of the nervous system cannot be ascribed to simple neuron circuits; rather, they depend on complex interactions established by the integrated functions of many neurons.

In the central nervous system, nerve cell bodies are present only in the gray matter. White matter contains neuronal processes but no nerve cell bodies. In the peripheral nervous system, cell bodies are found in ganglia and in some sensory regions (eg, olfactory mucosa).

CELL BODY, OR PERIKARYON

The cell body is the part of the neuron that contains the nucleus and surrounding cytoplasm, exclusive of the cell processes (Figure 9–2). It is primarily a trophic center, although it also has receptive capabilities. The perikaryon of most neurons receives a great number of nerve endings that convey excitatory or inhibitory stimuli generated in other nerve cells.

Most nerve cells have a spherical, unusually large, euchromatic (pale-staining) nucleus with a prominent nucleolus. Binuclear nerve cells are seen in sympathetic and sensory ganglia. The chromatin is finely dispersed, reflecting the intense synthetic activity of these cells.

The cell body (Figure 9–5) contains a highly developed rough endoplasmic reticulum organized into aggregates of parallel cisternae. In the cytoplasm between the cisternae are numerous polyribosomes, suggesting that these cells synthesize both structural proteins and proteins for transport. When appropriate stains are used, rough endoplasmic reticulum and free ribosomes appear under the light microscope as basophilic granular areas called **Nissl bodies** (Figures 9–2 and 9–6). The number of Nissl bodies varies according to neuronal type and functional state. They are particularly abundant in large nerve cells such as motor neurons (Figure 9–6). The **Golgi complex** is located only in the cell body and consists of multiple parallel arrays of smooth cisternae arranged around the periphery of the nucleus (Figure 9–5). Mitochondria are especially abundant in the axon terminals. They are scattered throughout the cytoplasm of the cell body.

Neurofilaments (intermediate filaments with a diameter of 10 nm) are abundant in perikaryons and cell processes. Neurofilaments bundle together as a result of the action of certain fixatives. When impregnated with silver, they form **neurofibrils** that are visible with the light microscope. The neurons also

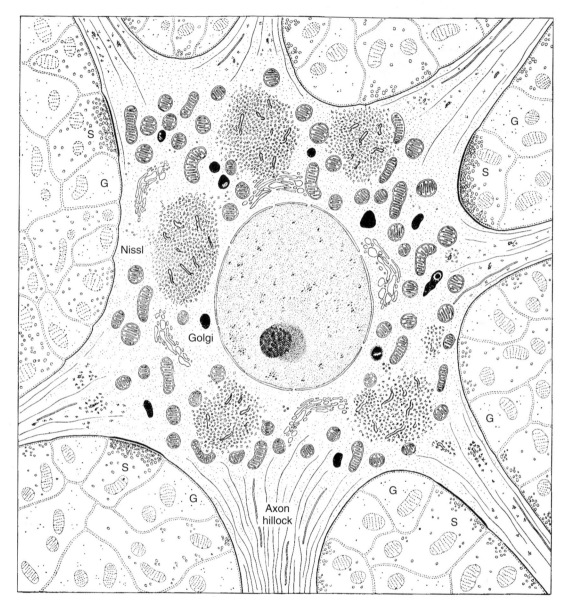

Figure 9–5. Ultrastructure of a neuron. The neuronal surface is completely covered either by synaptic endings of other neurons (S) or by processes of glial cells (G). At synapses, the neuronal membrane is thicker and is called the postsynaptic membrane. The neuronal process devoid of ribosomes (lower part of figure) is the axon hillock. The other processes of this cell are dendrites.

contain microtubules that are identical to those found in many other cells. Nerve cells occasionally contain inclusions of pigments, such as **lipofuscin,** which is a residue of undigested material by lysosomes.

DENDRITES & AXONS

Dendrites (Gr. *dendron,* tree) are usually short and divide like the branches of a tree (Figure 9–4). Most

nerve cells have numerous dendrites, which considerably increase the receptive area of the cell. The arborization of dendrites makes it possible for one neuron to receive and integrate a great number of axon terminals from other nerve cells. It has been estimated that up to 200,000 axonal terminations establish functional contact with the dendrites of the Purkinje cell found in the cerebellum (Figure 9–3). That number may be even higher in other nerve cells. Bipolar neurons, with only one dendrite, are uncom-

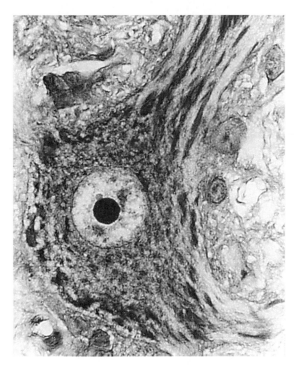

Figure 9–6. Photomicrograph of a motor neuron, a very large cell, from the spinal cord. The cytoplasm contains a great number of Nissl bodies. Note the large, round, light-stained nucleus, with a central dark-stained nucleolus. High magnification.

mon and are found only in special sites. Unlike axons, which maintain a constant diameter from one end to the other, dendrites become thinner as they subdivide into branches.

The composition of dendritic cytoplasm is similar to that of the perikaryon; however, dendrites are devoid of Golgi complexes.

Most neurons have only one axon; a very few have no axon at all. An axon is a cylindrical process that varies in length and diameter according to the type of neuron. Although some neurons have short axons, axons are usually very long processes. For example, axons of the motor cells of the spinal cord that innervate the foot muscles may have a length of up to 100 cm (about 40 inches). All axons originate from a short pyramid-shaped region, the **axon hillock,** that usually arises from the perikaryon (Figure 9–5). The plasma membrane of the axon is called the **axolemma** (*axon* + Gr. *eilema,* sheath); its contents are known as **axoplasm.**

In neurons that give rise to a myelinated axon, the portion of the axon between the axon hillock and the point at which myelination begins is called the **initial segment.** This is the site where various excitatory and inhibitory stimuli impinging on the neuron are algebraically summed, resulting in the decision to

propagate—or not to propagate—an action potential, or nerve impulse. It is known that several types of ion channels are localized in the initial segment and that these channels are important in generating the change in electrical potential that constitutes the action potential. In contrast to dendrites, axons have a constant diameter and do not branch profusely. Occasionally, the axon, shortly after its departure from the cell body, gives rise to a branch that returns to the area of the nerve cell body. All axon branches are known as **collateral branches** (Figure 9–2). Axonal cytoplasm (axoplasm) possesses mitochondria, microtubules, neurofilaments, and some cisternae of smooth endoplasmic reticulum. The absence of polyribosomes and rough endoplasmic reticulum emphasizes the dependence of the axon on the perikaryon for its maintenance. If an axon is severed, its peripheral parts degenerate and die.

AXONS & MOLECULAR MOVEMENT

There is a lively bidirectional transport of small and large molecules along the axon.

A. Anterograde Flow: Macromolecules and organelles are synthesized at the cell body and transported continuously along the axon to its terminals.

Anterograde flow occurs at three distinct speeds. A slow stream (a few millimeters per day) transports proteins and microfilaments. A flow of intermediate speed transports mitochondria, and a fast stream (100 times more rapid) transports the substances contained in vesicles that are needed at the axon terminal during neurotransmission.

B. Retrograde Flow: Simultaneously with anterograde flow, a flow in the opposite direction transports several molecules, including material taken up by endocytosis (including viruses and toxins). This process is used in neurology to study the pathways of neurons; peroxidase or another marker is injected in regions with axon terminals, and its distribution is followed after a certain period of time.

Proteins related to axon flow include **dynein,** a protein with ATPase activity present in microtubules (related to retrograde flow); and **kinesin,** a microtubule-activated ATPase that, when attached to vesicles, promotes anterograde flow in the axon.

SYNAPTIC COMMUNICATION

The synapse (Gr. *synapsis,* union) is responsible for the unidirectional transmission of nerve impulses.

Synapses are the sites where contact occurs between neurons or between neurons and other effector cells (eg, muscle and gland cells). The function of the synapse is to convert an electrical signal (impulse) from the presynaptic cell into a chemical signal that can be transferred to the **postsynaptic** cell. Most synapses transmit information by releasing **chemical messengers** during the signaling process. Chemical messengers can be separated into two types based on the effect they have on the postsynaptic cell: (1) **neurotransmitters** and (2) **neuromodulators.** Neurotransmitters are chemicals that, when combined with a receptor protein, either open or close ion channels or initiate second-messenger cascades. Neurotransmitters can be classified as **small-molecule transmitters, catecholamines,** or **neuroactive peptides** (Table 9–1). Neuromodulators are chemical messengers that modify the function of receptor proteins. Recently, neuroscientists have discovered that some chemical messengers, eg,. **nitric oxide,** may be able to function both as neurotransmitters and as neuromodulators. The synapse itself is formed by an axon terminal (**presynaptic terminal**) that delivers the signal; a region on the surface of another cell where a new signal is generated (**postsynaptic terminal**); and a thin intercellular space called the **synaptic cleft** (Figure 9–7). If an axon forms a synapse with a cell body, it is called an **axosomatic synapse;** with a dendrite, **axodendritic;** or with an axon, **axoaxonic** (Figure 9–8).

Table 9–1. Common neurotransmitters.

Small Molecules	Catecholamines	Neuroactive Peptides
Glutamate	Dopamine	Substance P
GABA (γ-amino-butyric acid)	Norepinephrine	Enkephalin
Glycine	Serotonin	Endorphin
Acetylcholine	Histamine	Vasopressin
		Vasoactive intestinal polypeptide

Although most synapses are **chemical synapses** and use chemical messengers, a few synapses transmit ionic signals through gap junctions that cross the pre- and postsynaptic membranes, thereby conducting neuronal signals directly. These synapses are called **electrical synapses.**

Synapses tend to be rigid structures; the plasma membranes at the pre- and postsynaptic regions are reinforced and appear thicker than the membranes adjacent to the synapse. In some instances pre- and postsynaptic membranes are bound by bridges between them.

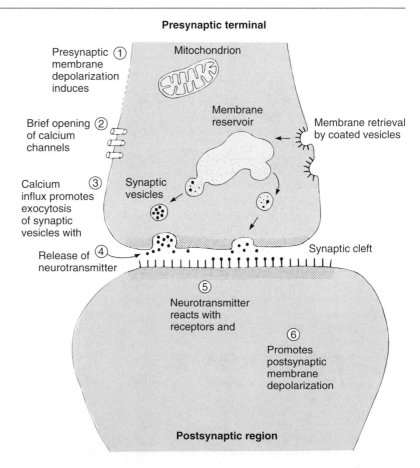

Presynaptic terminal

① Presynaptic membrane depolarization induces

Mitochondrion

Membrane reservoir

Membrane retrieval by coated vesicles

② Brief opening of calcium channels

③ Calcium influx promotes exocytosis of synaptic vesicles with

Synaptic vesicles

④ Release of neurotransmitter

Synaptic cleft

⑤ Neurotransmitter reacts with receptors and

⑥ Promotes postsynaptic membrane depolarization

Postsynaptic region

Figure 9–7. The main functional aspects of the two parts of the synapse: the presynaptic axon terminal and the postsynaptic region of the next neuron in the circuit. Numbers indicate the sequence of activity.

Types of synapses

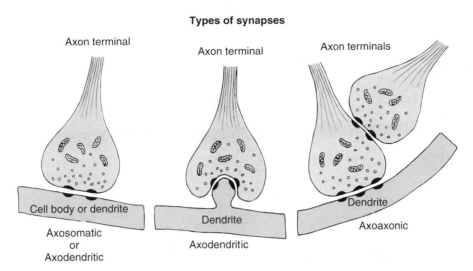

Figure 9–8. Types of synapses. The axon terminals usually transmit the nerve impulse to a dendrite or to a nerve cell body; less frequently, they make a synapse with another axon. (Redrawn, with permission, from Cormack DH: *Essential Histology.* Lippincott, 1993.)

The presynaptic terminal always contains **synaptic vesicles** and numerous **mitochondria** (Figures 9–7 and 9–9). The vesicles contain neurotransmitters; the mitochondria furnish energy for synaptic activity.

MEMBRANE POTENTIALS

The nerve cell and its effectors (muscle and gland cells) have their membranes decorated with molecules (pumps) that transport ions into and out of cells. The result of this transport creates a **membrane potential**—an unequal electrical charge on opposite sides of the cell membrane. The membrane is then considered to be **polarized.** When the nerve impulse is initiated, the unequal electrical charge (potential) returns to zero (**depolarization**). These rapid changes in potential are made possible by **ion channels,** a class of integral, transmembrane proteins. These channels have three important functions: (1) they conduct ions; (2) they recognize and select among specific ions; and (3) they open and close in response to specific electrical, mechanical, or chemical signals.

Neurotransmitters are generally synthesized in the cell body; they are then stored in vesicles in the presynaptic region of a synapse. During transmission of a nerve impulse, they are released into the synaptic cleft by **exocytosis.** The extra membrane that collects at the presynaptic region as a result of exocytosis of the synaptic vesicles is recycled by **endocytosis.** Recycled membrane is stored in a **membrane reservoir** (Figure 9–7). Some neurotransmitters are synthesized in the membrane reservoir, using enzymes and precursors brought by axonal transport.

The first neurotransmitters to be described were acetylcholine and norepinephrine. A norepinephrine-releasing axon terminal is shown in Figure 9–10. Further study of the chemical synapse has revealed more than 35 neurotransmitters, each with a different chemical composition. Most are amines, amino acids, or small peptides (neuropeptides). Inorganic substances such as nitric oxide have also been shown to act as neurotransmitters. Several peptides that act as neurotransmitters are used elsewhere in the body, eg, as hormones in the digestive tract. Neuropeptides are important in regulating feelings and drives, such as pain, pleasure, hunger, thirst, and sex (Figure 9–11).

Sequence of Events During Chemical Synapse Transmission

The events that take place during chemical synapse transmission are illustrated in Figure 9–7. Nerve impulses that sweep rapidly (in milliseconds) along the cell membrane promote an explosive electrical activity (depolarization) that is propagated along the cell membrane. This impulse briefly opens calcium channels in the presynaptic region, promoting a calcium influx that triggers the exocytosis of synaptic vesicles. The neurotransmitters released at the sites of exocytosis react with receptors present at the postsynaptic region, promoting a transient electric activity (depolarization) at the postsynaptic membrane. These synapses are called **excitatory,** because their activity promotes impulses in the postsynaptic cell membrane. In some synapses the neurotransmitter-receptor interaction has an opposite

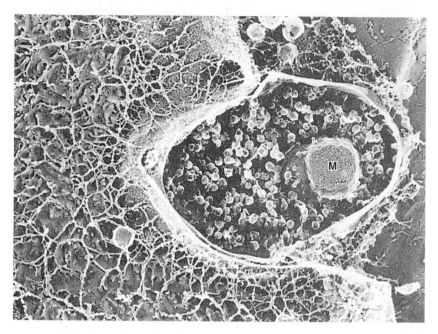

Figure 9–9. Electron micrograph of a rotary-replicated freeze-etched synapse. Synaptic vesicles surround a mitochondrion (M) in the axon terminal. × 25,000. (Reproduced, with permission, from Heuser JE, Salpeter SR: Organization of acetylcholine receptors in quick-frozen, deep-etched and rotary-replicated Torpedo postsynaptic membrane. J Cell Biol 1979;82:150.)

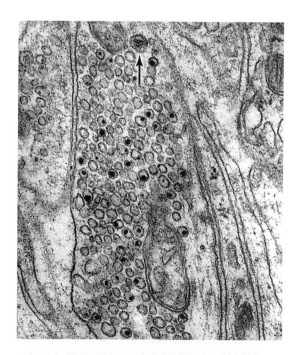

Figure 9–10. Adrenergic nerve ending. There are many 50-nm-diameter vesicles (arrow) with dark, electron-dense cores containing norepinephrine. × 40,000. (Courtesy of A Machado.)

effect, promoting **hyperpolarization** with no transmission of the nerve impulse. These are called **inhibitory** synapses. Thus, synapses can excite or inhibit impulse transmission and thereby regulate nerve activity (Figure 9–12).

Once used, neurotransmitters are removed quickly by enzymatic breakdown, diffusion, or endocytosis mediated by specific receptors on the presynaptic membrane. This removal of neurotransmitters is functionally important because it prevents an undesirable sustained stimulation of the postsynaptic neuron.

Local anesthetics are hydrophobic molecules that bind to sodium channels, inhibiting sodium transport and, consequently, also the action potential responsible for the nerve impulse.

GLIAL CELLS & NEURONAL ACTIVITY

Although neurons are the principal cells of nerve tissue, glial cells play an important supporting role. These cells are 10 times more abundant in the mammalian brain than neurons; they surround both cell bodies and their axonal and dendrite processes that occupy the interneuronal spaces.

Nerve tissue has only a very small amount of extracellular matrix, and glial cells (Table 9–2) furnish a microenvironment suitable for neuronal activity.

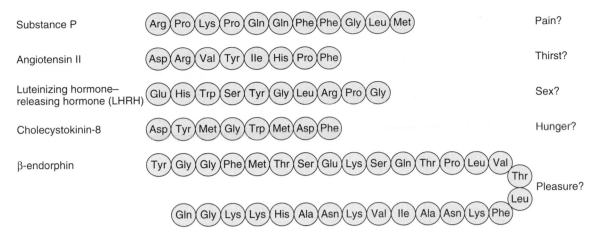

Figure 9–11. Amino acid sequence of some neuropeptides and the sensations and drives in which they probably participate. (Reproduced, with permission, from Alberts B et al: *Molecular Biology of the Cell.* 2nd ed. Garland Press, 1993.)

Oligodendrocytes

Oligodendrocytes (Gr. *oligos,* small, + *dendron* + *kytos,* cell) produce the myelin sheath that provides the electrical insulation of neurons in the central nervous system (Figures 9–13 and 9–14). These cells have a few small processes that wrap around axons, producing a myelin sheath as shown in Figure 9–15.

Schwann Cells

Schwann cells have the same function as oligodendrocytes but are located around axons in the periph-eral nervous system. One Schwann cell forms myelin around one axon, in contrast to the ability of oligodendrocytes to branch and serve more than one neuron and its processes. Figure 9–24 shows how the Schwann cell membrane wraps around the axon.

Astrocytes

Astrocytes (Gr. *astron,* star, + *kytos*) are star-shaped cells, because of their multiple radiating processes. These cells have bundles of intermediate filaments made of **glial fibrillary acid protein** that reinforce their structure. Astrocytes bind neurons to capillaries and to the pia mater (a thin connective tissue that covers the central nervous system; see below). Astrocytes with few long processes are called **fibrous astrocytes** and are located in the white matter; **protoplasmic astrocytes,** with many short-branched processes, are found in the gray matter (Figures 9–13 and 9–14). Astrocytes, compared to other glial cells, are by far the most numerous and exhibit an exceptional morphological and functional diversity.

In addition to their structural functions, astrocytes participate in controlling the ionic and chemical environment of neurons. One type of astrocyte develops processes with expanded **end-feet** that are linked to endothelial cells by junctional complexes. It is believed that through the end-feet, astrocytes transfer molecules and ions from the blood to the neurons. Expanded processes are also present at the external surface of the central nervous system, where they make a continuous layer (see Figure 9–20). Furthermore, when the central nervous system is damaged, astrocytes proliferate to form cellular scar tissue.

Astrocytes also play a role in regulating the numerous functions of the central nervous system. Astrocytes in vitro exhibit adrenergic receptors, amino acid receptors (eg, γ-aminobutyric acid [GABA]), and peptide receptors (including natriuretic peptide, angioten-

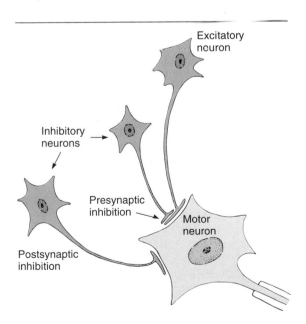

Figure 9–12. Examples of excitatory and inhibitory synapses in a motor neuron. (Redrawn, with permission, from Ganong WF: *Review of Medical Physiology.* 15th ed. Appleton & Lange, 1991.)

Table 9–2. Origin and principal functions of neuroglial cells.

Glial Cell Type	Origin	Location	Main Functions
Oligodendrocyte	Neural tube	Central nervous system	Myelin production, electric insulation
Schwann cell	Neural tube	Peripheral nerves	Myelin production, electric insulation
Astrocyte	Neural tube	Central nervous system	Structural support, repair processes Blood-brain barrier, metabolic exchanges
Ependymal cell	Neural tube	Central nervous system	Lining cavities of central nervous system
Microglia	Bone marrow	Central nervous system	Macrophagic activity

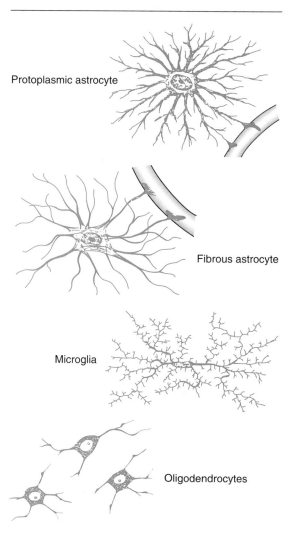

Figure 9–13. Drawings of neuroglial cells as seen in slides stained by metallic impregnation. Note that only astrocytes exhibit vascular end-feet, which cover the walls of blood capillaries.

sin II, endothelins, vasoactive intestinal peptide, and thyrotropin-releasing hormone). The presence of these and other receptors on astrocytes provides them with the ability to respond to several stimuli.

Astrocytes can influence neuronal survival and activity through their ability to regulate constituents of the extracellular environment, absorb local excess of neurotransmitters, and release metabolic and neuroactive molecules. The latter molecules include peptides of the angiotensinogen family, vasoactive endothelins, opioid precursors called **enkephalins,** and the potentially neurotrophic somatostatin. On the other hand, there is some evidence that astrocytes transport energy-rich compounds from the blood to the neurons and also metabolize glucose to lactate, which is then supplied to the neurons.

Finally, astrocytes are in direct communication with one another via gap junctions, forming a network through which information can flow from one point to another, reaching distant sites. For example, by means of gap junctions and the release of various cytokines, astrocytes can interact with oligodendrocytes to influence myelin turnover in both normal and abnormal conditions.

Ependymal Cells

Ependymal cells are low columnar epithelial cells lining the ventricles of the brain and central canal of the spinal cord. In some locations, ependymal cells are ciliated, which facilitates the movement of cerebrospinal fluid.

Microglia

Microglia (Gr. *micros,* small, + *glia*) are small elongated cells with short irregular processes (see Figures 9–13 and 9–14). They can be recognized in routine hematoxylin-and-eosin (H&E) preparations by their dense elongated nuclei, which contrast with the spherical nuclei of other glial cells. Microglia, phagocytic cells that represent the mononuclear phagocytic system in nerve tissue, are derived from precursor cells in the bone marrow. They are involved with inflammation and repair in the adult central nervous system, and they produce and release neutral proteases and oxidative radicals. When activated, microglia retract their processes and assume the morphologic characteristics

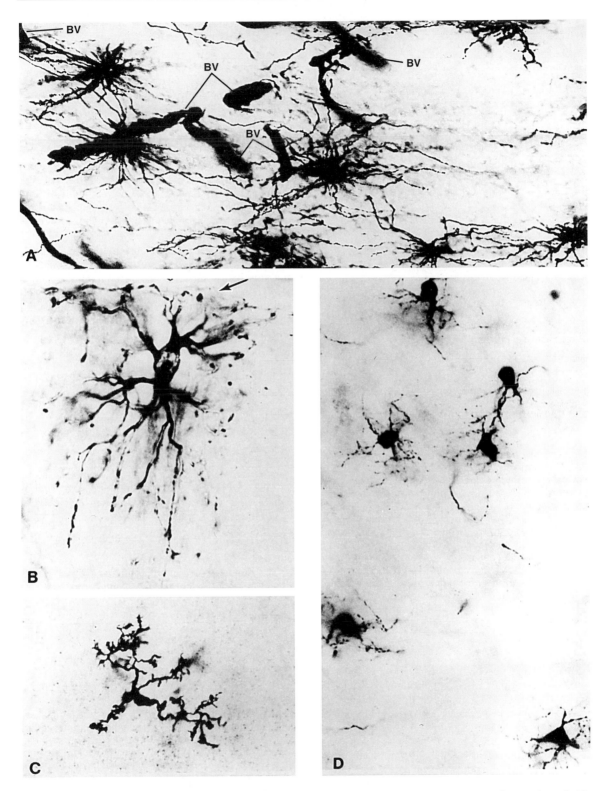

Figure 9–14. Photomicrographs (prepared with Golgi stain) of glial cells from the cerebral cortex of a monkey. **A:** Fibrous astrocytes, showing blood vessels (BV). × 1000. **B:** Protoplasmic astrocyte showing brain surface (arrow). × 1900. **C:** Microglial cell. × 1700. **D:** Oligodendrocytes. × 1900. (Reproduced, with permission, from Jones E, Cowan WM: The nervous tissue. In: *Histology: Cell and Tissue Biology,* 5th ed. Weiss L [editor]. Elsevier, 1983.)

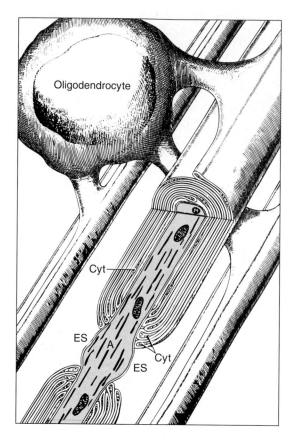

Figure 9–15. Myelin sheath of the central nervous system. The same oligodendrocyte forms myelin sheaths for several (3–50) nerve fibers. In the central nervous system, the nodes of Ranvier are sometimes covered by processes of other cells, or there is considerable extracellular space (ES) at that point. The axolemma shows a thickening where the cell membrane of the oligodendrocyte comes into contact with it. This limits the diffusion of materials into the periaxonal space between the axon and the myelin sheath. At upper left is a surface view of the cell body of an oligodendrocyte. Cyt, cytoplasm of glial cell; A, axon. (Redrawn and reproduced, with permission, from Bunge et al: J Biophys Biochem Cytol 1961;10:67.)

of macrophages, becoming phagocytic and acting as antigen-presenting cells (see Chapter 14). Microglia secrete a number of immunoregulatory cytokines and dispose of unwanted cellular debris caused by central nervous system lesions.

In multiple sclerosis, the myelin sheath is destroyed by an unknown mechanism with severe neurologic consequences. In this disease, microglia phagocytose and degrade myelin debris by receptor-mediated phagocytosis and lysosomal activity. In addition, AIDS dementia complex is caused by HIV-1 infection of the central

nervous system. Overwhelming experimental evidence indicates that perivascular and multinucleated microglia are infected by HIV-1. A number of cytokines, such as interleukin-1 and tumor necrosis factor-α, activate and enhance HIV replication in microglia.

THE CENTRAL NERVOUS SYSTEM

The central nervous system consists of the **cerebrum, cerebellum,** and **spinal cord.** It has virtually no connective tissue and is therefore a relatively soft, gel-like organ.

White & Gray Matter

When sectioned, the cerebrum, cerebellum, and spinal cord show regions of white (**white matter**) and gray (**gray matter**). The differential distribution of myelin in the central nervous system is responsible for these differences: The main component of white matter is myelinated axons (Figure 9–16) and

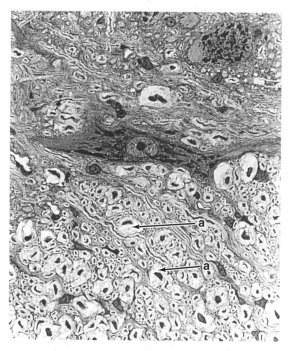

Figure 9–16. Boundary between white matter (below) and gray matter (above). White matter is composed of many myelinated axons (a), which appear in cross section in this photomicrograph. The cells seen in white matter are neuroglial cells, mainly oligodendrocytes responsible for myelin synthesis. Note the elongated neuron with its pale-stained nucleus and typically large, round nucleolus. The neuron cytoplasm contains many dark-stained granules, called Nissl bodies, formed by the precipitation of the rough endoplasmic reticulum and free polyribosomes during tissue processing. × 600.

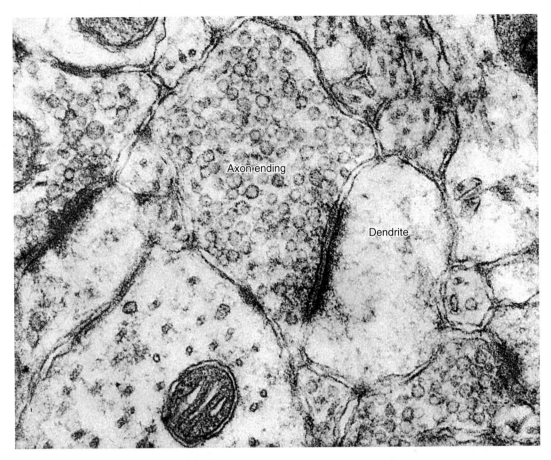

Figure 9–17. Electron micrograph of cerebral cortex. Near the center of the figure is a synapse between one axon ending and a dendrite. The postsynaptic (dendritic) membrane shows a greater accumulation of electron-dense material than does the presynaptic (axonal) membrane. This is an asymmetric synapse. The axon ending contains numerous synaptic vesicles. × 90,000. (Courtesy of A Peters.)

the myelin-producing oligodendrocytes. White matter does not contain neuronal cell bodies.

Gray matter contains neuronal cell bodies, dendrites, and the initial unmyelinated portions of axons and glial cells. This is the region where synapses occur (Figure 9–17). Gray matter is prevalent at the surface of the cerebrum and cerebellum, forming the **cerebral and cerebellar cortex,** whereas white matter is present in more central regions. Aggregates of neuronal cell bodies forming islands of gray matter embedded in the white matter are called **nuclei.** In the **cerebral cortex,** the gray matter has six layers of cells with different forms and sizes. Neurons of some regions of the cerebral cortex register **afferent (sensory)** impulses; in other regions, **efferent (motor)** neurons generate motor impulses that control voluntary movements. Cells of the cerebral cortex are related to the integration of sensory information and the initiation of voluntary motor responses.

The **cerebellar cortex** has three layers (Figures 9–18 and 9–19): an outer molecular layer, a central layer of large Purkinje cells, and an inner granule layer. The Purkinje cells have a conspicuous cell body and their dendrites are highly developed, assuming the aspect of a fan (Figure 9–3). These dendrites occupy most of the molecular layer and are the reason for the sparseness of nuclei. The granule layer is formed by very small neurons (the smallest in the body), which are compactly disposed, in contrast to the less cell-dense molecular layer (Figure 9–19).

In cross sections of the **spinal cord,** white matter is peripheral and gray matter is central, assuming the shape of an H (Figure 9–20). In the horizontal bar of this H is an opening, the **central canal,** which is a remnant of the lumen of the embryonic neural tube. It is lined by ependymal cells. The gray matter of the legs of the H forms the **anterior horns.** These contain motor neurons whose axons make up the ventral roots of the spinal nerves. Gray matter also forms the posterior horns (the arms of the H), which receive sensory fibers from neurons in the spinal ganglia (dorsal roots).

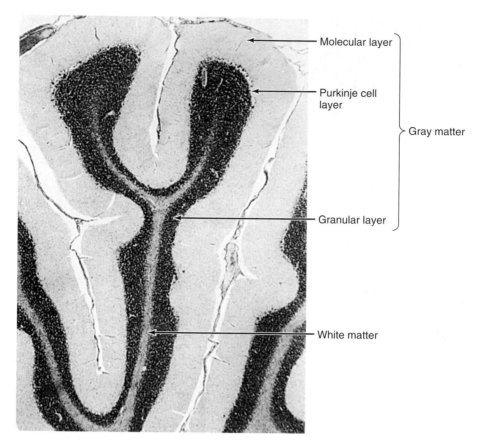

Figure 9–18. Photomicrograph of a portion of cerebellum. Each lobule contains a core of white matter and three layers of gray matter: granular, Purkinje cell, and molecular. H&E stain. × 28.

Spinal cord neurons are large and multipolar, especially in the anterior horns, where large motor neurons are found (Figure 9–20).

MENINGES

The central nervous system is protected by the skull and the vertebral column. It is also encased in membranes of connective tissue called the **meninges** (Figure 9–21). Starting with the outermost layer, the meninges are the **dura mater, arachnoid,** and **pia mater.** The arachnoid and the pia mater are linked together and are often considered a single membrane called the **pia-arachnoid.**

Dura Mater

The dura mater is the external layer (**meninx**) and is composed of dense connective tissue continuous with the periosteum of the skull. The dura mater that envelops the spinal cord is separated from the periosteum of the vertebrae by the epidural space, which contains thin-walled veins, loose connective tissue, and adipose tissue.

The dura mater is always separated from the arachnoid by the thin subdural space. The internal surface of all dura mater, as well as its external surface in the spinal cord, is covered by simple squamous epithelium of mesenchymal origin.

Arachnoid

The arachnoid (Gr. *arachnoeides,* cobweb-like) has two components: a layer in contact with the dura mater, and a system of trabeculae connecting the layer with the pia mater. The cavities between the trabeculae form the **subarachnoid space,** which is filled with cerebrospinal fluid and is completely separated from the **subdural space.** This space forms a hydraulic cushion that protects the central nervous system from trauma. The subarachnoid space communicates with the ventricles of the brain.

The arachnoid is composed of connective tissue devoid of blood vessels. Its surfaces are covered by the same type of simple squamous epithelium that

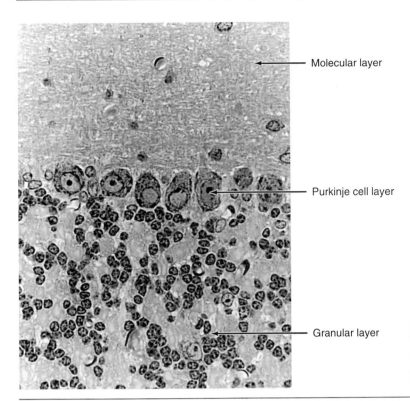

Molecular layer

Purkinje cell layer

Granular layer

Figure 9–19. Photomicrograph of cerebellar cortex. The staining procedure used does not reveal the unusually large dendritic arborization of the Purkinje cell, which is illustrated in Figure 9–3.

covers the dura mater. Since the arachnoid has fewer trabeculae in the spinal cord, it can be more cleanly distinguished from the pia mater in that area.

In some areas, the arachnoid perforates the dura mater, forming protrusions that terminate in venous sinuses in the dura mater. These protrusions, which are covered by endothelial cells of the veins, are called **arachnoid villi.** Their function is to reabsorb cerebrospinal fluid into the blood of the venous sinuses.

Pia Mater

The pia mater is a loose connective tissue containing many blood vessels. Although it is located quite close to the nerve tissue, it is not in contact with nerve cells or fibers. Between the pia mater and the neural elements is a thin layer of neuroglial processes, adhering firmly to the pia mater and forming a physical barrier at the periphery of the central nervous system. This barrier separates the central nervous system from the cerebrospinal fluid (Figure 9–21).

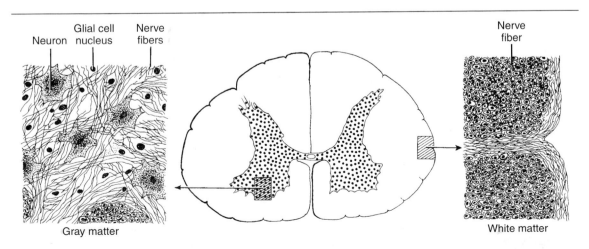

Neuron Glial cell nucleus Nerve fibers

Nerve fiber

Gray matter

White matter

Figure 9–20. Cross section through the spinal cord.

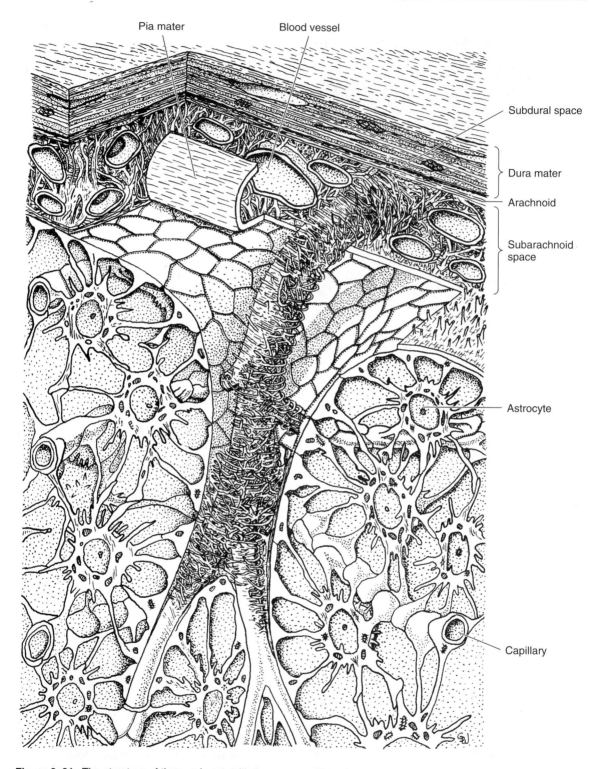

Pia mater

Blood vessel

Subdural space

Dura mater

Arachnoid

Subarachnoid space

Astrocyte

Capillary

Figure 9–21. The structure of the meninges, with the superposition of pia mater, arachnoid, and dura mater. Astrocytes form a three-dimensional net around the neurons (not shown). Note that the foot-like processes of the astrocytes form a continuous layer that involves the blood vessels that contribute to the blood-brain barrier. (Reproduced, with permission, from Krstić RV: *Microscopic Human Anatomy*. Springer-Verlag, 1991.)

The pia mater follows all the irregularities of the surface of the central nervous system and penetrates it to some extent along with the blood vessels. Pia mater is covered by squamous cells of mesenchymal origin.

Blood vessels penetrate the central nervous system through tunnels covered by pia mater—the **perivascular spaces.** The pia mater disappears before the blood vessels are transformed into capillaries. In the central nervous system, the blood capillaries are completely covered by expansions of the neuroglial cell processes (Figure 9–21).

Blood-Brain Barrier

The blood-brain barrier is a functional barrier that prevents the passage of some substances, such as antibiotics and chemical and bacterial toxic matter, from the blood to nerve tissue.

The blood-brain barrier results from the reduced permeability that is a property of blood capillaries of nerve tissue. Occluding junctions, which provide continuity between the endothelial cells of these capillaries, represent the main structural component of the barrier. The cytoplasm of these endothelial cells does not have the fenestrations found in many other locations, and very few pinocytotic vesicles are observed. The expansions of neuroglial cell processes that envelop the capillaries are partly responsible for their low permeability.

CHOROID PLEXUS & CEREBROSPINAL FLUID

The choroid plexus consists of invaginated folds of pia mater that penetrate the interior of the ventricles. It is found in the roofs of the third and fourth ventricles and in part in the walls of the lateral ventricles. It is a vascular structure made up of dilated fenestrated capillaries.

The choroid plexus is composed of loose connective tissue of the pia mater, covered by a simple cuboidal or low columnar epithelium (Figure 9–22) that has the cytologic characteristics of ion-transporting cells (see Chapter 4).

The main function of the choroid plexus is to elaborate cerebrospinal fluid, which contains only a small amount of solids and completely fills the ventricles, central canal of the spinal cord, subarachnoid space, and perivascular space. Cerebrospinal fluid is important for the metabolism of the central nervous system and acts as a protective device.

Cerebrospinal fluid is clear, has a low density (1.004–1.008 g/mL), and is very low in protein content. A few desquamated cells and two to five lymphocytes per milliliter are also present. Cerebrospinal fluid circulates through the ventricles, from which it passes into the subarachnoid space. There, arachnoid villi provide the main pathway for absorption of

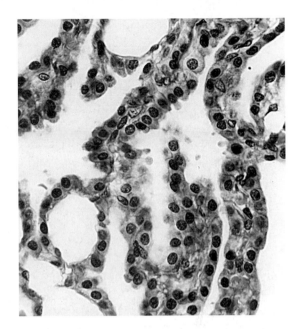

Figure 9–22. Photomicrograph of the choroid plexus. The numerous folds are covered by simple cuboidal epithelium. H&E stain. × 400.

cerebrospinal fluid into the venous circulation. (There are no lymphatic vessels in nerve tissue.)

A decrease in the absorption of cerebrospinal fluid or a blockage of outflow from the ventricles results in the condition known as **hydrocephalus** (Gr. *hydro,* water, + *kephale,* head), which promotes a progressive enlargement of the head followed by mental impairment and muscular weakness.

PERIPHERAL NERVOUS SYSTEM

The main components of the peripheral nervous system are the **nerves, ganglia,** and **nerve endings.** Nerves are bundles of nerve fibers surrounded by a series of connective tissue sheaths.

NERVE FIBERS

Nerve fibers consist of axons enveloped by a special sheath derived from cells of ectodermal origin. Groups of nerve fibers constitute the tracts of the brain, spinal cord, and peripheral nerves. Nerve fibers exhibit differences in their enveloping sheaths, related to whether the fibers are part of the central or the peripheral nervous system.

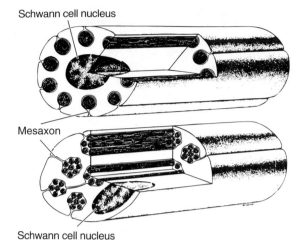

Schwann cell nucleus

Mesaxon

Schwann cell nucleus

Figure 9–23. Upper: The most frequent type of unmyelinated nerve fiber, in which isolated axons (shown in color) are surrounded by a Schwann cell and each axon has its own mesaxon. **Lower:** Many very thin axons are sometimes found together, surrounded by the Schwann cell. In such cases, there is one mesaxon for several axons.

Most axons in adult nerve tissue are covered by single or multiple folds of a sheath cell. In peripheral nerve fibers, the sheath cell is the **Schwann cell,** and in central nerve fibers it is the **oligodendrocyte.** Axons of small diameter are usually **unmyelinated nerve fibers** (Figures 9–23, 9–25, and 9–26). Pro-

gressively thicker axons are generally sheathed by increasingly numerous concentric wrappings of the enveloping cell, forming the **myelin sheaths.** These fibers are known as **myelinated nerve fibers** (Figures 9–24 and 9–25).

Myelinated Fibers

In myelinated fibers of the peripheral nervous system, the plasmalemma of the covering Schwann cell winds and wraps around the axon. The layers of membranes of the sheath cell unite and form **myelin,** a lipoprotein complex whose lipid component can be partly removed by standard histologic procedures (Figures 9–24 and 9–27).

> Myelin consists of many layers of modified cell membranes. These membranes have a higher proportion of lipids than do other cell membranes. Central nervous system myelin contains two major proteins: myelin basic protein and proteolipid protein. Several human demyelinating diseases are due to an insufficiency or lack of one or both of these proteins.

Each axon is surrounded by myelin formed by a sequential series of Schwann cells. The myelin sheath shows gaps along its path called the **nodes of Ranvier** (Figures 9–25 and 9–28); these represent the spaces between adjacent Schwann cells along the length of the axon. Interdigitating processes of Schwann cells partially cover the node. The distance between two nodes is called an **internode** and con-

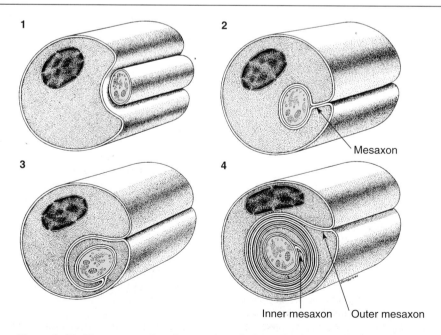

1

2

Mesaxon

3

4

Inner mesaxon   Outer mesaxon

Figure 9–24. Four consecutive phases of myelin formation in peripheral nerve fibers.

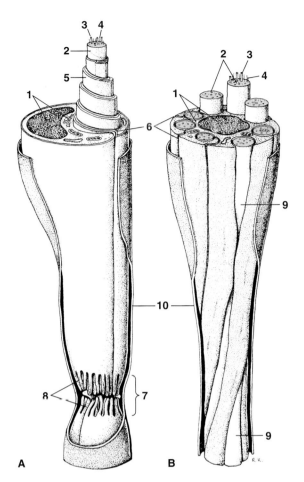

Figure 9–25. Ultrastructural features of myelinated (**A**) and an unmyelinated (**B**) nerve fibers. (1) Nucleus and cytoplasm of a Schwann cell; (2) axon; (3) microtubule; (4) neurofilament; (5) myelin sheath; (6) mesaxon; (7) node of Ranvier; (8) interdigitating processes of Schwann cells at the node of Ranvier; (9) side view of an unmyelinated axon; (10) basal lamina. (Slightly modified and reproduced, with permission, from Krstić RV: *Ultrastructure of the Mammalian Cell.* Springer-Verlag, 1979.)

sists of one Schwann cell. The length of the internode varies between 1 and 2 mm.

There are no Schwann cells in the central nervous system; there, the myelin sheath is formed by the processes of the oligodendrocytes. Oligodendrocytes differ from Schwann cells in that different branches of one cell can envelop segments of several axons (Figure 9–15).

Unmyelinated Fibers

In both the central and peripheral nervous systems, not all axons are sheathed in myelin. In the peripheral system, all unmyelinated axons are enveloped within simple clefts of the Schwann cells (Figure

9–23). Unlike their association with individual myelinated axons, each Schwann cell can sheathe many unmyelinated axons. Unmyelinated nerve fibers do not have nodes of Ranvier, because abutting Schwann cells are united to form a continuous sheath.

The central nervous system is rich in unmyelinated axons; unlike those in the peripheral system, these axons are not sheathed. In the brain and spinal cord, unmyelinated axonal processes run free among the other neuronal and glial processes.

NERVES

In the peripheral nervous system, the nerve fibers are grouped in bundles to form the nerves. Except for a few very thin nerves made up of unmyelinated fibers, nerves have a whitish, homogeneous, glistening appearance because of their myelin and collagen content.

Nerves (Figure 9–29) have an external fibrous coat of dense connective tissue called **epineurium,** which also fills the space between the bundles of nerve fibers. Each bundle is surrounded by the **perineurium,** a sleeve formed by layers of flattened epithelium-like cells. The cells of each layer of the perineurial sleeve are joined at their edges by tight junctions, an arrangement that makes the perineurium a barrier to the passage of most macromolecules and has the important function of protecting the nerve fibers from aggression. Within the perineurial sheath run the Schwann cell–sheathed axons and their enveloping connective tissue, the **endoneurium** (Figure 9–30). The endoneurium consists of a thin layer of reticular fibers. Endoneurial reticular fibers are produced by Schwann cells.

The nerves (Figure 9–29) establish communication between brain and spinal cord centers and the sense organs and effectors (muscles, glands, etc). They possess afferent and efferent fibers to and from the central nervous system. **Afferent** fibers carry the information obtained from the interior of the body and the environment to the central nervous system. **Efferent** fibers carry impulses from the central nervous system to the effector organs commanded by these centers. Nerves possessing only sensory fibers are called **sensory nerves;** those composed only of fibers carrying impulses to the effectors are called **motor nerves.** Most nerves have both sensory and motor fibers and are called **mixed nerves;** these nerves have both myelinated and unmyelinated axons (Figure 9–26).

GANGLIA

Ganglia are ovoid structures containing neuronal cell bodies and glial cells supported by connective

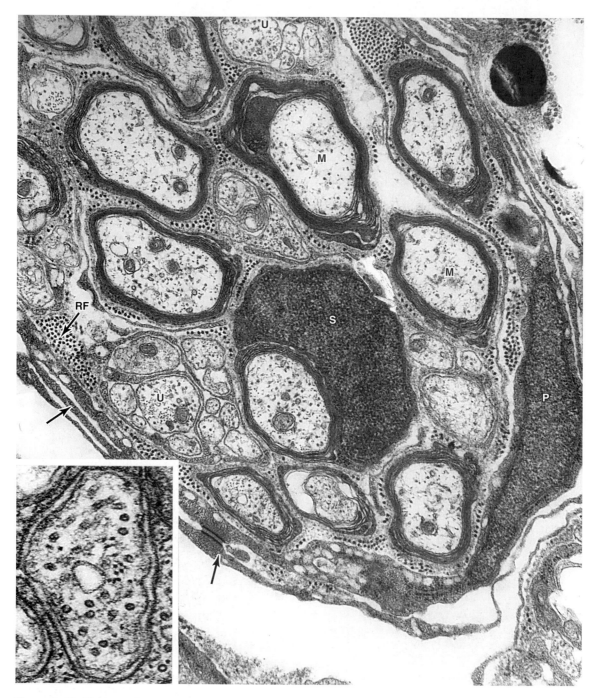

Figure 9–26. Electron micrograph of a peripheral nerve containing both myelinated (M) and unmyelinated (U) nerve fibers. The reticular fibers (RF) seen in cross section belong to the endoneurium. Near the center of the figure is a Schwann cell nucleus (S). The perineurial cells (P, arrows) form a barrier that controls access of materials to nerve tissue. × 30,000. **Inset:** Part of an axon, where numerous neurofilaments and microtubules are seen in cross section. × 60,000.

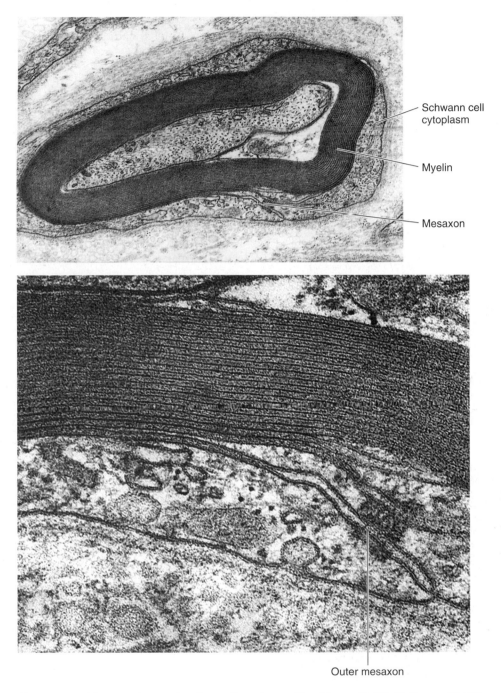

Figure 9–27. Electron micrographs of a myelinated nerve fiber. **Top:** × 20,000. **Bottom:** × 80,000.

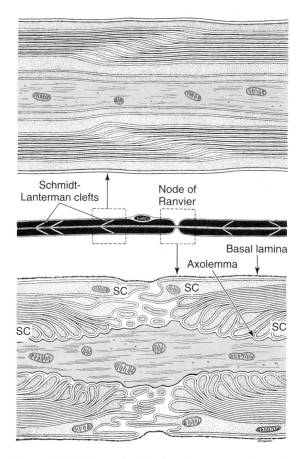

Figure 9–28. The center drawing shows a myelinated peripheral nerve fiber as seen under the light microscope. The process (shown in color) is the axon enveloped by the myelin sheath (black) and by the cytoplasm of Schwann cells. A Schwann cell nucleus, the Schmidt-Lanterman clefts, and a node of Ranvier are shown. The upper drawing shows the ultrastructure of the Schmidt-Lanterman cleft. The cleft is formed by Schwann cell cytoplasm that is not displaced to the periphery during myelin formation. The lower drawing shows the ultrastructure of a node of Ranvier. Note the appearance of loose interdigitating processes of the outer leaf of the Schwann cells' cytoplasm (SC) and the close contact of the inner leaf of the cytoplasm with the axolemma. This contact acts as a sort of barrier to the movement of materials in and out of the periaxonal space between the axolemma and the membrane of the Schwann cell. The basal lamina around the Schwann cell is continuous. Covering the nerve fiber is a connective tissue layer—mainly reticular fiber—that forms the endoneurial sheath of the peripheral nerve fibers.

tissue. Because they serve as relay stations to transmit nerve impulses, one nerve enters and another exits from each ganglion. The direction of the nerve impulse determines whether the ganglion will be a **sensory** or an **autonomic** ganglion.

Sensory Ganglia

Sensory ganglia receive afferent impulses that go to the central nervous system. Two types of sensory ganglia exist. Some are associated with cranial nerves (**cranial ganglia**); others are associated with the dorsal root of the spinal nerves and are called **spinal ganglia.** The latter comprise large neuronal cell bodies with prominent fine Nissl bodies surrounded by abundant small glial cells called **satellite cells** (Figure 9–31).

A connective tissue framework and capsule support the ganglion cells. The neurons of these ganglia are pseudounipolar and relay information from the ganglion's nerve endings to the gray matter of the spinal cord via synapses with local neurons.

Autonomic Ganglia

Autonomic ganglia appear as bulbous dilatations in autonomic nerves. Some are located within certain organs, especially in the walls of the digestive tract, where they constitute the **intramural ganglia.** These ganglia are devoid of connective tissue capsules, and their cells are supported by the stroma of the organ in which they are found.

Autonomic ganglia usually have multipolar neurons (Figure 9–32). As with craniospinal ganglia, autonomic ganglia have neuronal perikaryons with fine Nissl bodies.

The neurons of autonomic ganglia are frequently enveloped by a layer of satellite cells. In intramural ganglia, only a few satellite cells are seen around each neuron. Afferent nerve endings are associated with sensory receptors, discussed in Chapter 24. Efferent nerve endings to muscle tissue are discussed in Chapter 10.

AUTONOMIC NERVOUS SYSTEM

The autonomic (Gr. *autos,* self, + *nomos,* law) nervous system is related to the control of smooth muscle, the secretion of some glands, and the modulation of cardiac rhythm. Its function is to make adjustments in certain activities of the body to maintain a constant internal environment (**homeostasis**). Although the autonomic nervous system is by definition a motor system, fibers that receive sensation originating in the interior of the organism accompany the motor fibers of the autonomic system.

The term "autonomic" is not correct—although it is widely used—inasmuch as most of the functions of the autonomic nervous system are not autonomous at all; they are organized and regulated in the central

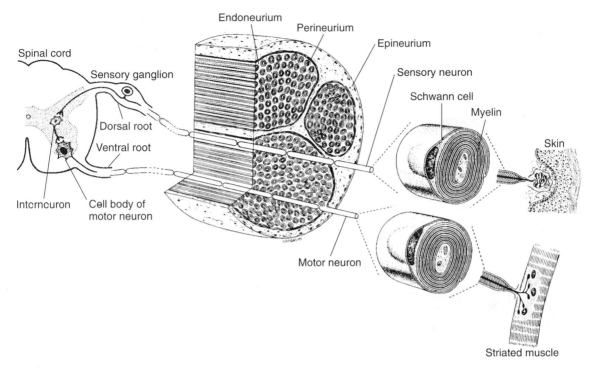

Figure 9–29. Schematic representation of a nerve and a reflex arc. In this example, the sensory stimulus starts in the skin and passes to the spinal cord via the dorsal root ganglion. The sensory stimulus then activates a motor neuron innervating skeletal muscle. Examples of the operation of this reflex are withdrawal of the finger from a hot surface and the knee-jerk reflex. (Slightly modified, redrawn, and reproduced, with permission, from Ham AW: *Histology,* 6th ed. Lippincott, 1969.)

nervous system. The concept of the autonomic nervous system is mainly functional. Anatomically, it is composed of collections of nerve cells located in the central nervous system, fibers that leave the central nervous system through cranial or spinal nerves, and nerve ganglia situated in the paths of these fibers. The term "autonomic" covers all the neural elements concerned with visceral function. In fact, the so-called autonomic functions are as dependent on the central nervous system as are the motor neurons that trigger muscle contractions.

The autonomic nervous system is a two-neuron network. The first neuron of the autonomic chain is located in the central nervous system. Its axon forms a synapse with the second multipolar neuron in the chain, located in a ganglion of the peripheral nervous system. The nerve fibers (axons) of the first neuron are called **preganglionic fibers;** the axons of the second neuron to the effectors—muscle or gland—are called **postganglionic fibers.** The chemical mediator present in the synaptic vesicles of all preganglionic endings and at anatomically parasympathetic postganglionic endings is **acetylcholine,** which is released from the terminals by nerve impulses.

The adrenal medulla is the only organ that receives preganglionic fibers, because the majority of the cells, after migration into the gland, differentiate into secretory cells rather than ganglion cells.

The autonomic nervous system is composed of two parts that differ both anatomically and functionally: the sympathetic system and the parasympathetic system (Figure 9–33). Nerve fibers that release acetylcholine are called **cholinergic.** Cholinergic fibers include all the preganglionic autonomic fibers (sympathetic as well as parasympathetic) and postganglionic parasympathetic fibers to smooth muscles, heart, and exocrine glands (Figure 9–33).

Sympathetic System

The nuclei (formed by a collection of nerve cell bodies) of the sympathetic system are located in the thoracic and lumbar segments of the spinal cord. Therefore, the sympathetic system is also called the **thoracolumbar division** of the autonomic nervous system. The axons of these neurons—preganglionic fibers—leave the central nervous system by way of the ventral roots and white communicating rami of the thoracic and lumbar nerves. The chemical media-

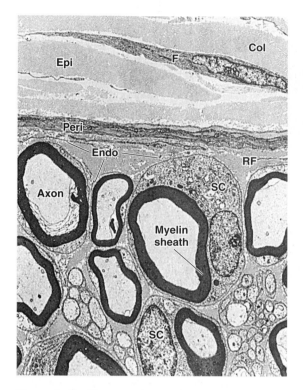

Figure 9–30. Electron micrograph of a cross section through a nerve, showing the epineurium (Epi), the perineurium (Peri), and the endoneurium (Endo). The epineurium is a dense connective tissue rich in collagen fibers (Col) and fibroblasts (F). The perineurium is made up of several layers of flat cells tightly joined together to form a barrier to the penetration of the nerve by macromolecules. The endoneurium is composed mainly of reticular fibers (RF) synthesized by Schwann cells. × 1200.

tor of the postganglionic fibers of the sympathetic system is **norepinephrine,** which is also produced by the adrenal medulla. Nerve fibers that release norepinephrine are called **adrenergic** (a word derived from noradrenalin, another term for norepinephrine). Adrenergic fibers innervate sweat glands and blood vessels of skeletal muscle. Cells of the adrenal medulla release a mixture of epinephrine and norepinephrine in response to preganglionic sympathetic stimulation.

Parasympathetic System

The parasympathetic system has its nuclei in the medulla and midbrain and in the sacral portion of the spinal cord. The preganglionic fibers of these neurons leave through four of the cranial nerves (III, VII, IX, and X) and also through the second, third, and fourth sacral spinal nerves. The parasympathetic system is therefore also called the craniosacral division of the autonomic system.

The second neuron of the parasympathetic series is found in ganglia smaller than those of the sympathetic system; it is always located near or within the effector organs. These neurons are usually located in the walls of organs (eg, stomach, intestines), in which case the preganglionic fibers enter the organs and form a synapse there with the second neuron in the chain.

The chemical mediator released by the pre- and postganglionic nerve endings of the parasympathetic system, **acetylcholine,** is readily inactivated by acetylcholinesterase—one of the reasons parasympathetic stimulation has both a more discrete and a more localized action than does sympathetic stimulation.

Distribution

Most of the organs innervated by the autonomic nervous system receive both sympathetic and parasympathetic fibers (Figure 9–33). Generally, in organs where one system is the stimulator, the other has an inhibitory action.

DEGENERATION & REGENERATION OF NERVE TISSUE

Although it has been shown that neurons can divide in the brain of adult birds, mammalian neurons usually do not divide, and their degeneration represents a permanent loss. Neuronal processes in the central nervous system are, within very narrow limits, replaceable by growth through the synthetic activity of their perikaryons. Peripheral nerve fibers can also regenerate if their perikaryons are not destroyed.

Death of a nerve cell is limited to its perikaryon and processes. The neurons functionally connected to the dead neuron do not die, except for those with only one link. In this latter instance, the isolated neuron undergoes **transneuronal degeneration.**

In contrast to nerve cells, neuroglia of the central nervous system—and Schwann cells and ganglionic satellite cells of the peripheral nervous system—are able to divide by mitosis. Spaces in the central nervous system left by nerve cells lost by disease or injury are invaded by neuroglia.

Since nerves are widely distributed throughout the body, they are often injured. When a nerve axon is transected, degenerative changes take place, followed by a reparative phase.

In a wounded nerve fiber, it is important to distinguish the changes occurring in the proximal segment from those in the distal segment. The proximal segment maintains its continuity with the trophic center (perikaryon) and frequently regenerates. The distal segment, separated from the nerve cell body, degenerates (Figure 9–34).

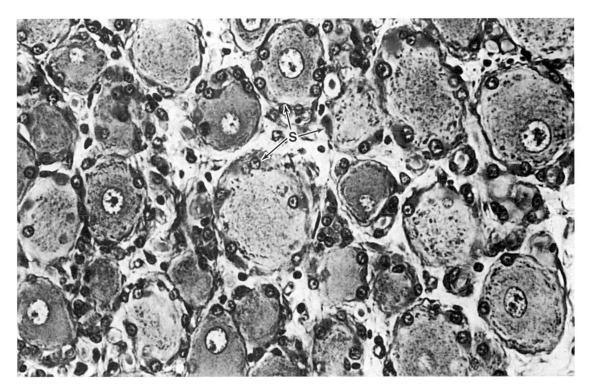

Figure 9–31. Photomicrograph of a spinal ganglion section showing neurons and satellite cells (S). Azan stain. × 300. (Reproduced, with permission, from Junqueira LC, Carneiro J: *Histologie.* Schiebler TH, Peiper U [translators]. Springer-Verlag, 1984.)

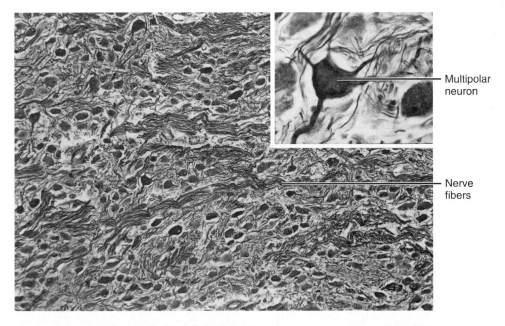

Multipolar
neuron

Nerve
fibers

Figure 9–32. Photomicrograph of a silver-stained section from an autonomic nerve ganglion. Neurons and nerve fibers appear black. × 80. **Inset:** A multipolar neuron. × 250.

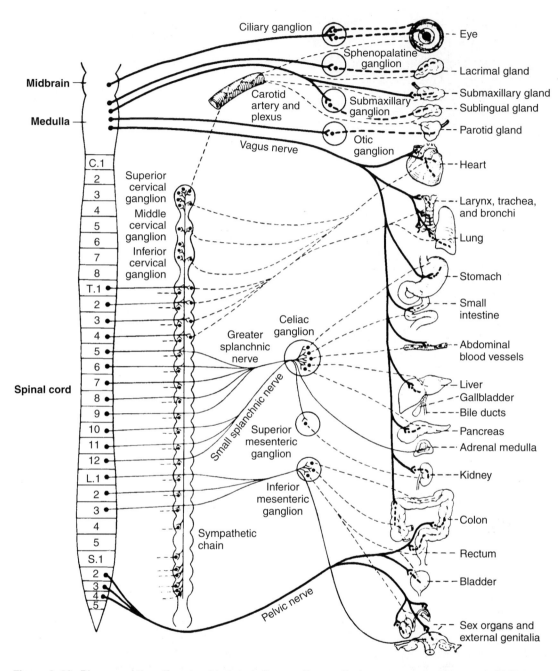

Figure 9–33. Diagram of the efferent autonomic pathways. Preganglionic neurons are shown as solid lines, postganglionic neurons as dotted lines. The heavy lines are parasympathetic fibers; the light lines are sympathetic fibers. (Slightly modified and reproduced, with permission, from Youmans W: *Fundamentals of Human Physiology,* 2nd ed. Year Book, 1962.)

Axonal injury causes several changes in the perikaryon: **chromatolysis,** ie, dissolution of Nissl substances with a consequent decrease in cytoplasmic basophilia; an increase in the volume of the perikaryon; and migration of the nucleus to a peripheral position in the perikaryon. The proximal segment of the axon degenerates close to the wound for a short distance, but growth starts as soon as debris is removed by macrophages. Macrophages produce interleukin-1, which stimulates Schwann cells to secrete substances that promote nerve growth.

In the nerve stub distal to the injury, both the axon (now separated from its trophic center) and the myelin sheath degenerate completely, and their rem-

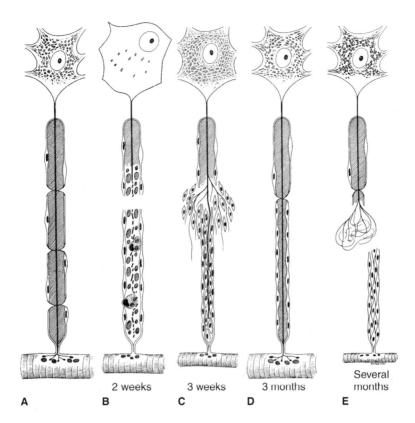

Figure 9–34. Main changes that take place in an injured nerve fiber. **A:** Normal nerve fiber, with its perikaryon and effector cell (striated skeletal muscle). Note the position of the neuron nucleus and the quantity and distribution of Nissl bodies. **B:** When the fiber is injured, the neuronal nucleus moves to the cell periphery, and Nissl bodies become greatly reduced in number. The nerve fiber distal to the injury degenerates along with its myelin sheath. Debris is phagocytosed by macrophages. **C:** The muscle fiber shows a pronounced denervation atrophy. Schwann cells proliferate, forming a compact cord penetrated by the growing axon. The axon grows at the rate of 0.5–3 mm/day. **D:** Here, the nerve fiber regeneration was successful. Note that the muscle fiber was also regenerated after receiving nerve stimuli. **E:** When the axon does not penetrate the cord of Schwann cells, its growth is not organized. (Redrawn and reproduced, with permission, from Willis RA, Willis AF: *The Principles of Pathology and Bacteriology,* 3rd ed. Butterworth, 1972.)

nants, excluding their connective tissue and perineurial sheaths, are removed by macrophages. While these regressive changes take place, Schwann cells proliferate within the remaining connective tissue sleeve, giving rise to solid cellular columns. These rows of Schwann cells serve as guides to the sprouting axons formed during the reparative phase.

After the regressive changes, the proximal segment of the axon grows and branches, forming several filaments that progress in the direction of the columns of Schwann cells. Only fibers that penetrate these Schwann cell columns will continue to grow and reach an effector organ (Figure 9–34).

When there is an extensive gap between the distal and proximal segments, or when the distal segment disappears altogether (as in the case of amputation of a limb), the newly grown nerve fibers may form a swelling, or **neuroma,** that can be the source of spontaneous pain (Figure 9–34).

Regeneration is functionally efficient only when the fibers and the columns of Schwann cells are directed to the correct place. The possibility is good, however, since each regenerating fiber gives origin to several processes, and each column of Schwann cells receives processes from several regenerating fibers. In an injured mixed nerve, however, if regenerating sensory fibers grow into columns connected to motor end-plates that were occupied by motor fibers, the function of the muscle will not be reestablished.

Neuronal Plasticity

Despite its general stability, the nervous system exhibits some plasticity in adults. Plasticity is very high during embryonic development, when an excess of nerve cells is formed and the ones that do not establish correct synapses with other neurons are eliminated. Several studies made in adult mammals have shown that, after an injury, the neuronal circuits may be reorganized by the growth of neuronal processes, forming new synapses to replace the ones lost by injury. Thus, new communications are established with some degree of functional recovery. This property of nerve tissue is known as **neuronal plasticity.** The regenerative processes in the nervous system are controlled by several growth factors produced by neu-

rons, glial cells, Schwann cells, and target cells. These growth factors form a family of molecules called **neurotrophins.**

Tumors of the Nervous System

Virtually all cells of the nerve tissue generate tumors. Glial cells produce gliomas, immature nerve cells produce **medulloblastomas,** and Schwann cells produce **schwannomas.** Because adult neurons do not divide, they do not produce tumors.

REFERENCES

Alberts B et al: *Molecular Biology of the Cell,* 3rd ed. Garland, 1994.

Axelrod J: Neurotransmitters. Sci Am 1974;230:58.

Bothwell M: Functional interactions of neurotrophins and neurotrophin receptors. Annu Rev Neurosci 1995;18:223.

Brightmann MW et al: The blood-brain barrier to proteins under normal and pathological conditions. J Neurol Sci 1970;10:215.

Giulian D, Carpuz M: Neuroglial secretion products and their impact on the nervous system. Adv Neurology 1993;59:315.

Heuser JE, Reese TS: Evidence for recycling of synaptic vesicle membrane during transmitter release at the frog neuromuscular junction. J Cell Biol 1973;57:315.

Heuser JE, Reese TS: Structural changes after transmitter release at the frog neuromuscular junction. J Cell Biol 1981;88:564.

Hubbard JI (editor): *The Peripheral Nervous System.* Plenum Press, 1974.

Jacobson M, Hunt RK: The origins of nerve-cell specificity. Sci Am 1973;228:26.

Kahn MA, de Vellis J: Growth factors in the CNS and their effects on oligodendroglia. Prog Brain Res 1995;105:145.

Keynes RD: Ion channels in the nerve-cell membrane. Sci Am 1979;240:126.

Lancaster IC Jr: Nitric oxide in cells. Am Sci 1992;80:248.

Landon DN (editor): *The Peripheral Nerve.* Chapman & Hall, 1976.

Morell P, Norton WT: Myelin. Sci Am 1980;242:88.

Murphy S (editor): *Astrocytes: Pharmacology and Function.* Academic Press, 1993.

Palay SL, Chan-Palay V: *Cerebellar Cortex, Cytology and Organization.* Springer-Verlag, 1974.

Patterson PH: Cytokines in Alzheimers disease and multiple sclerosis. Curr Opin Neurobiol 1995;5:642.

Peters A et al: *The Fine Structure of the Nervous System: The Neurons and Supporting Cells.* Saunders, 1976.

Reichardt LF, Kelly RB: A molecular description of nerve terminal function. Annu Rev Biochem 1983;52:871.

Rodgers RJ et al: Animal models of anxiety: an ethological perspective. Braz J Med Biol Res 1997;30:289.

Saffell JL et al: Axonal growth mediated by cell adhesion molecules requires activation of fibroblast growth factor receptors. Biochem Soc Trans 1995;23:469.

Schwartz JH: Axonal transport: components, mechanisms, and specificity. Annu Rev Neurosci 1979;2:467.

Sears TA (editor): *Neuronal-Glial Cell Interrelationships.* Springer-Verlag, 1982.

Shepherd GM: Microcircuits in the nervous system. Sci Am 1978;238:93.

Stevens CF: The neuron. Sci Am 1979;241:55.

Thoenen H: Neurotrophins and neuronal plasticity. Science 1995;270:593.

Muscle Tissue

10

Muscle tissue is composed of differentiated cells containing contractile proteins. The structural biology of these proteins generates the forces necessary for cellular contraction, which drives movement within certain organs and the body as a whole. Most muscle cells are of mesodermal origin, and they are differentiated mainly by a gradual process of lengthening, with simultaneous synthesis of myofibrillar proteins.

Three types of muscle tissue in mammals can be distinguished on the basis of morphologic and functional characteristics (Figure 10–1), and each type of muscle tissue has a structure adapted to its physiologic role. **Skeletal muscle** is composed of bundles of very long, cylindrical, multinucleated cells that show cross-striations. Their contraction is quick, forceful, and usually under voluntary control. It is caused by the interaction of thin actin filaments and thick myosin filaments whose molecular configuration allows them to slide upon one another. The forces necessary for sliding are generated by weak interactions in the bridges that bind actin to myosin. **Cardiac muscle** also has cross-striations and is composed of elongated, branched individual cells that lie parallel to each other. At sites of end-to-end contact are the **intercalated disks,** structures found only in cardiac muscle. Contraction of cardiac muscle is involuntary, vigorous, and rhythmic. **Smooth muscle** consists of collections of fusiform cells that do not show striations in the light microscope. Their contraction process is slow and not subject to voluntary control.

Some muscle cell organelles have names that differ from their counterparts in other cells. The cytoplasm of muscle cells (excluding the myofibrils) is called **sarcoplasm** (Gr. *sarkos,* flesh, + *plasma,* thing formed), and the smooth endoplasmic reticulum is called **sarcoplasmic reticulum.** The **sarcolemma** (*sarkos* + Gr. *lemma,* husk) is the cell membrane, or plasmalemma.

SKELETAL MUSCLE

Skeletal muscle consists of **muscle fibers,** bundles of very long (up to 30 cm) cylindrical multinucleated

cells with a diameter of 10–100 μm. Multinucleation results from the fusion of embryonic mononucleated myoblasts (muscle cell precursors). The oval nuclei are usually found at the periphery of the cell under the cell membrane. This characteristic nuclear location is helpful in distinguishing skeletal muscle from cardiac and smooth muscle, both of which have centrally located nuclei.

The variation in diameter of skeletal muscle fibers depends on such factors as the specific muscle and the age and sex, state of nutrition, and physical training of the individual. It is a common observation that exercise enlarges the musculature and decreases fat depots. The increase in muscle thus obtained is caused by formation of new myofibrils and a pronounced growth in the diameter of individual muscle fibers. This process, characterized by augmentation of cell volume, is called **hypertrophy** (Gr. *hyper,* above, + *trophe,* nourishment); tissue growth by an increase in the number of cells is termed **hyperplasia** (*hyper* + Gr. *plasis,* molding). Hyperplasia does not occur in either skeletal or cardiac muscle but does take place in smooth muscle, whose cells have not lost the capacity to divide by mitosis. Hyperplasia is rather frequent in organs such as the uterus, where both hyperplasia and hypertrophy occur during pregnancy.

Organization of Skeletal Muscle

The masses of fibers that make up the various types of muscle are not grouped in random fashion but are arranged in regular bundles surrounded by the **epimysium** (Gr. *epi,* upper, + *mys,* muscle), an external sheath of dense connective tissue surrounding the entire muscle (Figure 10–2). From the epimysium, thin septa of connective tissue extend inward, surrounding the bundles of fibers within a muscle. The connective tissue around each bundle of muscle fibers is called the **perimysium** (Gr. *peri,* around, + *mys*). Each muscle fiber is itself surrounded by a delicate layer of connective tissue, the **endomysium** (Gr. *endon,* within, + *mys*), composed mainly of a basal lamina and reticular fibers.

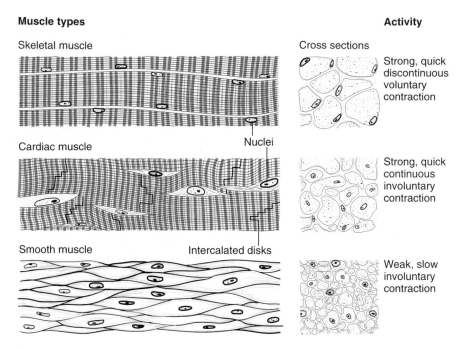

Figure 10–1. Structure of the three muscle types. The drawings at right show these muscles in cross section. Skeletal muscle is composed of large, elongated, multinucleated fibers. Cardiac muscle is composed of irregular branched cells bound together longitudinally by intercalated disks. Smooth muscle is an agglomerate of fusiform cells. The density of the packing between the cells depends on the amount of extracellular connective tissue present.

One of the most important roles of connective tissue is to mechanically transmit the forces generated by contracting muscle cells, because in most instances, individual muscle cells do not extend from one end of a muscle to the other.

Blood vessels penetrate the muscle within the connective tissue septa and form a rich capillary network that runs between and parallel to the muscle fibers. The capillaries are of the continuous type, and lymphatic vessels are found in the connective tissue.

Some muscles taper off at their extremities, where a myotendinous junction is formed. The electron microscope shows that in this transitional region, collagen fibers of the tendon insert themselves into complex infoldings of the plasmalemma of the muscle fibers.

Organization of Skeletal Muscle Fibers

As observed with the light microscope, longitudinally sectioned muscle cells or fibers show cross-striations of alternating light and dark bands (Figures 10–3 and 10–4). The darker bands are called **A bands (anisotropic,** ie, are birefringent in polarized light); the lighter bands are called **I bands (isotropic,** ie, do not alter polarized light). In the electron microscope, each I band is bisected by a dark transverse line, the **Z line.** The smallest repetitive subunit of the

contractile apparatus, the **sarcomere** (*sarkos* + Gr. *mere,* part), extends from Z line to Z line (Figures 10–5 and 10–6) and is about 2.5 µm long in resting muscle.

The sarcoplasm is filled with long cylindrical filamentous bundles called **myofibrils.** The myofibrils, which have a diameter of 1–2 µm and run parallel to the long axis of the muscle fiber, consist of an end-to-end chain-like arrangement of sarcomeres (Figures 10–5 and 10–6). The lateral registration of sarcomeres in adjacent myofibrils causes the entire muscle fiber to exhibit a characteristic pattern of transverse striations.

Studies with the electron microscope reveal that this sarcomere pattern is due mainly to the presence of two types of filaments—thick and thin—that lie parallel to the long axis of the myofibrils in a symmetric pattern.

The thick filaments are 1.6 µm long and 15 nm wide; they occupy the A band, the central portion of the sarcomere. The thin filaments run between and parallel to the thick filaments and have one end attached to the Z line (Figures 10–5 and 10–6). Thin filaments are 1.0 µm long and 8 nm wide. As a result of this arrangement, the I bands consist of the portions of the thin filaments that do not overlap the thick filaments. The A bands are composed mainly of thick filaments in addition to portions of overlapping

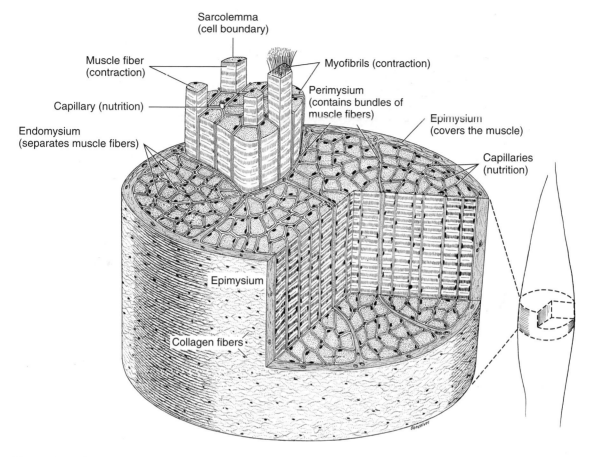

Figure 10–2. Structure and function of skeletal muscle. The drawing at right shows the area of muscle detailed in the enlarged segment. Color highlights endomysium, perimysium, and epimysium.

thin filaments. Close observation of the A band shows the presence of a lighter zone in its center, the **H band,** that corresponds to a region consisting only of the rod-like portions of the myosin molecule (Figures 10–5 and 10–6). Bisecting the H band is the **M line,** a region where lateral connections are made between adjacent thick filaments (Figure 10–6). The major protein of the M line is creatine kinase. Creatine kinase catalyzes the transfer of a phosphate group from phosphocreatine (a storage form of high-energy phosphate groups) to ADP, thus providing the supply of ATP necessary for muscle contraction.

Thin and thick filaments overlap for some distance within the A band. As a consequence, a cross section in the region of filament overlap shows each thick filament surrounded by six thin filaments in the form of a hexagon (Figures 10–6 and 10–7).

Striated muscle filaments contain several proteins; the four main proteins are actin, tropomyosin, troponin, and myosin. Thin filaments are composed of the first three proteins, whereas thick filaments con-

sist primarily of myosin. Myosin and actin together represent 55% of the total protein of striated muscle.

Actin is present as long filamentous (F-actin) polymers consisting of two strands of globular (G-actin) monomers, 5.6 nm in diameter, twisted around each other in a double helical formation (Figure 10–6). A notable characteristic of all G-actin molecules is their structural asymmetry. When G-actin molecules polymerize to form F-actin, they bind back to front, producing a filament with distinguishable polarity (Figure 10–8). Each G-actin monomer contains a binding site for myosin (Figure 10–9). Actin filaments, which anchor perpendicularly on the Z line, exhibit opposite polarity on each side of the line (Figure 10–6). The protein α-actinin, a major component of the Z line, is thought to anchor the actin filaments to this region. α-actinin and desmin (an intermediate filament protein) are believed to tie adjacent sarcomeres together, thus keeping the myofibrils in register.

Tropomyosin, a long, thin molecule about 40 nm

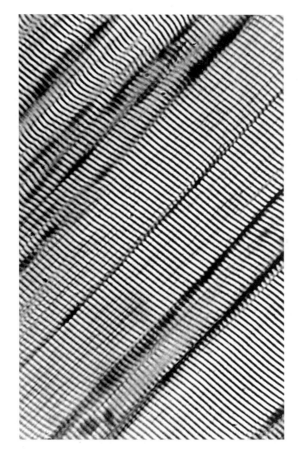

Figure 10–3. Photomicrograph of a section of skeletal muscle observed with the polarizing microscope. The appearance of the A bands as bright birefringement stripes is due to the highly ordered myosin molecules of the thick filaments. The I bands are dark. × 700.

tions at one end of each heavy chain form the heads, which have ATP binding sites as well as the enzymatic capacity to hydrolyze ATP (ATPase activity) and the ability to bind to actin. The four light chains are associated with the head (Figure 10–6). Several hundred myosin molecules are arranged within each thick filament with their rod-like portions overlapping and their globular heads directed toward either end (Figure 10–6).

Analysis of thin sections of striated muscle shows the presence of cross-bridges between thin and thick filaments. These bridges are known to be formed by the head of the myosin molecule plus a short part of its rod-like portion. These bridges are considered to be directly involved in the conversion of chemical energy into mechanical energy (Figure 10–9).

Sarcoplasmic Reticulum & Transverse Tubule System

The depolarization of the sarcoplasmic reticulum membrane, which results in the release of Ca^{2+} ions, is initiated at a specialized myoneural junction on the surface of the muscle cell. Surface-initiated depolarization signals would have to diffuse throughout the cell to effect the release of Ca^{2+} from internal sarcoplasmic reticulum cisternae. In larger muscle cells, the diffusion of the depolarization signal would lead to a wave of contraction, with peripheral myofibrils contracting before more centrally positioned myofibrils do. To provide for a uniform contraction, skeletal muscle possesses a system of **transverse (T) tubules** (Figure 10–10). These finger-like invaginations of the sarcolemma form a complex anastomosing network of tubules that encircle the boundaries of the A–I bands of each sarcomere in every myofibril (Figures 10–11 and 10–12).

Adjacent to opposite sides of each T tubule are expanded **terminal cisternae** of the sarcoplasmic reticulum. This specialized complex, consisting of a T tubule with two lateral portions of sarcoplasmic reticulum, is known as the **triad** (Figures 10–5, 10–11, and 10–12). At the triad, depolarization of the sarcolemma-derived T tubules is transmitted to the sarcoplasmic reticulum membrane.

As described above, muscle contraction depends on the availability of Ca^{2+} ions, and muscle relaxation is related to an absence of Ca^{2+}. The sarcoplasmic reticulum specifically regulates calcium flow, which is necessary for rapid contraction and relaxation cycles. The sarcoplasmic reticulum system consists of a branching network of smooth endoplasmic reticulum cisternae surrounding each myofibril (Figure 10–12). After a neurally mediated depolarization of the sarcoplasmic reticulum membrane, Ca^{2+} ions concentrated within the sarcoplasmic reticulum cisternae are passively released into the vicinity of the overlapping thick and thin filaments, whereupon they bind to troponin and allow bridging between actin and myosin. When the membrane depolarization

in length, contains two polypeptide chains. These molecules are bound head to tail, forming filaments that run over the actin subunits alongside the outer edges of the groove between the two twisted actin strands (Figure 10–8).

Troponin is a complex of three subunits: **TnT,** which strongly attaches to tropomyosin; **TnC,** which binds calcium ions; and **TnI,** which inhibits the actin-myosin interaction. A troponin complex is attached at one specific site on each tropomyosin molecule (Figure 10–8).

In thin filaments, each tropomyosin molecule spans seven G-actin molecules and has one troponin complex bound to its surface (Figure 10–8).

Myosin is a much larger complex (molecular mass ~ 500 kDa). Myosin can be dissociated into two identical heavy chains and two pairs of light chains. Myosin heavy chains are thin, rod-like molecules (150 nm long and 2–3 nm thick) made up of two heavy chains twisted together. Small globular projec-

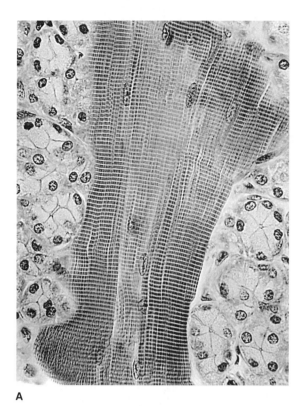 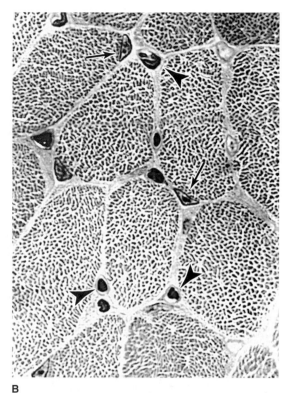

A   B

Figure 10–4. Photomicrographs of sections of skeletal muscle. **A:** Longitudinal section showing the transverse (cross) striations of the skeletal muscle fibers. The brightness of the striations in this figure is the reverse of that observed in Figure 10–3, owing to the polarization optics used for that figure. × 700. **B:** Transverse section. Note the individual myofibrils surrounded by a clear space that is occupied mainly by unstained smooth endoplasmic reticulum and mitochondria. The space between the fibers is occupied by blood capillaries (arrowheads) and the endomycium. Note the peripherally located muscle fiber nuclei (arrows) × 1000.

ends, the sarcoplasmic reticulum acts as a calcium sink and actively transports the Ca^{2+} back into the cisternae, resulting in the cessation of contractile activity.

Mechanism of Contraction

Resting sarcomeres consist of partially overlapping thick and thin filaments. During contraction, both the thick and thin filaments retain their original length. Since contraction is not caused by a shortening of individual filaments, it must be the result of an increase in the amount of overlap between the filaments. The **sliding filament** hypothesis of muscle contraction has received the most widespread acceptance.

The following is a brief description of how actin and myosin interact during a contraction cycle. At rest, ATP binds to the ATPase site on the myosin heads, but the rate of hydrolysis is very slow. Myosin requires actin as a cofactor to break down ATP rapidly and release energy. In a resting muscle,

myosin cannot associate with actin, because the binding sites for myosin heads on actin molecules are covered by the troponin-tropomyosin complex on the F-actin filament (Figure 10–9, top). When sufficiently high concentrations of calcium ions are available, however, they bind to the TnC subunit of troponin. The spatial configuration of the three troponin subunits changes and drives the tropomyosin molecule deeper into the groove of the actin helix (Figure 10–9). This exposes the myosin-binding site on the globular actin components, so that actin is free to interact with the head of the myosin molecule.

The binding of calcium ions to the TnC unit corresponds to the stage at which myosin-ATP is converted into the active complex. As a result of bridging between the myosin head and the G-actin subunit of the thin filament, the ATP is split into ADP and Pi, and energy is released. This activity leads to a deformation, or bending, of the head and a part of the rod-like portion (hinge region) of the myosin (Figure 10–9). Since the actin is bound to the myosin, move-

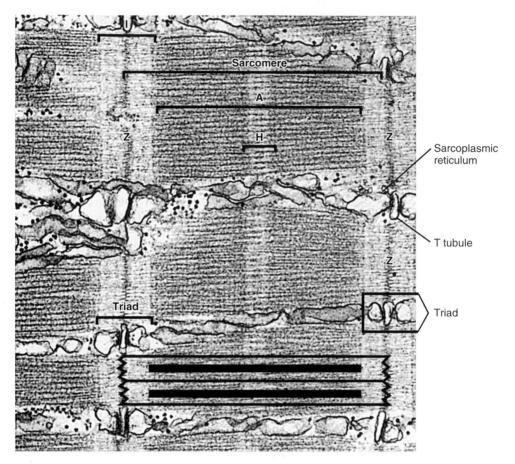

Figure 10–5. Electron micrograph of skeletal muscle of a tadpole. Note the sarcomere with its A, I, and H bands and Z line. The position of the thick and thin filaments in the sarcomere is shown schematically in the lower part of the figure. As illustrated here, triads in amphibian muscle are aligned with the Z line in each sarcomere. In mammalian muscle, however, each sarcomere exhibits two triads, one at each A–I band interface (see Figure 10–11). × 35,000. (Courtesy of KR Porter.)

ment of the myosin head pulls the actin past the myosin filament. The result is that the thin filament is drawn farther into the A band.

Although a large number of myosin heads extend from the thick filament, at any one time during the contraction only a small number of heads align with available actin-binding sites. As the bound myosin heads move the actin, however, they provide for alignment of new actin-myosin bridges. The old actin-myosin bridges detach only after the myosin binds a new ATP molecule; this action also resets the myosin head and prepares it for another contraction cycle. If no ATP is available, the actin-myosin complex becomes stable; this accounts for the extreme muscular rigidity (**rigor mortis**) that occurs after death. A single muscle contraction is the result of hundreds of bridge-forming and bridge-breaking cycles. The contraction activity that leads to a complete overlap between thin and thick filaments continues until Ca^{2+} ions are removed and the troponin-

tropomyosin complex again covers the myosin binding site.

During contraction, the I band decreases in size as thin filaments penetrate the A band. The H band— the part of the A band with only thick filaments—diminishes in width as the thin filaments completely overlap the thick filaments. A net result is that each sarcomere, and consequently the whole cell (fiber), is greatly shortened (Figure 10–13).

Innervation

Myelinated motor nerves branch out within the perimysial connective tissue, where each nerve gives rise to several terminal twigs. At the site of innervation, the nerve loses its myelin sheath and forms a dilated termination that sits within a trough on the muscle cell surface. This structure is called the **motor end-plate,** or **myoneural junction** (Figure 10–13). At this site, the axon is covered by a thin cytoplasmic layer of Schwann cells. Within the axon terminal are

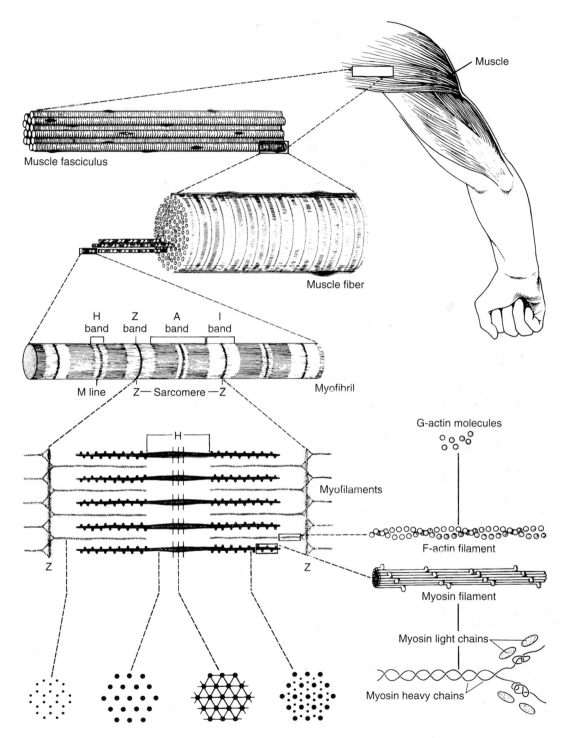

Figure 10–6. Structure and position of the thick and thin filaments in the sarcomere. The molecular structure of these components is shown at right. (Drawing by Sylvia Colard Keene. Reproduced, with permission, from Bloom W, Fawcett DW: *A Textbook of Histology,* 9th ed, Saunders, 1968.)

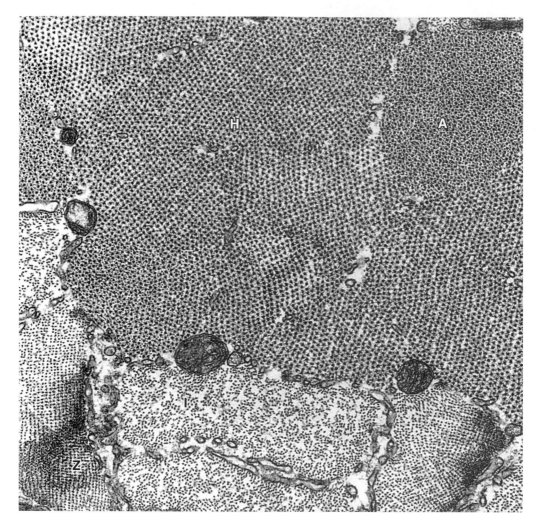

Figure 10–7. Transverse section of skeletal muscle myofibrils illustrating some of the features diagrammed in Figure 10–6. I, I band; A, A band; H, H band; Z, Z line. × 36,000.

numerous mitochondria and synaptic vesicles, the latter containing the neurotransmitter **acetylcholine** (see Chapter 9). Between the axon and the muscle is a space, the **synaptic cleft,** in which lies an amorphous basal lamina matrix. At the junction, the sarcolemma is thrown into numerous deep **junctional folds.** In the sarcoplasm below the folds lie several nuclei and numerous mitochondria, ribosomes, and glycogen granules.

When an action potential invades the motor endplate, acetylcholine is liberated from the axon terminal, diffuses through the cleft, and binds to acetylcholine receptors in the sarcolemma of the junctional folds. Binding of the transmitter makes the sarcolemma more permeable to sodium, which results in **membrane depolarization.** Excess acetylcholine is hydrolyzed by the enzyme cholinesterase bound to the synaptic cleft basal lamina. Acetylcholine break-

down is necessary to avoid prolonged contact of the transmitter with receptors present in the sarcolemma.

The depolarization initiated at the motor end-plate is propagated along the surface of the muscle cell and deep into the fibers via the transverse tubule system. At each triad, the depolarization signal is passed to the sarcoplasmic reticulum and results in the release of Ca^{2+}, which initiates the contraction cycle. When depolarization ceases, the Ca^{2+} is actively transported back into the sarcoplasmic reticulum cisternae, and the muscle relaxes.

Myasthenia gravis is an autoimmune disorder characterized by progressive muscular weakness caused by a reduction in the number of functionally active acetylcholine receptors in the sarcolemma of the myoneural junction. This reduction is caused by circulating antibodies that bind

Disassembled components of the thin filament

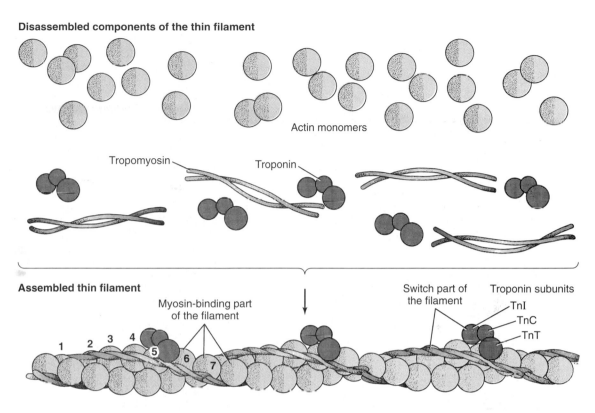

Actin monomers

Tropomyosin

Troponin

Assembled thin filament

Myosin-binding part of the filament

Switch part of the filament

Troponin subunits

TnI
TnC
TnT

1 2 3 4 5 6 7

Figure 10–8. Schematic representation of the thin filament, showing the spatial configuration of three major protein components—actin (shown in color), tropomyosin, and troponin (black). The individual components in the upper part of the drawing are shown in polymerized form in the lower part. The globular actin molecules are polarized (dark and light areas) and polymerize in one direction. Note that each tropomyosin molecule extends over seven actin molecules. TnI, TnC, and TnT are troponin subunits.

to the acetylcholine receptors in the junctional folds and inhibit normal nerve-muscle communication. As the body attempts to correct the condition, membrane segments with affected receptors are internalized, digested by lysosomes, and replaced by newly formed receptors. These receptors, however, are again made unresponsive to acetylcholine by the same antibodies, and the disease follows its progressive course.

A single nerve fiber (**axon**) can innervate one muscle fiber, or it may branch and be responsible for innervating 160 or more muscle fibers. In the case of multiple innervation, a single nerve fiber and all the muscles it innervates are called a **motor unit.** Individual striated muscle fibers do not show graded contraction—they contract either all the way or not at all. To vary the force of contraction, the fibers within a muscle bundle should not all contract at the same time. Since muscles are broken up into motor units, the firing of a single nerve motor axon will generate tension proportional to the number of muscle fibers innervated by that axon. Thus, the number of motor

units and the variable size of each unit can control the intensity of a muscle contraction. The ability of a muscle to perform delicate movements depends on the size of its motor units. For example, because of the fine control required by eye muscles, each of their fibers is innervated by a different nerve fiber. In larger muscles exhibiting coarser movements, such as those of the limb, a single, profusely branched axon innervates a motor unit that consists of more than 100 individual muscle fibers.

System of Energy Production

Skeletal muscle cells are highly adapted for discontinuous production of intense mechanical work through the release of chemical energy and must have depots of energy to cope with bursts of activity. The most readily available energy is stored in the form of ATP and phosphocreatine, both of which are energy-rich phosphate compounds. Chemical energy is also available in glycogen depots, which constitute about 0.5–1% of muscle weight. Muscle tissue obtains energy to be stored in phosphocreatine and ATP from the breakdown of fatty acids and glucose. In the

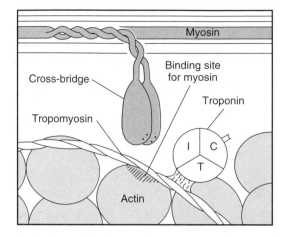

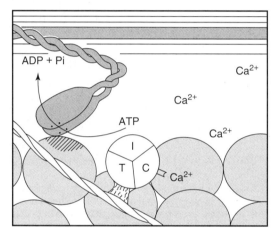

Figure 10–9. Muscle contraction, initiated by the binding of Ca^{2+} to the TnC unit of troponin, which exposes the myosin binding site on actin (cross-hatched area). In a second step, the myosin head binds to actin and the ATP breaks down into ADP, yielding energy, which produces a movement of the myosin head. As a consequence of this change in myosin, the bound thin filaments slide over the thick filaments. This process, which repeats itself many times during a single contraction, leads to a complete overlapping of the actin and myosin and a resultant shortening of the whole muscle fiber. I, T, C are troponin subunits. (Reproduced, with permission, from Ganong WF: *Review of Medical Physiology,* 14th ed. Appleton & Lange, 1989.)

resting muscle or during its recovery after contraction, the major substrate is fatty acids. Fatty acids are broken down to acetate by the enzymes of β-oxidation, located in the mitochondrial matrix. Acetate is then further oxidized by the citric acid cycle, with the resulting energy being conserved in the form of ATP. Fatty acids are the main energy source in the skeletal muscle of endurance athletes, such as long-distance runners. When skeletal muscles are subjected to a short-term (sprint) exercise, they rapidly metabolize glucose (coming mainly from muscle glycogen stores) to lactate, causing an oxygen debt that is repaid during the recovery period. The lactate formed during this type of exercise causes cramping and pain in skeletal muscles.

Based on their morphologic, histochemical, and biochemical characteristics, muscle fibers can be classified as type I (slow) and type II (quick). **Type I fibers** are rich in sarcoplasm, which contains myoglobin (accounting for the dark red color; see below). They are related to continuous contraction, and their energy is derived from oxidative phosphorylation of fatty acids. **Type II fibers** are related to rapid discontinuous contraction. They contain less myoglobin (producing a light red color). Type II fibers can be further divided into types IIA, IIB, and IIC, according to their activity and chemical characteristics (mainly, the stability of the actomyosin-ATPase they contain). Type IIB fibers have the fastest action and depend more than the others on glycolysis as a source of energy. The classification of muscle fibers has clinical significance for the diagnosis of muscle diseases, or myopathies (*mys* + Gr. *pathos,* suffering). In humans, skeletal muscles are frequently composed of mixtures of these various types of fibers, as shown in Figure 10–14.

The differentiation of muscle into red, white, and intermediate fiber types is controlled by its innervation. In experiments where the nerves to red and white fibers are cut, crossed, and allowed to regenerate, the myofibers change their morphologic and physiologic characteristics to conform to the innervating nerve. Simple denervation of muscle will lead to fiber atrophy and paralysis.

Other Components of the Sarcoplasm

Glycogen is found in abundance in the sarcoplasm in the form of coarse granules (Figure 10–10). It serves as a depot of energy that is mobilized during muscle contraction.

Another component of the sarcoplasm is **myoglobin;** this oxygen-binding protein, which is similar to hemoglobin, is principally responsible for the dark red color of some muscles. Myoglobin acts as an oxygen-storing pigment, which is necessary for the high oxidative phosphorylation level in this type of fiber. For obvious reasons, it is present in great amounts in the muscle of deep-diving ocean mammals (eg, seals, whales). Muscles that must maintain activity for prolonged periods usually are red and have a high myoglobin content.

Mature muscle cells have negligible amounts of rough endoplasmic reticulum and ribosomes, an observation that is consistent with the low level of protein synthesis in this tissue. Muscle spindles are described in Chapter 24.

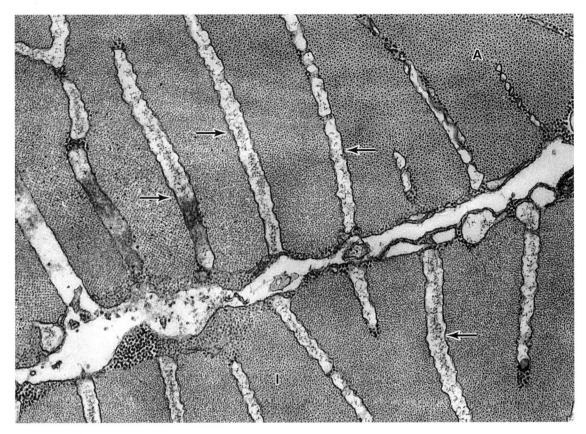

Figure 10–10. Electron micrograph of a transverse section of fish muscle, showing the surface of two cells limiting an intercellular space. Note the invaginations of the sarcolemma, forming the tubules of the T system (arrows). The dark, coarse granules in the cytoplasm (lower left) are glycogen particles. The section passes through the A band (upper right), showing thick and thin filaments. The I band is sectioned (lower left), showing only thin filaments. × 60,000. (Courtesy of KR Porter.)

CARDIAC MUSCLE

During embryonic development, the splanchnic mesoderm cells of the primitive heart tube align into chain-like arrays. Rather than fusing into syncytial (Gr. *syn,* together, + *kytos,* cell) cells, as in the development of skeletal muscle, cardiac cells form complex junctions between their extended processes. Cells within a chain often bifurcate, or branch, and bind to cells in adjacent chains. Consequently, the heart consists of tightly knit bundles of cells, interwoven in a fashion that provides for a characteristic wave of contraction that leads to a wringing out of the heart ventricles.

Mature cardiac muscle cells are approximately 15 μm in diameter and from 85 to 100 μm in length. They exhibit a cross-striated banding pattern identical to that of skeletal muscle. Unlike multinucleated skeletal muscle, however, each cardiac muscle cell possesses only one or two centrally located pale-staining nuclei. Surrounding the muscle cells is a delicate sheath of endomysial connective tissue containing a rich capillary network.

A unique and distinguishing characteristic of cardiac muscle is the presence of dark-staining transverse lines that cross the chains of cardiac cells at irregular intervals (Figure 10–15). These **intercalated disks** represent junctional complexes found at the interface between adjacent cardiac muscle cells (Figures 10–16, 10–17, and 10–18). The junctions may appear as straight lines or may exhibit a step-like pattern. Two regions can be distinguished in the step-like junctions—a **transverse portion,** which runs across the fibers at right angles, and a **lateral portion,** which runs parallel to the myofilaments. There are three main junctional specializations within the disk. **Fasciae adherentes,** the most prominent membrane specialization in transverse portions of the disk, serve as anchoring sites for actin filaments of the terminal sarcomeres. Essentially, they represent

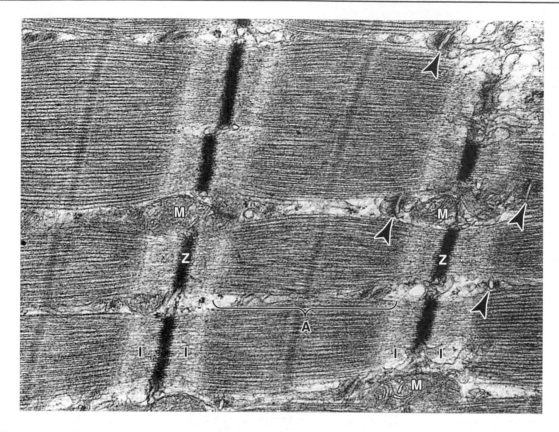

Figure 10–11. Electron micrograph of a longitudinal section of the skeletal muscle of a monkey. Note the mitochondria (M) between adjacent myofibrils. The arrowheads indicate triads—two for each sarcomere in this muscle—located at the A–I band junction. A, A band; I, I band; Z, Z line. × 40,000. (Reproduced, with permission, from Junqueira LCU, Salles LMM: *Ultra-Estrutura e Função Celular*. Edgard Blücher, 1975.)

hemi-Z bands. Maculae adherentes (desmosomes) are also present in the transverse portion and bind the cardiac cells together to prevent their pulling apart under constant contractile activity. On the lateral portions of the disk, **gap junctions** provide ionic continuity between adjacent cells (Figure 10–18). The significance of ionic coupling is that chains of individual cells act as a syncytium, allowing the signal to contract to pass in a wave from cell to cell.

The structure and function of the contractile proteins in cardiac cells are virtually the same as in skeletal muscle. The T-tubule system and sarcoplasmic reticulum, however, are not as regularly arranged in the cardiac myocytes. The T tubules are more numerous and larger in ventricular muscle than in skeletal muscle. Cardiac T tubules are found at the level of the Z band rather than at the A–I junction (as in mammalian skeletal muscle). The sarcoplasmic reticulum is not as well developed and wanders irregularly through the myofilaments. As a consequence, discrete myofibrillar bundles are not present.

Triads are not common in cardiac cells, because the T tubules are generally associated with only one lateral expansion of sarcoplasmic reticulum cisternae. Thus, heart muscle characteristically possesses **diads** composed of one T tubule and one sarcoplasmic reticulum cisterna.

Cardiac muscle cells contain numerous mitochondria, which occupy 40% or more of the cytoplasmic volume (Figure 10–19), reflecting the need for continuous aerobic metabolism in heart muscle. By comparison, only about 2% of skeletal muscle fiber is occupied by mitochondria. Fatty acids, transported to cardiac muscle cells by lipoproteins, are the major fuel of the heart. Fatty acids are stored as triglycerides in the numerous lipid droplets seen in cardiac muscle cells. A small amount of glycogen is present and can be broken down to glucose and used for energy production during periods of stress. Lipofuscin pigment granules (aging pigment), often seen in long-lived cells, are found near the nuclear poles of cardiac muscle cells.

A few differences in structure exist between atrial and ventricular muscle. The arrangement of myofilaments is the same in the two types of cardiac muscle, but atrial muscle has markedly fewer T tubules, and

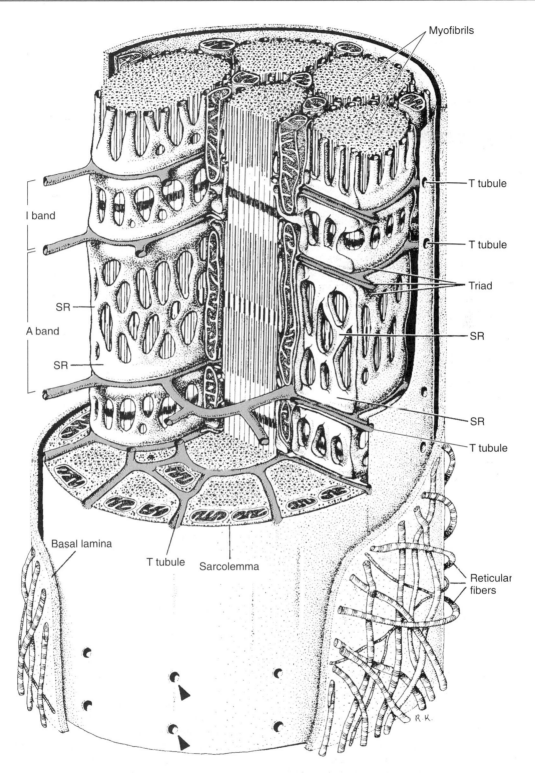

Figure 10–12. Segment of mammalian skeletal muscle. The sarcolemma and muscle fibrils are partially cut, showing the following components: The invaginations of the T system (shown in color) occur at the level of transition between the A and I bands twice in every sarcomere. They associate with terminal cisternae of the sarcoplasmic reticulum (SR), forming triads. Abundant mitochondria lie between the myofibrils. The cut surface of the myofibrils shows the thin and thick filaments. Surrounding the sarcolemma are a basal lamina and reticular fibers. (Reproduced, with permission, from Krsti RV: *Ultrastructure of the Mammalian Cell.* Springer-Verlag, 1979.)

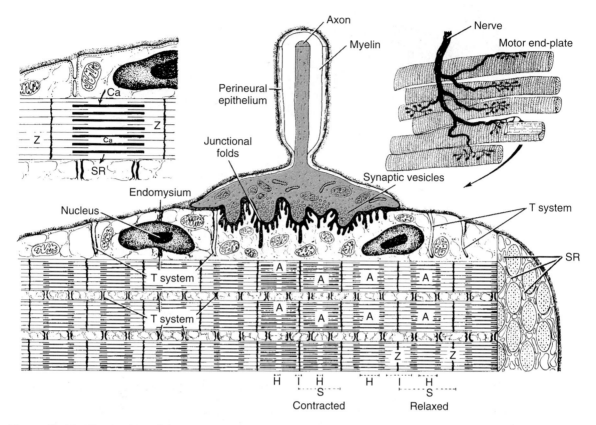

Figure 10–13. Ultrastructure of the motor end-plate and the mechanism of muscle contraction. The drawing at the upper right shows branching of a small nerve with a motor end-plate for each muscle fiber. The structure of one of the bulbs of an end-plate is highly enlarged in the center drawing. Note that the axon terminal bud contains synaptic vesicles. The region of the muscle cell membrane covered by the terminal bud has clefts and ridges called **junctional folds.** The axon (shown in color) loses its myelin sheath and dilates, establishing close, irregular contact with the muscle fiber. Muscle contraction begins with the release of acetylcholine from the synaptic vesicles of the end-plate. This neurotransmitter causes a local increase in the permeability of the sarcolemma. The process is propagated to the rest of the sarcolemma, including its invaginations (all of which constitute the T system), and is transferred to the sarcoplasmic reticulum (SR). The increase of permeability in this organelle liberates calcium ions (drawing at upper left) that trigger the sliding filament mechanism of muscle contraction. Thin filaments slide between the thick filaments and reduce the distance between the Z lines, thereby reducing the size of all bands except the A band. H, H band; S, sarcomere.

the cells are somewhat smaller. Membrane-limited granules, each about 0.2–0.3 μm in diameter, are found at both poles of cardiac muscle nuclei and in association with Golgi complexes in this region. These granules are most abundant in muscle cells of the right atrium (approximately 600 per cell), but they are also found in the left atrium, the ventricles, and several other places in the body (Figure 10–20). These atrial granules contain the high-molecular-weight precursor of a hormone known as **atrial natriuretic factor, auriculin,** or **atriopeptin.** Atrial natriuretic factor acts on the kidneys to cause sodium and water loss (natriuresis and diuresis). This hormone thus opposes the actions of aldosterone and antidiuretic hormone, whose effects on kidneys result in sodium and water conservation.

The rich autonomic nerve supply to the heart and the rhythmic impulse-generating and conducting structures are discussed in Chapter 11.

SMOOTH MUSCLE

Smooth muscle is composed of elongated, nonstriated cells (Figure 10–21), each of which is enclosed by a basal lamina and a network of reticular fibers (Figures 10–22 and 10–23). The last two components serve to combine the force generated by each smooth muscle fiber into a concerted action, eg, peristalsis in the intestine.

Smooth muscle cells are fusiform; ie, they are largest at their midpoints and taper toward their ends. They may range in size from 20 μm in small blood vessels to 500 μm in the pregnant uterus. During

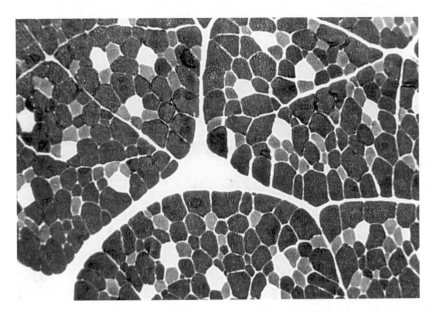

Figure 10–14. Transverse section of a striated muscle of the eye (rectus lateralis), stained by the histochemical technique for demonstrating myosin ATPase. Three types of fibers in the muscle are shown. Some thick fibers stain strongly for ATPase activity, and others stain very weakly. Thin fibers show intermediate activity. (Reproduced, with permission, from Khan MA et al: A calcium-citrophosphate technique for the histochemical localization of myosin ATPase. Stain Technol 1972;47:277.)

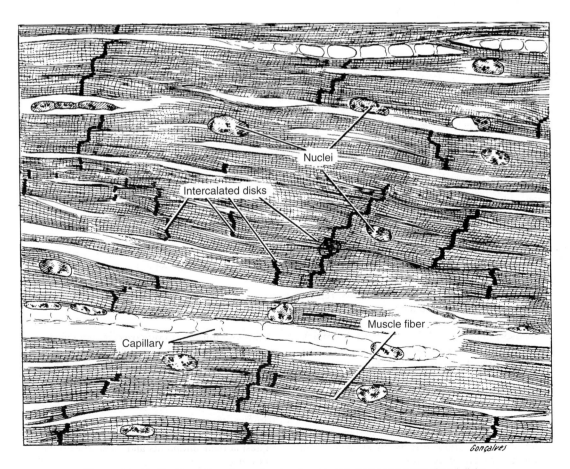

Figure 10–15. Section of heart muscle, showing central nuclei and intercalated disks.

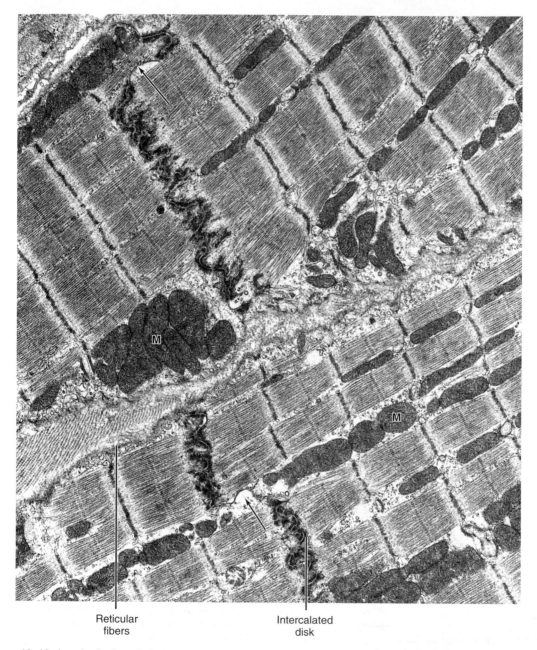

Reticular
fibers

Intercalated
disk

Figure 10–16. Longitudinal section of portions of two cardiac muscle cells. The transversely oriented parts of the intercalated disk consist of a fascia adherens and numerous desmosomes. The longitudinal parts (arrows) contain gap junctions. Mitochondria (M) are numerous. Reticular fibers are seen between the two cells. × 18,000. (Reproduced, with permission, from Junqueira LCU, Salles LMM: *Ultra-Estrutura e Função Celular*. Edgard Blücher, 1975.)

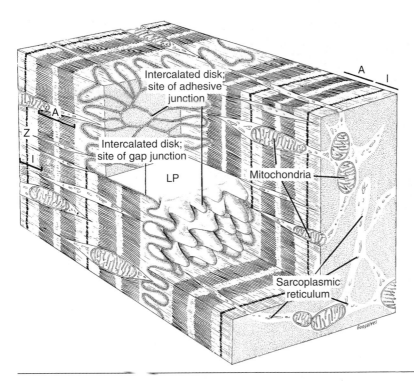

Intercalated disk; site of adhesive junction

Intercalated disk; site of gap junction

A

Z

I

LP

A   I

Mitochondria

Sarcoplasmic reticulum

Figure 10–17. Ultrastructure of heart muscle in the region of an intercalated disk. Contact between cells is accomplished by interdigitation in the transverse region; contact is broad and flat in the longitudinal plane (LP). A, A band; I, I band; Z, Z line. (Redrawn and reproduced, with permission, from Marshall JM: The heart. In: *Medical Physiology,* 13th ed, Vol 2, Mountcastle VB [editor]. Mosby, 1974. Based on the results of Fawcett DW, McNutt NS: J Cell Biol 1969;42:1, modified from Poche R, Lindner E: Zellforsch Mikrosk Anat 1955;43:104.)

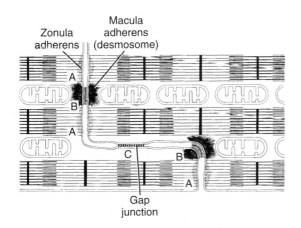

Zonula adherens

Macula adherens (desmosome)

A

B

A

C   B

A

Gap junction

Figure 10–18. Junctional specializations making up the intercalated disk. Fasciae (or zonulae) adherentes (A) in the transverse portions of the disk anchor actin filaments of the terminal sarcomeres to the plasmalemma. Maculae adherentes, or desmosomes (B), found primarily in the transverse portions of the disk, bind cells together, preventing their separation during contraction cycles. Gap junctions (C), restricted to longitudinal portions of the disk—the area subjected to the least stress—ionically couple cells and provide for the spread of contractile depolarization.

pregnancy, uterine smooth muscle cells undergo a marked increase in size and number. Each cell has a single nucleus located in the center of the broadest part of the cell. To achieve the tightest packing, the narrow part of one cell lies adjacent to the broad parts of neighboring cells (Figure 10–21). Such an arrangement viewed in cross section shows a range of diameters, with only the largest profiles containing a nucleus (Figures 10–21 and 10–22). The borders of the cell become scalloped when smooth muscle contracts, and the nucleus becomes folded or has the appearance of a corkscrew.

Concentrated at the poles of the nucleus are mitochondria, polyribosomes, cisternae of rough endoplasmic reticulum, and the Golgi complex. Pinocytotic vesicles are frequent near the cell surface (Figure 10–24).

A rudimentary sarcoplasmic reticulum is present; it consists of a closed system of membranes, similar to the sarcoplasmic reticulum of striated muscle. T tubules are not present in smooth muscle cells.

The characteristic contractile activity of smooth muscle is related to the structure and organization of its actin and myosin filaments, which do not exhibit the paracrystalline organization present in striated muscles. In smooth muscle cells, bundles of myofilaments crisscross obliquely through the cell, forming a lattice-like network. These bundles consist of thin filaments (5–7 nm) containing actin and tropomyosin and thick filaments (12–16 nm) consisting of myosin.

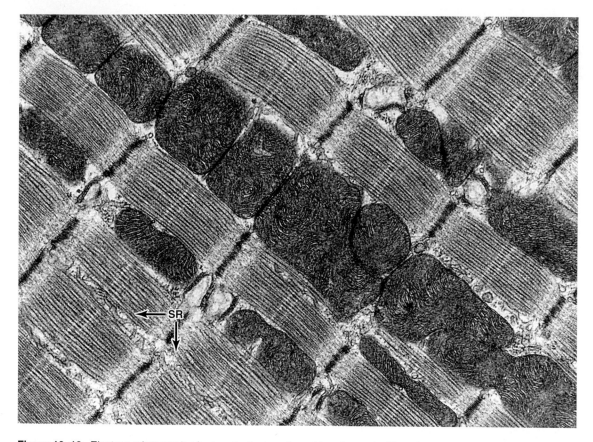

Figure 10–19. Electron micrograph of a longitudinal section of heart muscle. Note the striation pattern and the alternation of myofibrils and mitochondria rich in cristae. Note the sarcoplasmic reticulum (SR), which is the specialized calcium-storing smooth endoplasmic reticulum. × 30,000.

Both structural and biochemical studies reveal that smooth muscle actin and myosin contract by a sliding filament mechanism similar to that which occurs in striated muscles.

An influx of Ca^{2+} is involved in the initiation of contraction in smooth muscle cells. The myosin of smooth muscle, however, interacts with actin only when its light chain is phosphorylated. For this reason, and because the tropomyosin complex of skeletal muscle is absent, the contraction mechanism in smooth muscle differs somewhat from skeletal and cardiac muscle. Ca^{2+} in a smooth muscle complexes with **calmodulin,** a calcium-binding protein that is also involved in the contraction of nonmuscle cells. The Ca^{2+}-calmodulin complex activates myosin light-chain kinase, the enzyme responsible for the phosphorylation of myosin.

Factors other than calcium affect the activity of myosin light-chain kinase and thus influence the degree of contraction of smooth muscle cells. Contraction or relaxation may be regulated by hormones that act via cyclic AMP (cAMP). When levels of cAMP increase, myosin light-chain kinase is activated,

myosin is phosphorylated, and the cell contracts. A decrease in cAMP has the opposite effect, decreasing contractility. The action of sex hormones on uterine smooth muscle is another example of nonneural control. Estrogens increase cAMP and promote the phosphorylation of myosin and the contractile activity of uterine smooth muscle. Progesterone has the opposite effect: It decreases cAMP, promotes dephosphorylation of myosin, and relaxes uterine musculature.

Smooth muscle cells have an elaborate array of 10-nm intermediate filaments coursing through their cytoplasm. **Desmin (skeletin)** has been identified as the major protein of intermediate filaments in all smooth muscles, and **vimentin** is an additional component in vascular smooth muscle. Two types of **dense bodies** appear in smooth muscle cells. One is membrane-associated; the other is cytoplasmic. Both contain α-actinin and are thus similar to the Z lines of striated muscles. Both thin and intermediate filaments insert into dense bodies that transmit contractile force to adjacent smooth muscle cells and their surrounding network of reticular fibers.

The degree of innervation in a particular bundle of

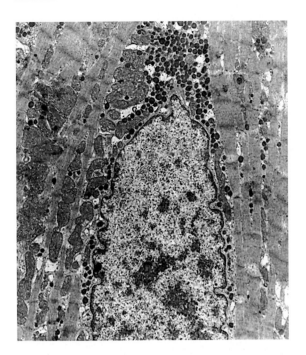

Figure 10–20. Electron micrograph of an atrial muscle cell showing the presence of natriuretic granules aggregated at the nuclear pole. (Courtesy of JC Nogueira.)

smooth muscle depends on the function and the size of that muscle. Smooth muscle is innervated by both sympathetic and parasympathetic nerves of the autonomic system. Elaborate neuromuscular junctions like those in skeletal muscle are not present in smooth muscle. Frequently, autonomic nerve axons terminate in a series of dilatations in the endomysial connective tissue.

In general, smooth muscle occurs in large sheets such as those found in the walls of hollow viscera, eg, the intestines, uterus, and ureters. Their cells possess abundant gap junctions and a relatively poor nerve supply. These muscles function in syncytial fashion and are called **visceral smooth muscles.** In contrast, the **multiunit smooth muscles** have a rich innervation and can produce such precise and graded contractions as those occurring in the iris of the eye.

Smooth muscle usually has spontaneous activity in the absence of nervous stimuli. Its nerve supply, therefore, has the function of modifying activity rather than, as in skeletal muscle, initiating it. Smooth muscle receives both adrenergic and cholinergic nerve endings that act antagonistically, stimulating or depressing its activity. In some organs, the cholinergic endings activate and the adrenergic nerves depress; in others, the reverse occurs.

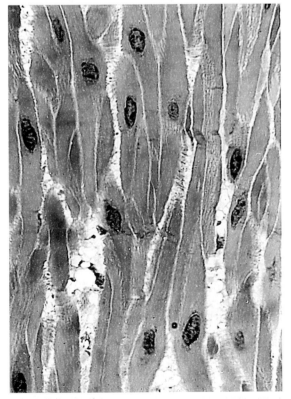

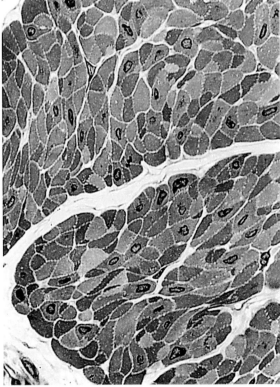

A

B

Figure 10–21. Photomicrographs of urinary bladder. Smooth muscle cells are sectioned longitudinally (**A**) and transversely (**B**). Note the reticular fibers around the bundles of smooth muscle cells.

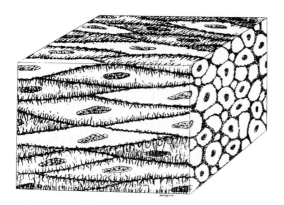

Figure 10–22. Segment of smooth muscle. All cells are surrounded by a net of reticular fibers. In cross section, these cells show various diameters.

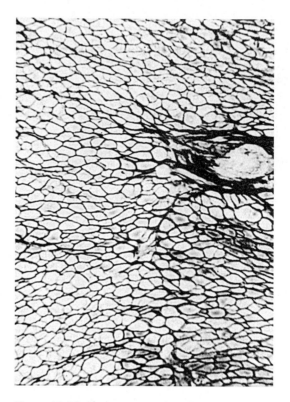

Figure 10–23. Transverse section of smooth muscle impregnated with silver to stain the reticular fibers. These fibers form a network that surrounds the muscle cells that are not stained by this method. At the right is an arteriole surrounded by thicker collagen fibers. × 300.

In addition to contractile activity, smooth muscle cells also synthesize collagen, elastin, and proteoglycans, which are extracellular products normally associated with the function of fibroblasts.

REGENERATION OF MUSCLE TISSUE

The three types of adult muscle have different potentials for regeneration after injury.

Cardiac muscle has virtually no regenerative capacity beyond early childhood. Defects or damage (eg, infarcts) in heart muscle are generally replaced by the proliferation of connective tissue, forming myocardial scars.

In skeletal muscle, although the nuclei are incapable of undergoing mitosis, the tissue can undergo limited regeneration. The source of regenerating cells is believed to be the **satellite cells.** The latter are a sparse population of mononucleated spindle-shaped cells that lie within the basal lamina surrounding each mature muscle fiber. Because of their intimate apposition with the surface of the muscle fiber, they can be identified only with the electron microscope. They are considered to be inactive myoblasts that persist after muscle differentiation. After injury or certain other stimuli, the normally quiescent satellite cells become activated, proliferating and fusing to form new skeletal muscle fibers. A similar activity of satellite cells has been implicated in muscle hypertrophy, where they fuse with their parent fibers to increase muscle mass after extensive exercise. The regenerative capacity of skeletal muscle is limited, however, after major muscle trauma or degeneration.

Smooth muscle is capable of an active regenerative response. After injury, viable mononucleated smooth muscle cells and pericytes from blood vessels (see Chapter 11) undergo mitosis and provide for the replacement of the damaged tissue.

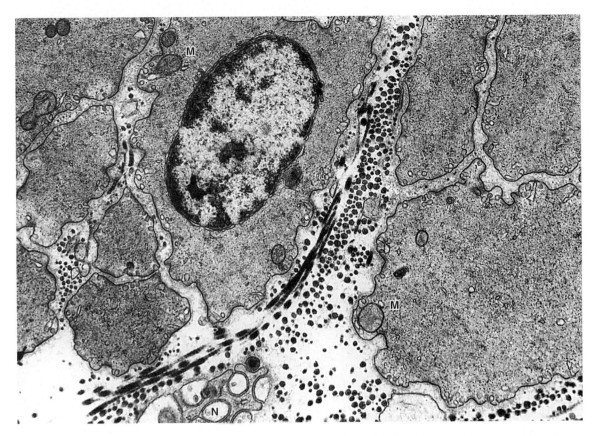

Figure 10–24. Electron micrograph of a transverse section of smooth muscle. The cells are sectioned at various diameters and have many subsurface vesicles in their cytoplasm. Thick and thin filaments are not organized into myofibrils, and there are few mitochondria (M). Note the collagen fibrils of the reticular fibers and a small unmyelinated nerve (N) between the cells. × 6650.

REFERENCES

Alberts B et al: *Molecular Biology of the Cell,* 3rd ed. Garland, 1994.

Bourne GH (editor): *The Structure and Function of Muscle.* Academic Press, 1972.

Bülbring E, Bolton TB (editors): Smooth muscle. Br Med Bull 1979;35:127.

Campion DR: The muscle satellite cell: a review. Int Rev Cytol 1984;87:225.

Cantin M, Genest J: The heart as an endocrine gland. Sci Am 1986;254:76.

Cohen C: The protein switch of muscle contraction. Sci Am 1975;233:36.

Gabella G, Blundell D: Nexuses between smooth muscle cells of the guinea-pig ileum. J Cell Biol 1979;82:239.

Heuser JE, Reese TS: Evidence for recycling of synaptic vesicle membrane during transmitter release at the frog neuromuscular junction. J Cell Biol 1973;57:315.

Huxley HE: Molecular basis of contraction in cross-striated muscles and relevance to motile mechanisms in other cells. In: *Muscle and Nonmuscle Motility.* Vol 1. Stracher A (editor). Academic Press, 1983.

Sommer JR, Johnson EA: A comparative study of Purkinje fibers and ventricular fibers. J Cell Biol 1968;36:497.

The Circulatory System

The circulatory system consists of the blood and lymphatic vascular systems. The blood vascular system is composed of the following structures:

The **heart,** whose function is to pump the blood.

The **arteries,** a series of efferent vessels that become smaller as they branch, and whose function is to carry the blood, with nutrients and oxygen, to the tissues.

The **capillaries,** a diffuse network of thin tubules that anastomose profusely and through whose walls the interchange between blood and tissues takes place.

The **veins,** which represent the convergence of the capillaries into a system of larger channels that convey products of metabolism (carbon dioxide, etc) toward the heart.

The **lymphatic vascular system** begins in the **lymphatic capillaries,** closed-ended tubules that anastomose to form vessels of steadily increasing size; these vessels terminate in the **blood vascular system** emptying into the large veins near the heart. The function of the lymphatic system is to return to the blood the fluid of the tissue spaces. Upon entering the lymphatic capillaries, this fluid contributes to the formation of the liquid part of the lymph; by passing through the lymphoid organs, it contributes to the circulation of lymphocytes and other immunologic factors.

By distributing hormones and nutrients to the cells and tissues of the body and transporting waste products to excretory organs, the circulatory system, along with the nervous system, contributes to the integrated functioning of the entire organism.

GENERAL STRUCTURE OF BLOOD VESSELS

All blood vessels have a number of structural features in common, although in the smallest vessels (capillaries and venules) the three tunics (described below) are greatly simplified. Blood vessels are structurally adapted according to physiologic requirements. Therefore, pulmonary arteries (low-pressure system) have thinner walls than do systemic arteries

(high-pressure system), such as the carotid or renal arteries.

There are no absolute criteria for distinguishing between large arteries, medium-sized arteries, and arterioles. Blood vessels constitute a continuous system, and some overlapping of classifications is to be expected. Generally, size or tissue composition (muscular, elastic, etc) is the basis for classification.

Tunics

Blood vessels are usually composed of the following layers, or tunics (L. *tunica,* coat), as shown in Figures 11–1 and 11–2:

A. Tunica Intima: The intima consists of a layer of **endothelial cells** lining the vessel's interior surface. These cells rest on a basal lamina and have a turnover rate of 1% per day. (See Capillaries, below, for a description of endothelial cells.) Beneath the endothelium is the **subendothelial layer,** consisting of loose connective tissue that may contain occasional smooth muscle cells. Both the connective tissue fibers and smooth muscle cells, when present, tend to be arranged longitudinally. In arteries, the intima is separated from the media by an **internal elastic lamina.** This lamina, composed of elastin, has gaps (**fenestrae**) that allow substances to diffuse to and nourish cells deep in the vessel wall.

B. Tunica Media: The media consists chiefly of concentric layers of helically arranged smooth muscle cells (Figure 11–2). Interposed among the smooth muscle cells are variable amounts of elastic fibers and lamellae, reticular fibers, and proteoglycans. Smooth muscle cells are the cellular source of this extracellular matrix. In larger arteries, a thinner **external elastic lamina** often separates the media from the outer tunica adventitia. In capillaries and postcapillary venules, the media is replaced by cells called **pericytes** (see Capillaries, below). In the media, rich in reticular fibers, collagen is mainly type III.

C. Tunica Adventitia: The adventitia consists principally of longitudinally oriented collagen and elastic fibers. Collagen in the adventitia is type I. The adventitial layer gradually becomes continuous with the enveloping connective tissue of the organ through which the vessel runs.

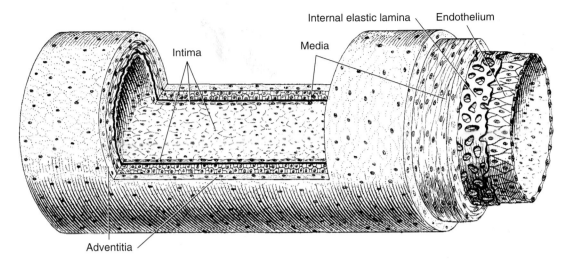

Figure 11–1. Drawing of a medium-sized muscular artery, showing its layers. Although the usual histologic preparations cause the layers to appear thicker than that shown here, the drawing is actually similar to the in vivo architecture of the vessel. After death, the vessel contracts, the layers become thicker, and the lumen becomes smaller and corrugated (as seen in Figures 11–2 and 11–9).

Vasa Vasorum

In large vessels, vasa vasorum ("vessels of the vessel") branch profusely in the adventitia and the outer part of the media (Figure 11–2). The vasa vasorum provide metabolites to the adventitia and the media in larger vessels, since the layers are too thick to be nourished solely by diffusion from the lumen.

These vessels are more frequent in veins than in arteries. This greater abundance of vasa vasorum can be attributed to the paucity of oxygen and nutritional substances in venous blood. Vasa vasorum can arise from branches of the artery they supply or from neighboring arteries.

Although **lymphatic capillaries** can penetrate the

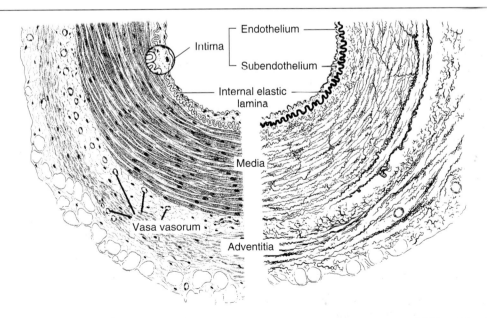

Figure 11–2. Comparative diagrams of a muscular artery prepared by hematoxylin-and-eosin (H&E) staining (**left**) and Weigert's staining method for elastic structures (**right**). The tunica media comprises a mixture of smooth muscle cells and reticular and elastic fibers. The adventitia and the outer part of the media have small blood vessels (vasa vasorum) and elastic and collagenous fibers.

media of veins, they are present in arteries only in the adventitia. This difference in distribution is probably related to differences in transmural pressures. The higher pressure across an arterial wall would tend to collapse a lymphatic capillary located near the arterial lumen, rendering it useless.

Innervation

Most blood vessels that contain smooth muscle in their walls are supplied with a profuse network of unmyelinated sympathetic nerve fibers (**vasomotor nerves**) whose neurotransmitter is norepinephrine. Discharge of norepinephrine from these nerves results in vasoconstriction. Because these efferent nerves generally do not enter the media of arteries, the neurotransmitter must diffuse for several micrometers to affect smooth muscle cells of the media. Gap junctions between smooth muscle cells of the media propagate the response to the neurotransmitter to the inner layers of muscle cells. In veins, nerve endings are found in both the adventitia and the media, but the overall density of innervation is less than that encountered in arteries. Arteries in skeletal muscle also receive a cholinergic vasodilator nerve supply. Acetylcholine released by these vasodilator nerves acts on the endothelium to produce nitric oxide, which diffuses into the smooth muscle cells, activating a cyclic GMP system of intracellular messengers. The muscle cells then relax, and the vessel lumen is dilated.

Afferent (sensory) nerve endings in arteries include the **baroreceptors** (pressure receptors [Gr. *baros,* weight, + L. *recipio,* to receive]) in the carotid sinus and the arch of the aorta as well as **chemoreceptors** of the carotid and aortic bodies.

SPECIFIC STRUCTURE OF BLOOD VESSELS

It is customary to divide the circulatory system into the **macrovasculature** (vessels more than 0.1 mm in diameter) and the **microvasculature** (vessels visible only with the light microscope). The microvasculature is particularly important because of its participation in the interchange between the circulatory system and surrounding tissues in both normal and inflammatory processes.

Capillaries

Capillaries have structural variations to permit different levels of metabolic exchange between blood and surrounding tissues.

Capillaries are composed of a single layer of **endothelial cells** of mesenchymal origin rolled up in the form of a tube. The average diameter of capillaries is small, varying from 7 to 9 μm. Their length usually varies from 0.25 mm to 1 mm, the latter being characteristic of muscle tissue. In a few instances

(eg, adrenal cortex, renal medulla), capillaries can be up to 50 mm long. The total length of capillaries in the human body has been estimated at 96,000 km (60,000 miles). When cut transversely, their walls are observed to consist of portions of one or more cells (Figure 11–3). The external surfaces of these cells usually rest on a basal lamina, a product of endothelial origin.

In general, endothelial cells are polygonal and about 10 × 30 μm when viewed face on; they are elongated in the direction of blood flow. The nucleus causes the cell to bulge into the capillary lumen. A small Golgi complex is present at the nuclear poles, a few mitochondria are evident, and free ribosomes as well as a few cisternae of rough endoplasmic reticulum are seen. Intermediate filaments (9–11 nm in diameter) are found in the perinuclear region. The presence of abundant microfilaments in endothelial cell cytoplasm is believed to be related to the proposed contractility of endothelial cells (Figure 11–4). The cell tapers toward the margins, where it can be 0.2 μm or less in thickness. Endothelial cells are held together by zonulae occludentes. Gap junctions are also present. Junctions of the zonula occludens type are present between most endothelial cells and are of physiologic importance. Such junctions offer variable permeability to the macromolecules that play a significant role in both normal physiologic and pathologic conditions.

Junctions between endothelial cells of venules are the loosest. At these locations there is a characteristic loss of fluid from the circulatory system during the inflammatory response, leading to edema.

There are **pericytes** (Gr. *peri,* around, + *kytos,* cell)—mesenchymal cells with long cytoplasmic processes that partly surround the endothelial cells—

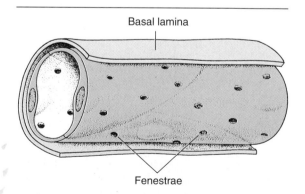

Figure 11–3. Structure of a capillary with fenestrae in its wall. (Not all capillaries have fenestrated walls.) The sectioned portion at left consists of two endothelial cells, and a basal lamina (lighter color) surrounds the capillary.

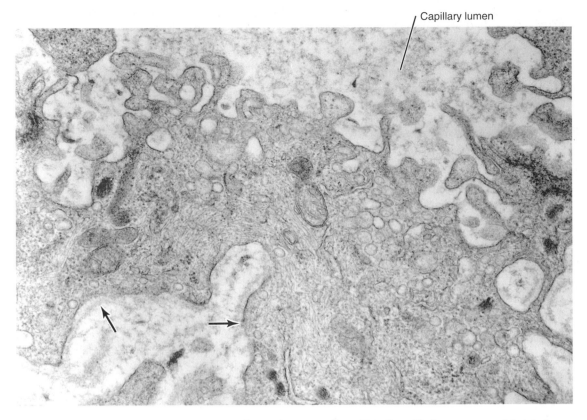

Figure 11–4. Electron micrograph of a section of a continuous capillary. Note the ruffled appearance of its interior surface, the large and small pinocytotic vesicles, and numerous microfilaments in the cytoplasm. Arrows show the basal lamina. Reduced slightly from × 30,000.

at various locations along capillaries and small venules (Figure 11–5). Enclosed in their own basal lamina, which may fuse with that of the endothelial cells, these perivascular cells have great potential for transformation into other cells. The presence of myosin, actin, and tropomyosin in pericytes strongly suggests that these cells also have a contractile function. After tissue injuries, pericytes proliferate and differentiate to form new blood vessels and connective tissue cells, thus participating in the repair process.

Capillaries can be grouped into four types, depending on the structure of the endothelial cells and the presence or absence of a basal lamina.

1. The **continuous,** or **somatic, capillary** (Figure 11–6) is characterized by the absence of fenestrae in its wall. This type of capillary is found in all kinds of muscle tissue, connective tissue, exocrine glands, and nervous tissue. Numerous pinocytotic vesicles, approximately 70 nm in their greatest diameter, are present on both sur-

faces of muscle capillaries; they also appear as isolated vesicles in the cytoplasm of these cells. These vesicles are responsible for the transport of macromolecules in both directions across the endothelial cell. Few or no pinocytotic vesicles are encountered in the continuous capillaries supplying most parts of the nervous system. This feature, in part, accounts for the existence of the **blood-brain barrier** (see Chapter 9).

2. **Fenestrated,** or **visceral, capillaries** are characterized by the presence of large fenestrae in the walls of endothelial cells. These fenestrae are 60–80 nm in diameter and are closed by a diaphragm that is thinner than a cell membrane (Figures 11–3 and 11–7) and does not have the trilaminar structure of a unit membrane (Figure 2–3). A continuous basal lamina is present. Fenestrated capillaries are encountered in tissues where rapid interchange of substances occurs between the tissues and the blood, as in the kidney, the intestine, and the endocrine glands. Macromolecules injected into the bloodstream can cross

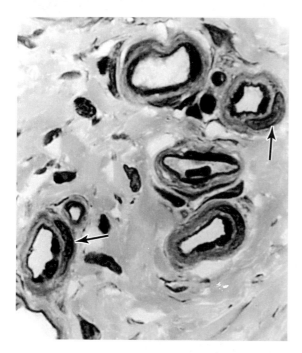

Figure 11–5. Photomicrograph showing small venules surrounded by connective tissue. Note the **pericytes** whose dark-stained elongated nuclei (arrows) are clearly seen around these small blood vessels. H&E stain.

the capillary wall through these fenestrae to enter the tissue spaces. This seems to be as important a mechanism of transcapillary transport as is pinocytotic transport (see Chapter 4).

3. The third type of capillary is also a fenestrated capillary, but in this case no diaphragms are present to close the openings (Figure 19–8). A very thick basal lamina separates this endothelium from the overlying epithelial cells (podocytes). This type of capillary is characteristic of the renal glomerulus (see Chapter 19).

4. The fourth type of capillary, the **discontinuous sinusoidal capillary** (Figure 16–14), has a tortuous path and greatly enlarged diameter (30–40 μm), which slows the circulation of blood. The endothelial wall is discontinuous, and the endothelial cells show multiple fenestrations without diaphragms (Figures 14–20 and 16–14). Macrophages are located either among or outside the cells of the endothelium. The basal lamina is often discontinuous. Sinusoidal capillaries are found mainly in the liver and in hematopoietic organs such as the bone marrow and spleen. The interchange between blood and tissues is greatly facilitated by the structure of the capillary wall.

As illustrated in Figure 11–8, capillaries anastomose freely, forming a rich network that interconnects the small arteries and veins. The arterioles branch into small vessels surrounded by a discontinuous layer of smooth muscle, the **metarterioles.** These branch into capillaries that form a network with a large surface area to facilitate the exchange of materials between the tissues and the blood. Constriction of metarterioles helps to regulate but does not completely stop the circulation in capillaries, and it maintains pressure differences in the arterial and venous systems. There is a simple ring of smooth muscle cells, or sphincter, at the point where capillaries originate from the metarteriole. This **precapillary sphincter** can completely stop the blood flow within the capillary. The entire network does not always function simultaneously, and the number of functional and open capillaries depends not only on the state of contraction of the metarterioles but also on arteriovenous anastomoses that enable the arterioles to empty directly into venules, as shown in Figure 11–8. These interconnections are abundant in skeletal muscle and the skin of the hands and feet. When vessels of the arteriovenous anastomosis contract, all the blood must pass through the capillary network. When they relax, some blood flows directly to a vein instead of circulating in the capillaries. Capillary circulation is controlled by neural and hormonal stimulation.

The richness of the capillary network is related to the metabolic activity of the tissues and represents a transition zone between the high-pressure system (arterial) and the low-pressure system (venous). Tissues with high metabolic rates, such as the kidney, liver, and cardiac and skeletal muscle, have an abundant capillary network; the opposite is true of tissues with low metabolic rates, such as smooth muscle and dense connective tissue.

An idea of the importance of the capillaries can be gained by noting that in the human body the surface area of the capillary network approaches 6000 m². Its total diameter is approximately 800 times larger than that of the aorta. A unit volume of fluid within a capillary is exposed to a larger surface area than is the same volume in the other parts of the system. The flow of blood in the aorta averages 320 mm/sec; in the capillaries, about 0.3 mm/sec. The capillary system can thus be compared to a lake that a full-flowing river enters and leaves; because of their thin walls and slow blood flow, the capillaries are a favorable place for the exchange of water, solutes, and macromolecules between blood and tissues.

Functions of Capillaries. Capillaries perform at least three important functions: They serve as a selective permeability barrier, a synthetic and metabolic system, and an antithrombogenic container for blood.

1.   **Permeability**—Capillaries (and postcapillary venules) are often referred to as **exchange vessels,** since it is at these sites that oxygen, carbon dioxide, substrates, and metabolites are transferred from blood to the tissues and from the tissues to blood.

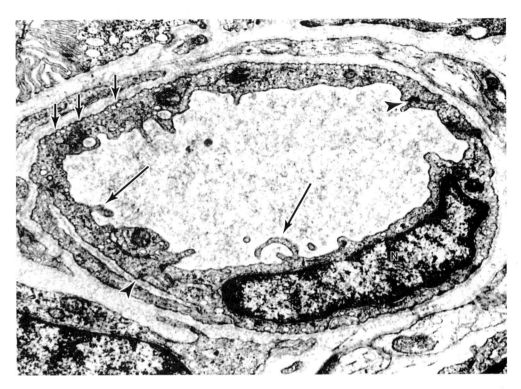

Figure 11–6. Electron micrograph of a transverse section of a continuous capillary. Note the nucleus (N) and the junctions between neighboring cells (arrowheads). Numerous pinocytotic vesicles are evident (arrows). The large arrows show large vesicles being formed by infoldings of broad sheets of the endothelial cell membrane. × 10,000.

Permeability of capillary walls varies with the size and charge of the permeating molecules and with the structure of the endothelial cell. The mechanism of the interchange of materials between blood and tissue is not known. Researchers have postulated the existence of two sizes of pores in capillary walls. The smaller pores are believed to have a diameter of 9–11 nm and the larger pores a diameter of 50–70 nm. Three possible morphologic equivalents of these physiologic pores are intercellular junctions and clefts between neighboring endothelial cells; fenestral diaphragms in fenestrated capillaries; and large numbers of pinocytotic vesicles that are believed to cross the endothelial cells of most capillaries.

Small hydrophobic and hydrophilic molecules (eg, oxygen, carbon dioxide, glucose) can diffuse or be actively transported across the plasmalemma of capillary endothelial cells. These substances are then transported by diffusion to the opposite cell surface, where they are discharged into the extracellular space. Water and some other hydrophilic molecules, less than 1.5 nm in diameter and below 10 kDa in molecular mass, can cross the capillary wall by diffusing through the intercellular junctions (paracellular pathway). The **intercellular junction** is now believed to be the morphologic counterpart of the **small pore** postulated in physiologic studies. The **large pore** is almost certainly represented morphologically by the **fenestrae** or **pinocytotic vesicles** of endothelial cells.

Abnormal states, such as inflammation induced by bacteria, chemical substances, and poisons (eg, snake or bee venom), apparently alter the permeability of the junctions between endothelial cells. Permeability of capillaries and postcapillary venules is greatly increased, and electron-dense colloidal substances pass from capillary and small venule lumens into surrounding tissues by traversing the endothelial cell junctions. Leukocytes leave the bloodstream by passing between endothelial cells and entering the tissue spaces through a process called **diapedesis.** The opening of these junctions seems to be mediated by locally liberated pharmacologically active substances, such as **histamine** and **bradykinin,** that increase vascular permeability and can also play a conspicuous role in inflammation.

The observation that some drugs, given intravenously, do not reach the brain, although such penetration occurs in almost all other tissues of the body, gave rise to the concept of the **blood-brain barrier.** This phenomenon was initially

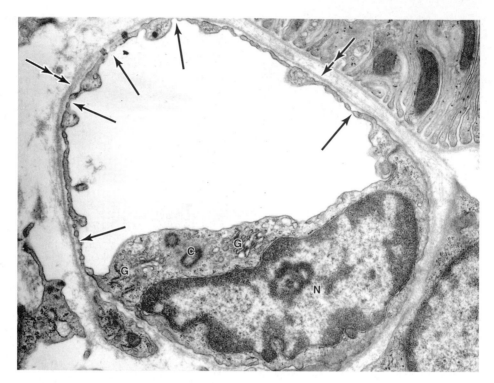

Figure 11–7. A fenestrated capillary in the kidney. Arrows indicate fenestrae closed by diaphragms. In this cell the Golgi complex (G), nucleus (N), and two centrioles (C) can be seen. Note the continuous basal lamina on the outer surface of the endothelial cell (double arrows). × 20,000. (Courtesy of J Rhodin.)

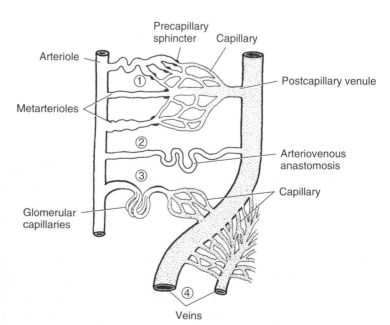

Figure 11–8. Types of microcirculation formed by small blood vessels. (**1**) The usual sequence of arteriole → metarteriole → capillary → venule and vein. (**2**) An arteriovenous anastomosis. (**3**) An arterial portal system as is present in the kidney glomerulus. (**4**) A venous portal system is present in the liver. (Reproduced, with permission, from Krstić RV: *Illustrated Encyclopedia of Human Histology.* Springer-Verlag, 1984.)

studied by means of intravenous administration of dyes that readily escape from capillaries to surrounding tissues. Careful study of brain capillaries showed that not only do they have few pinocytotic vesicles and no fenestrae, but occluding junctions between their endothelial cells do not permit the passage of macromolecules used as tracers. These properties apparently explain the barrier. Other blood-tissue barriers of physiologic and pathologic importance are the blood-ocular barrier, the blood-thymus barrier, the blood-nerve barrier, and the blood–testicular semiferous tubule barrier.

2. Metabolic functions—Capillary endothelial cells can metabolize a wide variety of substrates.

a. Activation—Conversion of angiotensin I (Gr. *angeion,* vessel, + *tendere,* to stretch) to angiotensin II (see Chapter 19).

b. Inactivation—Conversion of bradykinin, serotonin, prostaglandins, norepinephrine, thrombin, etc, to biologically inert compounds.

c. Lipolysis—Breakdown of lipoproteins, by enzymes located on the surface of endothelial cells, to yield triglycerides (energy) and cholesterol (substrates for steroid-hormone synthesis and membrane structure).

d. Production of vasoactive factors—Endothelial cells produce several substances that have an effect on vascular tone, eg, endothelins that are vasoconstrictive agents and nitric oxide, a relaxing factor.

3. Antithrombogenic function—When endothelial cells desquamate, the uncovered subendothelial connective tissue induces the aggregation of blood platelets. Subsequent fibrin coagulation forms solid masses called thrombi that can grow and obstruct vascular flow, a potentially life-threatening condition. Endothelial cells, when present, prevent contact of platelets with the subendothelial connective tissue, exerting an antithrombogenic effect (see Chapter 12).

Arteries

Arteries transport blood to the tissues. They resist changes in blood pressure in their initial portions and regulate blood flow in their terminal portions.

Arteries are usually classified, according to size, as arterioles, muscular arteries of medium or large diameter, or large, elastic arteries. In general, the walls of arteries are thicker than the walls of veins of the same overall diameter (Figure 11–9).

A. Arterioles: Arterioles are generally less than 0.5 mm in diameter and have relatively narrow lumens (Figure 11–12). The lumen is lined with endothelial cells similar to those in continuous capillaries.

An important characteristic of arterioles is the presence of rod-shaped granules, about 3 μm

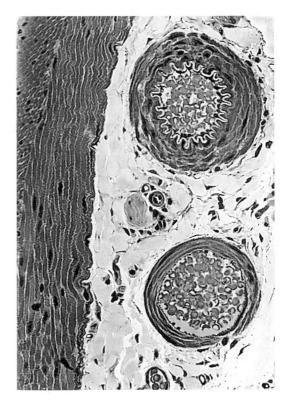

Figure 11–9. Photomicrograph of sections of a small muscular artery (above) and a venule (below). H&E stain.

long but only 0.1 μm wide. These are the **Weibel-Palade granules** found only in endothelial cells of vessels larger than capillaries. These granules contain a protein of the blood coagulation mechanism known as von Willebrand's factor (factor VIII). Deficiency of this group of proteins results in impaired adhesion of platelets to injured endothelium and in prolonged bleeding and is among the causes of **hemophilia.**

The subendothelial layer is very thin, and an internal elastic lamina is lacking except in the largest arterioles. The media is muscular and generally composed of one or two circularly arranged layers of smooth muscle cells; it shows no external elastic lamina (Figure 11–9). The adventitia is thin.

B. Muscular Arteries: Most of the named arteries in the human body are **muscular arteries** (Figures 11–2, 11–9, 11–10, and 11–11). The intima is similar to that of arterioles except that the subendothelial layer is somewhat thicker and a few smooth muscle cells may be present. An internal elastic lamina is prominent (Figures 11–10 and 11–11). The media may contain up to 40 layers of smooth muscle cells, although the number of layers diminishes as the artery becomes smaller. These cells are intermingled

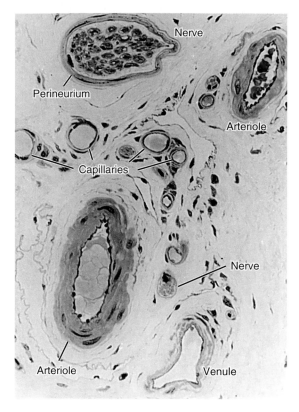

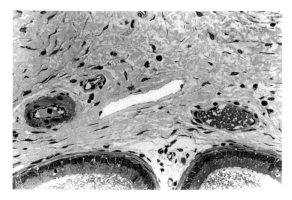

Figure 11–12. Photomicrograph of a small venule (right) and a small arteriole (left). Walls of the arteries are thicker than walls of the veins. A lymphatic vessel can be seen between the arteriole and the venule. Note the blood capillary next to the small arteriole and the field of loose connective tissue that surrounds the vessels.

Figure 11–10. Photomicrograph showing several types of small blood vessels and nerves. Note the perineurium in the larger nerve and the difference in wall thickness between arterioles and venules. Blood capillaries are also seen. Around these components is connective tissue, pale-stained. H&E stain.

with various numbers of elastic lamellae (depending on the size of the vessel) as well as reticular fibers and proteoglycans. An external elastic lamina is present in larger muscular arteries. The adventitia consists of collagen and elastic fibers, a few fibroblasts, and adipose cells. Lymphatic capillaries, vasa vasorum, and nerves are also found in the adventitia, and these structures may penetrate to the outer part of the media.

C. Large Elastic Arteries: Large elastic arteries include the aorta and its large branches. They have a yellowish color from the accumulation of elastin in the media. This type of artery has the following characteristics:

The intima is thicker than the corresponding tunic of a muscular artery. The subendothelial layer is thick. The connective tissue fibers of the subendothe-

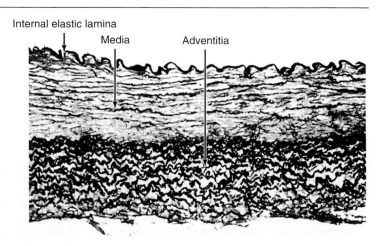

Figure 11–11. Photomicrograph of a section of muscular artery stained by Weigert's method for elastic structures. ×110.

lial layer display a longitudinal orientation and play an important role in the distortion of the endothelial layer of cells during rhythmic contractions and dilatations of the vessel. An internal elastic lamina, although present, may not be easily discerned, since it is similar to the elastic laminae of the next layer.

The media consists of a series of concentrically arranged, perforated elastic laminae whose number increases with age (there are 40 in the newborn, 70 in the adult). Once formed, elastic structures usually become metabolically inert (shown by autoradiographic studies), especially in older animals. These laminae become progressively thicker because of the deposit of elastin. Between the elastic laminae are smooth muscle cells, reticular fibers, and ground substance consisting mainly of chondroitin sulfate.

The tunica adventitia, which does not have an external limiting lamina, is relatively underdeveloped and contains elastic and collagen fibers.

D. Histophysiology of Arteries: The large arteries are called **conducting arteries,** because their major function is to transport blood away from the heart. These arteries also serve to smooth out the large fluctuations in pressure created by the heartbeat. During ventricular contraction (**systole**), the elastic laminae of conducting arteries are stretched and reduce the pressure change. During ventricular relaxation (**diastole**), ventricular pressure drops to a low level, but the elastic rebound of conducting arteries helps to maintain arterial pressure. As a consequence, arterial pressure and blood flow decrease and become less variable as the distance from the heart increases (Figure 11–13).

The function of medium-sized arteries, also known as **distributing arteries,** is to furnish blood to the various organs. The muscular layer in distributing arteries can control the flow of blood to various organs by contracting or not contracting, as a result of local chemical input or more generalized neural input.

Arteries undergo progressive and gradual changes from birth to death, and it is difficult to say where the normal growth processes end and the processes of involution begin. Each artery exhibits its own aging pattern. The coronary artery changes the most precociously, beginning at about 20 years of age. Other arteries begin to be modified only after age 40. When the media of an artery is weakened by an embryonic defect, disease, or lesion, the wall of the artery may dilate extensively. As this process of dilatation progresses, it becomes an **aneurysm** and can result in rupture of the wall. The importance of type III collagen in arterial structure is illustrated by Ehlers-Danlos syndrome type IV (a genetic deficiency of the synthesis of type III

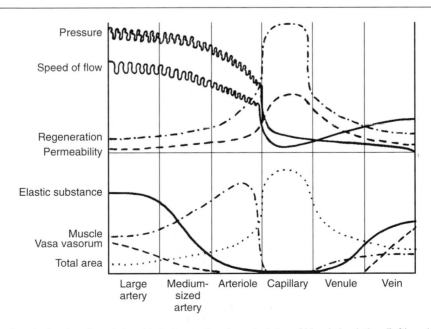

Figure 11–13. Graph showing the relationship between the characteristics of blood circulation (**left**) and the structure of the blood vessels (**bottom**). The arterial blood pressure and rapidity of flow decrease and become more constant as distance from the heart increases. This decrease coincides with a reduction in the number of elastic fibers and an increase in the number of smooth muscle cells in the arteries. The graph illustrates the gradual changes in the structure of vessels and their biophysical properties. Regeneration and permeability are highly developed in the capillaries. (Reproduced, with permission, from Cowdry EV: *Textbook of Histology.* Lea & Febiger, 1944.)

collagen), in which the main cause of death is spontaneous aortic rupture.

Atherosclerotic (Gr. *athere*, gruel, + *skleros*, hard) lesions are characterized by focal thickening of the intima, proliferation of smooth muscle cells and extracellular connective tissue elements, and the deposit of cholesterol in smooth muscle cells and macrophages. When heavily loaded with lipid, these cells are referred to as **foam cells** and form the macroscopically visible fatty streaks and plaques that characterize **atherosclerosis.** These changes may extend to the inner part of the tunica media, and the thickening may become so great as to occlude the vessel. Coronary arteries are among those most prone to atherosclerosis. Uniform thickening of the intima is believed to be a normal phenomenon of aging.

Certain arteries irrigate only definite areas of specific organs, and obstruction of the blood supply results in **necrosis** (death of tissues from a lack of metabolites). These **infarcts** occur commonly in the heart, kidneys, cerebrum, and certain other organs. In other regions (such as the skin), arteries anastomose frequently, and the obstruction of one artery does not lead to tissue necrosis, because the blood flow is maintained.

The polypeptide **angiotensin II** contributes to the regulation of blood pressure by binding initially to vascular endothelial cells. This endothelial stimulus is later transmitted to arterial smooth muscle cells, stimulating their contraction and thus causing an increase in blood pressure. Endothelial cells extend processes across the internal elastic lamina and communicate via gap junctions with smooth muscle cells.

Carotid Bodies

Small structures encountered near the bifurcation of the common carotid artery act as chemoreceptors sensitive to low oxygen tension, high carbon dioxide concentration, and low arterial blood pH. Carotid bodies consist of glomus cells (type I cells) and sheath cells (type II cells) surrounded by a rich vascular supply whose capillaries are of the fenestrated type. Most of the nerves of the carotid body (95% in the rat) are afferent fibers. The glomus cells contain numerous dense-core vesicles that store dopamine, norepinephrine, and serotonin. Whether the glomus cells or the afferent nerve endings are the principal chemoreceptor elements is controversial. Aortic bodies located on the arch of the aorta are similar in structure to the carotid body and are believed to have a similar function.

Carotid Sinuses

Carotid sinuses are slight dilatations of the internal carotid arteries. These sinuses contain **baroreceptors that detect changes in blood pressure and relay the information to the central nervous system. The arterial media of the sinus is thinner to permit changes according to the changes in blood pressure. The intima and the adventitia are very rich in nerve endings. The afferent nerve impulses are processed in the brain to control vasoconstriction and maintain normal blood pressure.**

Arteriovenous Anastomoses

Direct communication between arterial and venous circulation often takes place via interconnections called arteriovenous anastomoses, which are distributed throughout the body, generally in small vessels. The luminal diameters of anastomotic vessels vary with the physiologic condition of the organ. Changes in diameter of these vessels regulate blood pressure, flow, and temperature and the conservation of heat in particular areas (Figures 11–8 and 11–14). In addition to these direct connections, there are more complex structures, the **glomera** (plural of **glomus**)—

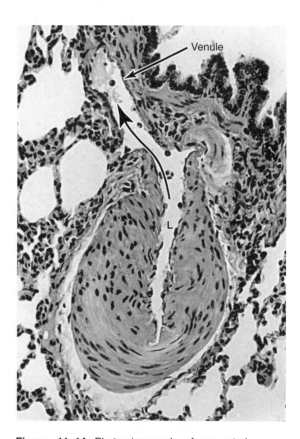

Venule

L

Figure 11–14. Photomicrograph of an arteriovenous anastomosis. Note that the arteriolar wall in the lower part of the figure shows several concentric layers of smooth muscle cells and is continuous with the venule. The arrow indicates the direction of blood flow. L, lumen. H&E stain.

mainly in fingerpads, fingernail beds, and ears. When the arteriole penetrates the connective tissue capsule of the glomus, it loses an internal elastic membrane and develops a thick muscular wall and small lumen. This arteriole is connected to a thin-walled vein. The glomera are believed to regulate blood flow and conservation of heat. They also participate in such physiologic phenomena as menstruation, erection, thermoregulation, and the regulation of blood pressure. All arteriovenous anastomoses are richly innervated by the sympathetic and parasympathetic nervous systems.

Veins

Veins return blood to the heart, aided by the action of smooth muscle and specialized valves.

When considered as a functional unit, the veins are **capacitance vessels,** because more than 70% of the total blood volume of the body is in this portion of the cardiovascular system at any one time. As with arteries, veins are arbitrarily classified into venules and veins of small, medium, and large size.

Venules have very thin walls. The adventitia is relatively thicker. The media in small venules may contain only contractile pericytes, but a few smooth muscle cells are usually present (Figure 11–14).

Venules with luminal diameters up to 50 μm have the structure and other biologic features of capillaries, eg, participation in inflammatory processes and interchange of cells and molecules between blood and tissues.

With the exception of the main trunks, most veins are **small** or **medium-sized,** with a diameter of 1–9 mm. The intima usually has a thin subendothelial layer, which may be absent at times. The media consists of small bundles of smooth muscle cells intermixed with reticular fibers and a delicate network of elastic fibers. The collagenous adventitial layer is well developed (Figure 11–15). Unlike arteries, small and medium-sized veins have valves in their interior. These structures consist of two semilunar folds of the tunica intima that project into the lumen. They are composed of elastic connective tissue and are lined on both sides by endothelium. The valves, which are especially numerous in veins of the limbs, direct the venous blood toward the heart. The propulsive force of the heart is reinforced by contraction of skeletal muscles that surround these veins.

Large veins have a well-developed tunica intima. The media is much thinner, with few layers of smooth muscle cells and abundant connective tissue. The adventitial layer is the thickest and best-devel-

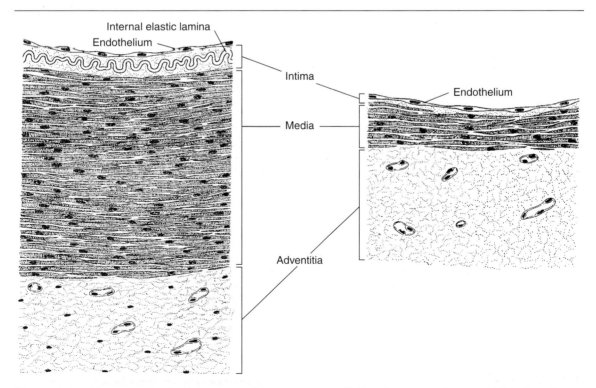

Figure 11–15. Diagram comparing the structure of a muscular artery (**left**) and accompanying vein (**right**). Note that the tunica intima and the tunica media are highly developed in the artery but not in the vein.

oped tunic in veins. Cardiac muscle is present in the adventitia of the venae cavae and pulmonary veins for a short distance before they empty into the heart. In large, unsupported abdominal veins (eg, mesenteric vein) or in other large veins that lie below the level of the heart, the adventitia frequently contains longitudinal bundles of smooth muscle (Figure 11–16). This adventitial muscle serves to strengthen the wall and prevent distention of the vessel. The circular and longitudinal arrangement of smooth muscle in these vessels may oppose the action of gravity by providing a peristaltic pumping of the blood up to the heart.

Heart

The heart is a muscular organ that contracts rhythmically, pumping the blood through the circulatory system. It is also responsible for producing a hormone called **atrial natriuretic factor.** Its walls consist of three tunics: the internal, or endocardium; the middle, or myocardium; and the external, or pericardium (*peri* + Gr. *kardia,* heart). The fibrous central region of the heart, the **fibrous skeleton,** serves as the base of the valves as well as the site of origin and insertion of the cardiac muscle cells.

A. Tunics: The **endocardium** is homologous with the intima of blood vessels. It consists of a single layer of squamous endothelial cells resting on a thin subendothelial layer of loose connective tissue that contains elastic and collagen fibers as well as some smooth muscle cells. Between the endocardium and the myocardium is a layer of connective tissue (often called the **subendocardial layer**), which consists of veins, nerves, and branches of the impulse-conducting system of the heart (Purkinje cells). The

myocardium is the thickest of the tunics of the heart and consists of cardiac muscle cells (see Chapter 10) arranged in layers that surround the heart chambers in a complex spiral. A large number of these layers insert themselves into the fibrous cardiac skeleton. The arrangement of these muscle cells is extremely varied, so that in histologic preparations of a small area, cells are seen to be oriented in many directions. The muscle cells of the heart are grouped into two populations: contractile cells and the impulse-generating and -conducting cells responsible for the electrical signal that initiates the heartbeat.

The **epicardium** is the serous covering of the heart, forming the visceral layer of the pericardium. It is covered externally by simple squamous epithelium (mesothelium) supported by a thin layer of connective tissue. A subepicardial layer of loose connective tissue contains veins, nerves, and nerve ganglia. The adipose tissue that generally surrounds the heart accumulates in this layer.

B. Fibrous Skeleton: The fibrous skeleton of the heart is composed of dense connective tissue. Its principal components are the **septum membranaceum,** the **trigona fibrosa,** and the **annuli fibrosi.** These structures consist of a dense connective tissue, with thick collagen fibers oriented in various directions. Certain regions contain nodules of fibrous cartilage.

C. Valves: The cardiac valves consist of a central core of dense fibrous connective tissue (containing both collagen and elastic fibers), lined on both sides by endothelial layers. The bases of the valves are attached to the annuli fibrosi of the fibrous skeleton.

D. Structures That Control Heartbeat: The impulse-generating and -conducting system of the heart consists of several structures that make it possible for the atria and ventricles to beat in succession and thus permit the heart to function as an efficient pump. The **sinoatrial node** is the pacemaker of the heart, in that it has the most rapid rhythmic activity (Figure 11–17). It is located close to the entrance of the superior vena cava into the right atrium. The nodal cells are modified cardiac muscle cells, smaller than atrial muscle cells and with fewer myofibrils. Nodal cells are concentrically arranged around a large nodal artery. Internodal tracts of specialized cells conduct the electrical depolarization of the sinoatrial node to the **atrioventricular node.** This mass of specialized cardiac muscle cells lies beneath the endocardium of the septal wall of the right atrium. The nodal cells are similar to those of the sinoatrial node. There are also large arterioles and considerable amounts of adipose tissue.

The **atrioventricular bundle of His** is formed by **Purkinje cells** (Figure 11–18) that penetrate the fibrous skeleton and then divide to form the **right** and **left bundle branches.** The left bundle again divides

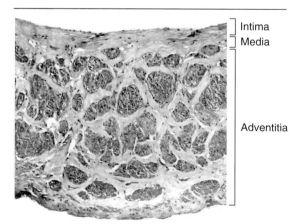

Figure 11–16. Photomicrograph of a section of a larger vein. Note the well-developed adventitia with characteristic longitudinal bundles of smooth muscle. H&E stain. × 100.

Intima
Media

Adventitia

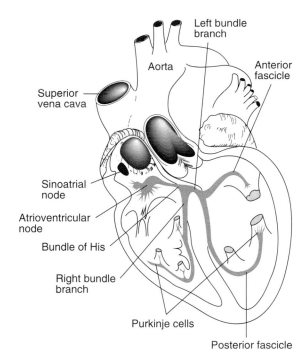

Figure 11–17. Diagram of the heart, showing the impulse-generating and -conducting system.

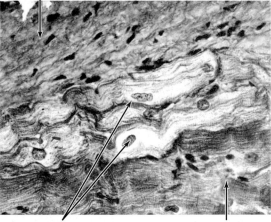

Connective tissue

Conducting (Purkinje) cells   Heart muscle

Figure 11–18. The Purkinje cells of the impulse-conducting system of the heart are characterized by a reduced number of myofibrils present mainly in the periphery of the muscle cell. Purkinje cells are held together by intercalated disks. The light area around the nuclei of the conducting cells is caused by a local accumulation of glycogen. H&E stain. × 400.

to form two fascicles. These bundles of Purkinje cells travel in the subendocardial layer to the apex of the heart, where they reverse their direction and begin giving off side branches that make contact with ordinary (working) cardiac muscle cells via gap junctions. This arrangement allows the stimulus for ventricular contraction to be rapidly conducted to the apex of the heart, which must contract first to eject blood from the ventricles. The wave of contraction then sweeps toward the base of the heart (pulmonary and aortic valves). Purkinje cells have a diameter considerably greater than that of ordinary cardiac muscle cells.

Both the parasympathetic and sympathetic divisions of the autonomic system contribute to innervation of the heart and form widespread plexuses at the base of the heart. Ganglionic nerve cells and nerve fibers are present in the regions close to the sinoatrial and atrioventricular nodes. Although these nerves do not affect generation of the heartbeat, a process attributed to the sinoatrial (pacemaker) node, they do affect heart rhythm. Stimulation of the parasympathetic division (vagus nerve) slows the heartbeat, whereas stimulation of the sympathetic nerve accelerates the rhythm of the pacemaker.

Lymphatic Vascular System

In addition to blood vessels, the human body has a system of endothelium-lined thin-walled channels

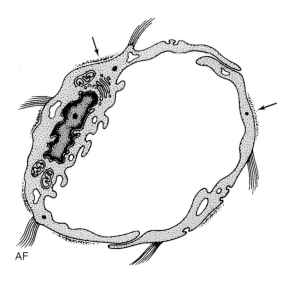

Figure 11–19. Structure of a lymphatic capillary at the electron microscope level. Note the overlapping free borders of endothelial cells, the discontinuous basal lamina (arrows), and the attachment of anchoring fibrils (AF). (Courtesy of J James.)

that collect fluid from the tissue spaces and return it to the blood. This fluid is called lymph; unlike the blood, it circulates in only one direction—toward the heart.

The **lymphatic capillaries** originate in the various tissues as thin, closed-ended vessels that consist of a single layer of endothelium. Lymphatic capillaries have no fenestrations in their endothelial cells, no zonula occludens between neighboring cells, and almost no basal lamina.

Lymphatic capillaries are held open by numerous microfibrils of the elastic fiber system (see Figure 5–16), which also bind them firmly to the surrounding connective tissue (Figure 11–19). Lymphatic capillaries absorb some of the electrolytes and proteins that continuously leave the blood capillaries. Contraction of the endothelial cells in the lymphatic capillaries permits large amounts of tissue fluid to enter the lymphatic system.

The thin lymphatic vessels gradually converge and ultimately end up as two large trunks—the **thoracic duct** and the **right lymphatic duct**—that empty into the junction of the left internal jugular vein with the left subclavian vein and into the confluence of the right subclavian vein and the right internal jugular vein. Interposed in the path of the lymphatic vessels are lymph nodes, whose morphologic characteristics and functions are discussed in Chapter 14. With rare exceptions, such as the central nervous system and the bone marrow, a lymphatic system is found in almost all organs.

The larger lymphatic vessels have a structure similar to that of veins except that they have thinner walls and lack a clear-cut separation between layers (intima, media, adventitia). They also have more numerous internal valves. The lymphatic vessels are dilated and assume a nodular, or beaded, appearance between the valves.

As in veins, lymphatic circulation is aided by the action of external forces (eg, contraction of surrounding skeletal muscle) on their walls. These forces act

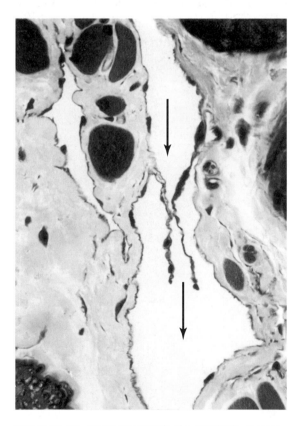

Figure 11–20. Photomicrograph of a lymphatic vessel in longitudinal section, showing a valve, the structure responsible for the unidirectional flow of lymph. Note the very thin wall of this vessel and its valve. Another lymphatic vessel can be seen in the upper left region of the figure. The arrows indicate the direction of lymph flow. H&E stain.

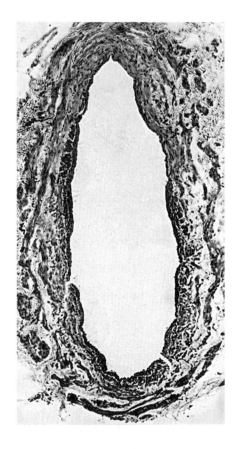

Figure 11–21. Section of the thoracic duct. H&E stain. × 200. (Reproduced, with permission, from Junqueira LC, Carneiro J: *Histologie,* Schiebler TH, Peiper U [translators]. Springer-Verlag, 1984.)

discontinuously, and unidirectional lymph flow is mainly a result of the presence of many valves in these vessels (Figure 11–20). Contraction of smooth muscle in the walls of larger lymphatic vessels also helps to propel lymph toward the heart.

The structure of the large **lymphatic ducts** (thoracic duct and right lymphatic duct) is similar to that of veins, with reinforced smooth muscle in the middle layer. In this layer, the muscle bundles are longitudinally and circularly arranged, with longitudinal fibers predominating (Figure 11–21). The adventitia is relatively underdeveloped. Like arteries and veins, large lymphatic ducts contain vasa vasorum and a rich neural network.

Tumors of Blood Vessels

Malignant tumors of blood vessels are infrequent. **Angiosarcomas** (*angeion* + Gr. *sarkos,* flesh, + *oma,* tumor) are rare malignant tumors believed to originate from endothelial cells. Hemangiopericytomas (Gr. *haima,* blood, + *angeion* + *peri* + *kytos* + *oma*) are usually benign and probably originate from pericytes. The presence of factor VIII, localized by immunohistochemical techniques, is characteristic of endothelial cell–derived tumors; tumors arising from pericytes do not contain this protein.

REFERENCES

Challice CE, Viragh S (editors): *Ultrastructure of the Mammalian Heart.* Academic Press, 1973.

Cliff WJ: *Blood Vessels.* Cambridge Univ Press, 1976.

Johnson PC: *Peripheral Circulation.* Wiley, 1978.

Joyce NE et al: Contractile proteins in pericytes. J Cell Biol 1985;100:1387.

Leak LV: Normal anatomy of the lymphatic vascular system. In: *Handbuch der Allgemeine Pathologie.* Meessen H (editor). Springer-Verlag, 1972.

Rhodin JAG: Architecture of the vessel wall. In: *Handbook of Physiology.* Section 2: *Cardiovascular System.* Vol 2. American Physiological Society, 1980.

Richardson JB, Beaulines A: The cellular site of action of angiotensin. J Cell Biol 1971;51:419.

Simionescu N: Cellular aspects of transcapillary exchange. Physiol Rev 1983;63:1536.

Thorgeirsson G, Robertson AL Jr: The vascular endothelium: pathobiologic significance. Am J Pathol 1978; 93:802.

Wagner D, Marder J: Biosynthesis of von Willebrand protein by human endothelial cells: processing steps and their intracellular localization. J Cell Biol 1984;99: 2123.

Blood Cells

Blood consists of the cells and fluid (about 5.5 L in a man) that flow in a regular unidirectional movement within the closed circulatory system. Blood is propelled mainly by the rhythmic contractions of the heart and is made up of two parts: **formed elements,** or blood cells, and **plasma** (Gr. *plasma,* thing formed), the liquid in which the formed elements are suspended. The formed elements are **erythrocytes** (red blood cells); **platelets;** and **leukocytes** (white blood cells).

If blood is removed from the circulatory system, it will clot. This clot contains formed elements and a clear yellow liquid called **serum,** which separates from the coagulum.

Blood that is collected and kept from coagulating by the addition of anticoagulants (heparin, citrate, etc) separates, when centrifuged, into layers that reflect its heterogeneity (Figure 12–1). The **hematocrit** is an estimate of the volume of packed erythrocytes per unit volume of blood. The normal value is 40–50% in the men and 35–45% in women.

The translucent, yellowish, somewhat viscous supernatant obtained when whole blood is centrifuged is the plasma. The formed elements of the blood separate into two easily distinguishable layers. The lower layer represents 42–47% of the entire volume of blood in the hematocrit tube. It is red and is made up of erythrocytes. The layer immediately above (1% of the blood volume), which is white or grayish in color, is called the **buffy coat** and consists of leukocytes. These elements separate because the leukocytes are less dense than the erythrocytes. Covering the leukocytes is a fine layer of platelets not distinguishable by the naked eye.

Leukocytes, which have diversified functions (Table 12–1), are one of the body's chief defenses against infection. They circulate throughout the body via the blood vascular system. Crossing the capillary wall, these cells become concentrated rapidly in the tissues, where they display their defensive capabilities. The blood vascular system is a distributing vehicle, transporting oxygen (O_2; see Figure 12–2), carbon dioxide (CO_2), metabolites, and hormones, among other substances. O_2 is bound mainly to the hemoglobin of the erythrocytes, whereas CO_2, in addition to being bound to the proteins of the erythrocytes (mainly hemoglobin), is carried in solution in the plasma as CO_2 or HCO_3^-.

The plasma transports nutrients from their site of absorption or synthesis, distributing them to various areas of the organism. It also transports metabolic residues, which are removed from the blood by the excretory organs. Blood, as the distributing vehicle for the hormones, permits the exchange of chemical messages between distant organs for normal cellular function. It further participates in the regulation of body temperature and in acid-base and osmotic balance.

Composition of Plasma

Plasma is an aqueous solution containing substances of low or high molecular weight that make up 10% of its volume. The plasma proteins account for 7% of the volume and the inorganic salts for 0.9%; the remainder of the 10% consists of several organic compounds—amino acids, vitamins, hormones, lipoproteins, etc—of various origins.

Through the capillary walls, the low-molecular-weight components of plasma are in equilibrium with the interstitial fluid of the tissues. The composition of plasma is usually an indicator of the mean composition of the extracellular fluids in general.

The main plasma proteins are **albumin; alpha, beta,** and **gamma globulins;** and **fibrinogen.** Albumin is the main component and has a fundamental role in maintaining the osmotic pressure of the blood. The gamma globulins are antibodies and are called **immunoglobulins.** Fibrinogen is necessary for the formation of fibrin in the final step of coagulation.

Several substances that are insoluble or only slightly soluble in water can be transported by the plasma because they combine with albumin or with the alpha and beta globulins. For example, lipids are insoluble in the plasma but combine with the hydrophobic portions of protein molecules. Since the protein molecules also have hydrophilic parts, the lipid-protein complex is soluble in water.

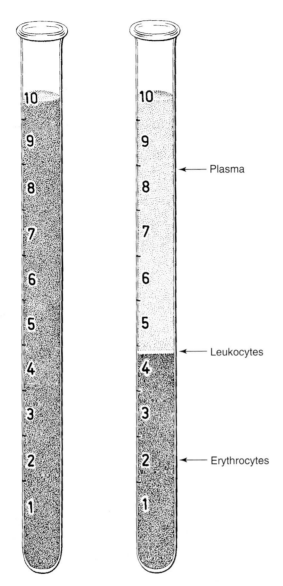

Figure 12–1. Hematocrit tubes with blood. **Left:** Before centrifugation. **Right:** After centrifugation. The erythrocytes represent 43% of the blood volume in the centrifuged tube. Between the sedimented erythrocytes and the supernatant light-colored plasma is a thin layer of leukocytes called the buffy coat.

Staining of Blood Cells

Blood cells are generally studied in smears or films prepared by spreading a drop of blood in a thin layer on a microscope slide. The blood should be evenly distributed over the slide and allowed to dry rapidly in air. In such films the cells are clearly visible and distinct from one another. Their cytoplasm is spread out, facilitating observation of their nuclei and cytoplasmic organization.

Blood smears are routinely stained with special mixtures of red (acidic) and blue (basic) dyes. These mixtures also contain **azures,** dyes that are useful in staining some structures of blood cells known as **azurophils** (azure + Gr. *philein,* to love). Some of these special mixtures are named (eg, Giemsa, Wright's, Leishman's) for the investigators who introduced their own modifications into the original mixture.

FORMED ELEMENTS OF BLOOD

Erythrocytes

Erythrocytes (red blood cells), which are anucleate, are packed with the O_2-carrying protein hemoglobin. Under normal conditions, these cells never leave the circulatory system.

Most mammalian erythrocytes are biconcave disks without nuclei (Figure 12–3). When suspended in an isotonic medium, human erythrocytes are 7.5 μm in diameter, 2.6 μm thick at the rim, and 0.8 μm thick in the center (Figure 12–4). The biconcave shape provides erythrocytes with a large surface-to-volume ratio, thus facilitating gas exchange.

The normal concentration of erythrocytes in blood is approximately 3.9–5.5 million per microliter in women and 4.1–6 million per microliter in men.

A decreased number of erythrocytes in the blood is usually associated with **anemia.** An increased number of erythrocytes (**erythrocytosis,** or **polycythemia**) may be a physiologic adaptation—it is found, for example, in people who live at high altitudes, where O_2 tension is low. Polycythemia (Gr. *polys,* many, + *kytos,* cell, + *haima,* blood), which is often associated with diseases of varying degrees of severity, increases blood viscosity; when severe, it can impair circulation of blood through the capillaries. Polycythemia might be better characterized as an increased hematocrit, ie, an increased volume occupied by erythrocytes.

Erythrocytes with diameters greater than 9 μm are called **macrocytes,** and those with diameters less than 6 μm are called **microcytes.** The presence of a high percentage of erythrocytes with great variations in size is called **anisocytosis** (Gr. *aniso,* uneven, + *kytos*).

The erythrocyte is quite flexible, a property that permits it to adapt to the irregular shapes and small diameters of capillaries. Observations in vivo show that when traversing the angles of capillary bifurcations, erythrocytes containing normal adult hemoglobin (HbA) are easily deformed and frequently assume a cup-like shape.

Table 12–1. Products and functions of the blood cells.

Cell Type	Main Products	Main Functions
Erythrocyte	Hemoglobin	CO_2 and O_2 transport
Leukocytes Neutrophil (terminal cell)	Specific granules and modified lysosomes (azurophilic granules)	Phagocytosis of bacteria
Eosinophil (terminal cell)	Specific granules, pharmacologically active substances	Defense against parasitic helminths; modulation of inflammatory processes
Basophil (terminal cell)	Specific granules containing histamine and heparin	Release of histamine and other inflammation mediators
Monocyte (not terminal cell)	Granules with lysosomal enzymes	Generation of mononuclear-phagocyte system cells in tissues; phagocytosis and digestion of protozoa and virus and senescent cells.
B lymphocyte	Immunoglobulins	Generation of antibody-producing terminal cells (plasmocytes)
T lymphocyte	Substances that kill cells. Substances that control the activity of other leukocytes (interleukins)	Killing of virus-infected cells
Natural killer cell (cytotoxic T cell)	Substances that promote perforations in the cell membrane of target cells (thereby killing them)	Killing of some tumor and virus-infected cells
Platelet	Blood-clotting factors	Clotting of blood

Erythrocytes are surrounded by a plasmalemma; because of its ready availability, this is the best-known membrane of any cell. It consists of about 40% lipid (phospholipids, cholesterol, glycolipids, etc), 50% protein, and 10% carbohydrate. About half the proteins span the lipid bilayer and are known as **integral membrane proteins** (see Chapter 2). Several peripheral proteins (see Figure 2–4A) are associ-

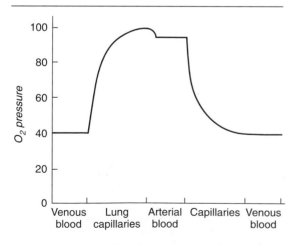

Figure 12–2. Blood O_2 content in each type of blood vessel. The amount of O_2 (O_2 pressure) is highest in arteries and lung capillaries; it decreases in tissue capillaries, where exchange takes place between blood and tissues.

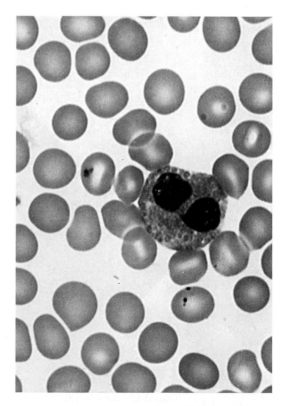

Figure 12–3. Photomicrograph of a Leishman-stained human blood smear, showing numerous erythrocytes and one granulocyte (eosinophil). × 1300.

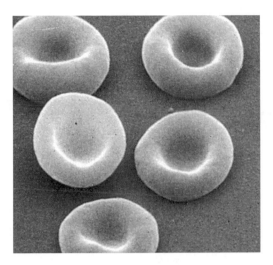

Figure 12–4. Scanning electron micrograph of normal human erythrocytes. Note their biconcave shape. × 3300.

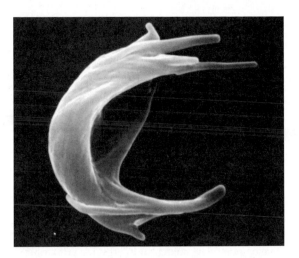

Figure 12–5. Scanning electron micrograph of a distorted erythrocyte from a person who is homozygous for the HbS gene (sickle cell disease). × 6500.

ated with the inner surface of the erythrocyte membrane. The peripheral proteins seem to serve as a membrane skeleton that determines the shape of the erythrocyte. They also permit the flexibility of the membrane necessary for the large changes in shape that occur when the erythrocyte passes through capillaries. Because erythrocytes are not rigid, the viscosity of blood normally remains low.

In their interiors, erythrocytes contain a 33% solution of hemoglobin, the O_2-carrying protein that accounts for their acidophilia. In addition, there are enzymes of the glycolytic and hexose-monophosphate-shunt pathways of glucose metabolism.

Inherited alterations in hemoglobin molecules are responsible for several pathologic conditions, of which **sickle cell disease** is an example. This inherited disorder is caused by a mutation of one nucleotide (**point mutation**) in the DNA of the gene for the β chain of hemoglobin. The triplet GAA (for glutamic acid) is changed to GUA, which specifies valine. As a result, the translated hemoglobin differs from the normal one by the presence of valine in the place of glutamic acid. The consequences of this substitution of a single amino acid are profound, however. When the altered hemoglobin (called HbS) is deoxygenated, it polymerizes and forms rigid aggregates that give the erythrocyte a characteristic sickle shape (Figure 12–5). The sickled erythrocyte is inflexible and fragile. It has a shortened life span that leads to anemia (a reduction in blood hemoglobin content and also increases the blood viscosity. Blood flow through the capillaries is retarded or even

stopped, leading to severe O_2 shortage (**anoxia**) in tissues.

Combined with O_2 or CO_2, hemoglobin forms **oxyhemoglobin** or **carbaminohemoglobin,** respectively. The reversibility of these combinations is the basis for the gas-transporting capability of hemoglobin. The combination of hemoglobin with carbon monoxide (**carboxyhemoglobin**) is irreversible, however, and causes a reduced capacity to transport O_2.

Anemia is a pathologic condition characterized by blood concentrations of hemoglobin below normal values. Although anemias are usually associated with a decreased number of erythrocytes, it is also possible for the number of cells to be normal—but for each cell to contain a reduced amount of hemoglobin (**hypochromic anemia**). Anemia may be caused by loss of blood (hemorrhage); insufficient production of erythrocytes by the bone marrow; production of erythrocytes with insufficient hemoglobin, usually related to iron deficiency in the diet; or accelerated destruction of blood cells.

Erythrocytes recently released by the bone marrow into the bloodstream often contain ribosomal RNA (rRNA), which, in the presence of supravital dyes (eg, brilliant cresyl blue), can be precipitated and stained. Under these conditions, the younger erythrocytes, called **reticulocytes** (see Figure 12–13), may have a few granules or a net-like structure in their cytoplasm. The process by which reticulocytes are released from the bone marrow into the circulation is not completely understood.

Reticulocytes normally constitute about 1% of the total number of circulating erythrocytes; this is the rate at which erythrocytes are replaced daily by the bone marrow. Increased numbers of reticulocytes indicate a demand for increased O_2-carrying capacity, which may be caused by such factors as hemorrhage or a recent ascent to high altitude.

Erythrocytes lose their mitochondria, ribosomes, and many cytoplasmic enzymes during maturation from reticulocytes to adult erythrocytes, a process that takes 24–48 hours. This breakdown of organelles and enzymes is not mediated by lysosomal enzymes. Instead, a group of ATP-dependent enzymes, present in the cytoplasm, are responsible for the disappearance of proteins and organelles during erythrocyte development. The source of energy for erythrocytes is glucose, which is anaerobically degraded to lactate. Because erythrocytes do not have a nucleus or other organelles necessary for protein synthesis, they do not synthesize hemoglobin.

Human erythrocytes survive in the circulation for about 120 days. Worn-out erythrocytes are removed from the circulation mainly by macrophages of the spleen and bone marrow. The signal for removal seems to be the appearance of defective complex oligosaccharides attached to integral membrane proteins of the plasmalemma.

Sometimes—mainly in disease states—nuclear fragments (containing DNA) remain in the erythrocyte after extrusion of its nucleus, which occurs late in its development (see Chapter 13).

Leukocytes

Leukocytes (white blood cells) migrate to the tissues, where they perform multiple functions.

On the basis of the presence and type of granule in their cytoplasm and the shape of the nucleus, leukocytes are classified into two groups: **granulocytes** (polymorphonuclear leukocytes) and **agranulocytes** (mononuclear leukocytes).

Granulocytes (L. *granulum,* granule, + Gr. *kytos*) possess two types of granules: the **specific** granules that bind either neutral or acidic components of the dye mixture and have specific functions and the **azurophilic granules.** Azurophilic granules stain purple and are lysosomes. Specific and azurophilic granules contain the enzymes listed in Table 12–2. Granulocytes have nuclei with two or more lobes and include the **neutrophils, eosinophils,** and **basophils.** All granulocytes have a life span of a few days, dying by apoptosis (programmed cell death) in the connective tissue. It is estimated that billions of neutrophils die by apoptosis (see Chapter 3) each day in the adult human. The resulting cellular debris is removed by macrophages and does not elicit an inflammatory response.

Agranulocytes do not have specific granules, but

Table 12–2. Granule composition in human granulocytes.

Cell Type	Specific Granules	Azurophilic Granules
Neutrophil	Alkaline phosphatase Collagenase Lactoferrin Lysozyme Several nonenzymatic antibacterial basic proteins (phagocytins)	Acid phosphatase α-mannosidase Arylsulfatase β-galactosidase β-glucuronidase Cathepsin 5′nucleotidase Elastase Collagenase Myeloperoxidase Lysozyme Acidic mucosubstances Cationic antibacterial proteins
Eosinophil	Acid phosphatase Arylsulfatase β-glucuronidase Cathepsin Phospholipase RNAase Eosinophilic peroxidase Major basic protein	
Basophil	Eosinophilic chemotactic factor Heparin Histamine Peroxidase	

they do contain various numbers of azurophilic granules (lysosomes) that bind the azure dyes of the stain. The nucleus is round or indented. This group includes the **lymphocytes** and **monocytes.**

The size and frequency (differential count) of blood leukocytes are presented in Table 12–3.

Leukocytes are involved in the cellular and humoral defense of the organism against foreign material. In suspension in the circulating blood, they are

Table 12–3. Size and number of human blood cells.

Cell Type	Size	Number*
Erythrocyte	6.5–8 μm (mean = 7.5 μm)	Male: 4.1–6 × 10^6/μL Female: 3.9–5.5 × 10^6/μL
Leukocyte		6000–10,000/μL
Neutrophil	12–15 μm	60–70%
Eosinophil	12–15 μm	2–4%
Basophil	12–15 μm	0–1%
Lymphocyte	6–18 μm	20–30%
Monocyte	12–20 μm	3–8%
Platelet	2–4 μm	200,000–400,000/μL

*Some publications give these values per cubic millimeter (mm^3). Microliters and cubic millimeters are identical units.

spherical, nonmotile cells, but they are capable of becoming flattened and motile on encountering a solid substrate. Leukocytes leave the capillaries by passing between endothelial cells and penetrating the connective tissue by means of a process called **diapedesis** (Gr. *dia,* through, + *pedesis,* to leap). Leukocytes are a normal cellular component of connective tissue. Diapedesis is a constant process, which accounts for the unidirectional flow of granulocytes and monocytes from the blood to the tissues. (Lymphocytes recirculate.) Diapedesis is increased in individuals infected by microorganisms.

The number of leukocytes in the blood varies according to age, sex, and physiologic conditions. In normal adults, there are roughly 6,000–10,000 leukocytes per microliter of blood.

Neutrophils (Polymorphonuclear Leukocytes)

Neutrophils constitute 60–70% of circulating leukocytes. They are 12–15 μm in diameter, with a nucleus consisting of 2–5 (usually 3) lobes linked by fine threads of chromatin (Figures 12–6, 12–7, and 12–8). The immature neutrophil (band form)

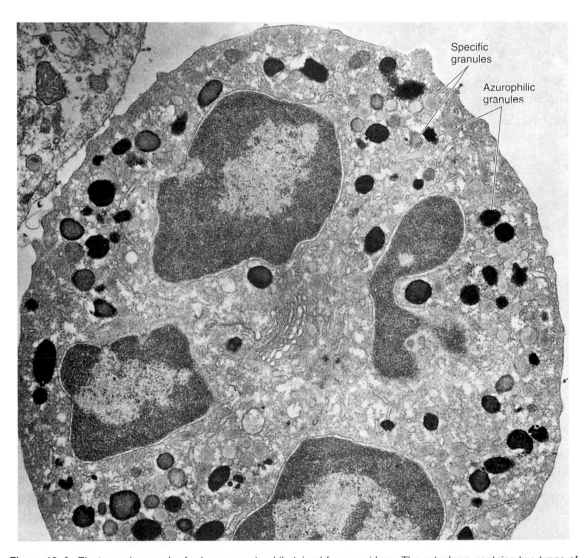

Figure 12–6. Electron micrograph of a human neutrophil stained for peroxidase. The cytoplasm contains two types of granules: the small, pale, peroxidase-negative specific granules and the larger, dense, peroxidase-positive azurophilic granules. The nucleus is lobulated (N^1-N^4), and the Golgi complex is small. Rough endoplasmic reticulum and mitochondria are not abundant, because this cell is in the terminal stage of its differentiation. × 27,000. Reproduced, with permission, from Bainton DF: Selective abnormalities of azurophil and specific granules of human neutrophilic leukocytes. Fed Proc 1981;40:1443.)

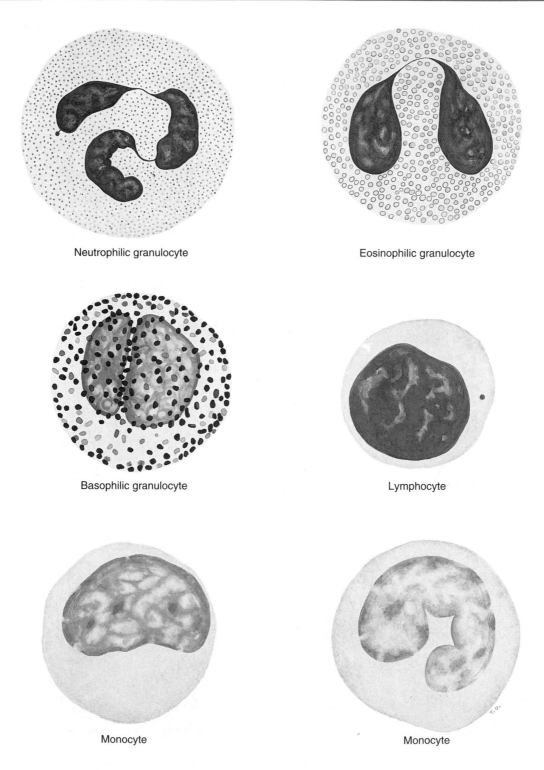

Neutrophilic granulocyte

Eosinophilic granulocyte

Basophilic granulocyte

Lymphocyte

Monocyte

Monocyte

Figure 12–7. The five types of human leukocytes. (See same figure reproduced in color plate.)

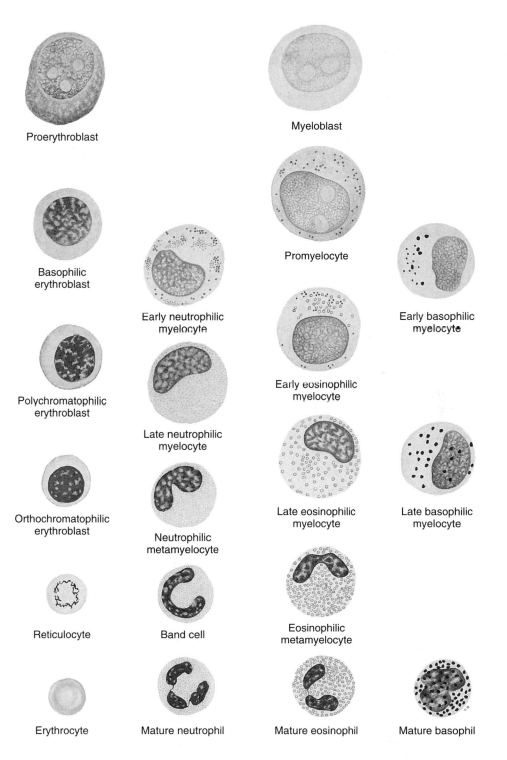

Figure 12–8. Stages of development of erythrocytes and granulocytes. (See same figure reproduced in color plate.)

has a nonsegmented nucleus in the shape of a horse-shoe.

The nuclei of all granulocytes have a similar chromatin pattern, in which dense masses of heterochromatin are distributed on the inner surface of the nuclear envelope. Zones of loosely arranged euchromatin are located mainly in the center of the nucleus.

Neutrophils with more than five lobes are called **hypersegmented** and are typically old cells. Although the maturation of the neutrophil parallels the increase in the number of nuclear lobes under normal conditions, this relationship is not absolute. In some pathologic conditions, young cells appear with five or more lobes.

In females, the inactive X chromosome appears as a drumstick-like appendage on one of the lobes of the nucleus (see Figure 12–7). However, this characteristic is not obvious in all neutrophils in a blood smear. The cytoplasm of the neutrophil contains two types of granules. The more abundant granules are the **specific granules,** which are small, near the limit of resolution of the light microscope (Figure 12–6).

The second granule population in neutrophils consists of **azurophilic granules** about 0.5 μm in diameter. These are primary lysosomes and contain the enzymes listed in Table 12–2. Neutrophils also contain glycogen in their cytoplasm.

Glycogen is broken down to yield energy via the glycolytic pathway of glucose oxidation. The citric acid cycle is less important, as might be expected in view of the paucity of mitochondria in these cells. The ability of neutrophils to survive in an anaerobic environment is highly advantageous, since they can kill bacteria and help clean up debris in poorly oxygenated regions, eg, inflamed or necrotic tissue.

Neutrophils are short-lived cells with a half-life of 6–7 hours in blood and a life span of 1–4 days in connective tissues, where they die by apoptosis.

Neutrophils constitute a defense against invasion by microorganisms, especially bacteria. They are active phagocytes of small particles and have sometimes been called **microphages** to distinguish them from **macrophages,** which are larger cells. Neutrophils are inactive and spherical while circulating but change shape upon adhering to a solid substrate, over which they migrate via pseudopodia.

Bacteria first adhere to the neutrophil surface and then are surrounded and engulfed by pseudopodia; in this way, bacteria eventually occupy vacuoles (phagosomes) delimited by a membrane derived from the cell surface. Immediately thereafter, specific granules fuse with and discharge their contents into the phagosomes. By means of proton pumps in the phagosome membrane, the pH of the vacuole is lowered to about 5.0, a favorable pH for maximal activity of lysosomal enzymes. Azurophilic granules then discharge their enzymes into the acid environment, killing and digesting the microorganisms.

During phagocytosis, a burst of O_2 consumption leads to the formation of superoxide (O_2^-) anions and hydrogen peroxide (H_2O_2). O_2^- is a short-lived free radical formed by the gain of one electron by O_2. It is a highly reactive radical that kills microorganisms ingested by neutrophils. Together with myeloperoxidase and halide ions, it forms a powerful killing system. Other strong oxidizing agents (eg, hypochlorite) can inactivate proteins. Lysozyme has the function of specifically cleaving a bond in the peptidoglycan that forms the cell wall of some gram-positive bacteria, thus causing their death. Lactoferrin avidly binds iron; because iron is a crucial element in bacterial nutrition, lack of its availability leads to bacterial death. The acid environment of phagocytic vacuoles can itself cause the death of certain microorganisms. A combination of these mechanisms will kill most microorganisms, which are then digested by lysosomal enzymes. Dead neutrophils, bacteria, semidigested material, and tissue fluid form a viscous, usually yellow collection of fluid called **pus.**

Several neutrophil hereditary dysfunctions have been described. In one of them, actin does not polymerize normally, and the neutrophils are sluggish. In another, there is a failure to produce O_2^-, H_2O_2, and hypochlorite, and microbial killing power is reduced. This dysfunction results from a deficiency of NADPH oxidase, leading to a deficient respiratory burst. Children with these dysfunctions are subject to persistent bacterial infections. More severe infections result when neutrophil dysfunction and macrophage dysfunction occur simultaneously.

Eosinophils

Eosinophils are far less numerous than neutrophils, constituting only 2–4% of leukocytes in normal blood. The cell has a diameter of 12–15 μm and contains a characteristic bilobed nucleus (Figure 12–7). The endoplasmic reticulum, Golgi complex, and mitochondria are poorly developed (Figure 12–9). Glycogen particles are relatively abundant. The main identifying characteristic is the presence of many large and elongated refractile specific granules (about 200 per cell) that are stained by eosin.

Eosinophilic specific granules have a crystalline core (**internum**) that lies parallel to the long axis of the granule (see Figure 12–9). It contains a protein—called the **major basic protein**—with a large number of arginine residues. This protein constitutes 50% of the total granule protein and accounts for the eosinophilia of these granules. The major basic protein also seems to function in the killing of parasitic

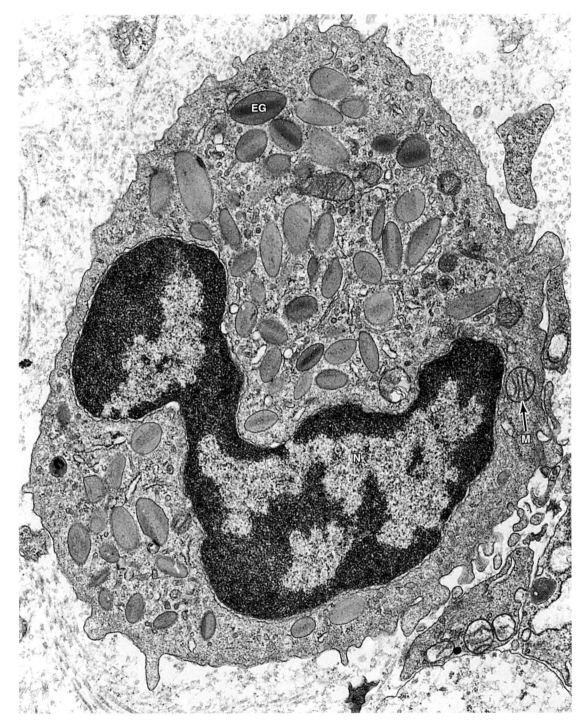

Figure 12–9. Electron micrograph of an eosinophil. Typical eosinophilic granules are clearly seen. Each granule has a disk-shaped electron-dense crystalline core that appears surrounded by a matrix enveloped by a unit membrane. EG, eosinophil granule; N, nucleus; M, mitochondria. × 20,000.

worms such as schistosomes. The less dense material surrounding the internum is known as the **externum,** or **matrix,** and consists of the enzymes listed in Table 12–2.

> An increase in the absolute number of eosinophils in blood (**eosinophilia**) is associated with allergic reactions and helminthic (parasitic) infections. In tissues, eosinophils are found in the connective tissues underlying epithelia of the skin, bronchi, gastrointestinal tract, uterus, and vagina, and surrounding the parasitic worms. In addition, these cells produce substances that modulate inflammation by inactivating the leukotrienes and histamine produced by other cells.

Corticosteroids (hormones from the adrenal cortex) produce a rapid decrease in the number of blood eosinophils, probably by interfering with the release of granulocytes from the bone marrow into the bloodstream.

Basophils

Basophils make up less than 1% of blood leukocytes and are therefore difficult to locate in smears of normal blood. They are about 12–15 μm in diameter and have a less heterochromatic nucleus than do other granulocytes. The nucleus is divided into irregular lobes, but the division is usually obscured by the overlying specific granules.

The specific granules (0.5 μm in diameter) stain metachromatically with the basic dye of the usual blood stains (Figures 12–7 and 12–8). This staining is due to the presence of heparin. Specific granules in basophils are fewer and more irregular in size and shape than the granules of the other granulocytes (Figure 12–10). Basophilic specific granules contain heparin and histamine and are capable of generating leukotrienes, which cause slow contraction of smooth

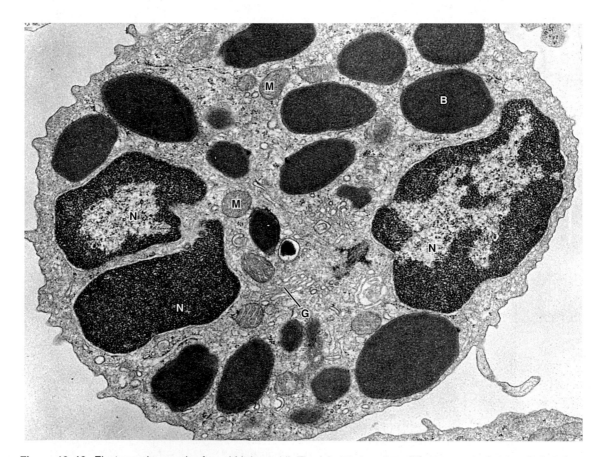

Figure 12–10. Electron micrograph of a rabbit basophil. The lobulated nucleus (N) appears as 3 separated portions. Note the basophilic granules (B), mitochondria (M), and Golgi complex (G). × 16,000. (Reproduced, with permission, from Terry RW et al: Lab Invest 1969;21:65.)

muscles. Basophils may supplement the functions of mast cells in immediate hypersensitivity reactions by migrating (under special circumstances) into connective tissues.

There is some similarity between granules of basophils and those of mast cells. Both are metachromatic and contain heparin and histamine. Basophils can liberate their granule content in response to certain antigens, as can mast cells (see Chapter 5). Despite the similarities they present, mast cells and basophils are not the same, for even in the same species they have different ultrastructural appearances, and they originate from different stem cells in the bone marrow.

In the dermatologic disease called **cutaneous basophil hypersensitivity,** basophils are the major cell type at the site of inflammation.

Lymphocytes

Lymphocytes constitute a family of spherical cells with similar morphologic characteristics. They can be classified into several groups according to distinctive surface molecules (markers), which can be distinguished only by immunocytochemical methods. They also have diverse functional roles, all related to immune reactions in defending against invading microorganisms, foreign macromolecules, and cancer cells (see Chapter 14).

Lymphocytes with diameters of 6–8 μm are known as **small lymphocytes.** A small number of **medium-sized lymphocytes** and **large lymphocytes** with diameters up to 18 μm are present in the circulating blood. This difference has functional significance in that some larger lymphocytes are believed to be cells activated by specific antigens. These cells differentiate into effector T or B lymphocytes. Both B and T lymphocytes possess specific antigen receptors on their surface, represented by monomeric IgM molecules in B cells and γδ or αβ heterodimeric receptors in T cells. In the periphery most T cells express the αβ T cell receptor (90%), and a small number express the γδ receptor. The αβ T cell receptor interacts with complexes of peptides associated with class I or class II MHC (major histocompatibility complex) molecules, but the specificity of the γδ T cell receptor is still unknown (see Chapter 14).

The small lymphocyte, which is predominant in the blood, has a spherical nucleus, sometimes with an indentation. Its chromatin is condensed and appears as coarse clumps, so that the nucleus is intensely stained in the usual preparations, a characteristic that facilitates identification of the lymphocyte. In blood smears, the nucleolus of the lymphocyte is not visible, but it can be demonstrated by special staining techniques and with the electron microscope.

The cytoplasm of the small lymphocyte is scanty, and in blood smears it appears as a thin rim around the nucleus. It is slightly basophilic, assuming a light blue color in stained smears (Figure 12–7). It may contain a few azurophilic granules. The cytoplasm of the small lymphocyte has a few mitochondria and a small Golgi complex associated with a pair of centrioles; it contains free polyribosomes (Figure 12–11).

Lymphocytes vary in life span; some live only a few days, and others survive in the circulating blood for many years. Lymphocytes are the only type of leukocytes that return from the tissues back to the blood, after diapedesis. (For lymphocyte recirculation, see Chapter 14.)

Monocytes

Monocytes are bone marrow–derived agranulocytes with diameters varying from 12 to 20 μm. The nucleus is oval, horseshoe- or kidney-shaped, and is generally eccentrically placed (see Figure 12–7). The chromatin is less condensed and has a more fibrillar arrangement than that in lymphocytes; this is the most consistent characteristic of the monocyte (see Figure 12–12). Because of their delicate chromatin distribution, the nuclei of monocytes stain lighter than do those of large lymphocytes.

The cytoplasm of the monocyte is basophilic and frequently contains very fine azurophilic granules (lysosomes), some of which are at the limit of the light microscope's resolution. These granules are distributed through the cytoplasm, giving it a bluish-gray color in stained smears. In the electron microscope, one or two nucleoli are seen in the nucleus, and a small quantity of rough endoplasmic reticulum, polyribosomes, and many small mitochondria are observed. A Golgi complex involved in the formation of the lysosomal granules is present in the cytoplasm. Many microvilli and pinocytotic vesicles are found at the cell surface.

Blood monocytes are precursor cells of the mononuclear phagocyte system (see Chapter 5). After crossing capillary walls and entering connective tissues, monocytes differentiate into macrophages.

Platelets

Blood platelets (**thrombocytes**) are nonnucleated, disk-like cell fragments 2–4 μm in diameter. Platelets originate from the fragmentation of giant polyploid **megakaryocytes** that reside in the bone marrow. Platelets promote blood clotting and help repair gaps in the walls of blood vessels, preventing loss of blood. Normal platelet counts range from 200,000 to 400,000 per microliter of blood. Platelets have a life span of about 10 days.

In stained blood smears, platelets often appear in clumps. Each platelet has a peripheral light blue–stained transparent zone, the **hyalomere,** and a central zone containing purple granules, called the **granulomere.**

Platelets contain a system of channels, the **open canalicular system,** that connect to invaginations of

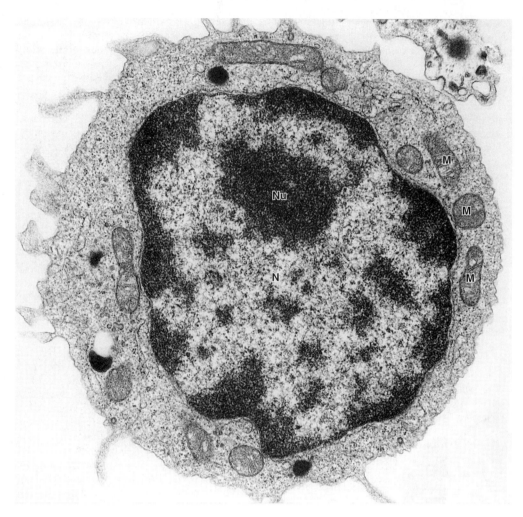

Figure 12–11. Electron micrograph of a human blood lymphocyte. This cell has little rough endoplasmic reticulum but a moderate quantity of free polyribosomes. Note the nucleus (N), the nucleolus (Nu) and the mitochondria (M). Reduced from × 22,000.

the platelet plasma membrane (Figure 12–13). This arrangement is probably of functional significance in facilitating the liberation of active molecules stored in platelets. Around the periphery of the platelet lies a **marginal bundle** of microtubules; this bundle helps to maintain the platelet's ovoid shape. In the hyalomere, there are also a number of electron-dense irregular tubes known as the **dense tubular system.** Actin and myosin molecules in the hyalomere can assemble to form a contractile system that functions in platelet movement and aggregation. A cell coat rich in glycosaminoglycans and glycoproteins, 15–20 nm thick, lies outside the plasmalemma and is involved in platelet adhesion.

The central granulomere possesses a variety of membrane-bound granules and a sparse population of mitochondria and glycogen particles (Figure 12–13). **Dense bodies (delta granules)**, 250–300 nm in di-

ameter, contain calcium ions, pyrophosphate, ADP, and ATP. These granules also take up and store serotonin (5-hydroxytryptamine) from the plasma. **Alpha granules** are a little larger (300–500 nm in diameter) and contain fibrinogen, platelet-derived growth factor, and several other platelet-specific proteins. Small vesicles, 175–250 nm in diameter, have been shown to contain only lysosomal enzymes and have been termed **lambda granules.** Most of the azurophilic granules seen with the light microscope in the granulomere of platelets are alpha granules.

Platelet functions. The role of platelets in controlling hemorrhage can be summarized as follows.

1. Primary aggregation—Discontinuities in the endothelium, produced by blood vessel lesions, are followed by absorption of plasma proteins on the subjacent collagen. Platelets immediately aggregate on this damaged tissue, forming a **platelet plug.**

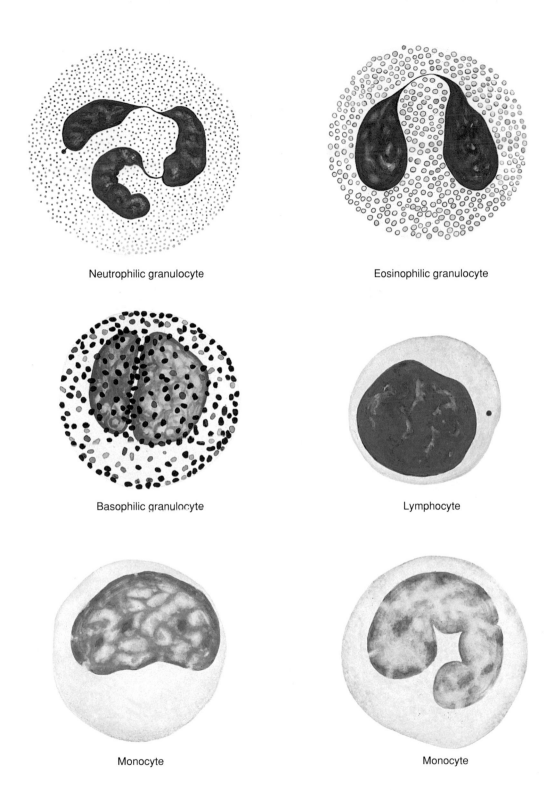

Neutrophilic granulocyte

Eosinophilic granulocyte

Basophilic granulocyte

Lymphocyte

Monocyte

Monocyte

Color Plate 1. The five types of human leukocytes. (See Figure 12–7.)

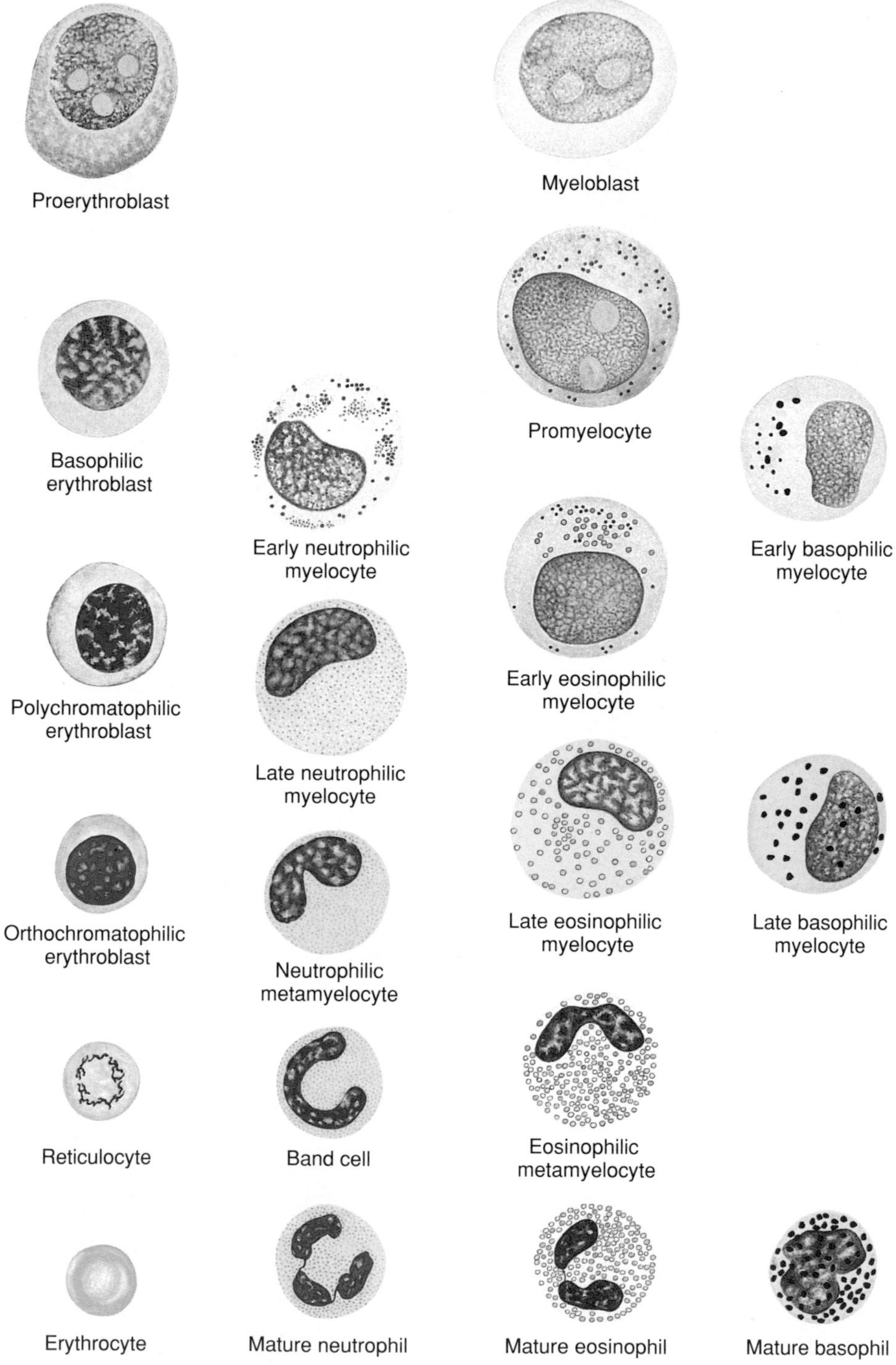

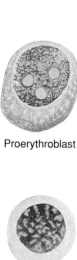

Proerythroblast

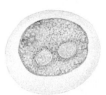

Myeloblast

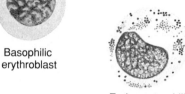

Basophilic
erythroblast

Early neutrophilic
myelocyte

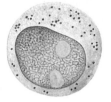

Promyelocyte

Early basophilic
myelocyte

Polychromatophilic
erythroblast

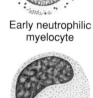

Late neutrophilic
myelocyte

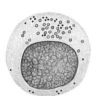

Early eosinophilic
myelocyte

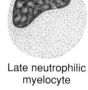

Orthochromatophilic
erythroblast

Neutrophilic
metamyelocyte

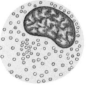

Late eosinophilic
myelocyte

Late basophilic
myelocyte

Reticulocyte

Band cell

Eosinophilic
metamyelocyte

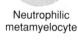

Erythrocyte

Mature neutrophil

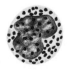

Mature eosinophil

Mature basophil

Color Plate 2. Stages of development of erythrocytes and granulocytes. (See Figure 12–8.)

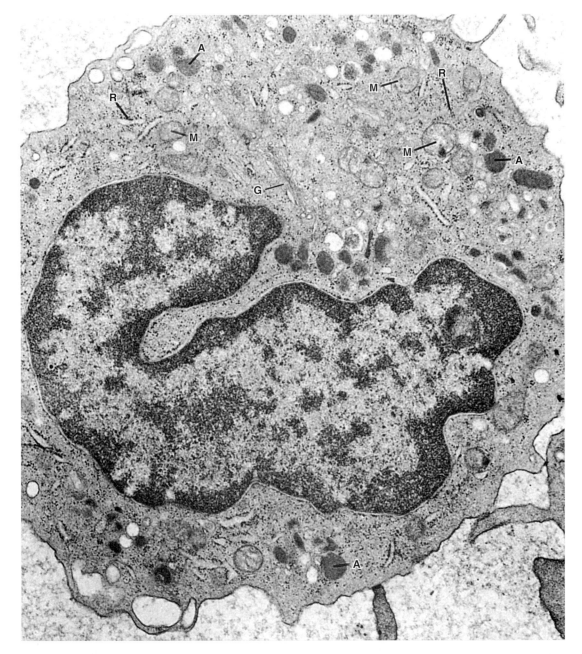

Figure 12–12. Electron micrograph of a human monocyte. Note the Golgi complex (G), the mitochondria (M), and the azurophilic granules (A). Rough endoplasmic reticulum is poorly developed. There are some free ribosomes (R). × 22,000. (Courtesy of DF Bainton and MG Farquhar.)

2. Secondary aggregation—Platelets in the plug release the content of their alpha and delta granules. ADP is a potent inducer of platelet aggregation.

3. Blood coagulation—During platelet aggregation, factors from the blood plasma, damaged blood vessels, and platelets promote the sequential interaction (**cascade**) of approximately 13 plasma proteins, giving rise to a polymer, **fibrin,** that forms a three-dimensional network of fibers trapping red cells, leukocytes, and platelets to form a **blood clot, or thrombus.**

4. Clot retraction—The clot that initially bulges into the blood vessel lumen contracts because of the interaction of platelet actin, myosin, and ATP.

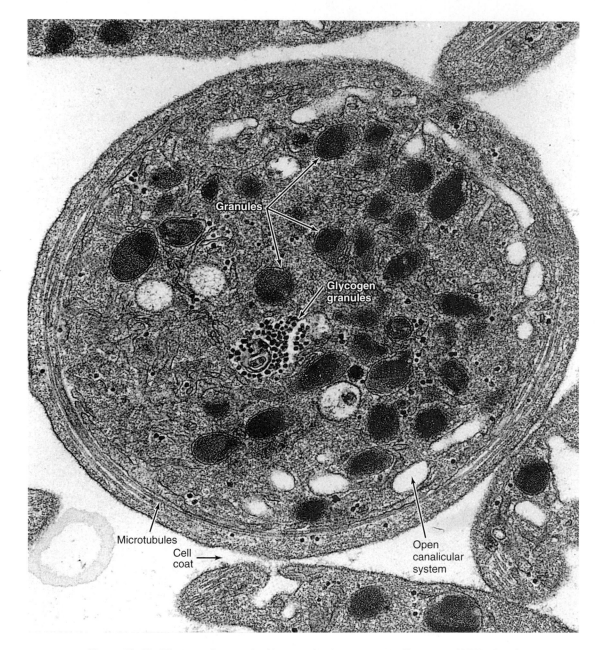

Figure 12–13. Electron micrograph of human platelets. × 40,740. (Courtesy of M Harrison.)

5. Clot removal—Protected by the clot, the vessel wall is restored by new tissue formation. The clot is then removed, mainly by the proteolytic enzyme **plasmin,** formed, through the activation of the plasma proenzyme **plasminogen,** by endothelium-produced **plasminogen activators.** Enzymes released from platelet lambda granules also contribute to clot removal.

REFERENCES

Bainton DF: Sequential degranulation of the 2 types of polymorphonuclear leukocyte granules during phagocytosis of microorganisms. J Cell Biol 1973;58:249.

Cline MJ: *The White Cell.* Harvard Univ Press, 1975.
Comenzo, RL, Berkman EM: Hematopoietic stem and progenitor cells from blood. Transfusion 1995;35:335.

Gowans JL: Differentiation of the cells which synthesize the immunoglobulins. Ann Immunol (Paris) 1974;125: 201.

Stites DP et al (editors): *Basic & Clinical Immunology,* 6th ed. Appleton & Lange, 1987.

Williams WJ et al: *Hematology,* 5th ed. McGraw-Hill, 1995.

Wintrobe MM et al: *Clinical Hematology,* 8th ed. Lea & Febiger, 1981.

Zucker-Franklin D et al: *Atlas of Blood Cells: Function and Pathology.* Vols 1 and 2. Lea & Febiger, 1981.

13   Hematopoiesis

Mature blood cells have a relatively short life span, and consequently the population must be continuously replaced with the progeny of stem cells produced in the **hematopoietic** (Gr. *haima,* blood, + *poiesis,* a making) organs. In the earliest stages of embryogenesis, blood cells arise from the yolk sac mesoderm. Sometime later, the liver and spleen serve as temporary hematopoietic tissues, but by the second month the clavicle has begun to ossify and begins to develop bone marrow in its core. As the prenatal ossification of the rest of the skeleton accelerates, the bone marrow becomes an increasingly important hematopoietic tissue.

After birth and on into childhood, erythrocytes, granular leukocytes, monocytes, and platelets are derived from stem cells located in bone marrow. The origin and maturation of these cells are termed, respectively, **erythropoiesis** (Gr. *erythros,* red, + *poiesis*), **granulopoiesis, monocytopoiesis,** and **megakaryocytopoiesis.** The bone marrow also produces cells that migrate to the lymphoid organs, producing the various types of lymphocytes discussed in Chapter 14.

Before attaining maturity and being released into the circulation, blood cells go through specific stages of differentiation and maturation. Because these processes are continuous, cells with characteristics that lie between the various stages are frequently encountered in smears of blood or bone marrow.

STEM CELLS, GROWTH FACTORS, & DIFFERENTIATION

Stem cells are **pluripotential** cells capable of self-renewal. Some of their daughter cells form specific, irreversibly differentiated cell types, and other daughter cells remain stem cells. A constant number of pluripotential stem cells is maintained in a pool, and cells recruited for differentiation are replaced with daughter cells from the pool.

Hematopoietic stem cells are isolated by using fluorescence-labeled antibodies to mark specific cell-surface antigens and a fluorescence-activated, cell-

sorting instrument. This technique is important in medical practice and research. Stem cells are also studied by means of experimental techniques that permit analysis of hematopoiesis in vivo and in vitro.

In vivo techniques include injecting the bone marrow of normal donor mice into lethally irradiated mice whose hematopoietic cells have been destroyed. In these animals, the transplanted bone marrow cells develop colonies of hematopoietic cells in the spleen.

In vitro techniques involve the use of a semisolid tissue culture medium made with a layer of cells derived from bone marrow stroma. This medium creates favorable microenvironmental conditions for hematopoiesis. Data from an extensive series of experiments show that under these favorable microenvironmental conditions, stimulation by growth factors influences the development of the various types of blood cells.

Pluripotential Hematopoietic Stem Cells. It is believed that all blood cells arise from a single type of stem cell in the bone marrow. Because this cell can produce all blood cell types, it is called a **pluripotential stem cell** (Figure 13–1). These cells proliferate and form one cell lineage that will become lymphocytes (**lymphoid cells**) and another lineage that will form the **myeloid cells** that develop in bone marrow (granulocytes, monocytes, erythrocytes, and megakaryocytes). Early in their development, lymphoid cells migrate from the bone marrow to the lymph nodes, spleen, and thymus, where they complete their differentiation into lymphocytes (Figure 13–1; see also Chapter 14).

Progenitor and Precursor Cells. The proliferating stem cells form daughter cells with reduced potentiality. These **unipotential** or **bipotential progenitor cells** generate **precursor cells** (**blasts**) in which the morphologic characteristics differentiate for the first time, suggesting the cell types they will become (see Figures 13–1 and 12–8). In contrast, stem and progenitor cells cannot be morphologically distinguished and resemble lymphocytes. Stem cells divide at a rate sufficient to maintain their relatively small population. The rate of cell division is accelerated in progenitor and precursor cells, and large numbers of

Phase	Stem Cells	Progenitor Cells	Precursor Cells (Blasts)	Mature Cells
Early morphologic	Not morphologically distinguishable; have the general aspect of lymphocytes		Beginning of morphologic differentiation	Clear morphologic differentiation
Mitotic activity	Low mitotic activity; self-renewing; scarce in bone marrow	High mitotic activity; self-renewing; common in marrow and lymphoid organs; mono- or bipotential	High mitotic activity; not self-renewing; common in marrow and lymphoid organs; monopotential	No mitotic activity; abundant in blood and hematopoietic organs

Figure 13-8 shows the morphologic differentiation of these cells.

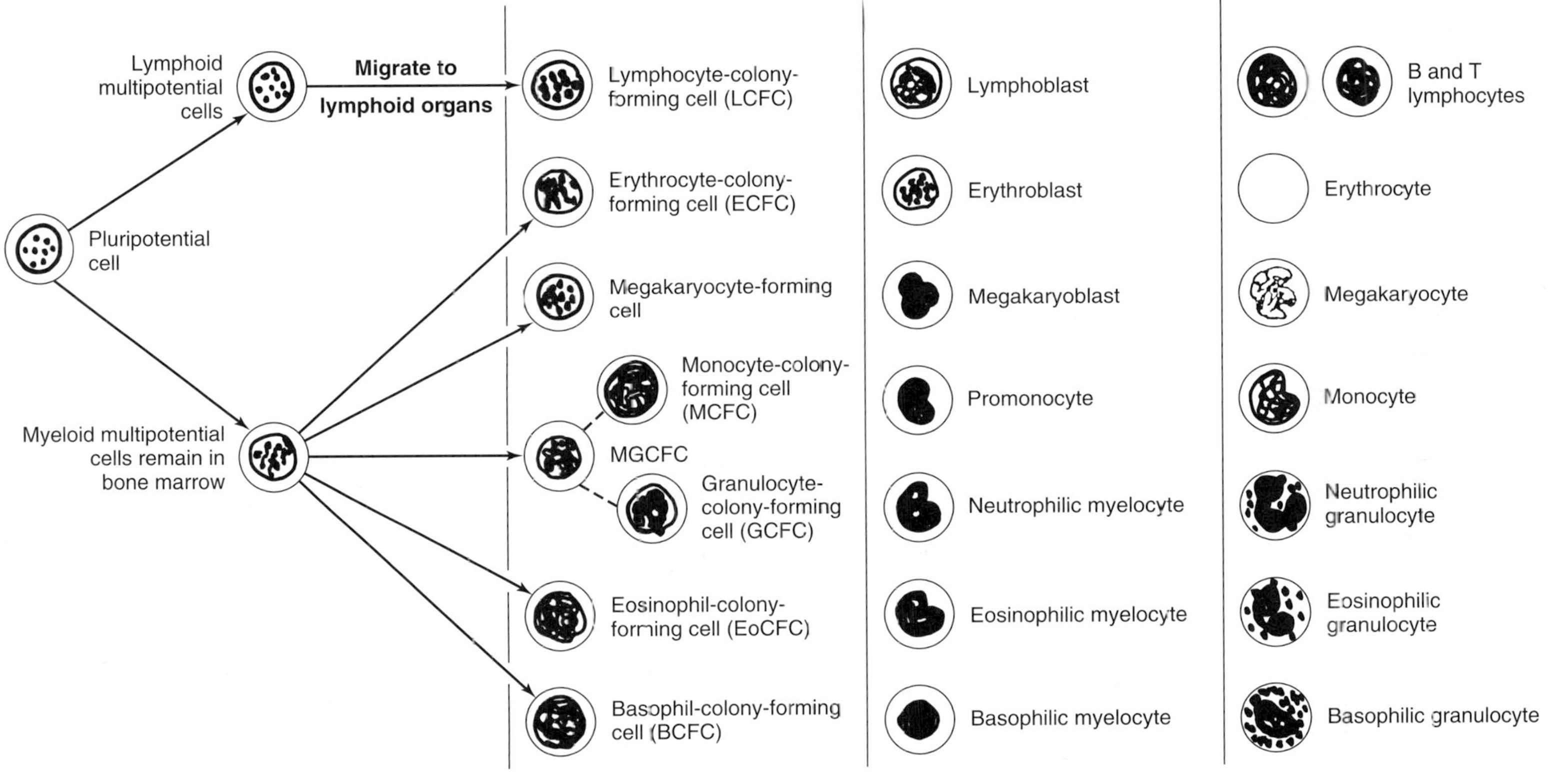

Figure 13–1. Differentiation of pluripotential stem cells during hematopoiesis. See also Figure 12–8.

differentiated, mature cells are produced (3×10^9 erythrocytes and 0.85×10^9 granulocytes/kg/day in human bone marrow). Whereas progenitor cells can divide and produce both progenitor and precursor cells, precursor cells produce only mature blood cells.

Hematopoiesis is therefore the result of simultaneous, continuous proliferation and differentiation of cells derived from stem cells whose potentiality is reduced as differentiation progresses. This process can be observed in both in vivo and in vitro studies, in which colonies of cells derived from stem cells with various potentialities appear. Colonies derived from a myeloid stem cell can produce erythrocytes, granulocytes, monocytes, and megakaryocytes, all in the same colony.

In these experiments, however, some colonies produce only red blood cells (erythrocytes). Other colonies produce granulocytes and monocytes. Cells forming colonies are called **colony-forming cells (CFC)**, or **colony-forming units (CFU)**. The convention in naming these various cell colonies is to use the initial letter of the cell each colony produces. Thus, MCFC denotes a monocyte-forming colony, ECFC forms erythrocytes, MGCFC forms monocytes and granulocytes, and so on.

Hematopoiesis depends on favorable microenvironmental conditions and the presence of growth factors. The microenvironmental conditions are furnished by cells of the stroma of hematopoietic organs, which produce an essential extracellular matrix. A general view of hematopoiesis shows that, as this process takes place, both the potential for differentiation and the self-renewing capacity of the initial cells gradually decrease. In contrast, the mitotic response to growth factors gradually increases, attaining its maximum in the middle of the process. From that point on, morphologic characteristics and functional activity develop, and mature cells form (Table 13–1). Once the necessary environmental conditions are present, the development of blood cells depends on factors that affect cell proliferation and differentiation. These substances are called **growth factors, colony-stimulating factors (CSF)**, or **hematopoietins (poietins)**. Growth factors, which have differing chemical compositions and complex, overlapping functions, act mainly by stimulating proliferation (mitogenic activity) of immature (mostly progenitor and precursor) cells, supporting the differentiation of maturing cells and enhancing the functions of mature cells.

The three functions just described may be present in the same growth factor, but they may be expressed with different levels of intensity in different growth factors. The isolation and cloning of genes for several growth factors permits both the mass production of growth factors and the study of their effects in vivo and in vitro. The main characteristics of the five best-characterized growth factors are presented in Table 13–2.

Growth factors have been used clinically to increase marrow cellularity and blood cell counts. The use of growth factors to stimulate the proliferation of leukocytes is opening broad new applications for clinical therapy. Potential therapeutic uses of growth factors include increasing the number of blood cells in diseases or induced conditions (eg, chemotherapy, irradiation) that result in low blood counts; increasing the efficiency of marrow transplants by enhancing cell proliferation; enhancing host defenses in patients with malignancies and infectious and immunodeficient diseases; and enhancing the treatment of parasitic diseases.

Hematopoietic diseases rarely result from the malfunctioning of hematopoietic organ stroma. They are usually caused by suppression or enhancement of undifferentiated cell production, with a consequent reduction or overproduction of hematopoietic cells. In some diseases, however, suppression and enhancement of proliferation of more than one type of stem cell can occur, sequentially or simultaneously. In such cases, there are reduced numbers of some cell types (eg, aplastic anemia, a disorder characterized by decreased production of hematopoietic cells) coinciding with increased numbers of others (eg, leukemia, the abnormal proliferation of leukocytes).

The initial experiments with normal bone marrow transplanted to lethally irradiated mice established the basis for bone marrow transplantation, now routinely used to treat some disorders of hematopoietic cell growth.

BONE MARROW

Bone marrow is one of the largest organs of the body and the main site of hematopoiesis. Under normal conditions, the production of blood cells by the marrow is perfectly adjusted to the organism's functions. It can adjust rapidly to the body's needs, increasing its activity several-fold in a very short time. Bone marrow is found in the medullary canals of long bones and in the cavities of cancellous bones (Figure 13–2). Two types of bone marrow have been described according to their appearance on gross examination: **red, or hematogenous, bone marrow,** whose color is produced by the presence of blood and blood-forming cells; and **yellow bone marrow,** whose color is produced by the presence of a great number of adipose cells. In newborns, all bone marrow is red and is therefore active in the production of blood cells. As the child grows, most of

Table 13–1. Changes in properties of hematopoietic cells during differentiation.

Stem Cells	Progenitor Cells	Precursor Cells (Blasts)	Mature Cells
Potentiality			
		Mitotic activity	
			Typical morphologic characteristics
Self-renewing capacity			
	Influence of growth factors		
			Differentiated functional activity

the bone marrow changes gradually into the yellow variety. Under certain conditions, such as severe bleeding or hypoxia, yellow bone marrow reverts to red bone marrow.

Red Bone Marrow

Red bone marrow (Figures 13–3 through 13–6) is composed of a **stroma** (from Greek, meaning bed), **hematopoietic cords,** and **sinusoidal capillaries.** The stroma is a three-dimensional meshwork of reticular cells and a delicate web of reticular fibers containing hematopoietic cells and macrophages. The matrix of bone marrow contains collagen types I and III, fibronectin, laminin, and proteoglycans. Laminin, fibronectin, and another cell-binding substance, **hemonectin,** interact with cell receptors to bind cells to the matrix. The sinusoids are formed by a continuous layer of endothelial cells. Some regions of the endothelium are thin and may be sites for migration of mature cells from the stroma into the sinusoid (Figure 13–6).

The sinusoidal capillaries are reinforced by an external discontinuous layer of reticular cells and a loose net of reticular fibers. The release of mature bone cells from the marrow is controlled by **releasing factors** produced in response to the needs of the organism. Several substances with releasing activity have been described, including the C3 component of **complement** (a series of immunologically active blood proteins), hormones (glucocorticoids and androgens), and some bacterial toxins. The release of cells from the marrow is illustrated in Figure 13–6.

The main functions of red bone marrow are the production of blood cells, destruction of red blood

Table 13–2. Main characteristics of the five best-know hematopoietic growth factors (colony-forming substances.)

Name	Human Gene Location and Producing Cells	Main Biologic Activity
Granulocyte (G-CSF)	Chromosome 17 Macrophages Endothelium Fibroblasts	Stimulates formation (in vitro and in vivo) of granulocytes. Enhances metabolism of granulocytes. Stimulates malignant (leukemic) cells.
Granulocyte + macrophage (GM-CSF)	Chrososome 5 T lymphocytes Endothelium Fibroblasts	Stimulates in vitro and in vivo production of granulocytes and macrophages.
Macrophage (M-CSF)	Chromosome 5 Macrophages Endothelium Fibroblasts	Stimulates formation of macrophages in vitro. Increases antitumor activity of macrophages.
Interleukin 3 (IL-3)	Chromosome 5 T lymphocytes	Stimulates in vivo and in vitro the production of all myeloid cells.
Erythropoietin (EPO)	Chromosome 7 Renal interstitial cells (outer cortex)	Stimulates red blood cell formation in vivo and in vitro.

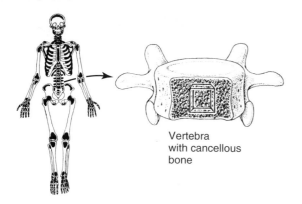

Figure 13–2. Distribution of red bone marrow (hematopoietic active) in the adult. This type of bone marrow tends to be located in cancellous bone tissue. (Reproduced, with permission, from Krstić RV: *Human Microscopic Anatomy.* Springer-Verlag, 1991.)

Vertebra with cancellous bone

cells, and storage (in macrophages) of iron derived from the breakdown of hemoglobin.

MATURATION OF ERYTHROCYTES

A **mature** cell is one that has differentiated to the stage at which it has the capability of carrying out all its specific functions. The basic process in matura-

tion is the synthesis of hemoglobin and the formation of an enucleated, biconcave, small corpuscle, the erythrocyte (see Figures 12–3 and 12–4). During maturation of the erythrocyte, several major changes take place. Cell volume decreases, and the nucleoli diminish in size until they become invisible in the light microscope. The nuclear diameter decreases, and the chromatin becomes increasingly more dense until the nucleus presents a pyknotic appearance (Figure 13–7) and is finally extruded from the cell. There is a gradual decrease in the number of polyribosomes (basophilia), followed by a simultaneous increase in the amount of hemoglobin (acidophilia) within the cytoplasm, and the mitochondria gradually disappear (Figures 13–8 and 13–9).

There are three to five intervening cell divisions between the proerythroblast and the mature erythrocyte. The development of an erythrocyte from the first recognizable cell of the series to the release of reticulocytes into the blood takes approximately 7 days. The hormone erythropoietin and substances such as iron, folic acid, and vitamin B_{12} are essential for the production of erythrocytes. **Erythropoietin** is a glycoprotein produced in the kidneys that stimulates the production of mRNA for **globin,** the protein component of the hemoglobin molecule.

Differentiation

The differentiation and maturation of erythrocytes involve the formation (in order) of proerythroblasts,

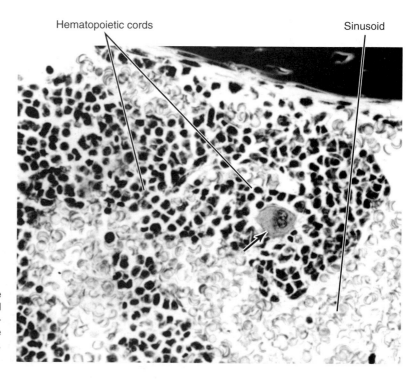

Hematopoietic cords

Sinusoid

Figure 13–3. Section of active bone marrow showing the cell cords separated by sinusoidal capillaries filled with erythrocytes. The arrow indicates a megakaryocyte. × 140.

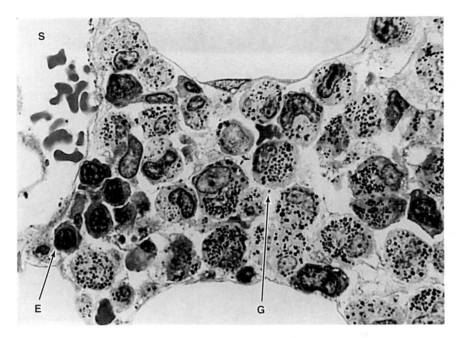

Figure 13–4. Photomicrograph of a section of red bone marrow. At the left is one sinusoid (S) with a group of erythrocyte precursors (E) nearby. Most of the figure is occupied by precursors of granulocytes (G), identified by the clearly visible cytoplasmic granules.

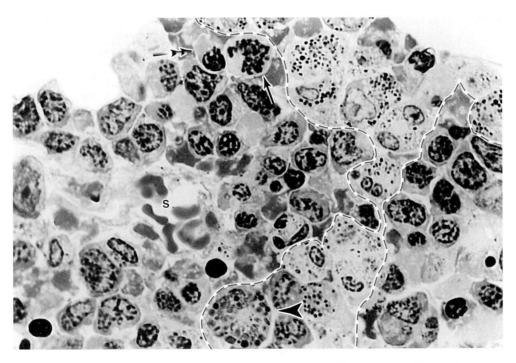

Figure 13–5. Photomicrograph (high-power magnification) of a section of red bone marrow. Close to the center and delimited by dotted lines are several granulocyte precursors with granules in their cytoplasm. The arrowhead indicates an immature eosinophil. The other cells with cytoplasmic granules are neutrophil precursors. The arrow shows a mitosis, and the double arrow indicates an erythroblast in the process of expelling its nucleus.

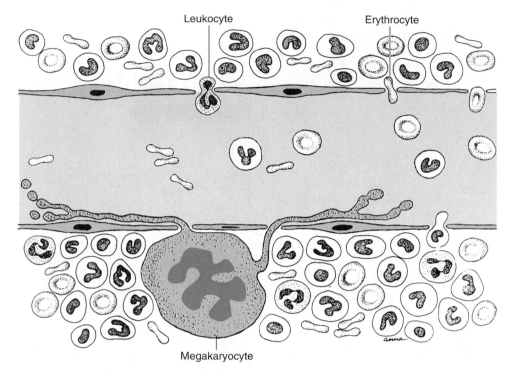

Figure 13–6. The passage of erythrocytes, leukocytes, and platelets across a sinusoid in bone marrow. Because immature erythrocytes (unlike leukocytes) do not have sufficient motility to cross the wall of the sinusoid, they are believed to enter the sinusoids by a pressure gradient that exists across its wall. Leukocytes, after the action of releasing substances (see text), are free to cross the wall of the sinusoid. Megakaryocytes form thin processes that cross the wall of the sinusoid and fragment at their tips, liberating the platelets.

basophilic erythroblasts, polychromatophilic erythroblasts, orthochromatophilic erythroblasts (normoblasts), reticulocytes, and erythrocytes (Figure 12–8).

The first recognizable cell in the erythroid series is the **proerythroblast.** It is a large cell with loose, lacy chromatin and clearly visible nucleoli; its cytoplasm is basophilic. The next stage is represented by the **basophilic erythroblast** (*erythros* + Gr. *blastos,* germ), with a strongly basophilic cytoplasm and a condensed nucleus that has no visible nucleolus. The basophilia of these two cell types is caused by the large number of polyribosomes involved in the synthesis of hemoglobin (Figure 12–8). During the next stage, polyribosomes decrease, and areas of the cytoplasm begin to be filled with hemoglobin. At this stage, staining causes several colors to appear in the cell—the **polychromatophilic** (Gr. *polys,* many, + *chroma,* color, + *philein,* to love) **erythroblast.** In the next stage, the nucleus continues to condense and no cytoplasmic basophilia is evident, resulting in a uniformly acidophilic cytoplasm—the **orthochromatophilic** (Gr. *orthos,* correct, + *chroma* + *philein*) **erythroblast.** At a given moment, this cell puts forth a series of cytoplasmic protrusions and expels its nu-

cleus, encased in a thin layer of cytoplasm. The remaining cell still has a small number of polyribosomes that, when treated with the supravital dye brilliant cresyl blue, aggregate to form a stained network. This cell is the **reticulocyte,** which soon loses its polyribosomes and becomes a mature erythrocyte.

MATURATION OF GRANULOCYTES

The **myeloblast** is the most immature recognizable cell in the myeloid series. It has a finely dispersed chromatin, and nucleoli can be seen. In the next stage, the **promyelocyte** (L. *pro,* before, + Gr. *myelos,* marrow, + *kytos,* cell) is characterized by its basophilic cytoplasm and azurophilic granules. These granules contain lysosomal enzymes and myeloperoxidase. The promyelocyte gives rise to the three known types of granulocyte. The first sign of differentiation appears in the myelocytes, in which specific granules gradually increase in quantity and eventually occupy most of the cytoplasm. These **neutrophilic, basophilic,** and **eosinophilic myelocytes** mature with further condensation of the nucleus and

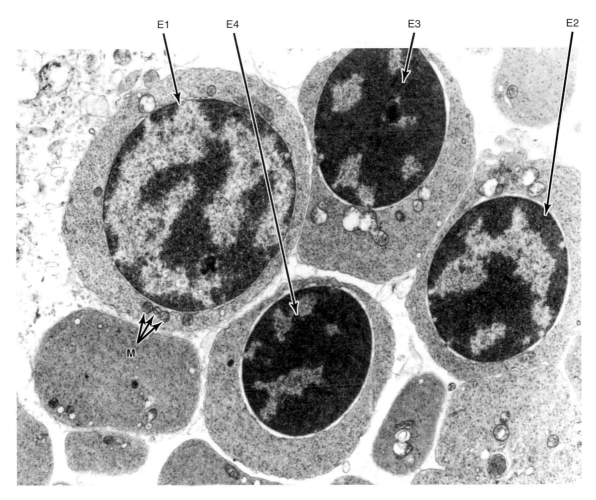

Figure 13–7. Electron micrograph of bone marrow. Four erythroblasts in successive stages of maturation are seen (E1, E2, E3, and E4). As the cell matures, its chromatin becomes gradually condensed, the accumulation of hemoglobin increases the electron density of the cytoplasm, and the mitochondria (M) decrease in number. × 11,000.

a considerable increase in their specific granule content (Figure 13–10). The neutrophilic granulocyte represents an intermediate stage, and its nucleus has the form of a curved rod (band cell). This cell appears in quantity in the blood after strong stimulation of hematopoiesis.

> The appearance of large numbers of immature neutrophils (band cells) in the blood is called a **shift to the left** and is clinically significant, usually indicating bacterial infection.

KINETICS OF NEUTROPHIL PRODUCTION

The total time taken for a myeloblast to emerge as a mature neutrophil in the circulation is about 11 days. Under normal circumstances, five mitotic divisions occur in the myeloblast, promyelocyte, and neutrophilic myelocyte stages of development.

Neutrophils pass through several functionally and anatomically defined compartments (Figure 13–11).

The **medullary formation compartment** can be subdivided into a mitotic compartment (~ 3 days) and a maturation compartment (~ 4 days).

A **medullary storage compartment** acts as a buffer system, capable of releasing large numbers of mature neutrophils on demand. Neutrophils remain in this compartment for about 4 days.

The **circulating compartment** consists of neutrophils suspended in plasma and circulating in blood vessels.

The **marginating compartment** is composed of neutrophils that are present in blood but do not circulate. These neutrophils are in capillaries and are temporarily excluded from the circulation by vasocon-

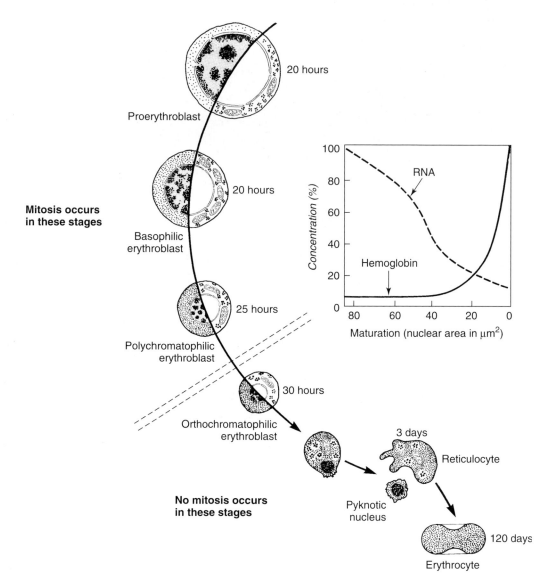

Figure 13–8. Summary of erythrocyte maturation. The stippled part of the cytoplasm (on the left) shows the continuous increase in hemoglobin concentration from proerythroblast to erythrocyte. There is also a gradual decrease in nuclear volume and an increase in chromatin condensation, followed by extrusion of a pyknotic nucleus. The times are the average life span of each cell type. In the graph, 100% represents the highest recorded concentrations of hemoglobin and RNA.

striction, or—especially in the lungs—they may be at the periphery of vessels, adhering to the endothelium, and not in the main bloodstream.

The marginating and circulating compartments are of about equal size, and there is a constant interchange of cells between them. The half-life of a neutrophil in these two compartments is 6–7 hours. The medullary formation and storage compartments to-gether are about 10 times as large as the circulating and marginating compartments.

Neutrophils and other granulocytes enter the connective tissues by passing through intercellular junctions found between endothelial cells of capillaries and postcapillary venules (**diapedesis**). The connective tissues form a fifth compartment for neutrophils, but its size is not known. Neutrophils reside here for

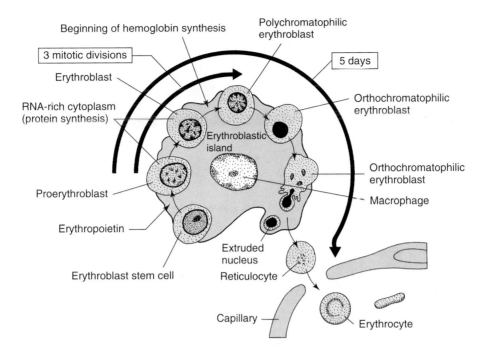

Figure 13–9. Sequence of events during the maturation of erythrocytes. Erythrocytes develop close to macrophages, forming an **erythroblastic island.** Through their phagocytic activity, macrophages destroy aged erythrocytes and transfer ferritin, an iron-containing protein complex, to the young erythroblasts. Macrophages also destroy the nuclei expelled by the erythroblasts and produce growth factors that influence hematopoiesis. (Redrawn, with permission, from Chandrasoma P, Taylor CR: *Concise Pathology.* Appleton & Lange, 1991.)

1–4 days and then die, whether or not they have performed their major function of phagocytosis.

Changes in the number of neutrophils in the peripheral circulation must be evaluated by taking all these compartments into consideration. Thus, **neutrophilia,** an increase in the number of neutrophils in the circulation, does not necessarily imply an increase in neutrophil production. Intense muscular activity or the administration of epinephrine causes neutrophils in the marginating compartment to move into the circulating compartment, causing an apparent neutrophilia even though neutrophil production has not increased.

Neutrophilia may also result from liberation of greater numbers of neutrophils from the medullary storage compartment. This type of neutrophilia is transitory and is followed by a recovery period during which no neutrophils are released.

The neutrophilia that occurs during the course of bacterial infections is due to an increase in production of neutrophils and a shorter duration of these cells in the medullary storage compartment.

In such cases, immature forms such as band cells, neutrophilic metamyelocytes, and even myelocytes may appear in the bloodstream. The neutrophilia that occurs during infection is of longer duration than that which occurs as a result of intense muscular activity.

MATURATION OF LYMPHOCYTES & MONOCYTES

Study of the precursor cells of lymphocytes and monocytes is difficult, because these cells do not contain specific cytoplasmic granules or nuclear lobulation, both of which facilitate the distinction between young and mature forms of granulocytes. Lymphocytes and monocytes are distinguished mainly on the basis of size, chromatin structure, and the presence of nucleoli in smear preparations. As lymphocyte cells mature, their chromatin becomes more compact, nucleoli become less visible, and the cells decrease in size. In addition, subsets of the lymphocyte series acquire distinctive cell-surface receptors during differentiation that can be detected by immunocytochemical techniques.

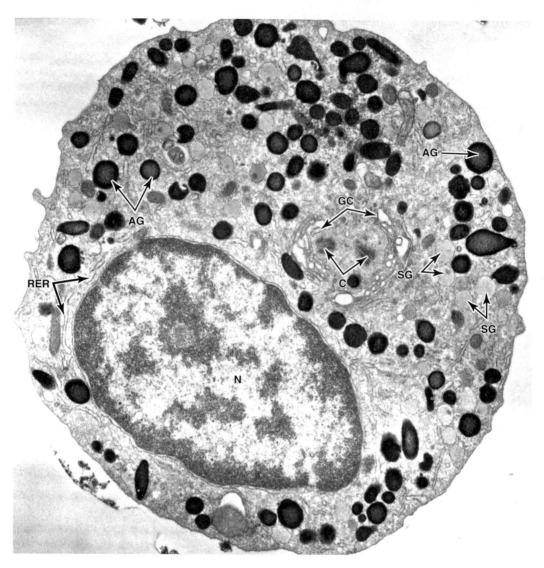

Figure 13–10. Neutrophilic myelocyte from normal human bone marrow treated with peroxidase. At this stage, the cell is smaller than the promyelocyte, and the cytoplasm contains two types of granules: large, peroxidase-positive azurophilic granules (AG), and smaller specific granules (SG), which do not stain for peroxidase. Note that the peroxidase reaction product is present only in azurophilic granules and is not seen in the rough endoplasmic reticulum (RER) or Golgi cisternae (GC), which are located around the centriole (C). N, nucleus. × 15,000. (Courtesy of DF Bainton.)

Lymphocytes

Circulating lymphocytes originate mainly in the thymus and the peripheral lymphoid organs (spleen, lymph nodes, tonsils, etc). However, all lymphocyte progenitor cells originate in the bone marrow. Some of these relatively undifferentiated lymphocytes migrate to the thymus, where they acquire the attributes of T lymphocytes. Subsequently, T lymphocytes populate specific regions of peripheral lymphoid organs. Other bone marrow lymphocytes differentiate into B lymphocytes in the bone marrow and then migrate to peripheral lymphoid organs, where they in-

habit and multiply in their own special compartments.

The first identifiable progenitor of lymphoid cells is the **lymphoblast,** a large cell capable of incorporating ^{3}H-thymidine and dividing two or three times to form **prolymphocytes.** Prolymphocytes are smaller and have relatively more condensed chromatin but none of the cell-surface antigens that mark prolymphocytes as T or B lymphocytes. In the thymus or bone marrow, these cells synthesize cell-surface receptors characteristic of their lineage, but they are not recognizable as distinct cell types in routine

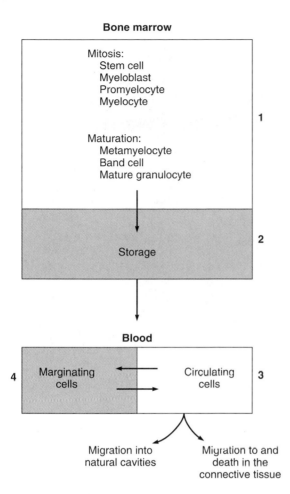

Figure 13–11. Functional compartments of neutrophils. **1:** Medullary formation compartment. **2:** Medullary storage (reserve) compartment. **3:** Circulating compartment. **4:** Marginating compartment. The size of each compartment is roughly proportional to the number of cells.

histologic procedures. The distinction is made by using immunocytochemical techniques.

Monocytes

The **monoblast** is a committed progenitor cell that is virtually identical to the **myeloblast** in its morphologic characteristics. Further differentiation leads to the **promonocyte,** a large cell (up to 18 μm in diameter) with a basophilic cytoplasm and a large, slightly indented nucleus. The chromatin is lacy, and nucleoli are evident. Promonocytes divide twice in the course of their development into **monocytes.** A large amount of rough endoplasmic reticulum is present, as is an extensive Golgi complex in which granule condensation can be seen to be taking place. These granules are **primary lysosomes,** which are observed as fine **azurophilic granules** in blood monocytes. Ma-

ture monocytes enter the bloodstream, circulate for about 8 hours, and then enter the connective tissues, where they mature into **macrophages** and function for several months.

> Abnormal bone marrow can produce diseases based on cells derived from that tissue. **Leukemias** are malignant clones of leukocyte precursors. They occur in lymphoid tissue (**lymphocytic leukemias**) and in bone marrow (**myelogenous** and **monocytic leukemias**). In these diseases, there is usually a release of large numbers of immature cells into the blood. The symptoms of leukemias are a consequence of this shift in cell proliferation, with a lack of some cell types and excessive production of others (which are often abnormal in function). The patient is usually anemic and prone to infection.
>
> A clinical technique that is helpful in the study of leukemias and other bone marrow disturbances is **bone marrow aspiration.** A needle is introduced through compact bone (usually the sternum), and a sample of marrow is withdrawn. The sample is spread on a microscope slide and stained. The use of labeled monoclonal antibodies specific to proteins in the membranes of precursor blood cells aids in identifying cell types derived from these stem cells and contributes to a more precise diagnosis of the various types of leukemia.

ORIGIN OF PLATELETS

In adults, platelets originate in the red bone marrow by fragmentation of the cytoplasm of mature **megakaryocytes** (Gr. *megas,* big, + *karyon,* nucleus, + *kytos*), which, in turn, arise by differentiation of **megakaryoblasts.**

Megakaryoblasts

The megakaryoblast is 15–50 μm in diameter and has a large ovoid or kidney-shaped nucleus (Figure 13–12) with numerous nucleoli. The nucleus becomes highly polyploid (ie, it contains up to 30 times as much DNA as a normal cell) before platelets begin to form. The cytoplasm of this cell is homogeneous and intensely basophilic.

Megakaryocytes

The megakaryocyte is a giant cell (35–150 μm in diameter) with an irregularly lobulated nucleus, coarse chromatin, and no visible nucleoli (Figures 13–13 and 13–14). The cytoplasm contains numerous mitochondria, a well-developed rough endoplasmic reticulum, and an extensive Golgi complex. Human platelets have conspicuous granules that contain biologically active substances, such as platelet-derived

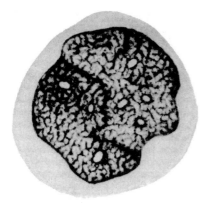

Megakaryoblast

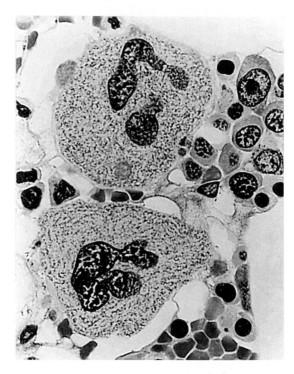

Figure 13–13. Photomicrograph of two megakaryocytes.

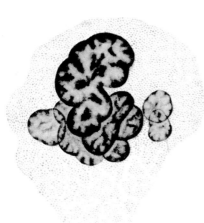

Megakaryocyte

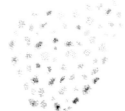

Platelets

Figure 13–12. Cells of the megakaryocyte series shown in a bone marrow smear. Note the formation of platelets at the lower end of the megakaryocyte.

growth factor, fibroblast growth factor, von Wille-brand's factor (which promotes adhesion of platelets to endothelial cells), and platelet factor IV (which stimulates blood coagulation). With maturation of the megakaryocyte, numerous invaginations of the plasma membrane ramify throughout the cytoplasm, forming the **demarcation membranes.** This system defines areas of a megakaryocyte's cytoplasm that can shed 4000–8000 platelets.

In certain forms of **thrombocytopenic purpura,** a disease in which the number of blood platelets is reduced, the platelets appear to be bound to the cytoplasm of the megakaryocytes, indicating a defect in the liberation mechanism of these corpuscles. The life span of platelets is approximately 10 days.

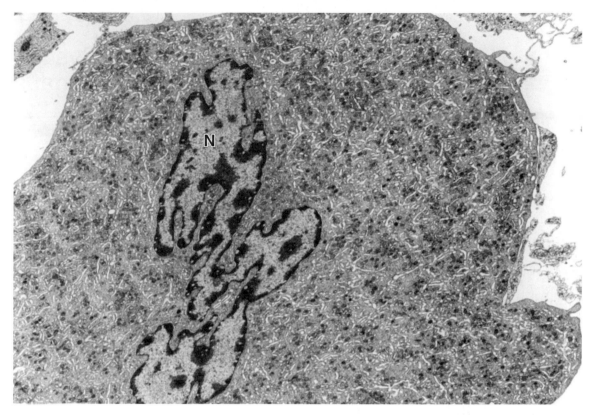

Figure 13–14. Electron micrograph of a megakaryocyte showing a lobulated nucleus (N) and numerous cytoplasmic granules. The demarcation membranes are visible as tubular profiles. × 4900. (Reproduced, with permission, from Junqueira LCU, Salles LMM: *Ultra-Estrutura e Função Celular.* Edgard Blücher, 1975.)

REFERENCES

Becker RP, DeBruyn PP: The transmural passage of blood cells into myeloid sinusoids and the entry of platelets into the sinusoidal circulation. Am J Anat 1976;145:183.

Berman I: The ultrastructure of erythroblastic islands and reticular cells in mouse bone marrow. J Ultrastruct Res 1967;17:291.

Chandrasoma P, Taylor CR: *Concise Pathology.* Appleton & Lange, 1991.

Evatt BL et al: *Megakaryocyte Biology and Precursors: In Vitro Cloning and Cellular Properties.* Elsevier/North-Holland, 1981.

Fleischmann RA et al: Totipotent hematopoietic stem cells: normal self-renewal and differentiation after transplantation between mouse fetuses. Cell 1982;30:351.

Foucar K: *Bone Marrow Pathology.* American Society of Clinical Pathologists (ASCP) Press, 1995.

Krstić RV: *Human Microscopic Anatomy.* Springer-Verlag 1991.

Pennington DG: The cellular biology of megakaryocytes. Blood Cells 1979;5:5.

Simmons PJ et al: The mobilization of primitive hemopoietic progenitors into the peripheral blood. Stem Cells 1994;12:187.

Tavassoli M, Yoffey JM: *Bone Marrow Structure and Function.* Liss, 1983.

Williams WJ et al (editors): *Hematology,* 5th ed. McGraw-Hill, 1995.

14 The Immune System & Lymphoid Organs

The immune system comprises structures and cells that are distributed throughout the body; their principal function is to protect the body from invasion and damage by microorganisms and foreign substances. Cells of the immune system have the ability to distinguish "self" (the organism's own macromolecules) from "nonself" (foreign substances) and to coordinate the destruction or inactivation of foreign substances (eg, individual molecules), parts of microorganisms, or even cancer cells that originate in the body. On occasion, the immune system reacts against normal body tissues, causing **autoimmune diseases.** The immune system includes both individual structures (eg, lymph nodes, spleen) and free cells (eg, lymphocytes, granulocytes, and cells of the mononuclear phagocyte system that are present in the blood, lymph, and connective tissues) that participate in immune responses. Another important component of the immune system is the **antigen-presenting cells,** found not only in the lymphoid tissues but also in other organs, such as the skin (which is heavily exposed to foreign antigens). The cells of the immune system communicate with each other and with cells of other systems through signaling proteins known as **cytokines.**

Lymphoid Organs

The main anatomical structures that participate in the immune response are the lymphoid organs: the thymus, spleen, and lymph nodes. Lymphoid nodules, smaller collections of lymphoid tissue that are formed mainly of nodular aggregates, are present in the mucosa of the digestive system (tonsils, Peyer's patches, and appendix), respiratory system, and urinary system, forming the mucosa-associated lymphoid tissue (**MALT**). The wide distribution of lymphoid structures and the constant circulation of lymphoid cells in the blood, lymph, and connective tissues provide the body with an elaborate, efficient system of surveillance and defense by immunocompetent cells (Figure 14–1).

All lymphocytes originate in the bone marrow; however, T lymphocytes mature further in the thy-

mus, whereas B lymphocytes leave the bone marrow as mature cells. For this reason, the bone marrow and the thymus are called the **primary** or **central lymphoid organs.** Lymphocytes migrate from these organs to the blood and **peripheral lymphoid organs** (spleen, lymph nodes, solitary nodules, tonsils, appendix, and Peyer's patches of the ileum) where they proliferate and complete their differentiation.

Basic Types of Immune Reactions

During evolution, two different but related types of specific immunity developed. The first was **cellular immunity,** in which **immunocompetent** cells react against and kill microorganisms, foreign cells (from tumors and transplants), and virus-infected cells. This category of immunity is mediated mainly by T lymphocytes, or T cells. The other type of immunity, **humoral immunity,** is related to the presence of circulating glycoproteins called **antibodies** that inactivate or destroy foreign substances. The antibodies are produced by plasma cells derived from B lymphocytes, or B cells.

Immunogens & Antigens

The foreign (nonself) substance encountered by the immune system acts as an **immunogen**—ie, a substance that elicits a response from the host. The response may be cellular, humoral, or (most commonly) both. Immunogens may be present in whole cells, such as bacteria or tumor cells, or in macromolecules, such as proteins, polysaccharides, or nucleoproteins. More specifically, an **antigen** (Gr. *anti,* against, + *genin,* to produce) is an immunogen that can react with an antibody, even if it is not capable of eliciting an immune reaction. Because most immunogens are also antigens, in this book the term "antigen" will be used. The specificity of the humoral immune response (B cells) is determined by small molecular domains—**antigenic determinants** or **epitopes**—of the antigen, whereas the specificity of the cellular immune response (T cells) is determined by small peptides associated with major histocompatibility complex (MHC) molecules on the membrane

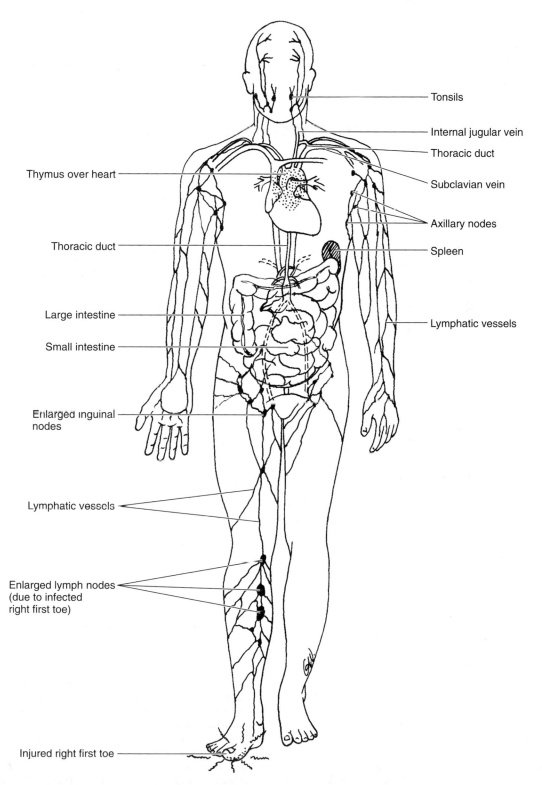

Figure 14–1. Distribution of lymphoid organs and lymphatic vessels in the body. As an example of the functions of lymphatic system, an infection of the first toe is shown with enlargement of the lymph nodes that collect lymph from the infected region. This enlargement is mainly due to the proliferation of B lymphocytes and their differentiation into antibody-secreting plasma cells. The infected toe becomes red, warm, painful, and swollen.

of antigen-presenting cells. An antigen that has many epitopes (eg, a bacterial cell) will elicit a wide spectrum of humoral and cellular responses.

Antibodies

Antibodies, also called **immunoglobulins,** are circulating plasma glycoproteins that interact specifically with the antigenic determinant that elicited their formation. Antibodies are secreted by plasma cells that arise by proliferation and differentiation of B lymphocytes. One important function of an antibody molecule is to combine specifically with the epitope it recognizes and then to signal other components of the immune system that this is a foreign invader to be eliminated. Some antibodies are able to agglutinate cells and to precipitate soluble antigens. Agglutination of microorganisms and harmful molecules localizes an invader and facilitates phagocytosis. Antigens bound to immunoglobulin (Ig) G or IgM activate the complement system, a group of plasma proteins, leading to lysis of microorganisms. The activated complement also stimulates phagocytosis of bacteria and other invaders' organisms. Neutrophils and macrophages have receptors for the Fc region of antigen-bound IgG; this antibody can attach the complex antigen-invader to these phagocytic cells.

Five classes of immunoglobulins are recognized in humans:

IgG, the most abundant class, constitutes 75% of serum immunoglobulins. Because it also serves as a model for the other classes, it will be described in detail. IgG consists of two identical light chains and two identical heavy chains (Figure 14–2), bound by disulfide bonds and noncovalent forces. When isolated, the two carboxyl-terminal portions of the heavy chains crystallize easily and are called **Fc** frag-

ments (fragment crystallizable). The Fc regions of several immunoglobulins react with specific receptors of many different cells. The four amino-terminal segments (two formed of light chains and two of heavy chains) constitute the **Fab** (fragment antigen-binding) fragments of the immunoglobulin. The Fab segments are variable in amino acid sequence and are thus responsible for the exquisite specificity of the immune response. IgG is the only immunoglobulin that crosses the placental barrier and is incorporated into the circulatory system of the fetus, protecting the newborn against infection.

IgA is found in small amounts in blood. It is the main immunoglobulin found in tears, colostrum, and saliva; in nasal, bronchial, intestinal, and prostatic secretions; and in the vaginal fluid. It is found in secretions as a dimer called **secretory IgA,** which is composed of two molecules of monomeric IgA united by a polypeptide chain called **protein J** and combined with another protein, the **secretory,** or **transport, component.** Because it is resistant to several enzymes, secretory IgA provides protection against the proliferation of microorganisms in body secretions. IgA monomers and protein J are secreted by plasma cells in the mucous membranes that line the digestive, respiratory, and urinary passages; the secretory component is synthesized by the mucosal epithelial cells (see Figure 15–2).

IgM constitutes 10% of blood immunoglobulins and usually exists as a pentamer with a molecular mass of 900 kDa. Together with IgD, it is the major immunoglobulin found on the surfaces of B lymphocytes. These two classes of immunoglobulins have both membrane-bound and circulating forms. Lymphocyte membrane-bound IgM and IgD serve as receptors for specific antigens. The result of this interaction is the proliferation and further differentiation of B lymphocytes, producing antibody-secreting plasma cells. Circulating IgM is also effective in activating the **complement system,** a group of plasma proteins that have the capacity to lyse cells, including bacteria.

IgE usually exists as a monomer. This immunoglobulin has a great affinity for receptors located in the plasma membranes of mast cells and basophils. Immediately after its secretion by plasma cells, IgE attaches to these cells and virtually disappears from the blood plasma. When the antigen that elicited the production of a specific IgE is again encountered, the antigen-antibody complex formed on the surface of a mast cell or basophil triggers the production and liberation of several biologically active substances, such as histamine, heparin, leukotrienes, and eosinophil-chemotactic factor of anaphylaxis (ECF-A). An **allergic reaction** is thus mediated by the activity of IgE and the antigens (**allergens**) that stimulate its production (see Mast Cells in Chapter 5).

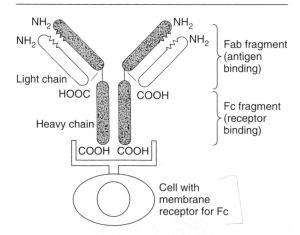

Figure 14–2. Structure and components of an immunoglobulin (antibody) molecule.

The properties and activities of **IgD** are not completely understood. It has a molecular mass of 180 kDa, and its concentration in blood plasma constitutes only 0.2% of the immunoglobulins. IgD is found on the plasma membranes of B lymphocytes (together with IgM) and is involved in the differentiation of these cells.

Switching of Immunoglobulin Classes

On its first encounter with an antigen, a B lymphocyte proliferates, serving as a stem cell for the development of a population of plasma cells that produce IgM. After subsequent stimulation by the same antigen, these plasma cells preferentially synthesize and secrete IgG, IgA, or IgE antibodies. This process is called **class switching.** IgM is apparently not very effective in killing microbes and is replaced by the more efficient IgG.

B & T Lymphocytes

A fundamental division of lymphocytes into two classes and several subclasses (Table 14–1) can be made on the basis of their site of differentiation and the presence of distinctive receptors in their membrane. Precursor cells originate in bone marrow in late fetal life, and slow proliferation of these cells continues during postnatal life. They differentiate into immunocompetent cells in the bone marrow and the thymus.

In the early 1960s, experiments using chicken embryos revealed one of the anatomic sites of lymphocyte differentiation. The **bursa of Fabricius** is a mass of lymphoid tissue near the cloaca of birds. When this tissue is destroyed in the embryo, chickens lack the ability to produce immunoglobulins. That is, humoral immunity, a process that requires the presence of immunoglobulins in the blood, is impaired. The number of lymphocytes found in specific regions of lymphoid tissue is profoundly reduced. The affected lymphocytes are known as **B lymphocytes** or **B cells.** In mammals, including humans, B cells acquire their differentiated characteristics in special microenvironments in the bone marrow.

Experimental removal of the thymus of newborn mice results in profound deficiencies in **cellular immune responses**—responses that require the presence of living cells—in contrast to humoral responses, which depend on circulating immunoglobulins. The cells involved are called **T lymphocytes,** or **T cells.** Early experiments in mice showed that the thymus has the same role in other mammals, including humans.

B lymphocytes derive from bone marrow and migrate to secondary nonthymic lymphoid structures, where they nest, proliferate when activated, and differentiate into antibody-secreting **plasma cells.** B cells constitute 5–10% of the circulating blood lymphocytes; each is covered by 150,000 molecules of IgM that are receptors for specific antigens. Some activated B cells do not become plasma cells; instead, they generate **B memory cells,** which react rapidly to a second exposure to the same antigen (Figure 14–3).

T cells constitute 65–75% of blood lymphocytes. They originate in the bone marrow and migrate to the thymus, where they proliferate and are carried by the blood to other lymphoid tissues. Four subpopulations of T cells have been recognized: **helper, suppressor, cytotoxic,** and **memory cells.** Helper cells stimulate the differentiation of B cells into plasma cells. Cytotoxic cells can act against foreign cells or virus-infected cells by means of two mechanisms. In one, they produce proteins called **perforins** that create holes in the cell membrane, with consequent cell lysis. In the other, they kill the cell by activating certain genes that induce programmed cell death, or **apoptosis** (see Chapter 3). Apoptosis is characterized by nuclear DNA degradation, nuclear degeneration, and condensation of cell membrane. Examination of tissues with apoptotic cells shows scant evidence of dying cells—explained by the rapid removal of apoptotic cells by macrophages. This removal process is specific; only apoptotic cells are rapidly phagocytosed before the integrity of the cell membrane is lost. Memory T cells react rapidly to the reintroduction of antigens and stimulate production of cytotoxic

Table 14–1. Lymphocyte types and main functions.*

Type	Main Function
B lymphocyte	Carries membrane receptors (IgM). When activated by specific antigens, proliferates by mitosis, differentiating into plasma cells that secrete large amounts of antibodies.
B memory lymphocyte	Activated B cell that is primed to respond more rapidly and to a greater extent upon subsequent exposure to the same antigen.
T cytotoxic lymphocyte	Carries TCRs, which are not immunoglobulins. Specialized to recognize antigens associated with MHC-I on the surface of other cells. Produces perforin and other proteins that kill foreign cells, virus-infected cells, and some tumor cells.
T helper lymphocyte	Carries TCRs. Modulates other T and B cells, stimulating their activities.
T suppressor lymphocyte	Carries TCRs. Modulates other T and B cells, decreasing their activities.
T memory lymphocyte	Carries TCRs. Is primed to respond more rapidly and to a greater extent upon subsequent exposure to the same antigen.
NK lymphocyte	Lacks T and B-cell receptors. Attacks virus-infected cells and cancer cells without previous stimulation.

*TCR, T-cell receptor; MHC-I, class I major histocompatibility complex; NK, natural killer.

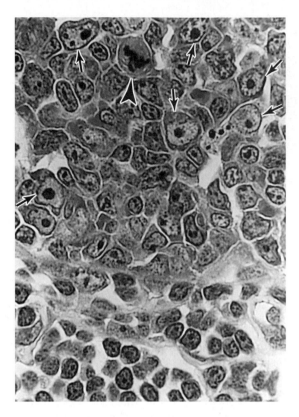

Figure 14–3. Photomicrograph showing immunoblasts (arrows) in the germinal center of a lymph nodule. These cells are large in size, with pale-stained nuclei, large nucleoli, and basophilic cytoplasm. The arrowhead indicates an immunoblast in mitotic division. In the lower part of the figure are numerous lymphocytes with typical dark-stained nuclei.

Table 14–2. Approximate percentage of lymphocytes in lymphoid organs.

Lymphoid Organ	T Lymphocytes, %	B Lymphocytes, %
Thymus	100	0
Bone marrow	10	90
Spleen	45	55
Lymph nodes	60	40
Blood	80	20

permit the identification and detection of differentiated subpopulations of these two types of cells. When stimulated by antigens, B and T cells produce large basophilic lymphoid cells called **immunoblasts** (Figure 14–3), whose cytoplasmic basophilia is due to large numbers of polyribosomes. These cells go through several mitotic cycles (clone selection and expansion) and may differentiate in several ways. B cells, for example, produce plasma cells, whose cytoplasm contains abundant rough endoplasmic reticulum synthesizing antibodies (glycoproteins), whereas stimulated T cells show numerous free polyribosomes in the cytosol.

In addition to B and T cells, there are **natural killer,** or **NK,** lymphocytes that lack the marker molecules characteristic of B and T cells. In the circulating blood, 10–15% of the lymphocytes are NK cells. They are called natural killer cells because they attack virus-infected cells and cancer cells, without previous stimulation.

Antigen-Presenting Cells

Antigen-presenting cells (**APCs**) are found in most tissues. APCs are derived from the bone marrow and constitute a heterogeneous cell population that includes dendritic cells, macrophages, Langerhans cells, B lymphocytes, and epithelial reticular cells of the thymus. In a process known as **antigen processing,** APCs have the capacity to partially digest proteins, reducing them to small peptides. Antigen processing is a necessary preliminary step for activation of T cells, because these cells are blind to native proteins and other antigens. Note that T cells can recognize only peptides associated with MHC molecules, whereas B cells can directly recognize proteins, peptides, lipids, polysaccharides, and many small molecules. Endocytosed exogenous proteins are digested in endosomes and lysosomes, and the resulting small peptides (10–30 amino acids) form a complex with class II MHC (MHC-II) molecules. Endogenous proteins in the cytosol are digested by proteosomes (multicatalytic proteases) to small peptides (8–11 amino acids) that are transported to the endoplasmic reticulum cisternae, where they form a complex with class I MHC (MHC-I) molecules. Both

T cells. Suppressor cells regulate both cellular and humoral immunity and inhibit the action of helper and cytotoxic cells. Helper and suppressor cells are also known collectively as **regulator cells.**

> Helper T cells are killed by the retrovirus that causes the immunodeficiency syndrome known as AIDS, crippling the immunity of infected patients and rendering them susceptible to opportunistic infections—microorganisms that usually do not infect healthy individuals.

B and T cells are not uniformly distributed in the lymphoid system (Table 14–2); they occupy special regions in nonthymic lymphoid structures. Although B and T cells are morphologically not distinguishable in either light or electron microscopes, they can be distinguished by immunocytochemical methods. They exhibit different surface proteins (markers) that class I and class II complexes are then transported to the cell membrane where they are inspected by T lymphocytes. CD4+ T cells interact with complexes of peptides with MHC-II molecules, whereas CD8+ T cells interact with complexes of peptides with MHC-I molecules.

Dendritic Cells

Dendritic cells, or interdigitating dendritic cells, arise from bone marrow precursors and may derive from monocytes. They are present in the interstitium of many organs, are abundant in T-cell areas of lymphoid organs, and are present in the epidermis as Langerhans cells. They are considered immunostimulatory cells, because they not only present antigens to T cells but are also able to stimulate naive T cells (T cells that have not yet had contact with antigen). Antigen-primed T cells can be stimulated by any APCs, including dendritic cells. After the discovery of dendritic cells as a minor cell type contained in adherent macrophage preparations, and with the development of techniques to isolate dendritic cells, their role as immunostimulatory cells was demonstrated. When dendritic cells were separated from macrophages and each cell type was tested for its ability to stimulate naive T cells, dendritic cells were able to do so whereas macrophages had little or no stimulatory capacity.

Dendritic cell precursors are seeded through the blood into nonlymphoid organs, where they lodge as immature dendritic cells. These cells are characterized by their high ability to capture and process antigens and their low ability to activate T cells. Inflammatory conditions induce the maturation of dendritic cells, which then migrate through the blood or afferent lymph to the peripheral lymphoid organs, where they proceed to the T cell areas. At this stage they undergo dramatic changes, losing the ability to capture antigens and acquiring an increased ability to activate T cells. In this way, mature dendritic cells are able to present T cells with antigen that has been captured in peripheral tissues. The ability of dendritic cells to be attracted to sites of antigen challenge and travel to peripheral organs is a crucial function of these APCs. For example, antigens entering via the skin are picked up by Langerhans cells and transported via lymph vessels to the satellite lymph node, where the immune reaction is initiated. Dendritic cells in other organs may also pick up antigens and take them to the spleen through the blood circulation.

Note that in the germinal center of lymph nodes, spleen, and other lymphoid tissues, there are cells with similar morphologic characteristics, called **follicular dendritic cells,** that are functionally different from interdigitating dendritic cells. Follicular dendritic cells are not derived from bone marrow and are unable to endocytose and process antigens. Thus, they do not function as APCs. However, they are very efficient in trapping antigens complexed to antibodies and complement factors, and they retain these antigens for long periods of time on their surface membrane, where the antigens are recognized by B cells.

Major Histocompatibility Complex

The immune system distinguishes self from non-self mainly by the presence on cell surfaces of major histocompatibility complex (MHC) molecules. In humans they are also called HLA, from human leukocyte antigen, because they were discovered in leukocytes. These molecules fall into two classes: MHC-I is present in all cells, whereas MHC-II is more restricted in distribution, being found in APCs such as macrophages, B cells, dendritic cells, and Langerhans cells. The MHC molecules constitute an intracellular system that places the MHC-peptide complex on the APC membrane for inspection by T lymphocytes. MHC molecules have a structure that is unique to each individual, which is the main reason that tissue grafts and organ transplants are often rejected if not made between identical twins who possess identical MHC and other molecules.

ORGAN TRANSPLANTATION

Tissue grafts and organ transplants are classified as **autografts** when the transplanted tissues or organs are taken from the individual receiving them; **isografts** when taken from an identical twin; **homografts** when taken from an individual (related or unrelated) of the same species; and **heterografts** when taken from an animal of a different species.

Autografts and isografts are readily accepted by the body as long as an efficient blood supply is established. There is no rejection in such cases, because the transplanted cells are genetically identical to those of the host and present the same MHC on their surfaces. The organism recognizes the grafted cells as self (same MHC) and produces no cellular or humoral reactions.

Homografts and heterografts, on the other hand, contain cells whose membranes have MHC-I molecules that are foreign to the host; they are therefore recognized and treated as such. Transplant rejection (Figure 14–4) is due mainly to the activity of NK lymphocytes and cytotoxic T lymphocytes that penetrate the transplant and destroy the transplanted cells.

Cytokines

Much recent work has focused on soluble factors—collectively called **cytokines**—that are made by, or act on, elements of the immune system and modulate the activities of this system. Cytokines are small protein molecules that are not antigen-specific, although their production is often antigen-driven. Cy-

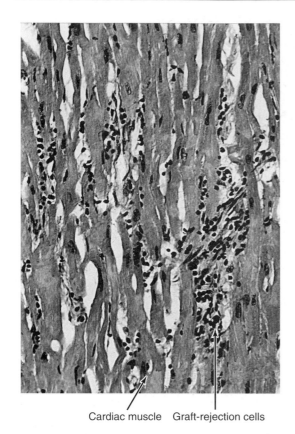

Cardiac muscle   Graft-rejection cells

Figure 14–4. Photomicrograph of human myocardium from a transplanted and rejected heart. Among the cardiac muscle fibers that show degenerative changes are many natural killer lymphocytes and cytotoxic T lymphocytes (graft-rejection cells). (Courtesy of T Brito.)

tokines produced by lymphocytes are called **lymphokines.** Some mediators that act between leukocytes are called **interleukins;** more than 10 interleukins have been described (Table 14–3). Other cytokines include a variety of **colony-stimulating factors** (see Table 13–2) made by T cells to stimulate lymphoid and hematopoietic organs. Other cytokines, eg, **tumor necrosis factors** (α and β) and **transforming growth factor-β**, are associated with inflammation, tumor defense, cell growth, and wound healing.

> The central nervous system also produces peptide hormones for which there are receptors on the surfaces of lymphocytes. This poorly understood communication system of chemical messengers between the brain and the immune system gives some biochemical support to the observation that the course of some diseases is influenced by the person's moods.

THYMUS

The thymus is a lymphoepithelial organ located in the mediastinum; it attains its peak development during youth. Whereas nonthymic lymphoid organs originate exclusively from mesenchyme (mesoderm), the thymus has a dual embryonic origin. Its lymphocytes arise from mesenchymal cells that invade an epithelial primordium that has developed from the endoderm of the third and fourth pharyngeal pouches.

The thymus has a connective tissue capsule that penetrates the parenchyma and divides it into lobules (Figure 14–5). Each lobule has a peripheral dark zone known as the **cortex** and a central light zone called the **medulla** (L. *medius,* middle).

Table 14–3. Interleukins*

	Origins	Some Functions
IL-1	Macrophages, keratinocytes, etc	Proinflammatory endogenous pyrogen; activates fibroblasts, granulocytes. osteoclasts; makes T cells responsive to signals
IL-2	T cells	Proliferation of T, B, and natural killer cells
IL-3	T cells	Proliferation of early hematopoietic cells (multi-CSF)
IL-4	T cells, mast cells	Governs B-cell isotype switching to IgG and IgE
IL-5	T cells, mast cells, possibly B cells	Eosinophil differentiation and proliferation; IgA production
IL-6	Macrophages, T cells, fibroblasts	Proinflammatory; B-cell differentiation; thymocyte growth
IL-7	Bone marrow stroma	B-cell differentiation and maturation
IL-8	Keratinocytes, fibroblasts, monocytes	Neutrophil chemotaxis and activation
IL-9	T cells	Proliferation of T cells, thymocytes, mast cells
IL-10	T cells, mast cells, possibly B cells	Inhibition of cytokine synthesis in various cells; proliferation of mast cells

*IL, interleukin; CSF, colony-stimulating factor.

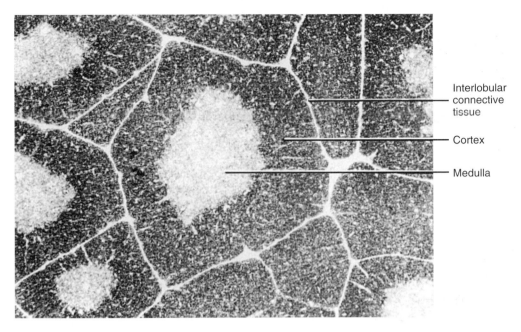

Interlobular connective tissue

Cortex

Medulla

Figure 14–5. Photomicrograph of the thymus. Hematoxylin-and-eosin (H&E) stain. × 32.

The **cortex** is composed of an extensive population of T lymphocytes, dispersed epithelial reticular cells, and few macrophages. Because the cortex is richer in small lymphocytes than the medulla, it stains more darkly. The epithelial reticular cells are stellate cells with light-staining oval nuclei. Usually, they are joined to similar adjacent cells by desmosomes (Figure 14–6). Bundles of intermediate keratin filaments (tonofibrils) in their cytoplasm are evidence of the epithelial origin of these cells (Figure 14–7).

Some investigators have described several types of thymic epithelial reticular cells according to their location and structure. The functions of each type of epithelial reticular cell are still not completely understood.

Because of the proliferation of lymphocytes in the cortex, immature T lymphocytes are produced in quantity and accumulate in this region. Although most of these lymphocytes die in the cortex by apoptosis and are removed by macrophages, a small number migrate to the medulla and enter the bloodstream through the walls of venules. These cells migrate to nonthymic lymphoid structures and accumulate in specific sites as T lymphocytes.

The **medulla** contains **Hassall's corpuscles,** which are characteristic of this region (Figure 14–8). These structures are concentrically arranged, flattened epithelial reticular cells that become filled with keratin filaments, degenerate, and sometimes calcify. Their function is unknown. The medulla has the same cell population as the cortex, with a larger number of epithelial reticular cells.

Vascularization

Arteries enter the thymus through the capsule; they branch and penetrate the organ more deeply, following the septa of connective tissue. Arterioles leave the septa to penetrate the parenchyma along the border between the cortical and medullary zones. These arterioles give off capillaries that penetrate the cortex in an arched course; they finally reach the medulla, where they drain into venules. The medulla is supplied with capillary branches of the arterioles in the medullary-cortical border. The capillaries of the medulla drain into venules, which also receive capillaries returning from the cortical zone.

Thymic capillaries have a nonfenestrated endothelium and a very thick basal lamina (Figure 14–9). Endothelial cells have thin processes that perforate the basal lamina and may come in contact with epithelial reticular cells. Small vessels of the cortical parenchyma are surrounded by a sheath of epithelial reticular cells that form a **blood-thymus barrier.** The blood-thymus barrier consists of pericytes, the capillary basal lamina, the basal lamina of the epithelial reticular cell, cells of the nonfenestrated endothelium, and the epithelial reticular cells themselves. This barrier prevents circulating antigens from reaching the thymic cortex where T lymphocytes are being formed.

Medullary veins penetrate the connective tissue septa and leave the thymus through its capsule. There is no blood-thymus barrier in the medulla.

The thymus has no afferent lymphatic vessels and does not constitute a filter for the lymph, as do lymph nodes. The few lymphatic vessels encountered in the

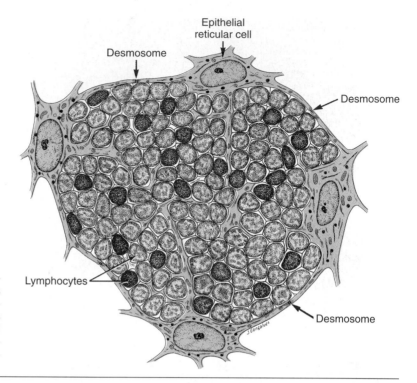

Figure 14–6. The relationship between epithelial reticular cells (shown in color) and thymic lymphocytes. Note the desmosomes and the long processes of epithelial reticular cells extending among the lymphocytes. Note also the absence of reticular fibers.

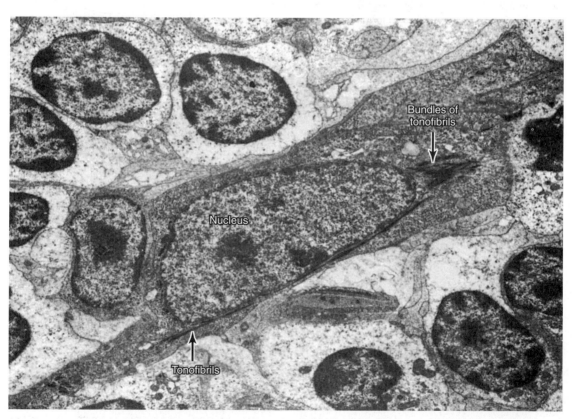

Figure 14–7. Thymic medulla seen under the electron microscope. An epithelial reticular cell runs diagonally across the figure. The nucleus has fine chromatin, and cytokeratin fibers (tonofibrils) are present in the cytoplasm. × 7100.

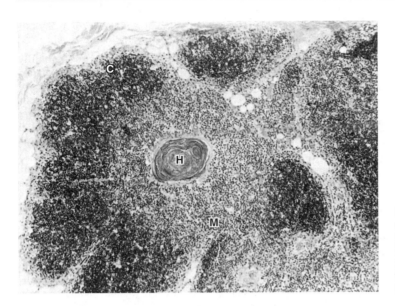

Figure 14–8. Photomicrograph of a human thymus, showing the dense cortical (C) and lighter medullary (M) zones. Near the center, one Hassall's corpuscle (H) appears in the medulla. Connective tissue septa form incomplete lobules. H&E stain. × 118.

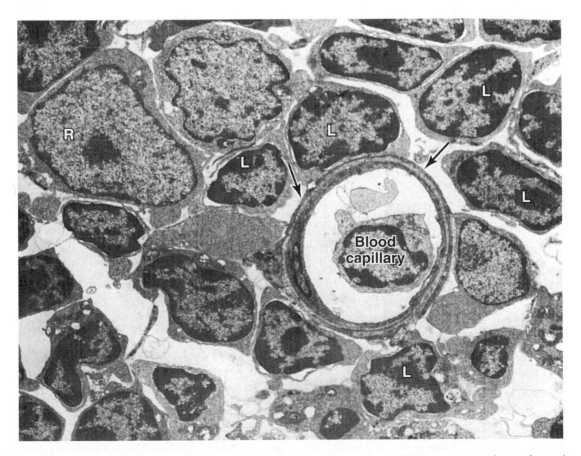

Figure 14–9. Electron micrograph of the thymic cortex. A blood capillary shows a thick basement membrane. Arrows indicate the epithelial reticular cells covering it. These components surrounding the capillary are responsible for the blood-thymus barrier. Note the lymphocytes (L) and the reticular cell (R). × 28,500.

thymus are all efferent; they are located in the walls of blood vessels and in the connective tissue of the septa and the capsule.

Histophysiology

The thymus shows its maximum development in relation to body weight immediately after birth; it undergoes involution after puberty. It is continually repopulated by cells derived from the bone marrow. Stem cells committed to originate T cells arise in the bone marrow and migrate to the thymus during both fetal and adult life. After penetrating the thymus, the developing T cells or thymocytes initially populate the cortex. Surface molecules that are expressed on these immature thymocytes include the CD44 and CD1 markers, whose functions are unknown. The first T-cell receptor (TCR) gene rearrangement occurs at the fetal stage and involves the γ and δ genes. The γδ TCR is the first TCR to be expressed during T-cell development. A few days after its expression, the αβ TCR overtakes the expression of the γδ TCR, and by birth most thymocytes express the αβ TCR. This sequence is in agreement with the observation that more than 90% of mature T cells in the periphery express the αβ TCR, whereas the γδ T cells constitute a minor population of the cells in lymphoid organs. Although γδ cells are a conspicuous T-cell population within the epithelium of skin, intestine, and respiratory ducts, our knowledge of their function and specificity is far behind our understanding of αβ T cells.

Almost simultaneously with the expression of the αβ TCR, the thymocytes begin to express the accessory molecules CD4 and CD8 and are designated double-positive cells (Figure 14–10). At this stage they are submitted to the process of positive and neg-

ative selection. The cortical double positive thymocytes interact with cortical epithelial cells and bone marrow–derived cells expressing MHC molecules and undergo positive and negative selection processes that shape the T-cell repertoire for self-restriction and self-tolerance. **Positive selection** involves the interaction of double-positive thymocytes with self-peptide-MHC complexes on thymic epithelial cells, leading to survival of these cells. **Negative selection** involves the interaction of double-positive thymocytes with self-peptide complexes on thymic APCs, resulting in the death of these thymocytes. As the surviving thymocytes mature, they move on to the medulla and become either CD4+ helper cells or CD8+ cytotoxic T cells. At this stage they migrate to peripheral lymphoid tissues.

During their development in the thymus, more than 95% of the thymocytes die owing to three main causes: by negligence when their TCRs are not directed to MHC molecules expressed in the thymus; by the expression of TCRs with high affinity for self-MHC molecules (negative selection), and by unproductive TCR gene rearrangement. Thus, self-tolerance is mostly acquired in the thymus during the development of T cells. The large majority of immature thymocytes die by apoptosis in the cortical region, and all apoptotic thymocytes are localized within thymic macrophages. However, a small number of T cells escape the central negative-selection process and pass to the periphery. Peripheral mature T cells with autoreactivity are tolerated when these cells are exposed to self-antigens under determined conditions that lead to T-cell deletion or inactivation (anergy). Failure of one of these mechanisms results in autoimmunity.

In contrast to T cells, whose specificity is acquired

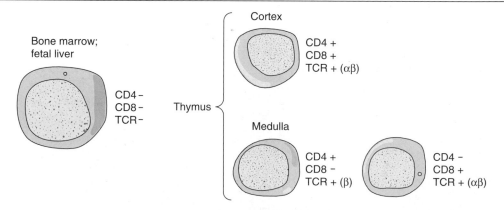

Figure 14–10. Maturation of T cells in the thymus. Double-negative cells in bone marrow and fetal liver migrate to the thymus cortex, where they express the TCR (initially γδ, later αβ) and CD4 and CD8 accessory molecules (double-positive cells). The double-positive cells lose one of the accessory molecules and migrate to the thymus medulla as CD4+ CD8– (helper T-cell precursors) or CD4– CD8+ (cytotoxic T-cell precursors). From the medulla, T cells pass to the periphery.

only in the thymus, B cells acquire their specificity not only in the bone marrow but also in the peripheral lymphoid organs owing to the phenomenon of affinity maturation. Affinity maturation changes the affinity and may even change the specificity of the B-cell antigen receptor. These changes are due to somatic mutations in the immunoglobulin genes involving primarily genes of the variable segments of both heavy and light chains that occur in the B-cell antigen receptor after antigen stimulation. Thus, B-cell tolerance must occur both in the bone barrow and in the lymphoid organs.

In mammals, the main thymus-dependent areas (rich in T cells) are the paracortical zones of lymph nodes, some parts of Peyer's patches, and the periarterial sheaths in the white pulp of the spleen.

The thymus produces several protein growth factors that stimulate proliferation and differentiation of T lymphocytes. They seem to be paracrine secretions, acting in the thymus. Four factors have been identified: thymosin-α, thymopoietin, thymolin, and thymic humoral factor. The thymus is also subject to the effects of several hormones. Injections of some adrenocorticosteroids cause a reduction in lymphocyte number and mitotic rate and atrophy of the cortical layer of the thymus. **Adrenocorticotropic hormone (ACTH)**, produced by the anterior pituitary, achieves the same effect by stimulating the activity of the adrenal cortex. Male and female sex hormones also accelerate thymic involution, whereas castration has the opposite effect.

LYMPH NODES

Lymph nodes are encapsulated spherical or kidney-shaped organs composed of lymphoid tissue that are distributed throughout the body along the course of the lymphatic vessels. The nodes are found in the axilla and the groin, along the great vessels of the neck, and in large numbers in the thorax and abdomen, especially in mesenteries. Lymph nodes constitute a series of in-line filters that are important in the body's defense against microorganisms and the spread of tumor cells. All tissue fluid–derived lymph is filtered by at least one node before returning to the circulation. Lymph nodes have a convex side and a concave depression, the **hilum** (sometimes spelled "hilus"), through which arteries and nerves enter and veins and lymphatic vessels leave the organ (Figure 14–11). The shape and internal structure of lymph nodes vary greatly, but all have the basic pattern of organization illustrated in Figures 14–12 and 14–13.

A connective tissue **capsule** surrounds the lymph

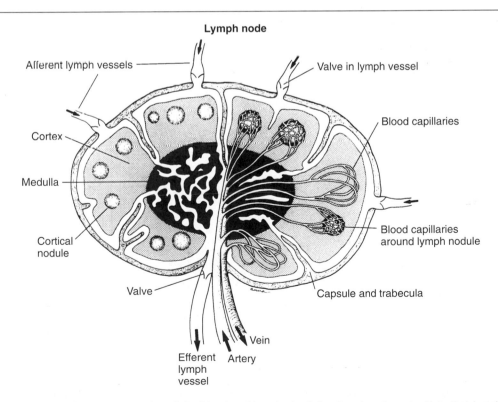

Figure 14–11. Schematic representation of the blood and lymph circulation in a lymph node. Note that lymph enters through the convex side of the node and leaves through the hilum. Blood enters and leaves the node by the hilum.

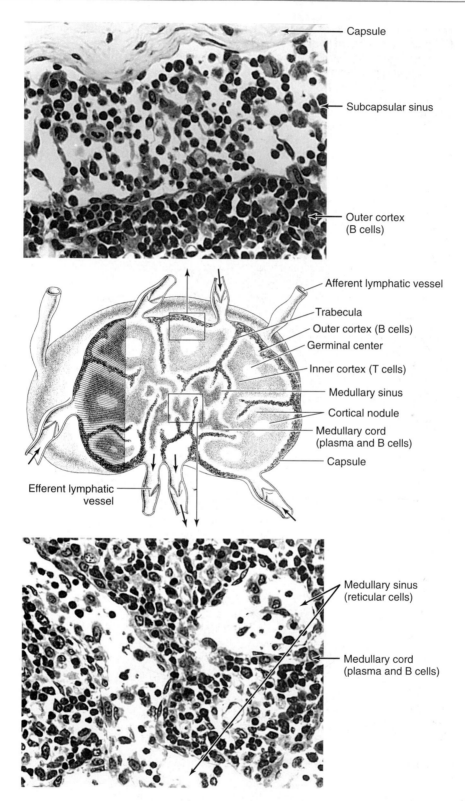

Figure 14–12. Histologic structure of a lymph node. The rectangular areas in the center drawing are magnified in the upper and lower photographs. The cortical layer is composed mainly of lymphoid nodules, whose germinal centers (lightly stained core of each nodule) are clearly seen in the center of the drawing.

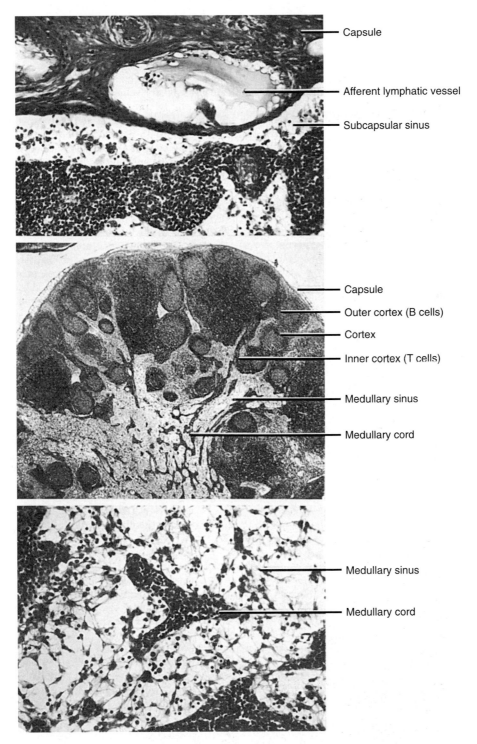

Figure 14–13. Photomicrographs of lymph nodes, reduced from × 30 (middle) and × 200 (top and bottom) magnification. H&E stain.

node, sending trabeculae into its interior. Each node contains an **outer cortex,** an **inner cortex,** and a **medulla** (see Figure 14–12). Large branched follicular dendritic cells are found throughout the lymph node and function as APCs.

Cortices

A. Outer Cortex: At the surface of the outer cortex is the **subcapsular sinus,** which is limited on its outer boundary by the capsule and on its inner boundary by the outer cortex. It is formed of a loose network of macrophages and reticular cells and fibers. The subcapsular sinus communicates with the medullary sinuses through **intermediate sinuses** that run parallel to the capsular trabeculae. The **outer cortex** is formed of a network of reticular cells and fibers whose meshwork is populated by B cells. Within the cortical lymphoid tissue are spherical structures called **lymphoid nodules.**

B. Inner Cortex: The inner cortex is a continuation of the outer cortex and contains few, if any, nodules but many T lymphocytes.

Medulla

The medulla is composed of the **medullary cords,** which are branched extensions of the inner cortex that contain B lymphocytes and some plasma cells. The medullary cords are separated by dilated, capillary-like structures called **medullary lymphoid sinuses** (see Figures 14–12 and 14–13). These sinuses are irregular spaces containing lymph; like the subcapsular and intermediate sinuses, they are partially lined by reticular cells and macrophages. Reticular cells (Figure 14–14) and fibers frequently bridge the sinus in a loose network.

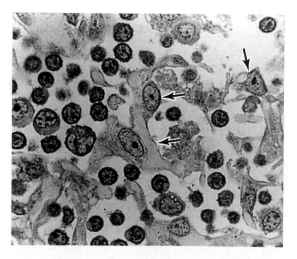

Figure 14–14. Photomicrograph of the medulla of a lymph node shown in the reticular cells (arrows) around and across the medullary sinuses. The sparse small, round cells with dark-stained nuclei and a very small amount of cytoplasm are lymphocytes. H&E stain.

The functions of B and T lymphocytes are most notable in immunodeficiency diseases, which are caused by defects in the B cells, T cells, or both. Figure 14–15 illustrates the correlation between pathologic conditions and changes in the lymph nodes.

Lymph and Blood Circulation

Afferent lymphatic vessels cross the capsule of each node and pour lymph into the subcapsular sinus. From there, lymph passes through intermediate sinuses that run parallel to the trabeculae of the capsule and into the interior of the node, where they reach the medullary sinuses. The complex architecture of both the subcapsular and the medullary sinuses slows the flow of lymph through the node, facilitating the uptake and digestion of foreign materials by macrophages and APCs. Lymph also infiltrates lymphoid tissue, flows slowly from cortex to medulla, and is collected by **efferent lymphatic vessels** at the hilum of each node. Valves in both the afferent and efferent vessels aid the unidirectional flow of lymph (Figure 14–11).

Penetration of blood vessels into lymph nodes is limited to small arteries that enter at the hilum and form capillaries in the lymphoid nodules. In the nodules, small veins originate and exit at the hilum.

Histophysiology

Lymph flows through the lymph nodes to be cleared of foreign particles before its return to the blood circulation. Because the nodes are distributed throughout the body, lymph formed in tissues must cross at least one node before entering the bloodstream.

Each node receives lymph from, and is said to be a **satellite node** of, a limited region of the body. Malignant tumors often metastasize via these nodes.

As lymph flows through the sinuses, 99% or more of the antigens and other debris are removed by the phagocytotic activity of macrophages. Infection and antigenic stimulation cause the affected lymph nodes to enlarge and form multiple germinal centers (Figure 14–16) with active cell proliferation. Although plasma cells constitute only 1–3% of the cell population in resting nodes, their numbers increase greatly in stimulated lymph nodes and partially account for the enlargement of those structures.

Recirculation of Lymphocytes: A Communication System

Lymphocytes leave the lymph nodes by efferent lymphatic vessels and eventually reach the bloodstream—all lymph formed in the body drains back into the blood. Lymphocytes return to the lymph nodes by leaving the blood through specific blood vessels, the **postcapillary,** or **high endothelial,**

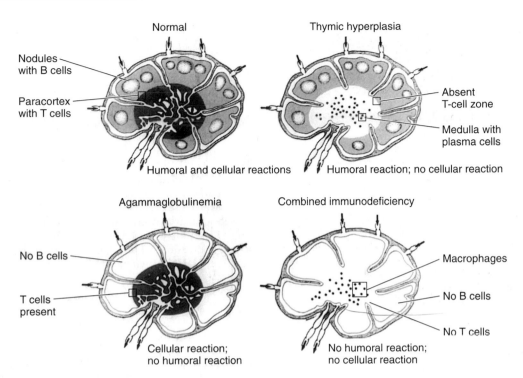

Figure 14–15. Pathologic conditions in lymph nodes related to deficiency of B cells, T cells, or both. (Redrawn, with permission, from Chandrasoma P, Taylor CR: *Concise Pathology.* Appleton & Lange, 1991.)

venules (Figure 14–17). These venules have an unusual endothelial lining of tall cuboidal cells, and lymphocytes are capable of traveling between them. Some lymphocytes are long-living cells and can recirculate many times in this way. High endothelial venules are also present in other lymphoid organs, such as the appendix, tonsils, and Peyer's patches, but not in the spleen. Although recirculation of lymphocytes also occurs there, it is most prominent in the lymph nodes.

The homing behavior of lymphocytes is due to complementary molecules on their surface and on the tall endothelial cells of postcapillary venules. Through recirculation, locally stimulated lymphocytes (eg, in an infected finger) from satellite lymph nodes will inform other lymphoid organs and prepare the organism for a generalized immune response against the infection. The continuous recirculation of lymphocytes results in a constant monitoring of all parts of the body by cells that inform the immune system of the presence of foreign antigens. During passage through the lymphoid organs, lymphocytes meet antigens on the membrane of APCs that have migrated there from infected sites.

SPLEEN

The spleen is the largest accumulation of lymphoid tissues in the body. Because of its abundance of phagocytotic cells and the close contact between these cells and circulating blood, the spleen is an important defense against microorganisms that penetrate the circulation. It is also the site of destruction of many erythrocytes. As is true of all other lymphoid organs, the spleen is a production site for activated lymphocytes, which pass into the blood. The spleen reacts promptly to antigens carried in the blood and is an important immunologic blood filter and antibody-forming organ.

General Structure

The spleen is surrounded by a capsule of dense connective tissue that sends out trabeculae that divide the **parenchyma,** or **splenic pulp,** into incomplete compartments (Figure 14–18). At the hilum on the medial surface of the spleen, the capsule gives rise to a number of trabeculae that carry nerves and arteries into the splenic pulp. Veins derived from the parenchyma and lymphatic vessels that originate in the trabeculae leave through the hilum. The splenic pulp has no lymphatic vessels.

In humans, the connective tissue of the capsule and trabeculae contains only a few smooth muscle cells. The spleen, like other lymphoid structures, is formed of a network of reticular tissue that contains lymphoid cells, macrophages, and APCs.

Splenic Pulp

On the surface of a cut through an unfixed spleen,

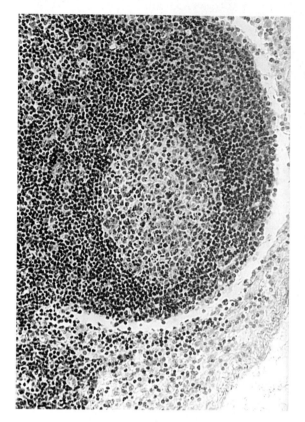

Figure 14–16. Photomicrograph of a lymphoid nodule with a germinal center (the lightly stained central area, containing many immunoblasts).

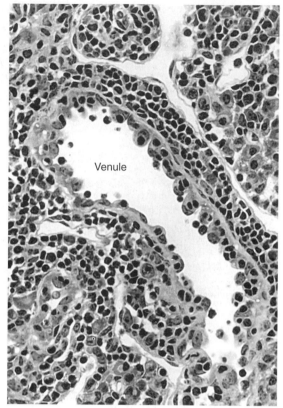

Venule

Figure 14–17. Photomicrograph of a lymphoid nodule showing a high endothelial venule being crossed by lymphocytes. Molecules at the lymphocyte surface are recognized by receptors in endothelial cells. This recognition determines the homing of the lymphocytes.

one can observe white spots in the parenchyma. These are lymphoid nodules and are part of the **white pulp.** The nodules appear within the **red pulp,** a dark red tissue that is rich in blood (Figures 14–19 and 14–20). Examination under a low-power microscope reveals that the red pulp is composed of elongated structures, the splenic cords (**Billroth's cords**), that lie between the sinusoids.

Blood Circulation

The splenic artery divides as it penetrates the hilum, branching into **trabecular arteries,** vessels of various sizes that follow the course of the connective tissue trabeculae. When they leave the trabeculae to enter the parenchyma, the arteries are immediately enveloped by a sheath of lymphocytes called the **periarterial lymphatic sheath** (**PALS**). These vessels are known as **central arteries** or **white pulp arteries** (Figure 14–21). Although the lymphocytic sheath (white pulp) thickens along its course to form a number of lymphoid nodules in which the vessel occupies an eccentric position (Figures 14–22 and 14–23), the

vessel is still called the central artery. During its course through the white pulp, the artery also divides into numerous radial branches that supply the surrounding lymphoid tissue.

After leaving the white pulp, the central artery subdivides to form straight **penicillar arterioles** with an outside diameter of approximately 24 μm. Near their termination, some of the penicillar arterioles are surrounded by a sheath of reticular cells, lymphoid cells, and macrophages.

Beyond the sheath, the vessels continue as simple arterial capillaries that carry blood to the sinusoids (red pulp sinuses). These sinusoids occupy the spaces between the red pulp cords (Figure 14–19). The manner in which blood flows from the arterial capillaries of the red pulp to the interior of the sinusoids has not yet been completely explained. Some investigators suggest that the capillaries open directly into the sinusoids, and others maintain that the blood passes through the spaces between the red pulp cord cells and then moves on to be collected by the sinusoids (Figures 14–22 and 14–24). The first theory suggests

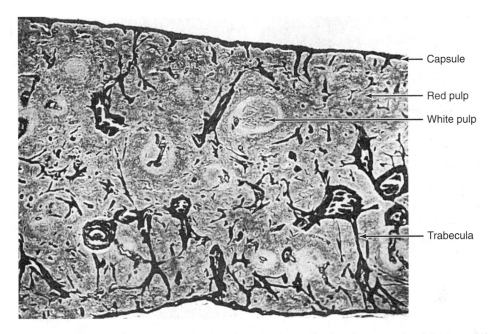

Figure 14–18. Photomicrograph of a silver-stained section of spleen, showing the general architecture of the organ. × 30.

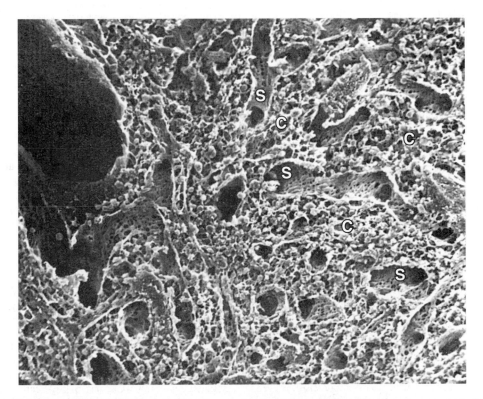

Figure 14–19. General view of splenic red pulp with a scanning electron microscope. Note the sinusoids (S) and the splenic cords (C). × 360. (Reproduced, with permission, from Miyoshi M, Fujita T: Stereo-fine structure of the splenic red pulp. A combined scanning and transmission electron microscope study on dog and rat spleen. Arch Histol Jpn 1971;33:225.)

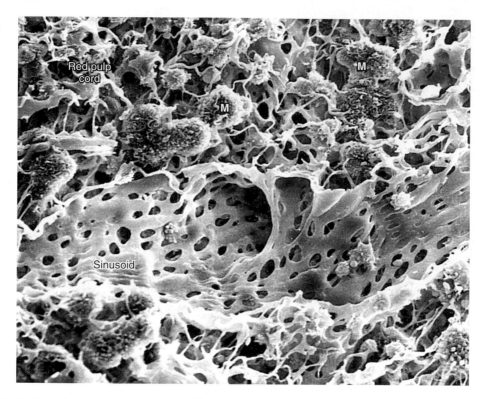

Figure 14–20. Scanning electron micrograph of the red pulp of the spleen showing sinusoids, red pulp cords, and macrophages (M). Note the multiple fenestrations in the endothelial cells of the sinusoids. × 1600. (Reproduced, with permission, from Miyoshi M, Fujita T: Stereo-fine structure of the splenic red pulp. A combined scanning and transmission electron microscope study on dog and rat spleen. Arch Histol Jpn 1971;33:225.)

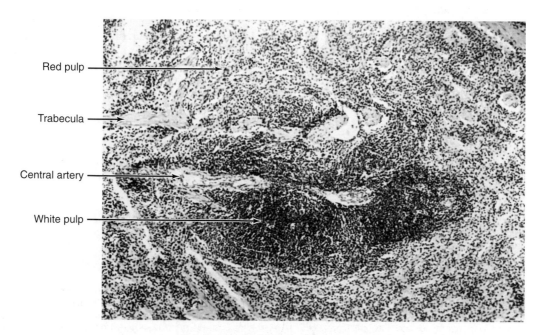

Figure 14–21. Photomicrograph of splenic white and red pulp. H&E stain. × 100.

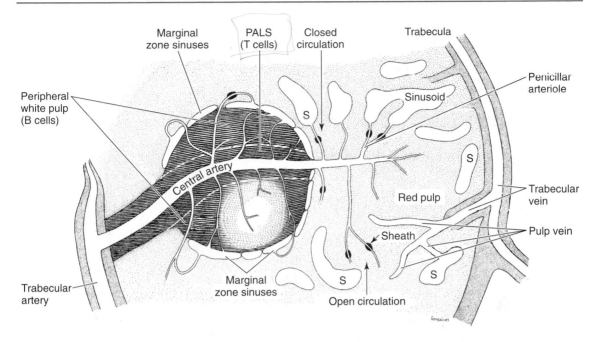

Figure 14–22. Schematic view of the blood circulation of the spleen. Theories of open and closed circulation are represented. Splenic sinuses (S) are indicated. PALS, periarterial lymphatic sheath. (Redrawn and reproduced, with permission, from Greep RO, Weiss L: *Histology,* 3rd ed. McGraw-Hill, 1973.)

a **closed circulation;** ie, the blood always remains inside the vessels. According to the second theory, the circulation would open into the parenchyma of the red pulp (Billroth's cords), and the blood would pass through the space between the cells to reach the sinusoids (**open circulation**). Current evidence suggests that blood circulation in the human spleen is of the open type.

From the sinusoids, blood proceeds to the red pulp veins that join together and enter the trabeculae, forming the **trabecular veins** (Figure 14–22). The splenic vein originates from these vessels and emerges from the hilum of the spleen. The trabecular veins do not have individual muscle walls; their walls are composed of trabecular tissue. They can be considered channels hollowed out in the trabecular connective tissue and lined by endothelium.

White Pulp

White pulp consists of lymphoid tissue that sheathes both the central arteries and the lymphoid nodules appended to the sheaths. The lymphoid cells surrounding the central arteries are mainly T lymphocytes and form the PALS (Figure 14–25). Lymphoid nodules consist mainly of B lymphocytes.

Between the white pulp and the red pulp lies a **marginal zone** consisting of many sinuses and loose lymphoid tissue. Few lymphocytes but many active

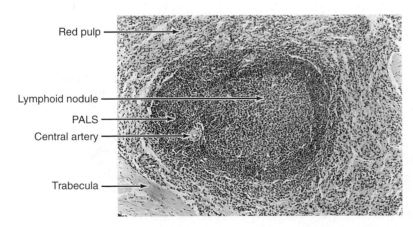

Figure 14–23. Photomicrograph of the spleen showing a lymphoid nodule (white pulp) surrounded by red pulp. PALS, periarterial lymphatic sheath. × 150.

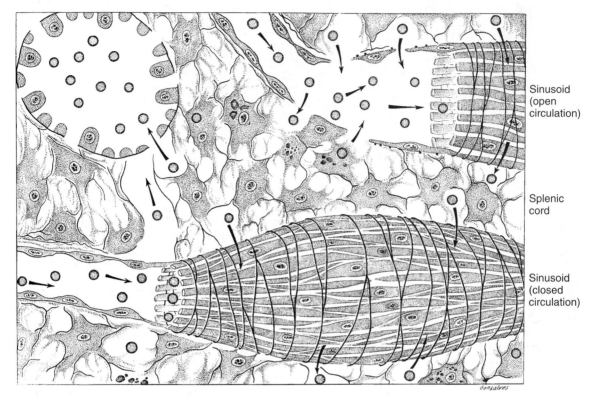

Figure 14–24. Structure of the red pulp of the spleen, showing splenic sinusoids and splenic cords with reticular and phagocytic cells (some with ingested material). The disposition of the reticular fibers in the red pulp is illustrated. In the splenic cords they form a three-dimensional network; in the sinusoids they are mainly perpendicular to the long axis of the sinusoid. Both the open and closed theories of circulation are illustrated. Arrows indicate blood flow and options for movement of blood cells.

macrophages can be found there. The marginal zone contains an abundance of blood antigens and thus plays a major role in the immunologic activities of the spleen. Many of the pulp arterioles derived from the central artery extend out and away from the white pulp but then turn back and drain into sinuses of the marginal zone that encircles the nodules. As a consequence of this drainage, which includes the added blood flow from vessels within the white pulp that also terminate in the marginal zone, this area plays a significant role in filtering the blood and initiating an immune response. In addition, large numbers of macrophages remove antigenic debris.

Interdigitating dendritic cells (which are APCs) in the marginal zone trap and present antigens to immunologically competent cells. The marginal zone removes not only antigens but also T and B lymphocytes from the blood. As lymphocytes leave the systemic circulation to penetrate the white pulp, they pass dendritic cells, which may have antigen fragments in their surfaces. If the appropriate B cells, T cells, and antigen are present, an immune response will be initiated. Activated B cells migrate to the center of the white pulp nodule and give rise to plasma

cells and memory B cells. Plasma cells migrate to the splenic cords and release antibodies into the blood in the sinuses.

The lymphocytes of the central portion of the PALS are **thymus-dependent,** whereas the marginal zones and the nodules—the **peripheral white pulp**—are populated by B lymphocytes (Figure 14–25).

Red Pulp

The red pulp contains splenic cords and sinusoids. The splenic cords are composed of a loose network of reticular cells supported by reticular fibers (collagen type III). In addition, the splenic cords contain macrophages, T and B lymphocytes, plasma cells, and many blood cells (erythrocytes, platelets, and granulocytes).

The sinusoids of the spleen are lined by elongated endothelial cells with long axes parallel to the long axes of the sinusoids. These cells are enveloped in reticular fibers set mainly in a transverse direction, much like the hoops on a barrel (Figure 14–24). The transverse and longitudinal fibers join to form a network enveloping the sinusoid cells and macrophages

Lymph node

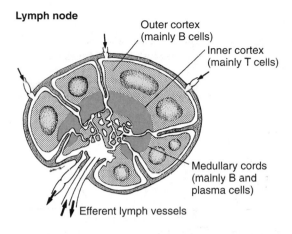

Spleen

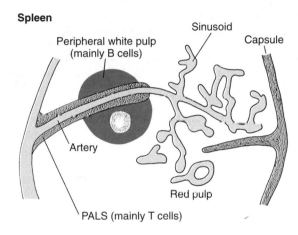

Figure 14–25. Distribution of B and T cells in lymph nodes and spleen. PALS, periarterial lymphatic sheath.

that occupy the spaces between neighboring endothelial cells. Around the sinusoid is an incomplete basal lamina.

Because the spaces between endothelial cells of the splenic sinusoids are 2–3 μm in diameter or smaller (Figure 14–20), only flexible cells are able to pass easily from the red pulp cords to the lumen of the sinusoids.

As already stated, the secondary lymphoid structures have regions that are populated by cells of the T or B family. Figure 14–25 gives a general idea of their distribution in the lymph nodes and the spleen.

Histophysiology

The best-known functions of the spleen are the production of lymphocytes, the destruction of erythrocytes, the defense of the organism against invaders that enter the bloodstream, and the storage of blood.

A. Production of Lymphocytes: The white pulp of the spleen produces lymphocytes that migrate to the red pulp and reach the lumens of the sinusoids, where they are incorporated into the blood.

> In certain pathologic conditions (eg, leukemia), the spleen may reinitiate the production of granulocytes and erythrocytes, a function present during fetal life, and undergo a process known as **myeloid metaplasia** (the occurrence of myeloid tissues in extramedullary sites). In leukemia, there is splenomegaly (enlarged spleen), anemia, and the presence of immature granulocytes and nucleated erythrocytes.

B. Destruction of Erythrocytes: Erythrocytes have an average life span of 120 days, after which they are destroyed, mainly in the spleen. A reduction in their flexibility and changes in their membrane seem to be the signals for destruction of erythrocytes. Degenerating erythrocytes are also removed in the bone marrow.

Macrophages in the splenic cords engulf and digest the erythrocytes that frequently fragment in the extracellular space. The hemoglobin they contain is broken down into several parts. The protein, globin, is hydrolyzed to amino acids that are reused in protein synthesis. Iron is released from heme and, together with transferrin, is transported in blood to the bone marrow, where it is reused in erythropoiesis. Iron-free heme is metabolized to **bilirubin,** which is excreted in the bile by liver cells. After surgical removal of the spleen (splenectomy), there is an increase in abnormal erythrocytes, seen to have deformed shapes in blood smears. There is also an increase in the number of blood platelets, suggesting that the spleen normally removes aged platelets.

C. Defense Against Invaders: Because it contains both B and T lymphocytes as well as APCs and phagocytic cells, the spleen is important in the immune defense of the body. In the same way that lymph nodes are a filter for the lymph, the spleen is a filter for the blood. Of all the phagocytotic cells of the organism, those of the spleen are most active in the phagocytosis of living organisms (bacteria and viruses) and inert particles that find their way into the bloodstream.

UNENCAPSULATED LYMPHOID TISSUE

Lymphoid nodules—also called **lymphoid follicles**—are isolated or aggregated in the loose connective tissues of several organs, mainly in the lamina propria of the digestive tract, upper respiratory tract, and urinary passages. Unencapsulated nodules have the same microscopic structure as do nodules in the cortex of a lymph node. They are composed of densely packed lymphocytes (mainly B lymphocytes) that differentiate into plasma cells after appropriate antigenic stimulation.

Primary lymphoid nodules are spherical or

ovoid, with no clear central region. **Secondary nodules** have a clear zone, the **germinal center,** in their interior (Figure 14–16). The germinal center is a collection of activated cytoplasm-rich lymphocytes (lymphoblasts) that appear only after birth in response to exposure to antigens.

Peyer's patches are aggregates of unencapsulated nodules found in the lamina propria of the ileum (see Chapter 15).

Lymphoid nodules (usually in the form of loose infiltrates of lymphocytes) found in the mucosa of several organs are collectively called mucosa-associated lymphoid tissue, or **MALT.** The best-studied components of the MALT are the lymphoid tissue found in the mucosa of the digestive system (gut-associated lymphoid tissue, or **GALT**) and its counterpart in the bronchial ducts, **BALT.**

TONSILS

Tonsils are organs composed of aggregates of incompletely encapsulated lymphoid tissues that lie beneath, and in contact with, the epithelium of the initial portion of the digestive tract. Depending on their location, tonsils in the mouth and pharynx are called **palatine, pharyngeal,** or **lingual tonsils.** They produce lymphocytes, many of which infiltrate the epithelium.

Palatine Tonsils

The two palatine tonsils are located in the lateral walls of the oral part of the pharynx. Under the squamous stratified epithelium, the dense lymphoid tissue in these tonsils forms a band that contains lymphoid nodules, generally with germinal centers (Figure 14–26). Each tonsil has 10–20 epithelial invaginations that penetrate the parenchyma deeply, forming **crypts,** whose lumens contain desquamated epithelial cells, live and dead lymphocytes, and bacteria (Figure 14–27). Crypts may appear as purulent spots in tonsillitis. Separating the lymphoid tissue from subjacent structures is a band of dense connective tissue, the **capsule** of the tonsil. This capsule usually acts as a barrier against spreading tonsillar infections.

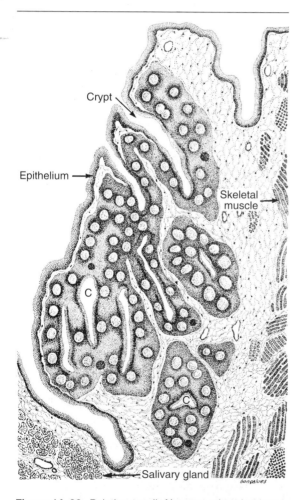

Figure 14–26. Palatine tonsil. Numerous lymphoid nodules can be seen near the stratified squamous epithelium of the oropharynx. The light areas in the lymphoid tissue are germinal centers. Note the sections through the epithelial crypts (C).

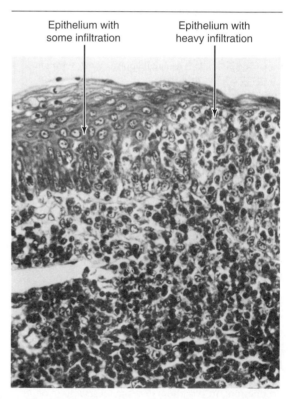

Figure 14–27. Photomicrograph of a palatine tonsil. The stratified squamous epithelium is infiltrated by lymphocytes. H&E stain. × 400.

Pharyngeal Tonsil

The pharyngeal tonsil is a single tonsil situated in the superior-posterior portion of the pharynx. It is covered by ciliated pseudostratified columnar epithelium typical of the respiratory tract, and areas of stratified epithelium can also be observed.

The pharyngeal tonsil is composed of pleats of mucosa and contains diffuse lymphoid tissue and nodules. It has no crypts, and its capsule is thinner than those of the palatine tonsils.

Hypertrophy of the pharyngeal tonsil resulting from chronic inflammation is called **adenoids.**

Lingual Tonsils

The lingual tonsils are smaller and more numerous than the palatine and pharyngeal tonsils. They are situated at the base of the tongue (see Figure 15–3) and are covered by stratified squamous epithelium. Each lingual tonsil has a single crypt.

REFERENCES

Abbas AK et al: *Cellular and Molecular Immunology.* Saunders, 1994.

Alberts B et al: The immune system. In: *Molecular Biology of the Cell,* 3rd ed. Garland, 1994.

Austyn JM, Wood KJ: *Principles of Cellular and Molecular Immunology.* Oxford Univ Press, 1993.

Balfour BM et al: Antigen-presenting cells, including Langerhans cells, veiled cells, and interdigitating cells. Ciba Found Symp 1981;84:281.

Cella M et al: Origin, maturation and antigen presenting function of dendritic cells. Curr Opin Immunol 1997;9:10.

Claman HN: The biology of the immune response. JAMA 1992;268:2790.

Darnell J et al: Immunity. In: *Molecular Cell Biology,* 2nd ed. Scientific American Books, 1990.

Douglas SD: Development and structure of cells in the immune system. In: *Basic & Clinical Immunology,* 4th ed. Stites DP et al (editors). Lange, 1982.

Rajewsky K: B-cell differentiation: clonal selection and learning in the antibody system. Nature 1996;381:751.

Raviola E, Karnovsky MJ: Evidence for a blood-thymus barrier using electron opaque tracers. J Exp Med 1972;136:466.

Sainte-Marie G, Peng FS: High endothelial venules of the rat lymph node, a review and a question: Is their activity antigen specific? Anat Rec 1996;245:593.

Smith CA, Wood EJ: Immunological defence. In: *Cell Biology,* 2nd ed. Chapmann and Hall, 1996.

Steinman RM: The dendritic cell system and its role in immunogenicity. Annu Rev Immunol 1991;9:271.

Stevens SK et al: Differences in the migration of B and T lymphocytes: organ-selective localization in vivo and the role of lymphocyte-endothelial cell recognition. J Immunol 1982;128:844.

Tough DF, Sprent J: Lifespan of lymphocytes. Immunol Res 1995;14:252.

Volk P, Meyer LM: The histology of reactive lymph nodes. Am J Surg Pathol 1987;11:866.

Weigent DA, Blalock JE: Interactions between the neuroendocrine and immune systems: common hormones and receptors. Immunol Rev 1987;100:79.

Digestive Tract

The digestive system consists of the digestive tract—oral cavity, mouth, esophagus, stomach, small and large intestines, rectum, and anus—and its associated glands—salivary glands, liver, and pancreas. Its function is to obtain from ingested food the molecules necessary for the maintenance, growth, and energy needs of the body. Large molecules such as proteins, fats, complex carbohydrates, and nucleic acids are broken down into small molecules that are easily absorbed through the lining of the digestive tract. Water, vitamins, and minerals are also absorbed from ingested food. In addition, the inner layer of the digestive tract is a protective barrier between the content of the tract's lumen and the internal milieu of the body.

The first step in the complex process known as digestion occurs in the mouth, where food is moistened by saliva and ground by the teeth into smaller pieces; saliva also initiates the digestion of carbohydrates. Digestion continues in the stomach and small intestine, where the food—transformed into its basic components (amino acids, monosaccharides, free fatty acids, monoglycerides, etc)—is absorbed. Water absorption occurs in the large intestine, causing the undigested contents to become semisolid.

GENERAL STRUCTURE OF THE DIGESTIVE TRACT

The entire gastrointestinal tract presents certain common structural characteristics. It is a hollow tube composed of a lumen whose diameter varies, surrounded by a wall made up of four principal layers: the **mucosa, submucosa, muscularis,** and **serosa.** The structure of these layers is summarized below and illustrated in Figure 15–1.

The **mucosa** comprises an **epithelial lining;** a **lamina propria** of loose connective tissue rich in blood and lymph vessels and smooth muscle cells, sometimes also containing glands and lymphoid tissue; and the **muscularis mucosae,** usually consisting of a thin inner circular layer and an outer longitudinal layer of smooth muscle cells separating the mucosa

from the submucosa. The mucosa is frequently called a **mucous membrane.**

The **submucosa** is composed of dense connective tissue with many blood and lymph vessels and a **submucosal** (also called **Meissner's**) **nerve plexus.** It may also contain glands and lymphoid tissue.

The **muscularis** contains smooth muscle cells that are spirally oriented and divided into two sublayers according to the main direction the muscle cells follow. In the internal sublayer (close to the lumen), the orientation is generally circular; in the external sublayer, it is mostly longitudinal. The muscularis also contains the **myenteric** (or **Auerbach's**) **nerve plexus,** which lies between the two muscle sublayers, and blood and lymph vessels in the connective tissue between the muscle sublayers.

The **serosa** is a thin layer of loose connective tissue, rich in blood and lymph vessels and adipose tissue, and a simple squamous covering epithelium (**mesothelium**).

The main functions of the epithelial lining of the digestive tract are to provide a selectively permeable barrier between the contents of the tract and the tissues of the body, to facilitate the transport and digestion of food, to promote the absorption of the products of this digestion, and to produce hormones that affect the activity of the digestive system. Cells in this layer produce mucus for lubrication and protection.

The abundant lymphoid nodules in the lamina propria and the submucosal layer protect the organism (in association with the epithelium) from bacterial invasion. The necessity for this immunologic support is obvious, because the entire digestive tract—with the exception of the oral cavity, esophagus, and anal canal—is lined by a simple thin, vulnerable epithelium. The lamina propria, located just below the epithelium, is a zone rich in macrophages and lymphoid cells, some of which actively produce antibodies. These antibodies are mainly immunoglobulin A (IgA) and are bound to a secretory protein produced by the epithelial cells of the intestinal lining and secreted into the intestinal lumen (Figure 15–2). This complex protects against viral and bacterial invasion.

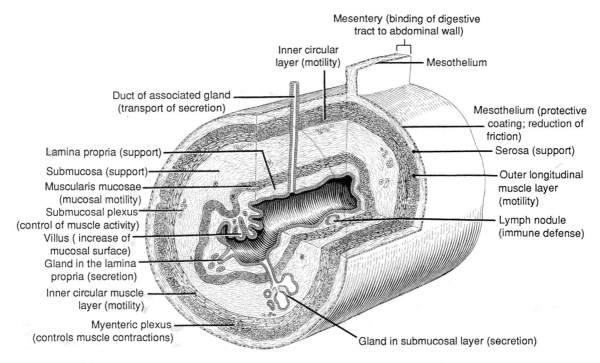

Figure 15–1. Schematic structure of a portion of the digestive tract with various components and their functions. (Redrawn and reproduced, with permission, from Bevelander G: *Outline of Histology,* 7th ed. Mosby, 1971.)

As discussed in Chapter 14, the IgA present in the respiratory, digestive, and urinary tracts is resistant to proteolytic enzymes and can therefore coexist with the proteases present in the intestinal lumen.

The muscularis mucosae promotes the movement of the mucosa independent of other movements of the digestive tract, increasing its contact with the food. The contractions of the muscularis, generated and coordinated by nerve plexuses, propel and mix the food in the digestive tract. These plexuses are composed mainly of nerve cell aggregates (multipolar visceral neurons) that form small parasympathetic ganglia. A rich network of pre- and postganglionic fibers of the autonomic nervous system and some visceral sensory fibers in these ganglia permit communication between them. The number of these ganglia along the digestive tract is variable; they are more numerous in regions of greatest motility.

In certain diseases, such as **Hirschsprung disease** (congenital megacolon) or **Chagas disease** (*Trypanosoma cruzi* infection), the plexuses in the digestive tract are severely injured and most of their neurons are destroyed. This results in disturbances of digestive tract motility, with frequent dilatations in some areas. The abundant innervation from the autonomic nervous system

that the digestive tract receives provides an anatomic explanation of the widely observed action of emotional stress on the digestive tract—a phenomenon of importance in psychosomatic medicine.

THE ORAL CAVITY

The oral cavity is lined with nonkeratinized stratified squamous epithelium. Its superficial cells are nucleated, with scanty granules of keratin in their interiors. In the lips, a transition from nonkeratinized to keratinized epithelium can be observed. The lamina propria has papillae, similar to those in the dermis of the skin, and is continuous with a submucosa containing diffuse small salivary glands.

The roof of the mouth consists of the hard and soft palates, both covered with the same type of stratified squamous epithelium. In the hard palate, the mucous membrane rests on bony tissue. The soft palate has a core of skeletal muscle and numerous mucous glands in its submucosa.

The palatine **uvula** is a small conical process that extends downward from the center of the lower border of the soft palate. It has a core of muscle and areolar connective tissue covered by typical oral mucosa.

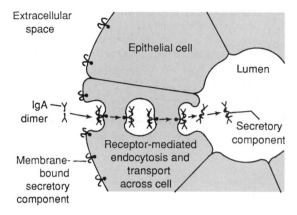

Figure 15–2. The mechanism by which the secretory component mediates the transport of a dimeric IgA molecule across an epithelial cell. The IgA dimer is synthesized by plasma cells of the lamina propria. The secretory component is synthesized by the epithelial cell as a transmembrane glycoprotein and serves as a receptor on its basolateral surface for binding the IgA dimer. The secretory component–IgA complex enters the cell and is exposed at the apical surface. The part of the secretory component that is bound to the IgA dimer is then cleaved from its transmembrane tail (black dot), releasing the IgA dimer into the intestinal lumen. The IgA dimer is adsorbed to the surface of epithelial cells, where it inhibits bacterial and viral adherence, a process called **immunoexclusion.** (Reproduced, with permission, from Alberts B et al: *Molecular Biology of the Cell,* Garland, 1983.)

1. TONGUE

The tongue is a mass of striated muscle covered by a mucous membrane whose structure varies according to the region. The muscle fibers cross one another in three planes; they are grouped in bundles, usually separated by connective tissue. Because the connective tissue of the lamina propria penetrates the spaces between the muscular bundles, the mucous membrane is strongly adherent to the muscle. The mucous membrane is smooth on the lower surface of the tongue. The tongue's dorsal surface is irregular, covered anteriorly by a great number of small eminences called **papillae.** The posterior one third of the dorsal surface of the tongue is separated from the anterior two thirds by a V-shaped boundary. Behind this boundary, the surface of the tongue shows small bulges composed mainly of two types of small lymphoid aggregations: small collections of lymphoid nodules; and the lingual tonsils, where lymphoid nodules aggregate around invaginations (crypts) of the mucous membrane (Figure 15–3).

Papillae

Papillae are elevations of the oral epithelium and lamina propria that assume various forms and functions. There are four types (see Figure 15–3):

A. Filiform Papillae: Filiform papillae have an elongated conical shape; they are quite numerous and are present over the entire surface of the tongue. Their epithelium, which does not contain taste buds, is frequently partly keratinized.

B. Fungiform Papillae: Fungiform papillae resemble mushrooms in that they have a narrow stalk and a smooth-surfaced, dilated upper part. These

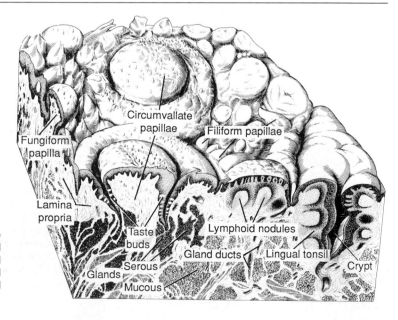

Figure 15–3. Surface of the tongue on the region close to its V-shaped boundary, between the anterior and posterior portions. Note the lymphoid nodules, lingual tonsil, glands, and papillae.

papillae, which contain scattered taste buds on their upper surfaces, are irregularly interspersed among the filiform papillae.

C. Foliate Papillae: Foliate papillae are poorly developed in humans. They consist of two or more parallel ridges and furrows on the dorsolateral surface of the tongue. Ducts from serous glands drain into the bases of the furrows.

D. Circumvallate Papillae: Circumvallate papillae are 7–12 extremely large circular papillae whose flattened surfaces extend above the other papillae. They are distributed in the V region in the posterior portion of the tongue. Numerous serous (von Ebner's) glands drain their contents into the deep groove that encircles the periphery of each papilla. This moat-like arrangement provides a continuous flow of fluid over the great number of taste buds present along the sides of these papillae. The glands also secrete a lipase that probably prevents the formation of a hydrophobic layer over the taste buds that would hinder their function. This flow of secre-

tions is important in removing food particles from the vicinity of the taste buds so that they can receive and process new gustatory stimuli. Along with this local role, lingual lipase is active in the stomach and can digest up to 30% of dietary triglycerides. Other small mucous and serous glands dispersed throughout the lining of the oral cavity act in the same way as the serous glands associated with this type of papilla to prepare the taste buds in other parts of the oral cavity—epiglottis, pharynx, palate, etc—to respond to taste stimuli (see Chapter 24).

2. PHARYNX

The pharynx, a transitional space between the oral cavity and the respiratory and digestive systems, forms an area of communication between the nasal region and the larynx. The pharynx is lined by stratified squamous epithelium of the mucous type, except in those regions of the respiratory portions that are not subject

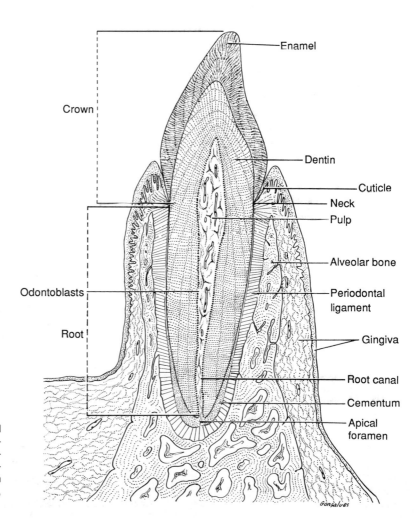

Figure 15–4. Diagram of a sagittal section from an incisor tooth in position in the mandibular bone. (Redrawn and reproduced, with permission, from Leeson TS, Leeson CR: *Histology,* 2nd ed. Saunders, 1970.)

Crown

Odontoblasts

Root

Enamel

Dentin

Cuticle

Neck

Pulp

Alveolar bone

Periodontal ligament

Gingiva

Root canal

Cementum

Apical foramen

to abrasion. These latter areas have a ciliated pseudostratified columnar epithelium with goblet cells.

The pharynx contains the tonsils (described in Chapter 14). The mucosa of the pharynx also has many small mucous glands in its dense connective tissue layer. The constrictor and longitudinal muscles of the pharynx are located outside this layer.

3. TEETH & ASSOCIATED STRUCTURES

In adult humans, there are normally 32 **permanent teeth.** These teeth are disposed in two bilaterally symmetric arches in the maxillary and mandibular bones, with eight teeth in each quadrant: two incisors, one canine, two premolars, and three permanent molars. Twenty of the permanent teeth are preceded by **deciduous (baby) teeth;** the remainder (the permanent molars) have no deciduous precursors.

Each tooth is composed of a portion that projects above the **gingiva (gum)**—the **crown**—and one or more **roots** below the gingiva that hold the teeth in bony sockets called **alveoli,** one for each tooth (Figure 15–4). The crown is covered by the extremely hard **enamel** and the roots by **cementum.** These two coverings meet at the **neck (cervix)** of the tooth. The interior of a tooth contains another calcified material, **dentin,** which surrounds a tissue-filled space known as the **pulp cavity** (Figure 15–4). The pulp cavity extends to the apex of the root (the root canal), where an orifice (**apical foramen**) permits the entrance and exit of blood vessels, lymphatics, and nerves of the pulp cavity. The **periodontal ligament** (or **membrane**) is a collagenous, fibrous structure that fixes the tooth firmly in its bony socket (alveolus).

Dentin

Dentin is a calcified tissue like bone but is harder because of its higher content of calcium salts (70% of dry weight). It is composed mainly of type I collagen fibrils, glycosaminoglycans, and calcium salts in the form of **hydroxyapatite** crystals. The organic matrix of dentin is secreted by **odontoblasts,** cells that line the internal surface of the tooth, separating it from the pulp cavity (Figures 15–5 and 15–7). The odontoblast is a slender polarized cell that produces organic matrix only at the dentinal surface. These cells have the structure of polarized protein-secreting cells with secretion granules containing procollagen; the cytoplasm of each odontoblast contains a nucleus at its base. Odontoblasts have slender, branched cytoplasmic extensions that penetrate perpendicularly through the width of the dentin—the **odontoblast processes** (Tomes' fibers). These processes gradually become longer as the dentin becomes thicker, running in small canals called **dentinal tubules** that are extensively branched near the junction between dentin and enamel (Figure 15–6). Odontoblast processes have a diameter of 3–4 μm near the cell

body but gradually become thinner at their distal ends.

The matrix produced by odontoblasts is initially unmineralized and is called **predentin** (Figure 15–5). The mineralization of developing dentin begins when membrane-limited vesicles—**matrix vesicles**—appear. They contain fine crystals of hydroxyapatite that grow and serve as nucleation sites for further mineral deposition on the surrounding collagen fibrils.

Unlike bone, dentin persists as a mineralized tissue long after destruction of the odontoblasts. It is therefore possible to maintain teeth whose pulp and odontoblasts have been destroyed by infection. In adult teeth, destruction of the covering enamel by erosion from use or dental caries (tooth decay) usually triggers a reaction in the dentin that causes it to resume the synthesis of its components.

Enamel

Enamel is the hardest component of the human body and the richest in calcium. It consists of about 95% calcium salts (mainly hydroxyapatite), 0.5% or-

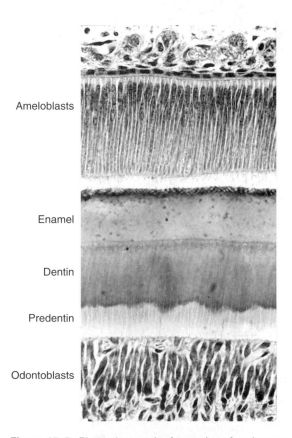

Figure 15–5. Photomicrograph of a section of an immature tooth, showing predentin and enamel. The ameloblasts and odontoblasts are both disposed as palisades. Masson's stain. × 350.

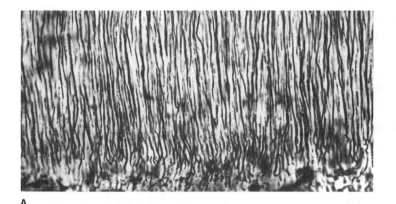

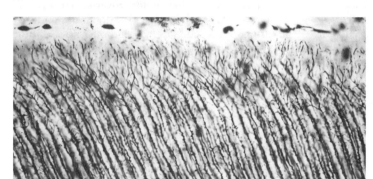

Figure 15–6. Photomicrograph of a section of a tooth, showing the odontoblast processes of the dentin. **A:** Initial portion. **B:** Terminal portion. These processes gradually get thinner and terminate by branching into delicate extensions. × 400.

ganic material, and water as the remainder. Enamel is produced by cells of ectodermal origin, whereas most of the other structures of teeth derive from mesodermal or neural crest cells. The organic enamel matrix is not composed of collagen fibrils but of at least two heterogeneous classes of proteins called **amelogenins** and **enamelins.** The roles of these proteins in the organization of the mineral component of enamel are under intensive investigation.

Enamel consists of elongated rods or columns of hydroxyapatite crystals—**enamel rods (prisms)**—that are bound together by **interrod enamel.** Both interrod enamel and enamel rods are formed of hydroxyapatite crystals; they differ only in the orientation of the crystals. Each rod extends through the entire thickness of the enamel layer.

Enamel matrix is secreted by cells called **ameloblasts** (Figure 15–5). These tall columnar cells possess numerous mitochondria in the region below the nucleus. Rough endoplasmic reticulum and a well-developed Golgi complex are found above the nucleus. Each ameloblast has an apical extension, known as a **Tomes' process,** containing numerous secretory granules that contain the proteins that make up the enamel matrix.

Pulp

Tooth pulp consists of loose connective tissue. Its main components are odontoblasts, fibroblasts, thin collagen fibrils, and a ground substance that contains glycosaminoglycans (Figure 15–7).

Pulp is a highly innervated and vascularized tissue. Blood vessels and myelinated nerve fibers enter the apical foramen and divide into numerous branches. Some nerve fibers lose their myelin sheaths and extend for a short distance into the dentinal tubules. These fibers are sensitive to pain, the only sensory modality recognized in teeth.

Associated Structures

The structures responsible for maintaining the teeth in the maxillary and mandibular bones consist of the **cementum, periodontal ligament, alveolar bone,** and **gingiva.**

A. Cementum: Cementum covers the dentin of the root and is similar in composition to bone, although haversian systems and blood vessels are absent. It is thicker in the apical region of the root, where there are **cementocytes,** cells with the appearance of osteocytes. Like osteocytes, they are encased in lacunae that communicate through canaliculi. Like

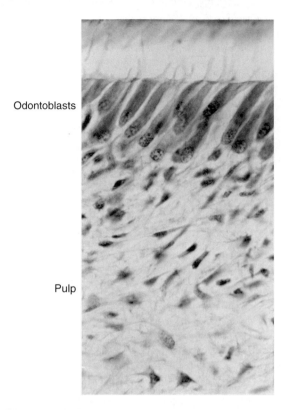

Odontoblasts

Pulp

Figure 15–7. Photomicrograph of dental pulp, in which fibroblasts are abundant. In the upper region are the odontoblasts, from which the odontoblast processes derive. Hematoxylin-and-eosin (H&E) stain. × 400.

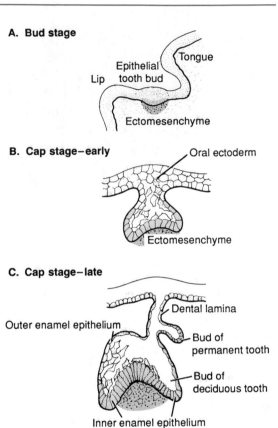

A. Bud stage

Tongue

Epithelial
tooth bud

Lip

Ectomesenchyme

B. Cap stage–early

Oral ectoderm

Ectomesenchyme

C. Cap stage–late

Dental lamina

Outer enamel epithelium

Bud of
permanent tooth

Bud of
deciduous tooth

Inner enamel epithelium

D. Bell stage

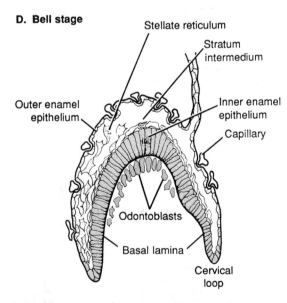

Stellate reticulum

Stratum
intermedium

Outer enamel
epithelium

Inner enamel
epithelium

Capillary

Odontoblasts

Basal lamina

Cervical
loop

Figure 15–8. Stages of bud development. The epithelium (lighter color) of a tooth bud (**A**) proliferates and invades the underlying mesenchyme to form a cap-shaped structure (**B** and **C**). In the cap stage, the epithelium differentiates into the inner enamel epithelium, which will give rise to ameloblasts. In the bell stage (**D**), neural crest–derived cells (darker color) differentiate into odontoblasts. (Modified and reproduced, with permission, from Warshawsky H: *Histology: Cell and Tissue Biology,* 5th ed. Weiss L [editor]. Elsevier, 1983.)

bone tissue, cementum is labile and reacts to the stresses to which it is subjected by resorbing old tissue or producing new tissue. When the periodontal ligament is destroyed, cementum undergoes necrosis and may be resorbed. Continuous production of cementum compensates for the normal growth that teeth undergo and maintains close contact between the roots of the teeth and their sockets.

B. Periodontal Ligament: The periodontal ligament is composed of a special type of dense connective tissue whose fibers penetrate the cementum of the tooth and bind it to the bony walls of its socket while permitting limited movement of the tooth. It serves as the periosteum of the alveolar bone. Its fibers are organized to support the pressures exerted during mastication. This avoids transmission of pressure directly to the bone—a process that would cause the bone's localized resorption.

Collagen of the periodontal ligament has characteristics that resemble those of immature tissue. It has a high protein turnover rate (as demonstrated by autoradiography) and a large soluble collagen content. The space between its fibers is filled with glycosaminoglycans.

The high rate of collagen renewal in the periodontal ligament allows processes affecting protein or collagen synthesis—eg, protein or vitamin C deficiency (**scurvy**)—to cause atrophy of this ligament. As a consequence, teeth become loose in their sockets; in extreme cases they fall out. This relative plasticity of the periodontal ligament is important because it allows orthodontic intervention, which can produce extensive changes in the disposition of teeth in the mouth.

C. Alveolar Bone: The alveolar bone is in immediate contact with the periodontal ligament. It is an immature type of bone (primary bone) in which the collagen fibers are not arranged in the typical lamellar pattern of adult bone. Many of the collagen fibers of the periodontal ligament are arranged in bundles that penetrate this bone and the cementum, forming a connecting bridge between the two structures. The bone closest to the roots of the teeth forms the socket. Vessels and nerves run through the alveolar bone to the apical foramen of the root to enter the pulp.

D. Gingiva: The gingiva is a mucous membrane firmly bound to the periosteum of the maxillary and mandibular bones. It is composed of stratified squamous epithelium and numerous connective tissue papillae. This epithelium is bound to the tooth enamel by means of a cuticle that resembles a thick basal lamina and forms the **epithelial attachment of Gottlieb.** The epithelial cells are attached to this cuticle by hemidesmosomes. Between the enamel and the epithelium is the **gingival crevice**—a small deepening surrounding the crown.

Development of Teeth

At about 6 weeks of gestation, the basal layer of the oral epithelium (ectoderm) proliferates and bulges into the underlying **ectomesenchyme** derived from the neural crest (Figure 15–8A). A horseshoe-shaped band known as the **dental lamina** is formed in each jaw. A little later, 10 regions of intensified mitotic activity are present in each dental lamina. These ectodermal outgrowths form caps over clumps of ectomesenchyme, and each collection of cells (tooth bud) will develop into a deciduous tooth. The ectomesenchyme is formed by mesenchymal cells (see Chapter 5) associated with neural crest cells that originate from the ectoderm. The intervening ectodermal cells later degenerate and disappear. The ectodermal component of a tooth bud forms the **enamel organ** responsible for the secretion of enamel (Figure 15–8B and C). The ectomesenchymal component forms the **dental papilla** from which will differentiate odontoblasts (cells that secrete dentin) and other structures of the dental pulp (Figure 15–8D). Mesenchyme also condenses around the enamel organ and will eventually differentiate into **cementoblasts**

(cells that form cementum) and the periodontal ligament.

The enamel organ continues to enlarge and assumes a bell shape at about 8 weeks of gestation. The **outer (external) enamel epithelium,** which is continuous with the dental lamina, is indented by numerous capillary vessels. Cells immediately adjacent to the dental papilla assume a columnar shape and form the **inner (internal) enamel epithelium.** These cells differentiate into **ameloblasts** (cells that will secrete enamel). Other epithelial cells between the outer and inner layers form the **stellate reticulum** and the **stratum intermedium;** the functions of these layers are not well defined (Figure 15–8D).

A continuous basal lamina separates the outer enamel epithelium from the surrounding connective tissues. This basal lamina then curves around and separates the inner enamel epithelium from ectomesenchymal cells of the dental papilla. The point where the outer enamel epithelium meets the inner enamel epithelium is called the **cervical loop** (Figure 15–8D).

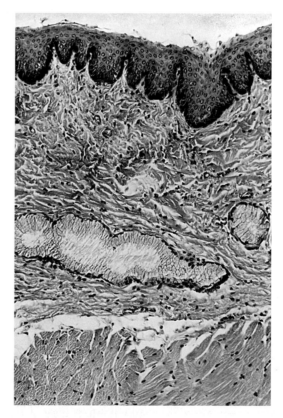

Figure 15–9. Photomicrograph of a section of the upper region of the esophagus. Mucous glands are in the submucosa; striated muscle is in the muscularis. H&E stain. × 20.

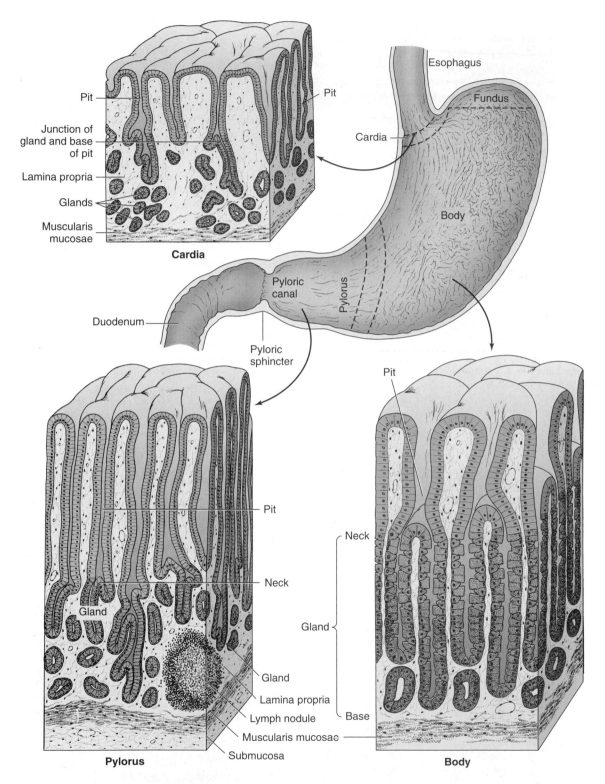

Figure 15–10. Regions of the stomach and their histologic structure.

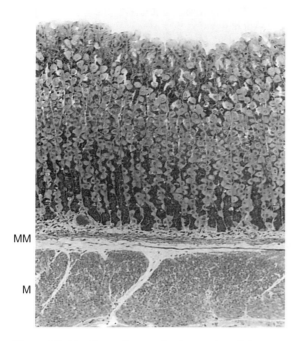

Figure 15–11. Photomicrograph of a section of the gastric glands in the fundus of the stomach. Parietal cells (light-stained) predominate in the mid and upper regions of the glands; chief (zymogenic) cells (dark-stained) predominate in the lower region of the gland. MM, muscularis mucosae; M, muscular layer.

Ameloblast differentiation is induced by ectomesenchymal cells of the dental papilla. Before ameloblasts begin to secrete enamel, they cause a superficial layer of cells of the dental papilla to elongate and differentiate into odontoblasts. Odontoblasts begin to secrete predentin, which in turn stimulates the secretion of enamel by ameloblasts. Thus, a wave of reciprocal inductions passes from the future occlusal surface of the crown toward the neck of the tooth.

A. Formation of Dentin: Odontoblasts secrete procollagen, which becomes organized into the collagen fibrils of predentin. These cells also mediate the mineralization of collagen fibrils, leading to the formation of dentin. The cell bodies of odontoblasts retreat into the pulp cavity as dentin accumulates, but their processes remain in dentinal tubules that span the entire thickness of the dentin.

B. Formation of Enamel: Ameloblasts are unusual epithelial cells in that their bases, adjacent to the basal lamina, become their secretory surfaces. Tight junctions are found around both the histologic apex (functional base) and the histologic base (functional apex) of each cell. Rough endoplasmic reticulum and an elaborate Golgi complex are found in the cytoplasm between the nucleus and the functional apex of these cells. Ameloblasts are responsible for the breakdown of the basal lamina that separates these cells from odontoblasts and dentin. Tomes'

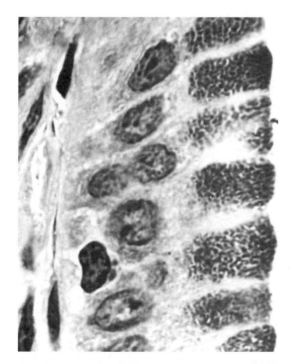

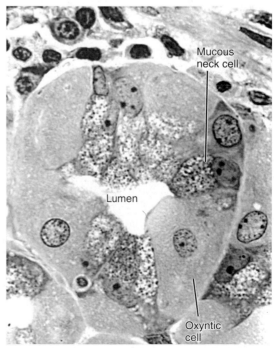

Mucous
neck cell

Lumen

Oxyntic
cell

Figure 15–12. Photomicrograph of a mucus-secreting surface epithelium (**left**) and mucous neck cells intercalated between parietal cells (**right**).

processes, the short, conical extensions of amelo-blasts, are the sites of secretion of enamel matrix. The lateral surfaces of these processes secrete the organic matrix of the interrod enamel, whereas the apical surface is responsible for deposition of the matrix of enamel rods. The role of ameloblasts in mineralization is not clear, but hydroxyapatite crystals are formed on the organic matrix. This matrix is later almost completely removed, probably by the ameloblasts. After enamel formation is complete, the enamel organ consists of a stratified squamous epithelium that erodes rapidly when the tooth erupts into the oral cavity.

C. Root Development: After the crown is completely developed, and just before its eruption, the cervical loop grows apically to envelop the dental papilla and forms **Hertwig's root sheath,** which is composed of the fused outer and inner enamel epithelia. The inner layer induces formation of odontoblasts that produce the dentin of the tooth root. When the dentin has been formed, the root sheath breaks up, and the newly formed dentin induces the differentiation of cementoblasts from mesenchymal cells of the surrounding dental sac. Cementoblasts form cementum, the bone-like tissue covering the roots of teeth.

D. Permanent Teeth: On the labial side of each dental lamina, a mass of ectodermal cells pushes out to form the **successional lamina** bud of the permanent tooth (Figure 15–8C). Here, too, are 20 regions of intensified mitotic activity, one corresponding to each of the permanent counterparts of the deciduous teeth. In addition, dental lamina cells burrow backward, and the tooth germs of the permanent molars are budded off in succession. The tooth germs for the second and third molars are not formed until after birth.

ESOPHAGUS

The part of the gastrointestinal tract called the **esophagus** is a muscular tube whose function is to transport foodstuffs from the mouth to the stomach. It is covered by nonkeratinized stratified squamous epithelium (Figure 15–9). In general, it has the same layers as the rest of the digestive tract. In the submucosa are groups of small mucus-secreting glands, the **esophageal glands.** In the lamina propria of the region near the stomach are groups of glands, the **esophageal cardiac glands,** that also secrete mucus. At the distal end of the esophagus, the muscular layer

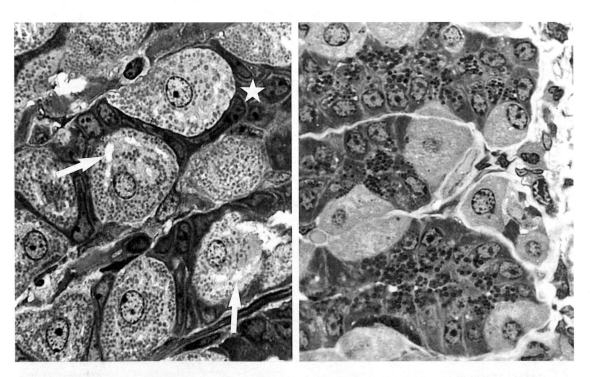

Figure 15–13. Photomicrographs of stomach mucosa in the fundus. **Left:** A section of the neck region showing parietal cells rich in mitochondria and their characteristic intracellular canaliculi (arrows). The star indicates stem cells. **Right:** The basal portion of the gland contains chief cells (characterized by basophilic cytoplasm) and pepsin-containing secretory granules. A few parietal cells are also present. × 900.

consists of only smooth muscle cells; in the mid portion, a mixture of striated and smooth muscle cells; and at the proximal end, only striated muscle cells. Only that portion of the esophagus that is in the peritoneal cavity is covered by serosa. The rest is covered by a layer of loose connective tissue, the adventitia, which blends into the surrounding tissue.

STOMACH

The stomach is a mixed exocrine-endocrine organ that digests food and secretes hormones. It is a dilated segment of the digestive tract whose main functions are to continue the digestion of carbohydrates initiated in the mouth, add an acidic fluid to the ingested food, transform it by muscular activity into a viscous mass (**chyme**), and promote the initial digestion of proteins with the enzyme **pepsin**. It also produces a gastric lipase that digests triglycerides with the help of lingual lipase. Gross inspection reveals four regions: **cardia, fundus, body,** and **pylorus** (Figure 15–10). Because the fundus and body are identical in microscopic structure, only three histologic regions are recognized. The mucosa and submucosa of the undistended stomach lie in longitudi-

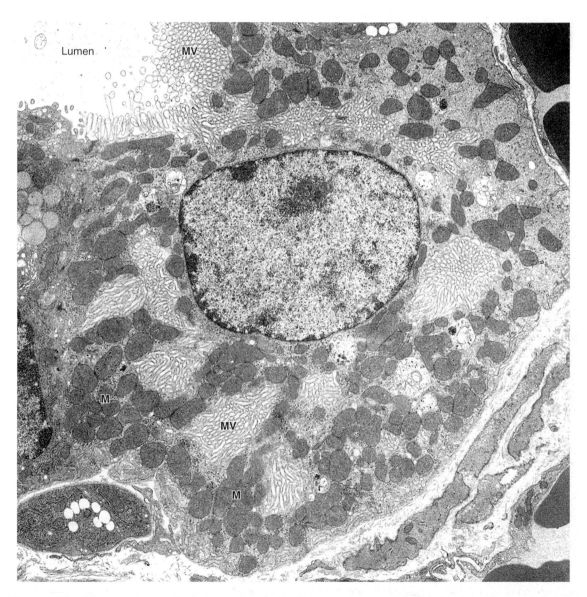

Figure 15–14. Electron micrograph of an active parietal cell. Note the microvilli (MV) protruding into the intracellular canaliculi and the abundant mitochondria (M). × 10,200. (Courtesy of S Ito.)

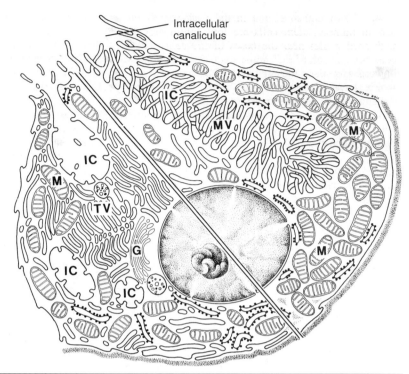

Intracellular
canaliculus

Figure 15–15. Composite diagram of a parietal cell, showing the ultrastructural differences between a resting cell (**left**) and an active cell (**right**). Note that the tubulovesicles (TV) in the cytoplasm of the resting cell fuse to form microvilli (MV) that fill up the intracellular canaliculi (IC). G, Golgi complex; M, mitochondria; MV, microvilli. (Based on the work of Ito S, Schofield GC. J Cell Biol 1974;63:364.)

nally directed folds known as **rugae.** When the stomach is filled with food, these folds flatten out.

Mucosa

The gastric mucosa consists of a **surface epithelium** that invaginates to various extents into the lamina propria, forming **gastric pits.** Emptying into the gastric pits are branched, tubular glands (cardiac, gastric, and pyloric) characteristic of each region of the stomach. The **lamina propria** of the stomach is composed of loose connective tissue interspersed with smooth muscle and lymphoid cells. Separating the mucosa from the underlying submucosa is a layer of smooth muscle, the **muscularis mucosae.**

When the luminal surface of the stomach is viewed under low magnification, numerous small circular or ovoid invaginations of the lining epithelium are observed. These are the openings of the gastric pits (Figures 15–10 and 15–11). The epithelium covering the surface and lining the pits is a simple columnar epithelium, and all the cells secrete mucus (Figure 15–12). When released from these cells, the mucus forms a thick layer that protects them from the effects of the strong acid secreted by the stomach.

Tight junctions around surface and pit cells also form part of the barrier to acid. Stress and other psychosomatic factors, or such substances as aspirin that cause gastric irritation, can disrupt this epithelial layer and lead to ulceration. The initial ulceration may heal, or it may be further aggravated by the local action of pepsin and hydrochloric acid, leading to additional gastric and duodenal ulcers.

Cardia

The cardia is a narrow circular band, 1.5–3 cm in width, at the transition between the esophagus and the stomach (Figure 15–10). Its lamina propria contains simple or branched tubular cardiac glands. The terminal portions of these glands are frequently coiled, often with large lumens. Most of the secretory cells produce mucus and lysozyme (an enzyme that attacks bacterial walls), but a few hydrochloride-producing parietal cells can be found. These glands are similar in structure to the cardiac glands of the terminal portion of the esophagus.

Fundus & Body

The lamina propria of the fundus and body is filled with branched, tubular **gastric (fundic) glands,** three to seven of which open into the bottom of each gastric pit. The distribution of epithelial cells in gastric glands is not uniform (Figures 15–10 and 15–11). The **neck** of the glands consists of stem, mucous neck, and oxyntic (parietal) cells (Figure 15–12); the **base** of the glands contains parietal, chief (zymogenic), and enteroendocrine cells.

A. Stem Cells: Found in the neck region but few in number, stem cells are low columnar cells with oval nuclei near the bases of the cells. These cells have a high rate of mitosis; some of them move upward to replace the pit and surface mucous cells, which have a turnover time of 4–7 days. Other daughter cells migrate more deeply into the glands and differentiate into mucous neck cells and parietal, chief, and enteroendocrine cells. These cells are replaced much more slowly than are surface mucous cells.

B. Mucous Neck Cells: Mucous neck cells are present in clusters or as single cells between parietal cells in the necks of gastric glands. Their mucus secretion is quite different from that of the surface epithelial mucous cells. They are irregular in shape,

with the nucleus at the base of the cell. Their secretory granules are near the apical surface and stain intensely with periodic acid–Schiff.

C. Oxyntic (Parietal) Cells: Parietal cells are present mainly in the upper half of gastric glands; they are scarce in the base. They are rounded or pyramidal cells, with one centrally placed spherical nucleus and intensely eosinophilic cytoplasm (Figures 15–10, 15–11, and 15–13). The most striking features seen in the electron microscope are an abundance of mitochondria and a deep, circular invagination of the apical plasma membrane, forming the **intracellular canaliculus** (Figure 15–14). In the resting cell, a number of tubulovesicular structures can be seen in the apical region just below the plasmalemma (Figure 15–15, left). At this stage, the cell

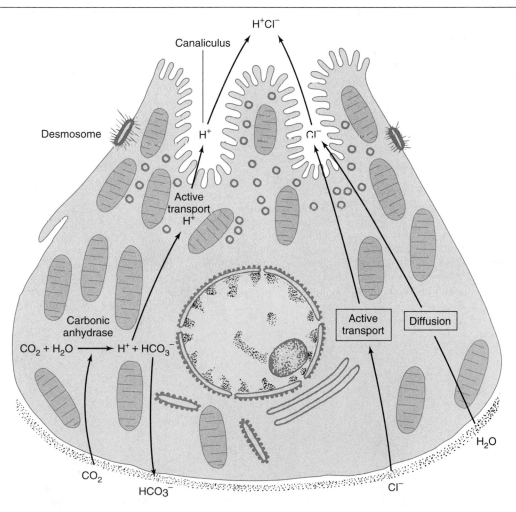

Figure 15–16. Diagram of a parietal cell, showing the main steps in the synthesis of hydrochloric acid. Under the action of carbonic anhydrase, blood CO_2 produces carbonic acid. Carbonic acid dissociates into a bicarbonate ion and a proton H^+, which is pumped to the stomach lumen. The tubulovesicles of the cell apex are seen to be related to hydrochloric acid secretion, because their number decreases after parietal cell stimulation. The bicarbonate ion returns to the blood and is responsible for a measurable increase in blood pH during digestion.

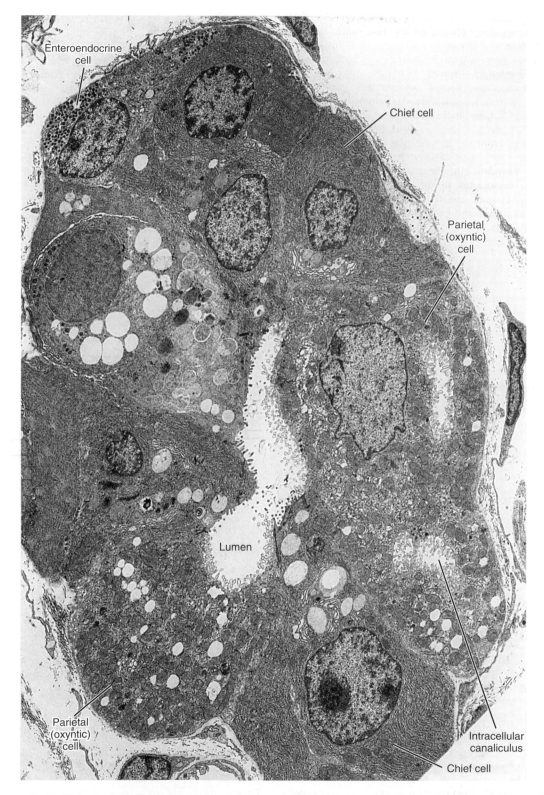

Figure 15–17. Electron micrograph of a section of gastric gland in the fundus of the stomach. Note the lumen and the parietal cells, containing abundant mitochondria; chief cells, with extensive rough endoplasmic reticulum; and enteroendocrine cells, with basal secretory granules. × 5300.

has few microvilli. When stimulated to produce hydrochloric acid, tubulovesicles fuse with the cell membrane to form more microvilli, thus providing a generous increase in the surface of the cell membrane (Figure 15–15, right).

Parietal cells secrete hydrochloric acid, 0.16 mol/L; potassium chloride, 0.07 mol/L; traces of other electrolytes; and gastric intrinsic factor (see below). A major secretion of parietal cells is H^+, which originates from the dissociation of the H_2CO_3 produced by the action of **carbonic anhydrase,** an enzyme abundant in these cells. Once produced, H_2CO_3 dissociates in the cytoplasm into H^+ and $H_2CO_3^-$ (Figure 15–16). The presence of abundant mitochondria in the parietal cells indicates that their metabolic processes, particularly the pumping of H^+, are highly energy consuming.

In cases of atrophic gastritis, both parietal and chief cells are much less numerous, and the gastric juice has little or no acid or pepsin activity. In humans, oxyntic cells are the site of production of **intrinsic factor,** a glycoprotein that binds avidly to vitamin B_{12}. In other species, however, the intrinsic factor may be produced by other cells.

The complex of vitamin B_{12} with intrinsic factor is absorbed by pinocytosis into the cells in the ileum—which explains why a lack of intrinsic factor can lead to vitamin B_{12} deficiency. This condition results in a disorder of the erythrocyte-forming mechanism known as **pernicious anemia;** it is usually caused by **atrophic gastritis.** In a certain percentage of cases, pernicious anemia seems to be an autoimmune disease, because antibodies against parietal cell proteins are often detected in the blood of patients with the disease.

The secretory activity of parietal cells is initiated by various mechanisms. One mechanism is through the cholinergic nerve endings. Histamine and a polypeptide called **gastrin,** both secreted in the gas-

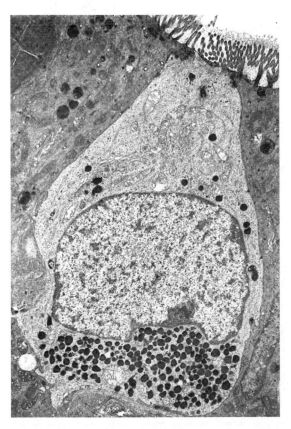

Figure 15–18. Electron micrograph of an enteroendocrine cell (open type) of the human duodenum. Note the microvilli in its apex. × 6900. (Courtesy of AGE Pearse.)

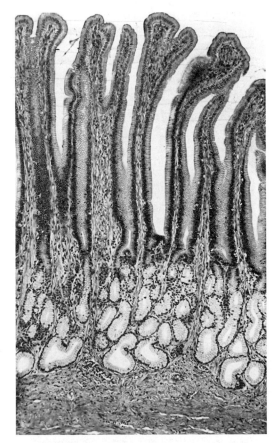

Figure 15–19. Photomicrograph of a section of the pyloric region of the stomach. Note the deep gastric pits with short pyloric glands in the lamina propria. H&E stain. × 40.

tric mucosa, act strongly to stimulate the production of hydrochloric acid.

D. Chief (Zymogenic) Cells: Chief cells predominate in the lower region of the tubular glands (Figure 15–17) and have all the characteristics of protein-synthesizing and -exporting cells. Their basophilia is due to the abundant rough endoplasmic reticulum (see Chapter 4). The granules in their cytoplasm contain the inactive enzyme **pepsinogen.** When inactive pepsinogen is released into the acid environment of the stomach, the proenzyme is converted into the highly active proteolytic enzyme **pepsin.** In humans, these cells also produce the enzyme **lipase.**

E. Enteroendocrine Cells: Enteroendocrine cells, discussed more extensively below, are found near the bases of gastric glands (Figures 15–17 and 15–18).

In the fundus of the stomach, **5-hydroxytryptamine** (serotonin) is one of the principal secretory products. Tumors called **carcinoids,** which arise from these cells, are responsible for the clinical symptoms caused by overproduction of serotonin.

Pylorus

The pylorus (from Latin, meaning a gatekeeper) has deep gastric pits into which the branched, tubular **pyloric glands** open. These glands are similar to the glands of the cardiac region. In the pyloric region, however, long pits and short coiled glands are found—the reverse of the situation in the cardiac region (Figure 15–19). These glands secrete mucus as well as appreciable amounts of the enzyme lysozyme. **Gastrin (G) cells** (which release **gastrin**) are intercalated among the mucous cells of pyloric glands. Gastrin stimulates the secretion of acid by the parietal cells of gastric glands. Other enteroendocrine cells (**D cells**) secrete **somatostatin,** which inhibits the release of some other hormones, including gastrin.

Other Layers of the Stomach

The **submucosa** is composed of dense connective tissue and blood and lymph vessels; it is infiltrated by lymphoid cells, macrophages, and mast cells. The **muscularis** is composed of smooth muscle fibers ori-

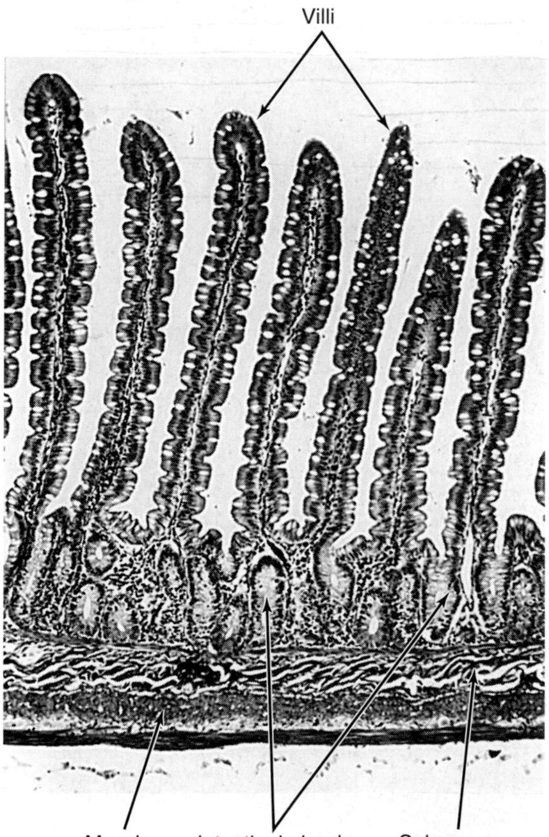

Figure 15–20. Photomicrograph of the small intestine. Note the villi, intestinal glands, submucosa, and muscle layers. H&E stain. × 40.

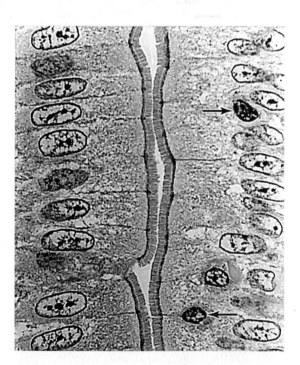

Figure 15–21. Photomicrograph of the epithelium covering the ileum. Note the numerous absorptive cells with their brush borders, the clearly visible intercellular limits, and the junctional complexes, seen at this magnification as dots between the apical portions of adjacent cells.

Mitochondria   Microvilli   Nucleus

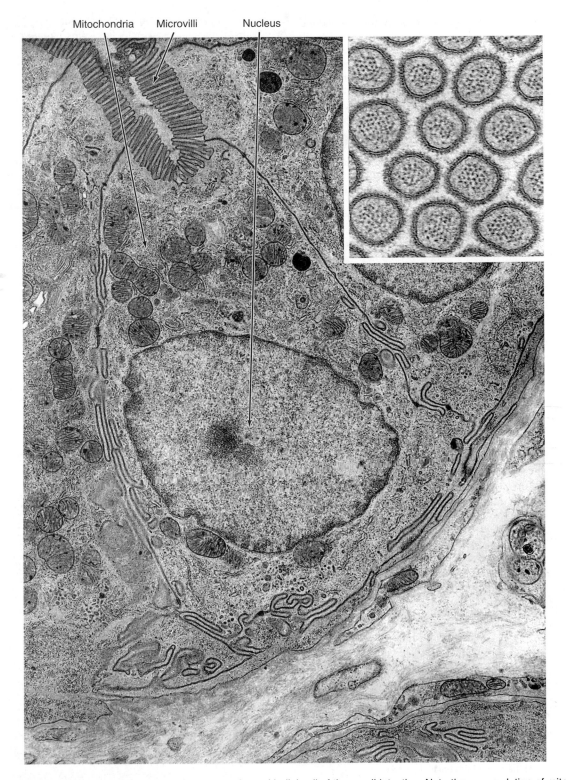

Figure 15–22. Electron micrograph of an absorptive epithelial cell of the small intestine. Note the accumulation of mitochondria in its apex. The luminal surface is covered with microvilli (shown in transverse section in the **inset**). Actin filaments, sectioned transversely, constitute the principal structural feature in the core of the microvilli. × 6300. (Courtesy of KR Porter.)

ented in three main directions. The external layer is longitudinal, the middle layer is circular, and the internal layer is oblique. At the pylorus, the middle layer is greatly thickened to form the **pyloric sphincter.** The **serosa** is thin and covered by mesothelium.

SMALL INTESTINE

The small intestine is the site of terminal food digestion, nutrient absorption, and endocrine secretion.

The processes of digestion are completed in the small intestine, and the products of digestion are absorbed. The small intestine is relatively long—approximately 5 m—permitting prolonged contact between food and digestive enzymes, as well as between the digested products and the absorptive cells of the epithelial lining. The small intestine consists of three segments: **duodenum, jejunum,** and **ileum,** which have many characteristics in common and will be discussed together.

Mucous Membrane

Viewed with the naked eye, the lining of the small intestine shows a series of permanent folds, **plicae circulares (Kerckring's valves),** consisting of mucosa and submucosa and having a semilunar, circular, or spiral form. The plicae are most developed in, and consequently a characteristic of, the jejunum. They do not constitute a significant feature of the duodenum and ileum, although they are frequently present. **Intestinal villi** are 0.5–1.5 mm long outgrowths of the mucosa (epithelium plus lamina propria) projecting into the lumen of the small intestine. In the duodenum they are leaf-shaped, gradually assuming finger-like shapes as they reach the ileum (Figures 15–20 and 15–24).

Between the villi are small openings of simple tubular glands called **intestinal glands** (also inappropriately called **crypts**), or **glands of Lieberkühn** (Figures 15–20 and 15–24).

The epithelium of the villi is continuous with that of the glands. The intestinal glands contain stem cells, some absorptive cells, goblet cells, Paneth's cells, and enteroendocrine cells.

Absorptive cells are tall columnar cells, each with an oval nucleus in the basal half of the cell. At the apex of each cell is a homogeneous layer called the **striated (brush) border** (Figure 15–21). When viewed with the electron microscope, the striated border is seen to be a layer of densely packed **microvilli** (Figures 15–22 and 15–23). Each microvillus is a cylindrical protrusion of the apical cytoplasm that is approximately 1 μm tall by 0.1 μm in diameter and consists of the cell membrane enclosing a core of actin microfilaments associated with other proteins (Figure 15–21). Each absorptive cell is estimated to have an average of 3000 microvilli, and 1 mm^2 of mucosa contains about 200 million of these structures. Microvilli have the important physiologic function of increasing the area of contact between the intestinal surface and food. Disaccharidases and peptidases bound to microvilli hydrolyze the disaccha-

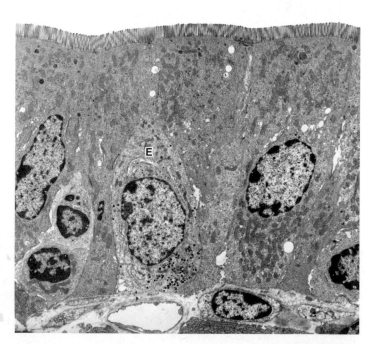

Figure 15–23. Electron micrograph of epithelium of the small intestine. Abundant microvilli at the cell apex can be seen to form the brush border. At the left are two lymphocytes migrating in the epithelium. In the center is an enteroendocrine cell (E) with its basal secretory granules. × 1850.

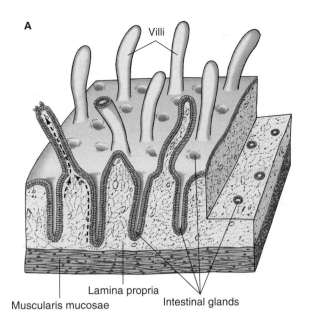

A

Villi

Lamina propria

Muscularis mucosae

Intestinal glands

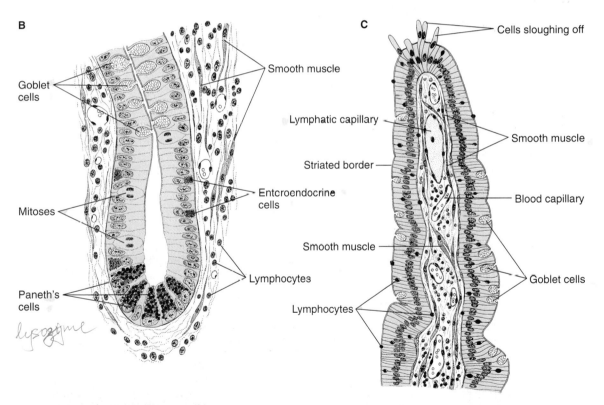

B

Goblet
cells

Smooth muscle

Entcroendocrine
cells

Mitoses

Lymphocytes

Paneth's
cells

lysozyme

C

Cells sloughing off

Lymphatic capillary

Smooth muscle

Striated border

Blood capillary

Smooth muscle

Goblet cells

Lymphocytes

Figure 15–24. Schematic diagrams illustrating the structure of the small intestine. **A:** The small intestine under low magnification. In the villus to the left, note the desquamation of epithelial cells. Because of constant mitotic activity of the cells from the closed end of the glands and the upward migration of these cells (dashed arrows), the intestinal epithelium is continuously renewed. Note the intestinal glands of Lieberkühn. **B:** The intestinal glands have a lining of intestinal epithelium and goblet cells (upper portion). At the lower level, the immature epithelial cells are frequently seen in mitosis; note also the presence of Paneth's and enteroendocrine cells. As the immature cells progress upward, they differentiate and develop microvilli, seen as a brush border in the electron microscope. (See Figure 15–23.) Cell proliferation and cell differentiation occur simultaneously in the closed end of these glands. **C:** A villus tip showing the columnar covering epithelium with its striated border and a moderate number of goblet cells. Blood capillaries, a lymphatic capillary, smooth muscle cells, and lymphocytes can be seen in the connective tissue core of the villus. Great numbers of lymphocytes are in the epithelial layer. Cells are sloughing off at the apex of the villus. (Redrawn and reproduced, with permission, from Ham AW: *Histology,* 6th ed. Lippincott, 1969.)

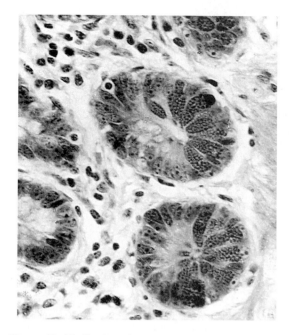

Figure 15–25. Section of the basal portion of the intestinal glands showing the Paneth's cells with their typical large secretory granules. × 600.

rides and dipeptides into monosaccharides and amino acids that are easily absorbed.

Deficiencies of these disaccharidases have been described in human diseases characterized by digestive disturbances. Some of the enzymatic deficiencies seem to be of genetic origin.

A more important function of the columnar intestinal cells is to absorb the nutrient molecules produced by the digestive process (discussed below).

Goblet cells are interspersed between the absorptive cells (Figures 15–21 and 15–24). They are less abundant in the duodenum and increase in number as they approach the ileum. These cells produce acid glycoproteins that are hydrated and form mucus, whose main function is to protect and lubricate the lining of the intestine.

Paneth's cells in the basal portion of the intestinal glands are exocrine cells with secretory granules in their apical cytoplasm. Researchers using immunocytochemical methods have detected lysozyme—an enzyme that digests the cell walls of some bacteria—in the large eosinophilic secretory granules of these cells (Figures 15–24 through 15–27). Lysozyme has

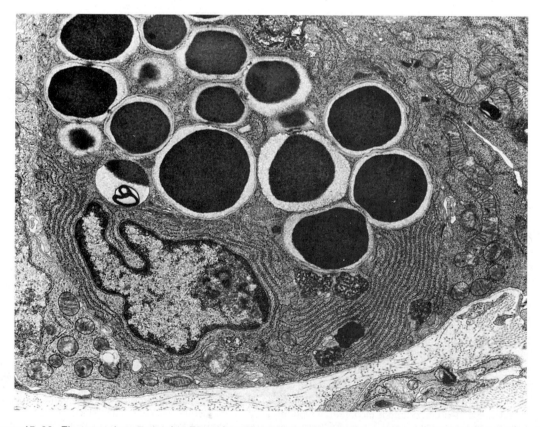

Figure 15–26. Electron micrograph of a Paneth's cell. Note the basal nucleus with prominent nucleolus, abundant rough endoplasmic reticulum, and large secretory granules with a protein core surrounded by a halo of polysaccharide-rich material. These granules contain lysozyme, a lytic enzyme involved in the regulation of intestinal bacteria. × 3000.

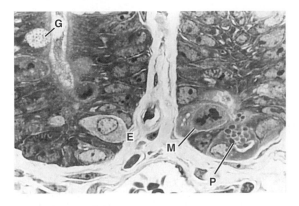

Figure 15–27. Photomicrograph of the basal portion of two glands (crypts) of the small intestine. Enteroendocrine cell (E), Paneth's cell (P), goblet cell (G), and a cell in mitosis (M) are seen.

antibacterial activity and may play a role in controlling the intestinal flora.

M (microfold) cells are specialized epithelial cells overlying the lymphoid follicles of Peyer's patches. These cells are characterized by the presence of numerous membrane invaginations that form pits containing many intraepithelial lymphocytes and antigen-presenting cells (macrophages). M cells can endocytose antigens and transport them to the underlying macrophages and lymphoid cells, which then migrate to other compartments of the lymphoid system (nodes), where immune responses to foreign antigens are initiated. M cells represent an important link in the intestinal immunologic system (Figures 15–28 and 15–30). The basement membrane under M cells is discontinuous, facilitating transit between the lamina propria and M cells (Figure 15–29).

The very large mucosal surface of the gastrointestinal tract is exposed to many potentially invasive microorganisms. Secretory immunoglobulins of the IgA class (discussed earlier) are the first line of defense. Another protective device is the intercellular tight junctions that make the epithelial cells a barrier to the penetration of microorganisms. In addition—

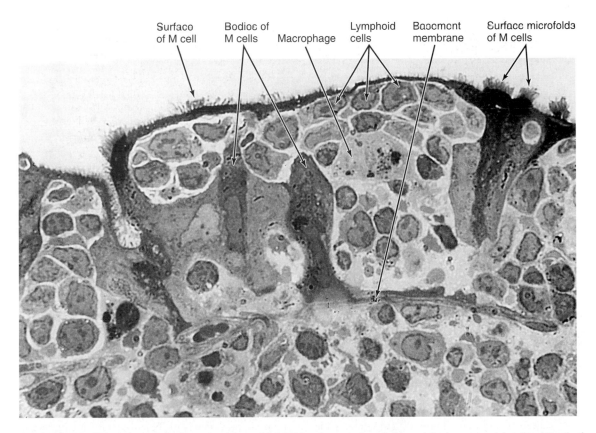

Figure 15–28. Photomicrograph from a region of intestine where a lymphoid nodule is covered by the intestinal mucosa. Note the presence of M cells that form a special compartment containing lymphoid cells. A macrophage (an antigen-presenting cell) is also in the compartment. (Courtesy of M Neutra.)

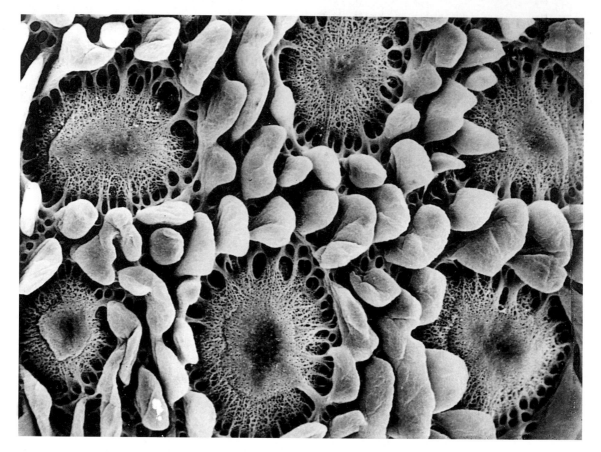

Figure 15–29. Scanning electron micrograph of the intestinal surface after removal of the mucosal epithelium, showing the basement membrane. Note that this layer is continuous when covering the remnants of the intestinal villi but assumes the structure of a sieve when covering the lymphoid follicles above Peyer's patches. This configuration permits an easier means for immunogenic materials to reach underlying lymphoid tissues. (Courtesy of S McClugage.)

and probably serving as the main protective barrier— the gastrointestinal tract contains antibody-secreting plasma cells, macrophages, and a very large number of lymphocytes (Figure 15–30), located in both the mucosa and the submucosa. Together, these cells are called the gut-associated lymphatic tissue (GALT).

Endocrine Cells of the Gastrointestinal Tract

In addition to the cells discussed above, the gastrointestinal tract contains some widely distributed cells with characteristics of the **diffuse neuroendocrine system** (see Chapter 4). The main results obtained so far are summarized in Figure 15–31 and Table 15–1. Figure 15–31 shows that the distribution of these cells in the digestive tract is not uniform.

Polypeptide-secreting cells of the digestive tract fall into two classes: the **open type,** in which the apex of the cell presents microvilli and contacts the lumen of the organ (Figure 15–18); and the **closed type,** in which the cellular apex is covered by other epithelial cells (Figure 15–17). It has been suggested that in the open type, the chemical contents of the digestive tract might act on its microvilli and thereby influence secretion of these cells. Although the picture of gastrointestinal endocrinology is still incomplete, the activity of the digestive system is clearly controlled by the nervous system and modulated by a complex system of locally produced peptide hormones.

Lamina Propria Through Serosa

The lamina propria of the small intestine is composed of loose connective tissue with blood and lymph vessels, nerve fibers, and smooth muscle cells.

The lamina propria penetrates the core of the intestinal villi, taking along blood and lymph vessels, nerves, connective tissue, and smooth muscle cells. The smooth muscle cells are responsible for the rhythmic movements of the villi, which are important for absorption (see Figure 15–24).

The muscularis mucosae does not present any pe-

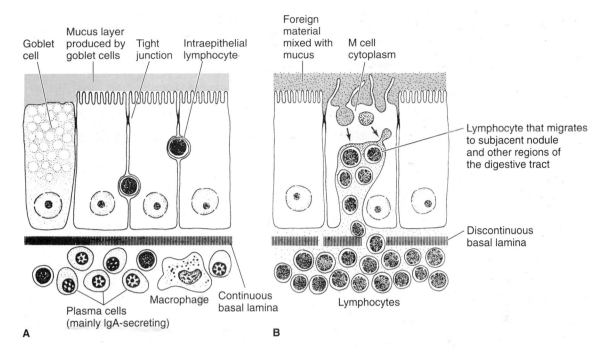

Figure 15–30. Some aspects of immunologic protection of the intestine. **A:** A condition that is more frequent in the upper tract, such as in the jejunum. There are many IgA-secreting plasma cells, scattered lymphocytes, and some macrophages. Note the lymphocytes in the lining epithelium but located outside the epithelial cells, and below the tight junctions. **B:** A condition that is more frequent in the ileum, where aggregates of lymphocytes are located under M cells. The M cells transfer foreign material (microorganisms and macromolecules) to lymphocytes located deep in the cavities of the M cells. Lymphocytes spread the information received from this foreign material to other regions of the digestive tract, and probably to other organs, through blood and lymph.

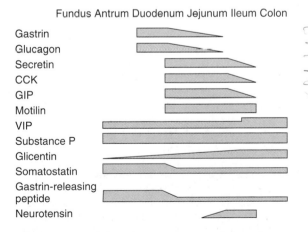

Figure 15–31. Distribution of gastrointestinal peptides along the gastrointestinal tract. The thickness of each bar is proportionate to the concentration of the peptide in the mucosa. CCK, cholecystokinin; GIP, gastric inhibitory polypeptide; VIP, vasoactive intestinal polypeptide. (Reproduced, with permission, from Ganong WF: *Review of Medical Physiology,* 15th ed. Appleton & Lange, 1991.)

culiarities in this organ. The **submucosa** contains, in the initial portion of the duodenum, clusters of ramified, coiled tubular glands that open into the intestinal glands. These are the **duodenal** (or **Brunner's**) **glands** (Figure 15–32). Their cells are of the mucous type. The product of secretion of the glands is distinctly alkaline (pH 8.1–9.3). It acts to protect the duodenal mucous membrane against the effects of the acid gastric juice and to bring the intestinal contents to the optimum pH for pancreatic enzyme action.

The lamina propria and the submucosa of the small intestine contain aggregates of lymphoid nodules known as **Peyer's patches,** an important component of the GALT. Each patch consists of 10–200 nodules and is visible to the naked eye as an oval area on the antimesenteric side of the intestine. There are about 30 patches in the human, most of them in the ileum. When viewed from the luminal surface, each Peyer's patch appears as a dome-shaped area devoid of villi. Instead of absorptive cells, its covering epithelium consists of **M cells.**

Table 15–1. Principal enteroendocrine cells in the gastrointestinal tract.

Cell Type and Location	Hormone Produced	Major Action
A–stomach	Glucagon	Hepatic glycogenolysis
G–pylorus	Gastrin	Stimulation of gastric acid secretion
S–small intestine	Secretin	Pancreatic and biliary bicarbonate and water secretion
K–small intestine	Gastric inhibitory polypeptide	Inhibition of gastric acid secretion
L–small intestine	Glucagon-like substance (glicentin)	Hepatic glycogenolysis
I–small intestine	Cholecystokinin	Pancreatic enzyme secretion, gallbladder contraction
D–pylorus, duodenum	Somatostatin	Local inhibition of other endocrine cells
Mo–small intestine	Motilin	Increased gut motility
EC–digestive tract	Serotonin, substance P	Increased gut motility
D_1–digestive tract	Vasoactive intestinal polypeptide	Ion and water secretion, increased gut motility

Vessels & Nerves

The blood vessels that nourish the intestine and remove absorbed products of digestion penetrate the muscularis and form a large plexus in the submucosa (Figure 15–33). From the submucosa, branches extend through the muscularis mucosae and lamina propria and into the villi. Each villus receives, according to its size, one or more branches that form a capillary network just below its epithelium. At the tips of the villi, one or more venules arise from these capillaries and run in the opposite direction, reaching the veins of the submucosal plexus. The lymph vessels of the intestine begin as closed tubes in the core of the villi. These capillaries, despite being larger than the blood capillaries, are difficult to observe because their walls are so close together that they appear to be collapsed. These vessels (**lacteals**) run to the region of lamina propria above the muscularis mucosae, where they form a plexus. From there they are directed to the submucosa, where they surround lymphoid nodules. Lacteals anastomose repeatedly and leave the intestine along with the blood vessels.

The innervation of the intestines is formed by both an **intrinsic component** and an **extrinsic component.** The intrinsic component comprises groups of neurons that form the myenteric (Auerbach's) nerve plexus (Figure 15–34) between the outer longitudinal and inner circular layers of the muscularis and the **submucosal (Meissner's) plexus** in the submucosa. The plexuses contain some sensory neurons that receive information from nerve endings near the epithelial layer and in the smooth muscle layer regarding the composition of the intestinal content (chemoreceptors) and the degree of expansion of the intestinal wall (mechanoreceptors). The other nerve cells are effectors and innervate the muscle layers

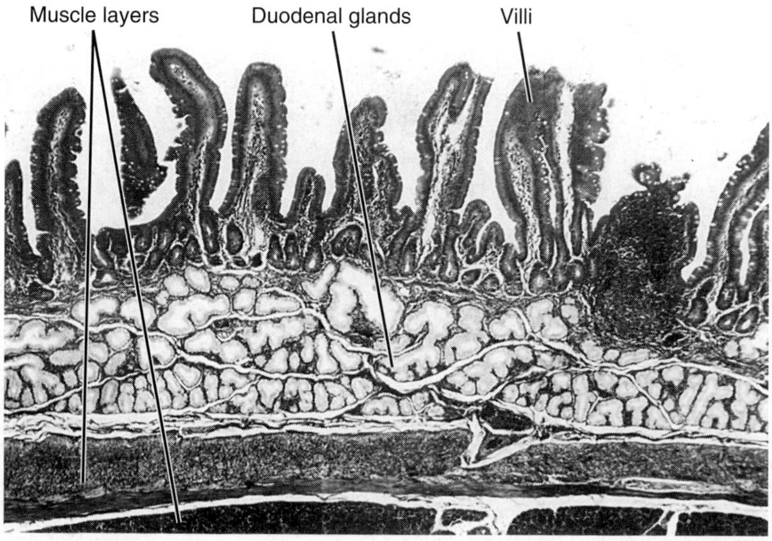

Figure 15–32. Photomicrograph of the duodenum, showing villi and duodenal glands in the submucosa. The dark structure at the right is a lymphoid nodule; at the bottom are two smooth muscle layers of the muscularis. H&E stain. × 30.

Muscle layers   Duodenal glands   Villi

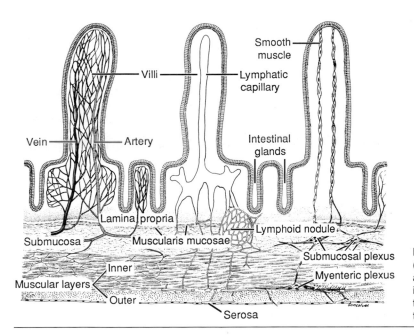

Figure 15–33. Blood circulation (left), lymphatic circulation (center), and innervation (right) of the small intestine. The smooth muscle system for contracting the villi is illustrated in the villus on the right.

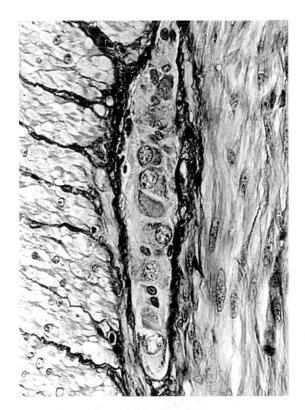

Figure 15–34. Photomicrograph of a group of neurons (with large nuclei) and satellite cells (with small nuclei) constituting a component of the myenteric plexus between two smooth muscle layers. Note the dark-stained collagen fibers.

and hormone-secreting cells. The intrinsic innervation formed by these plexuses is responsible for the intestinal contractions that occur in the total absence of the extrinsic innervation. The extrinsic innervation is formed by parasympathetic cholinergic nerve fibers that stimulate the activity of the intestinal smooth muscle and by sympathetic adrenergic nerve fibers that depress intestinal smooth muscle activity.

Histophysiology

The presence of plicae, villi, and microvilli greatly increases the surface of the intestinal lining—an important characteristic in an organ in which absorption occurs so intensely. It has been calculated that plicae increase the intestinal surface 3-fold, the villi increase it 10-fold, and the microvilli increase it 20-fold. Together, these processes are responsible for a 600-fold increase in the intestinal surface, resulting in a total area of 200 m².

When the digestive process is completed, its products are absorbed in the small intestine. Lipid digestion occurs mainly as a result of the action of pancreatic lipase and bile. In humans, most of the lipid absorption takes place in the duodenum and upper jejunum. Figures 15–35 and 15–36 illustrate current concepts of this process of absorption.

The amino acids and monosaccharides derived from the digestion of proteins and carbohydrates are absorbed by the epithelial cells through active transport.

The absorption of nutrients is greatly hindered in disorders marked by atrophy of the intestinal

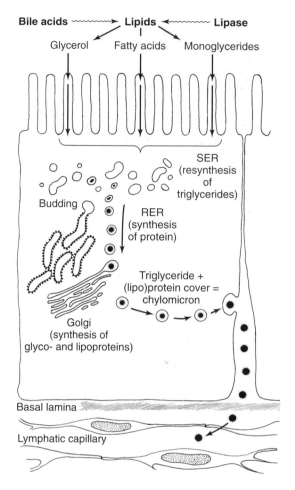

Figure 15–35. Lipid absorption in the small intestine. Lipase promotes the hydrolysis of lipids to monoglycerides and fatty acids in the intestinal lumen. These compounds are stabilized in an emulsion by the action of bile acids. The products of hydrolysis cross the microvilli membranes passively and are collected in the cisternae of the smooth endoplasmic reticulum (SER), where they are resynthesized to triglycerides. These triglycerides are surrounded by a thin layer of proteins that form particles called chylomicrons (0.2–1 μm in diameter). Chylomicrons are transferred to the Golgi complex and then migrate to the lateral membrane, cross it by a process of membrane fusion (exocytosis), and flow into the extracellular space in the direction of the blood and lymphatic vessels. Most chylomicrons go to the lymph; a few go to the blood vessels. The long-chain lipids (>C12) go mainly to the lymphatic vessels. Fatty acids of fewer than 10–12 carbon atoms are not re-esterified to triglycerides - but leave the cell directly and enter the blood vessels. RER, rough endoplasmic reticulum. (Based on results of Friedman HI, Cardell RR Jr: Anat Rec 1977;188:77.)

mucosa caused by infections or nutritional deficiencies, producing the **malabsorption syndrome.**

Another process important for intestinal function is the rhythmic movement of the villi. This movement is the result of the contraction of smooth muscle cells running vertically between the muscularis mucosae and the tip of the villi (see villus at right in Figure 15–33). These contractions occur at the rate of several strokes per minute and have a pumping action on the villi that propel the lymph to the mesenteric lymphatics. The surface area of the villi is increased by the microvilli, which have a cytoskeleton containing many actin microfilaments that are associated with other proteins with a supporting function (Figure 15–37).

LARGE INTESTINE

The large intestine consists of a mucosal membrane with no folds except in its distal (rectal) portion. No villi are present in this portion of the intestine (Figure 15–38). The intestinal glands are long and characterized by a great abundance of goblet and absorptive cells and a small number of enteroendocrine cells (Figure 15–39). The absorptive cells are columnar and have short, irregular microvilli (Figure 15–40). The large intestine is well suited to its main functions: absorption of water, formation of the fecal mass, and production of mucus. Mucus is a highly hydrated gel that not only lubricates the intestinal surface but also covers bacteria and particulate matter. The absorption of water is passive, following the active transport of sodium out of the basal surfaces of the epithelial cells (Figure 15–40).

The lamina propria is rich in lymphoid cells and in nodules that frequently extend into the submucosa. This richness in lymphoid tissue (GALT) is related to the abundant bacterial population of the large intestine. The muscularis comprises longitudinal and circular strands. This layer differs from that of the small intestine, because fibers of the outer longitudinal layer congregate in three thick longitudinal bands called **teniae coli.** In the intraperitoneal portions of the colon, the serous layer is characterized by small, pendulous protuberances composed of adipose tissue—the **appendices epiploicae** (Figure 15–41).

In the anal region, the mucous membrane forms a series of longitudinal folds, the **rectal columns of Morgagni.** About 2 cm above the anal opening, the intestinal mucosa is replaced by stratified squamous epithelium. In this region, the lamina propria contains a plexus of large veins that, when excessively dilated and varicose, produce hemorrhoids.

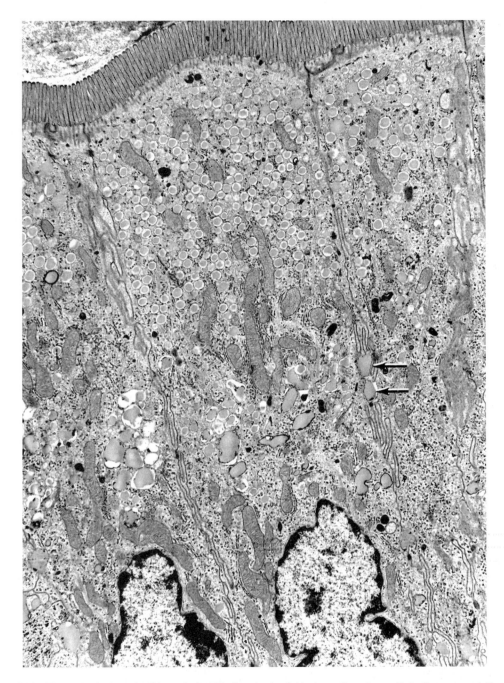

Figure 15–36. Electron micrograph of intestinal epithelium in the lipid-absorption phase. Note the accumulation of lipid droplets in vesicles of the smooth endoplasmic reticulum. (Compare with Figure 15–22.) These vesicles fuse near the nucleus, forming larger lipid droplets that migrate laterally and cross the cell membrane to the extracellular space (arrows). × 5000. (Courtesy of HI Friedman.)

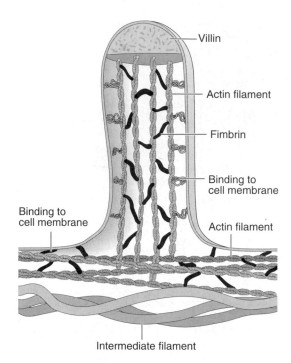

Figure 15–37. Structure of a microvillus. A cytoskeleton of actin filaments, associated with other proteins, keeps the shape of the microvillus. The actin filaments are continuous with the microfilaments of the terminal web (see Chapter 4), which also contains intermediate filaments. Note that in this location actin filaments have a structural role and are not related to movement, as is usually the case when these microfilaments are present. To fulfill its supportive role, actin is associated with other proteins that link the microfilaments to one another and to the cell membrane.

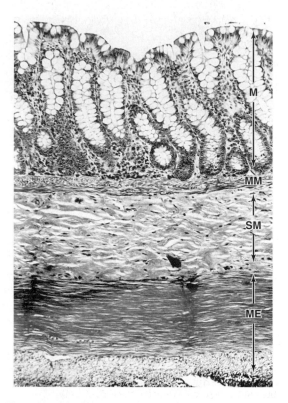

Figure 15–38. Photomicrograph of a section of large intestine with its various layers. Note the absence of villi. M, mucosa; MM, muscularis mucosae; SM, submucosa; ME, muscularis externa. H&E stain. × 30.

Cell Renewal
in the Gastrointestinal Tract

The epithelial cells of the entire gastrointestinal tract are constantly being cast off and replaced with new ones formed through mitosis of stem cells. These stem cells are located in the basal layer of the esophageal epithelium, the neck of gastric glands, the lower half of the intestinal glands (Figure 15–42), and the bottom third of the crypts of the large intestine. From this proliferative zone in each region, cells move to the maturation area, where they undergo structural and enzymatic maturation, providing the functional cell population of each region. In the small intestine the cells die by apoptosis (see Chapter 3) in the tip of the villi.

The high rate of cell renewal explains why the intestine is affected promptly by the administration of antimitotic drugs, as in cancer chemotherapy. The epithelial cells continue to be lost at the tips of the villi, but the drugs inhibit cell proliferation. This inhibition promotes atrophy of the epithelium, which results in defective absorption of nutrients, excessive fluid loss, and diarrhea. Paneth's cells of the intestinal glands have a much slower turnover rate, living about 30 days before being replaced.

APPENDIX

The appendix is an evagination of the cecum; it is characterized by a relatively small, narrow, and irregular lumen that is caused by the presence of abundant lymphoid follicles in its wall. Although its general structure is similar to that of the large intestine, it contains fewer and shorter intestinal glands and has no teniae coli (Figure 15–43).

Because the appendix is closed-ended, its contents are not renewed rapidly, and it frequently becomes a site of inflammation (**appendicitis**). The inflammation can progress to the point of destruction of this structure, with consequent infection of the peritoneal cavity.

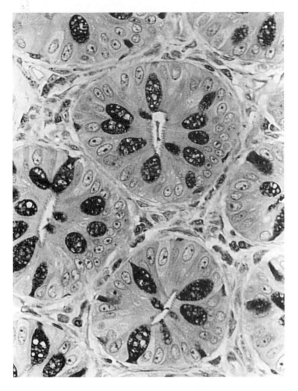

Figure 15–39. Photomicrograph of a section of large intestine. Note the intestinal glands in cross section, with abundant goblet cells. Periodic acid–Schiff stain.

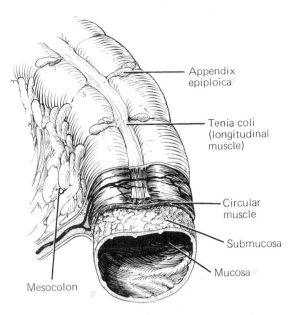

Figure 15–41. Cross section of colon. (Reproduced, with permission, from Way LW [editor]: *Current Surgical Diagnosis & Treatment,* 8th ed. Appleton & Lange, 1988.)

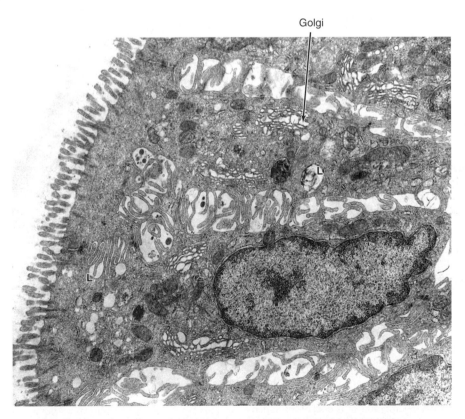

Figure 15–40. Electron micrograph of epithelial cells of the large intestine. Note the microvilli at the luminal surface, the well-developed Golgi complex, and dilated intercellular spaces filled by interdigitating membrane leaflets, a sign of active water transport. × 3900.

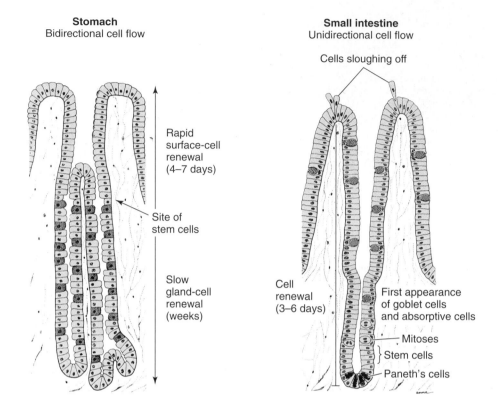

Figure 15–42. Regeneration of the epithelial lining of the stomach and small intestine. Note differences in the location of stem cells.

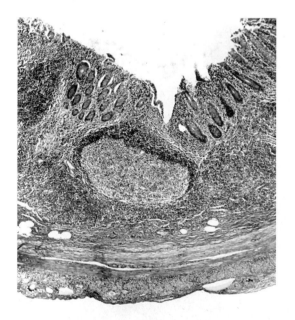

Figure 15–43. Photomicrograph of a section of appendix, with a few glands and numerous lymphoid nodules. H&E stain. × 20.

Cancer of the Digestive Tract

Approximately 90–95% of malignant tumors of the digestive system are derived from intestinal or gastric epithelial cells. Malignant tumors of the large bowel are derived almost exclusively from its glandular epithelium (**adenocarcinomas**) and are the second most common cause of cancer deaths in the United States.

REFERENCES

Cheng H, Leblond CP: Origin, differentiation and renewal of the four main epithelial cell types in the mouse small intestine. 5. Unitarian theory of the origin of the four epithelial cell types. Am J Anat 1974;141:537.

Forte JG: Mechanism of gastric H^+ and Cl^- transport. Annu Rev Physiol 1980;42:111.

Friedman HL, Cardell RR Jr: Alterations in the endoplasmic reticulum and Golgi complex of intestinal epithelial cells during fat absorption and after termination of this process: a morphological and morphometric study. Anat Rec 1977;188:77.

Gabella G: Innervation of the gastrointestinal tract. Int Rev Cytol 1979;59:130.

Grube D: The endocrine cells of the digestive system: amines, peptides and modes of action. Anat Embryol (Berl) 1986;175:151.

Hoedemseker PJ et al: Further investigations about the site of production of Castles gastric intrinsic factor. Lab Invest 1966;15:1163.

Ito S: Functional gastric morphology. In: *Physiology of the Gastrointestinal Tract.* Vol 1. Johnson LR (editor). Raven Press, 1981.

Jankowski A et al: Maintenance of normal intestinal mucosae: function, structure and adaptation. Gut 1994;35: S1.

Klockars M, Reitamo S: Tissue distribution of lysozyme in man. J Histochem Cytochem 1975;23:932.

McClugage SG et al: Porosity of the basement membrane overlying Peyer's patches in rats and monkeys. Gastroenterology 1986;91:1128.

Moog F: The lining of the small intestine. Sci Am 1981; 245:154.

Mooseker MS, Tilney LG: Organization of an actin filament-membrane complex: Filament polarity and membrane attachment in the microvilli of intestinal epithelial cells. J Cell Biol 1975;67:725.

Owen D: Normal histology of the stomach. Am J Surg Pathol 1986;10:48.

Pabst R: The anatomical basis for the immune function of the gut. Anat Embryol (Berl) 1986;176:135.

Pfeiffer CJ et al: *Gastrointestinal Ultrastructure.* Academic Press, 1974.

Glands Associated with the Digestive Tract

The glands associated with the digestive tract include the salivary glands, the pancreas, the liver, and the bile-depot gallbladder. The functions of the salivary glands are to wet and lubricate the oral cavity and its contents, to initiate the digestion of carbohydrates, and to secrete such protective substances as the immunoglobulin IgA, lysozyme, and lactoferrin. The main functions of the pancreas are to produce digestive enzymes that act in the small intestine and to secrete the hormones insulin and glucagon into the bloodstream. The liver produces bile, an important fluid in the digestion of fats. The liver plays a major role in lipid, carbohydrate, and protein metabolism and inactivates and metabolizes many toxic substances and drugs. It also participates in iron metabolism and the synthesis of blood proteins and the factors necessary for blood coagulation. The gallbladder absorbs water from the bile and stores the bile in a concentrated form.

SALIVARY GLANDS

Exocrine glands in the mouth produce saliva, which has digestive, lubricating, and immunologic functions. In addition to the small glands scattered throughout the oral cavity (described in Chapter 15), there are three pairs of large salivary glands: the **parotid, submandibular (submaxillary)**, and **sublingual glands.** These glands consist of two general types of secretory cells—serous and mucous (Figure 16–1)—and a duct system.

Serous cells are usually pyramidal in shape, with a broad base resting on the basal lamina and a narrow apical surface with short, irregular microvilli facing the lumen (Figures 16–2 and 16–3). They exhibit characteristics of polarized protein-secreting cells (Figures 4–20 and 4–25). Adjacent secretory cells are joined together by junctional complexes consisting of zonulae occludentes (tight junctions), zonulae adherentes (adhering junctions), desmosomes, and gap junctions. Serous cells usually form a spherical mass of cells called an **acinus (alveolus)** with a lumen in the center.

This structure can be likened to a grape attached to its stem; the stem corresponds to the duct system.

Mucous cells are usually cuboidal to columnar in shape; their nuclei are oval and pressed toward the bases of the cells. They exhibit the characteristics of mucus-secreting cells (Figures 4–23, 4–25, 16–3, and 16–4). Mucous cells are most often organized as **tubules,** consisting of cylindrical arrays of secretory cells surrounding a lumen.

In the human **submandibular gland,** serous and mucous cells are arranged in a characteristic pattern. The mucous cells form tubules, but their ends are capped by serous cells, which constitute the **serous demilunes** (Figures 16–1 and 16–4).

Myoepithelial cells, described in Chapter 4, are found within the basal lamina of glandular and ductal epithelia of salivary glands. Myoepithelial cells surrounding serous acini are highly branched cells (sometimes called **basket cells**); those associated with mucous tubules and intercalated ducts are spindle-shaped and lie parallel to the length of the duct.

In the **duct system,** secretory end-pieces empty into **intercalated ducts** lined by cuboidal epithelial cells. Several of these ducts join to form an **intralobular duct,** the **striated duct** (Figure 16–1).

Striated ducts are characterized by radial striations that extend from the bases of the cells to the level of the nuclei. When viewed in the electron microscope, the striations are seen to consist of infoldings of the basal plasma membrane with numerous elongated mitochondria that are aligned parallel to the infolded membranes; this structure is characteristic of ion-transporting cells (Figure 4–18; see Chapter 4).

The striated ducts of each lobule converge and drain into ducts in the connective tissue septae separating the lobules, where they become **interlobular,** or **excretory, ducts.** They are initially lined with stratified cuboidal epithelium, but more distal parts of the excretory ducts are lined with stratified columnar epithelium. The main duct of each major salivary gland ultimately empties into the oral cavity and is lined with nonkeratinized stratified squamous epithelium.

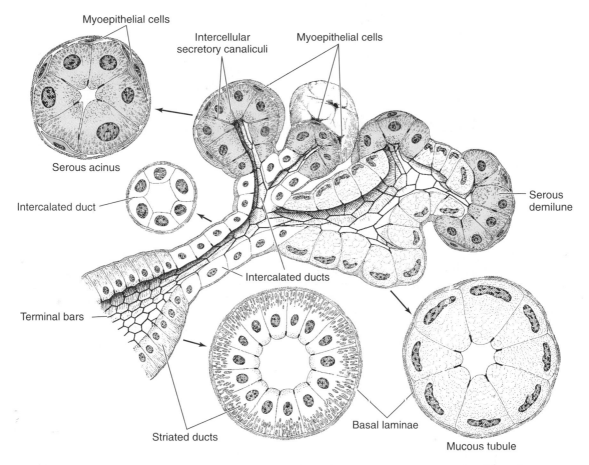

Figure 16–1. The structure of the submandibular (submaxillary) gland. The secretory portions are composed of pyramidal serous (lighter color) and mucous (stippled) cells. The nuclei of serous cells are euchromatic and rounded, and an accumulation of rough endoplasmic reticulum is evident in the basal third of the cell. The apex of the cell is filled with protein-rich secretory granules. The nuclei of mucous cells, flattened with condensed chromatin, are located near the bases of the cells. Mucous cells have little rough endoplasmic reticulum and contain distinct secretory granules. The short intercalated ducts are lined with cuboidal epithelium. The striated ducts are composed of columnar cells with characteristics of ion-transporting cells (see Chapter 4) such as basal membrane invaginations and mitochondrial accumulation. Myoepithelial cells are shown in a darker color.

The large salivary glands are surrounded by a capsule of connective tissue, rich in collagen fibers. From this capsule, septa of connective tissue penetrate the gland, dividing it into lobules. Vessels and nerves enter the gland at the hilum and gradually branch into the lobules. A rich vascular and nerve plexus surrounds the secretory and ductal components of each lobule.

Parotid Gland

The parotid gland is a branched acinar gland; its secretory portion is composed almost exclusively of serous cells (Figure 16–2). In humans, in addition to having the characteristics of serous cells, the secretory granules of these cells exhibit a positive periodic acid–Schiff (PAS) reaction that indicates the presence of polysaccharides. The secretory granules are rich in proteins and have a high amylase activity. The encapsulating connective tissue contains many plasma cells and lymphocytes. The plasma cells secrete IgA (Figure 15–2), which forms a complex with a **secretory component** synthesized by the serous acinar, intercalated duct, and striated duct cells. The IgA-rich secretory complex released into the saliva is resistant to enzymatic digestion and constitutes an immunologic defense mechanism against pathogens in the oral cavity.

Submandibular (Submaxillary) Gland

The submandibular gland is a branched tubuloacinar gland (Figures 16–3 and 16–4); its secretory portion contains both mucous and serous cells. The serous cells contain protein secretory granules that

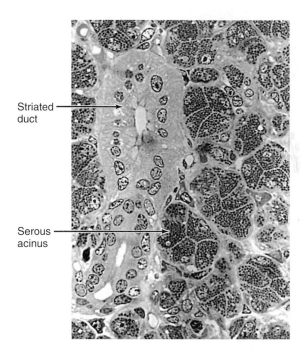

Striated duct

Serous acinus

Figure 16–2. Photomicrograph of a parotid gland. Its secretory portion consists of serous amylase-producing cells that store this enzyme in secretory granules.

are PAS-positive because of the presence of carbohydrate moieties. Serous cells are the main component of this gland and are easily distinguished from mucous cells by their rounded nuclei and basophilic cytoplasm. The presence of extensive lateral and basal membrane infoldings toward the vascular bed increases the ion-transporting surface area 60 times, facilitating electrolyte and water transport. Because of these folds, the cell boundaries are indistinct. Serous cells are responsible for the weak amylolytic activity present in this gland and its saliva. The cells that form the demilunes in the submandibular gland secrete the enzyme **lysozyme,** whose main activity is to hydrolyze the walls of certain bacteria.

Sublingual Gland

The sublingual gland, like the submandibular gland, is a branched tubuloacinar gland formed of serous and mucous cells, although it contains no acini formed exclusively of serous cells. Mucous cells predominate in this gland; serous cells are present only on demilunes of mucous acini (Figure 16–5). As in the submandibular gland, cells that form the demilunes in this gland secrete lysozyme.

Histophysiology

The moistening and lubricating functions of the salivary glands are performed by the water and gly-

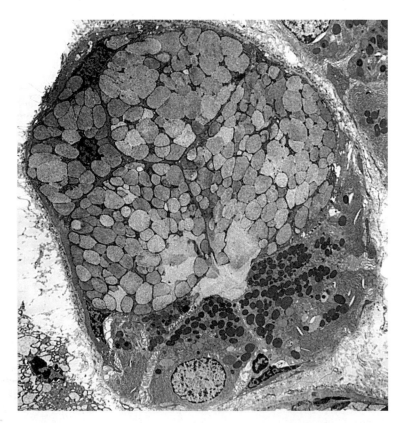

Figure 16–3. Electron micrograph of a mixed acinus from a human submandibular gland. Note the difference between the serous (lower part) and mucous (upper part) secretory granules. × 2500. (Courtesy of JD Harrison.)

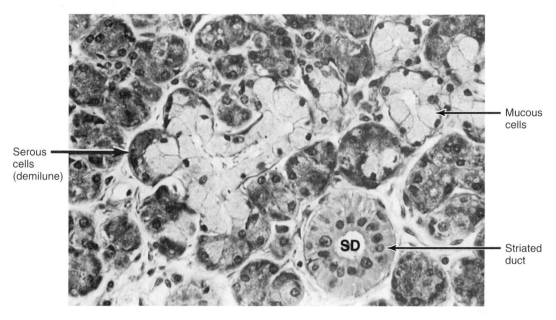

Figure 16–4. Photomicrograph of a section of human submandibular gland. Note the presence of dense serous cells forming acini and demilunes. The pale-staining mucous cells are grouped along the tubular portion of this tubuloacinar gland. In the lower right region is a striated duct demilune (SD) where serous cells are eccentrically displaced, assuming the form of a crescent. H&E stain. × 360.

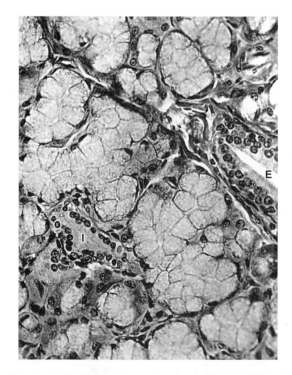

Figure 16–5. Photomicrograph of a human sublingual gland showing the predominance of mucous cells. An intralobular duct (I) and an interlobular (excretory) duct sheathed with connective tissue (E) duct are also present. H&E stain. × 600.

coproteins of saliva. Glycoproteins are synthesized mainly by the mucous cells and to a lesser degree by the serous cells of the glands. These fluids also provide solvents for substances that stimulate the taste buds. Human saliva consists of secretions from the parotid glands (25%), the submandibular glands (70%), and the sublingual glands (5%).

Another function of these glands is the digestion of carbohydrates. Most of the hydrolysis of ingested carbohydrates is the result of salivary amylase activity. This digestion, which begins in the mouth, also takes place in the stomach before the gastric juice acidifies the food and thus decreases amylase activity considerably.

In addition to synthesizing the secretory component necessary for the transport of secretory IgA from the connective tissues, across the acinar and duct cells, and into the saliva, acinar and intercalated duct cells also secrete lactoferrin and lysozyme. Lactoferrin binds iron, a nutrient necessary for bacterial growth, and lysozyme hydrolyzes the cell walls of certain bacteria. Thus, saliva is important in defending the oral cavity against pathogens.

Parasympathetic stimulation of the salivary glands, usually through the smell or taste of food, provokes a copious watery secretion with relatively little organic content. Sympathetic nerve stimulation produces small amounts of viscous saliva, rich in organic material.

PANCREAS

The pancreas is a mixed exocrine-endocrine gland that produces digestive enzymes and hormones. The enzymes are stored and released by cells of the exocrine portion. The hormones are synthesized in clusters of cells of the endocrine tissue known as *islets of Langerhans* (see Chapter 21). The exocrine portion of the pancreas is a compound acinar gland (Figure 16–6), similar in structure to the parotid gland. In histologic sections, a distinction between the two glands can be made based on the absence of striated ducts and the presence of the islets of Langerhans in the pancreas. Another characteristic detail is that the initial portions of intercalated ducts penetrate the lumens of the acini. Nuclei, surrounded by a pale cytoplasm, belong to **centroacinar cells** that constitute the intra-acinar portion of the intercalated duct (Figures 16–7 and 16–8). These cells are found only in pancreatic acini. Intercalated ducts are tributaries of larger interlobular ducts lined by columnar epithelium. There are no striated ducts in the pancreatic duct system.

The exocrine pancreatic acinus is composed of several serous cells surrounding a lumen (Figures 16–9 and 16–10). These cells are highly polarized, with a spherical nucleus, and are typical protein-secreting cells. The number of zymogen granules pre-

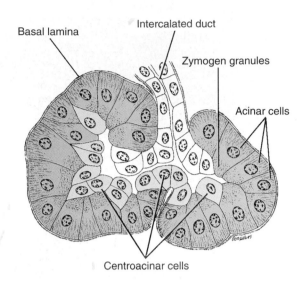

Figure 16–7. Schematic drawing of the structure of pancreatic acini. Acinar cells (darker color) are pyramidal, with granules at their apex and rough endoplasmic reticulum at their base. The intercalated duct partly penetrates the acini. These duct cells are known as centroacinar cells (lighter color). Note the absence of myoepithelial cells.

sent in each cell varies according to the digestive phase and attains its maximum in animals that have fasted.

The pancreas is covered by a thin capsule of connective tissue that sends septa into it, separating the pancreatic lobules. The acini are surrounded by a basal lamina that is supported by a delicate sheath of reticular fibers. The pancreas has a rich capillary network.

In addition to water and ions, the human exocrine pancreas secretes the following digestive enzymes and proenzymes: **trypsinogen, chymotrypsinogen, carboxypeptidase, ribonuclease, deoxyribonuclease, triacylglycerol lipase, phospholipase A$_2$, elastase,** and **amylase.**

Pancreatic secretion is controlled mainly through two hormones—**secretin** and **cholecystokinin** (previously called **pancreozymin**)—that are produced by enteroendocrine cells of the duodenal mucosa. Stimulation of the vagus nerve will also produce pancreatic secretion.

Secretin promotes secretion of an abundant fluid, poor in enzyme activity and rich in bicarbonate. It is probably secreted by the duct cells, not by the acinar cells. This secretion serves to neutralize the acidic **chyme** (partially digested food) so that pancreatic enzymes can function at their optimal neutral pH range. Cholecystokinin promotes secretion of a less abundant but enzyme-rich fluid. This hormone acts mainly in the extrusion of zymogen granules. The in-

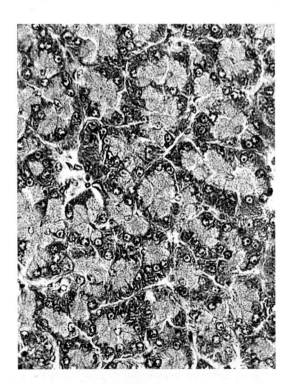

Figure 16–6. Photomicrograph of the acinar portion of the pancreas with its secretory cells. H&E stain. × 400.

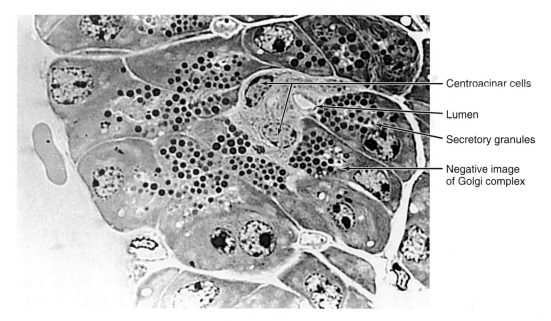

Centroacinar cells

Lumen

Secretory granules

Negative image
of Golgi complex

Figure 16–8. Photomicrograph of a pancreatic acinus showing secretory granules at the cell apex and two centroacinar cells at the margin of a small lumen.

tegrated action of both these hormones provides for a heavy secretion of enzyme-rich pancreatic juice.

> In conditions of extreme malnutrition such as **kwashiorkor,** pancreatic acinar cells and other active protein-secreting cells atrophy and lose much of their rough endoplasmic reticulum. The production of digestive enzymes is also hindered.

LIVER

The liver is the organ in which nutrients absorbed in the digestive tract are processed and stored for use by other parts of the body. It is thus an interface between the digestive system and the blood.

The liver is the second-largest organ of the body (the largest is the skin) and the largest gland, weighing about 1.5 kg. It is situated in the abdominal cavity beneath the diaphragm. Most of its blood (70–80%) comes from the portal vein; the smaller percentage is supplied by the hepatic artery. All the materials absorbed via the intestines reach the liver through the portal vein, except the complex lipids (**chylomicrons**), which are transported mainly by lymph vessels. The position of the liver in the circulatory system is optimal for gathering, transforming, and accumulating metabolites and for neutralizing and eliminating toxic substances. Elimination occurs in the bile, an exocrine secretion of the liver that is important in lipid digestion.

1. STRUCTURE

Stroma

The liver is covered by a thin connective tissue capsule (**Glisson's capsule**) that becomes thicker at the **hilum,** where the portal vein and the hepatic artery enter the liver and where the right and left hepatic ducts and lymphatics exit. These vessels and ducts are surrounded by connective tissue all the way to their termination (or origin) in the portal spaces between classic liver lobules. At this point, a delicate reticular fiber network that supports the hepatocytes and sinusoidal endothelial cells of the liver lobules is formed.

The Liver Lobule

The basic structural component of the liver is the liver cell, or **hepatocyte** (Gr. *hepar,* liver, + *kytos,* cell). These epithelial cells are grouped in interconnected plates. In light-microscope sections, structural units called **classic liver lobules** can be seen (Figure 16–11). The liver lobule is formed of a polygonal mass of tissue about 0.7 × 2 mm in size (Figures 16–11 and 16–12). In certain animals (eg, pigs), lobules are separated from each other by a layer of connective tissue. This is not the case in humans, where the lobules are in close contact along most of their length, making it difficult to establish the exact limits between different lobules. In some regions, the lobules are demarcated by connective tissue containing bile ducts, lymphatics, nerves, and blood vessels.

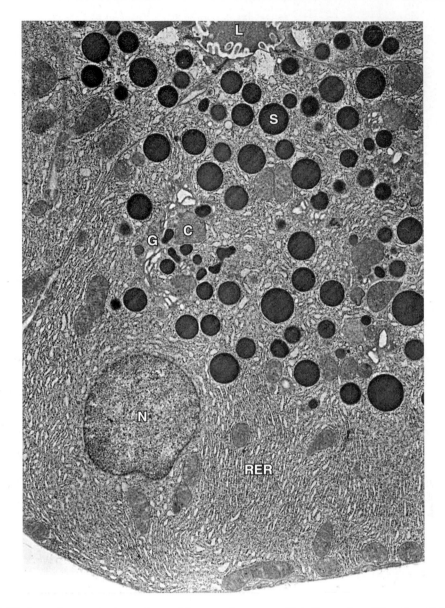

Figure 16–9. Electron micrograph of an acinar cell from a rat pancreas. Note the nucleus (N) surrounded by numerous cisternae of rough endoplasmic reticulum (RER) near the base of the cell. The Golgi complex (G) is situated at the apical pole of the nucleus and is associated with several condensing vacuoles (C) and numerous mature secretory (zymogen) granules (S). The lumen (L) contains proteins recently released from the cell by exocytosis. × 8000.

These regions, the **portal spaces,** are present at the corners of the lobules and are occupied by the **portal triads.** The human liver contains three to six portal triads per lobule, each with a venule (a branch of the portal vein), an arteriole (a branch of the hepatic artery), a duct (part of the bile duct system), and lymphatic vessels. The venule is usually the largest of these structures, containing blood from the superior and inferior mesenteric and splenic veins. The arteriole contains blood from the celiac trunk of the abdominal aorta. The duct, lined by cuboidal epithelium, carries bile from the parenchymal cells

(hepatocytes) and eventually empties into the hepatic duct. One or more lymphatics carry lymph, which eventually enters the blood circulation. All these structures are embedded in a sheath of connective tissue (Figure 16–13).

The hepatocytes in the liver lobule are radially disposed. They form a layer one or two cells thick, arranged like the bricks of a wall. These cellular plates are directed from the periphery of the lobule to its center and anastomose freely, forming a labyrinthine and sponge-like structure (Figure 16–12). The space between these plates contains capillaries, the

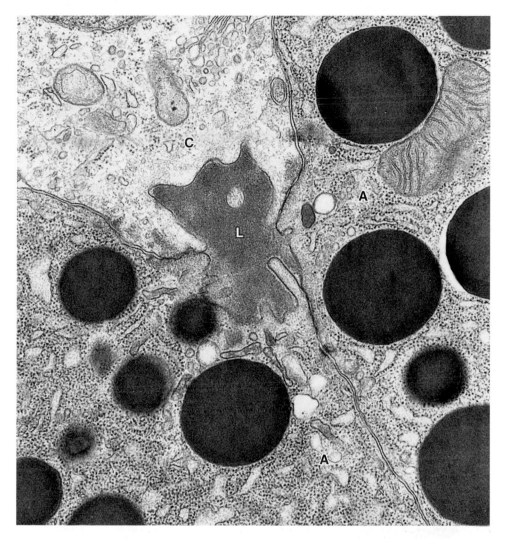

Figure 16–10. Electron micrograph of the apex of two pancreatic acinar cells (A) and a centroacinar cell (C) from a rat pancreas. Note the lack of secretory granules and the very scant rough endoplasmic reticulum in the centroacinar cell as compared with the acinar cell. L, acinar lumen. × 30,000.

liver sinusoids (Figures 16–11, 16–12, and 16–13). As discussed in Chapter 11, sinusoidal capillaries are irregularly dilated vessels composed solely of a discontinuous layer of fenestrated endothelial cells. The fenestrae are about 100 nm in diameter and are grouped in clusters that form "sieve plates" (Figure 16–14).

The endothelial cells are separated from the underlying hepatocytes by a subendothelial space known as the **space of Disse,** which contains microvilli of the hepatocytes (see Figures 16–18 and 16–21). Blood fluids readily percolate through the endothelial wall and make intimate contact with the surface of the hepatocytes, permitting an easy exchange of macromolecules from the sinusoidal lumen to the hepatocytes and vice versa. This exchange is physiologically important not only because of the large

number of macromolecules (eg, lipoproteins, albumin, fibrinogen) secreted into the blood by hepatocytes but also because the liver takes up and catabolizes many of these large molecules. The sinusoid is surrounded and supported by a delicate sheath of reticular fibers. In addition to the endothelial cells, the sinusoids contain phagocytotic cells of the mononuclear phagocyte system known as **Kupffer cells.** These cells are found on the luminal surface of the endothelial cells. Kupffer cells are typical macrophages. Their main functions are to metabolize aged erythrocytes, digest hemoglobin, and secrete proteins related to immunologic processes. Myofibroblasts, described in Chapter 5, are found in the walls of liver blood vessels, including the wall of sinusoids (space of Disse).

The sinusoids arise in the periphery of the lobule,

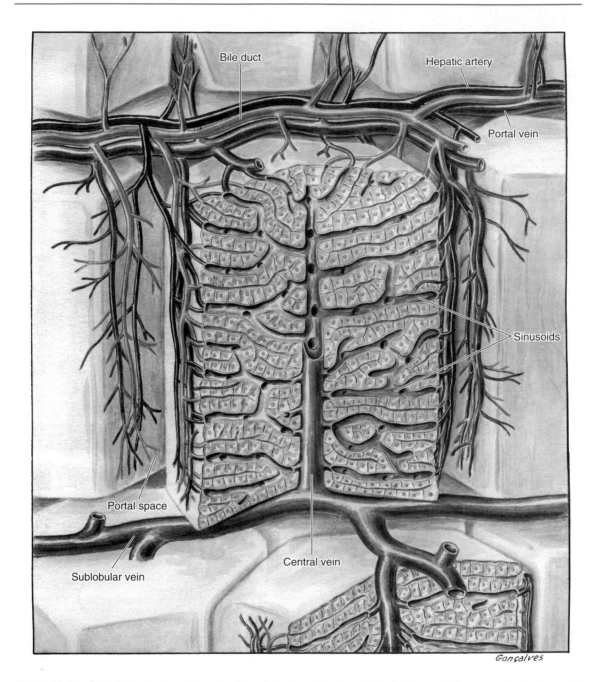

Figure 16–11. Schematic drawing of the structure of the liver. The liver lobule in the center is surrounded by the portal space (dilated here for clarity). Arteries, veins, and bile ducts occupy the portal spaces. Nerves, connective tissue, and lymphatic vessels are also present but are (again, for clarity) not shown in this illustration. In the lobule, note the radial disposition of the plates formed by hepatocytes; the sinusoidal capillaries separate the plates. The bile canaliculi can be seen between the hepatocytes. The sublobular (intercalated) veins drain blood from the lobules. (Redrawn and reproduced, with permission, from Bourne G: *An Introduction to Functional Histology.* Churchill, 1953.)

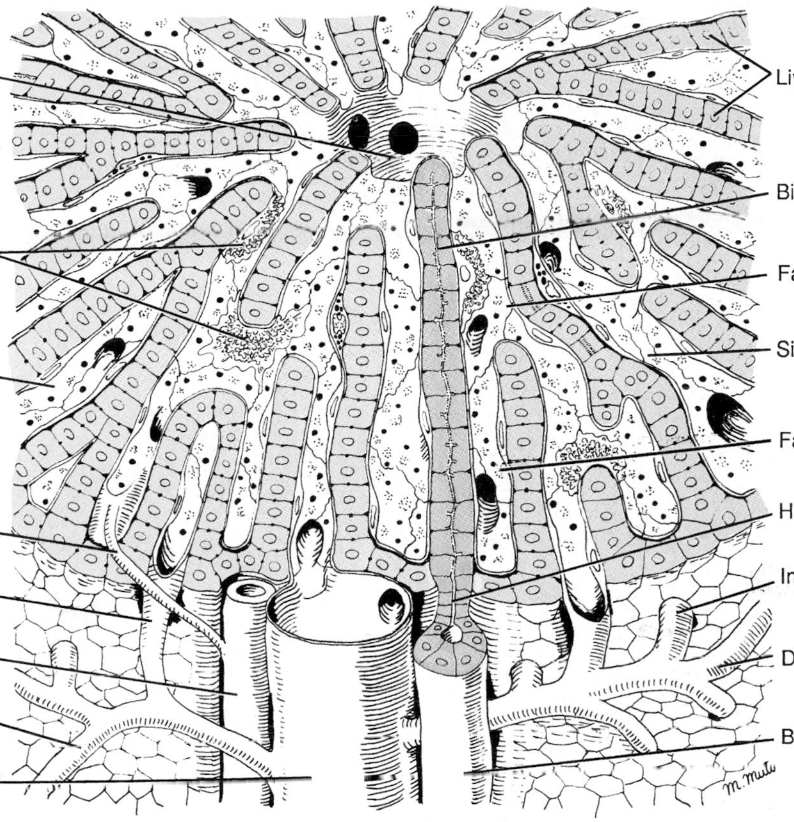

Figure 16–12. Three-dimensional aspect of the normal liver. In the upper center is the central vein; in the lower center, the portal vein. Note the bile canaliculus (darker color), liver plates (lighter color), Hering's canal, Kupffer cells, sinusoid, fat-storing cell, and sinusoid endothelial cells. (Courtesy of M Muto.)

fed by the inlet venules, the terminal branches of the portal veins, and the hepatic arterioles. They run in the direction of the lobular center, where they drain into the central vein (Figures 16–11 and 16–12).

> **Cirrhosis** of the liver, a diffuse process characterized by collagen infiltration, is one of the leading causes of death in Western countries. The prevailing hypothesis to explain the genesis of cirrhosis suggests that hepatic cell injury (caused by several agents, including alcohol) triggers an intense collagen secretion in the myofibroblasts in the liver.

Blood Supply

The liver is unusual in that it receives blood from two sources: 80% of the blood derives from the **portal vein,** which carries oxygen-poor, nutrient-rich blood from the abdominal viscera, and 20% derives from the **hepatic artery,** which supplies oxygen-rich blood (Figures 16–11 and 16–12).

A. Portal Vein System: The portal vein branches repeatedly and sends small **portal venules**

to the portal triads. The portal venules, sometimes called the **interlobular branches,** branch into the **distributing veins** that run around the periphery of the lobule. From the distributing veins, small **inlet venules** empty into the **sinusoids.** The sinusoids run radially, converging in the center of the lobule to form the **central,** or **centrolobular, vein.** This vessel has thin walls consisting only of endothelial cells supported by a sparse population of collagen fibers. As the central vein progresses along the lobule, it receives more and more sinusoids and gradually increases in diameter. At its end, it leaves the lobule at its base by merging with the larger **sublobular vein** (Figure 16–11). The sublobular veins gradually converge and fuse, forming the two or more large **hepatic veins** that empty into the inferior vena cava.

The portal system conveys blood from the pancreas and spleen and blood containing nutrients absorbed in the intestines. Nutrients are accumulated and transformed in the liver. Toxic substances are also neutralized and eliminated in the liver.

B. Arterial System: The hepatic artery branches repeatedly and forms the **interlobular ar-**

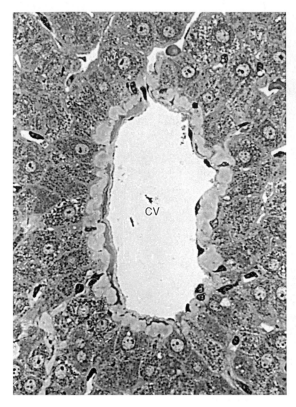 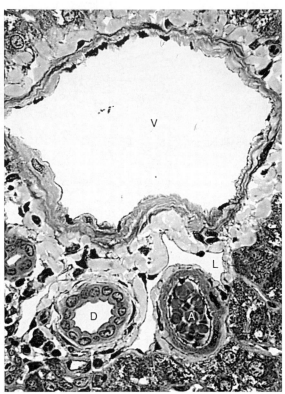

Figure 16–13. Photomicrograph of the liver. **Left:** A central vein (CV). Note the liver plates that anastomose freely, limiting the space occupied by the sinusoids. H&E stain. × 200. **Right:** A portal space with its characteristic artery (A), vein (V), and bile duct (D) surrounded by connective tissue. × 300.

teries. Some of these arteries irrigate the structures of the portal and others form arterioles (inlet arterioles; see Figure 16–12) that end directly in the sinusoids at various distances from the portal spaces, thus providing a mixture of arterial and portal venous blood in the sinusoids. The main function of the arterial system is to supply an adequate amount of oxygen to hepatocytes.

Blood flows from the periphery to the center of the **classic liver lobule.** Consequently, oxygen and metabolites, as well as all other toxic or nontoxic substances absorbed in the intestines, reach first the peripheral cells and then the central cells of the lobule. This direction of blood flow partly explains why the behavior of the perilobular cells differs from that of the centrolobular cells (Figure 16–15). This duality of behavior of the hepatocyte is particularly evident in pathologic specimens, where changes are seen in either the central cells or the peripheral cells of the lobule.

This description corresponds to the classic concept of liver lobule, in which the centrolobular vein constitutes the axis of the lobule. Figure 16–16 shows

the hexagons, limited by portal spaces, with a central vein.

Other points of reference can be used in analyzing possible functional units of the liver's structure. Another unit that can be visualized—the **portal lobule**—has at its center the portal triad and at its periphery the regions of adjoining hepatic lobules. All of these lobules drain bile into the bile duct of the central portal triad. A portal lobule is triangular, as opposed to the polygonal appearance of the classic liver lobule. It has a central vein at the tip of each of its angles, and it contains parts of three adjoining liver lobules, as indicated by the dashed triangle in Figure 16–16, with the portal space at its center.

Another way of subdividing the liver into functional lobules is to regard the region that is irrigated by a terminal branch of the distributing veins as a unit of liver parenchyma. This unit, called the **hepatic acinus** (of Rappaport), appears diamond-shaped in section (Figure 16–16). In addition to the terminal branches of the portal vein, an arterial branch and a bile ductule are in the center of this sub-

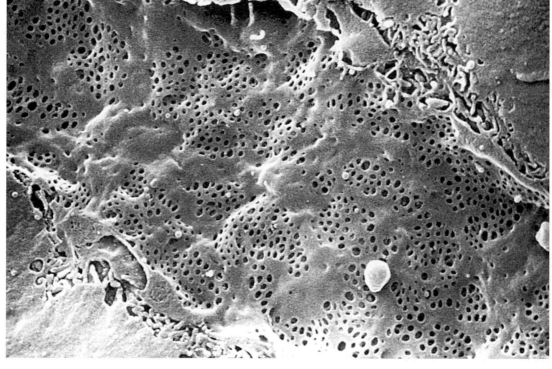

Figure 16–14. Scanning electron micrograph of the endothelial lining of a sinusoidal capillary in rat liver, showing the grouped fenestrations in its wall. At the borders, edges of cut hepatocytes are present, with their villi protruding into spaces of Disse. × 6500. (Courtesy of E Wisse.)

division of liver parenchyma, which is situated in adjacent areas of two liver lobules (Figure 16–16).

Based on their proximity to the distributing veins, cells in the hepatic acinus can be subdivided into zones (Figure 16–16). Cells in zone I are those closest to the vessel and consequently the first to alter the incoming blood or to be affected by it. Cells in zone II are the next to respond to the blood, and those in zone III see portal vein blood that has already been altered by cells in zones I and II. For example, after feeding, cells in zone I are the first to receive incoming glucose and to store it as glycogen. Any glucose passing the cells in zone I would likely be picked up by cells in zone II. In the fasting state, cells in zone I would be the first to respond to glucose-poor blood by breaking down glycogen and releasing it as glucose. In this event, the cells in zones II and III would not respond to the fasting condition until the glycogen in zone I cells was depleted. This zonal arrangement would account for some of the differences in the selective damage of hepatocytes caused by various noxious agents or disease conditions.

The Hepatocyte

Hepatocytes are polyhedral, with six or more surfaces, and have a diameter of 20–30 μm. In sections stained with hematoxylin and eosin (H&E), the cytoplasm of the hepatocyte is eosinophilic, mainly because of the large number of mitochondria and some smooth endoplasmic reticulum. Hepatocytes located at different distances from the portal triads show differences in structural, histochemical, and biochemical characteristics. The surface of each hepatocyte is in contact with the wall of the sinusoids, through the space of Disse, and with the surfaces of other hepatocytes. Wherever two hepatocytes abut, they delimit a tubular space between them known as the **bile canaliculus** (Figures 16–12, 16–17, 16–18, and 16–19).

The canaliculi, the first portions of the bile duct system, are tubular spaces 1–2 μm in diameter. They are limited only by the plasma membranes of two hepatocytes and have a small number of microvilli in their interiors (Figures 16–18 and 16–19). The cell membranes near these canaliculi are firmly joined by tight junctions (described in Chapter 4). Gap junc-

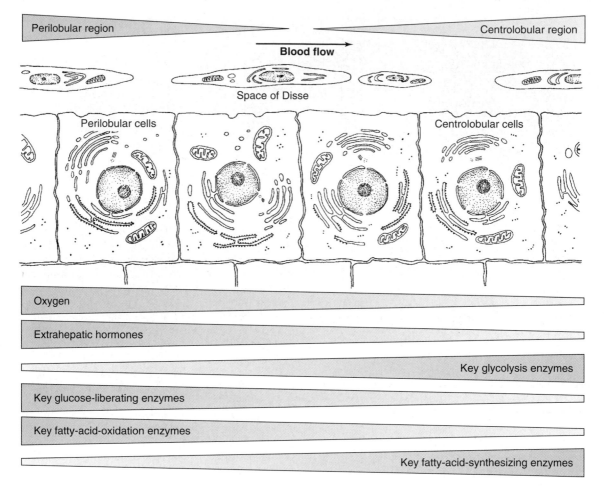

Figure 16–15. The heterogeneity of hepatocytes from the perilobular to the centrolobular regions. (Courtesy of A Brecht.)

tions are frequent between hepatocytes and are sites of intercellular communication, an important process in the coordination of these cells' physiologic activities. The bile canaliculi form a complex anastomosing network progressing along the plates of the liver lobule and terminating in the region of the portal spaces (Figure 16–12). The bile flow therefore progresses in a direction opposite to that of the blood, ie, from the center of the classic liver lobule to its periphery. At the periphery, bile enters the **bile ductules,** or **Hering's canals** (Figures 16–12 and 16–20). These ductules are composed of cuboidal cells with clear cytoplasm and few organelles. After a short distance, the ductules cross the limiting hepatocytes of the lobule and end in the **bile ducts** in the portal triads (Figures 16–11 and 16–20). Bile ducts are lined by cuboidal or columnar epithelium and have a distinct connective tissue sheath. They gradu-

ally enlarge and fuse, forming right and left **hepatic ducts,** which subsequently leave the liver.

The surface of the hepatocyte that faces the space of Disse bears many microvilli that protrude into that space, but there is always a space between them and the cells of the sinusoidal wall (Figures 16–18 and 16–21). The hepatocyte has one or two rounded nuclei with one or two typical nucleoli. Some of the nuclei are polyploid; ie, they contain some even multiples of the haploid number of chromosomes. Polyploid nuclei are characterized by their greater size, which is proportional to their ploidy. The hepatocyte has an abundant endoplasmic reticulum—both smooth and rough (Figures 16–18 and 16–22). In the hepatocyte, the rough endoplasmic reticulum forms aggregates dispersed in the cytoplasm; these are often called **basophilic bodies.** Several proteins (eg, blood albumin, fibrinogen) are synthesized on polyri-

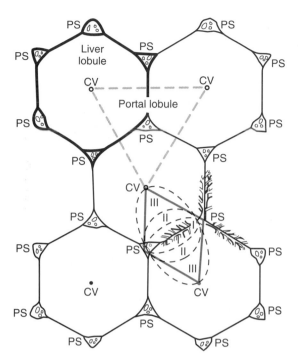

Figure 16–16. The territories of the classic liver lobules, hepatic acini, and portal lobules. In the drawing, the classic lobule has a central vein (CV) and is outlined by the solid lines that connect the portal spaces (PS). The portal lobules (lighter color) have their centers in the portal spaces; they are outlined by lines that connect the central veins (upper triangle). The portal lobules constitute the portion of the liver from which bile flows to a portal space. The hepatic acinus (darker color) is the region irrigated by a single distributing vein (diamond-shaped figure). Zones of the hepatic acinus are indicated by I, II, and III. (Redrawn and reproduced, with permission, from Leeson TS, Leeson CR: *Histology,* 2nd ed. Saunders, 1970.)

bile. When bilirubin or bilirubin glucuronide is not excreted, various diseases characterized by jaundice can result (see Figure 16–25). One of the frequent causes of jaundice in newborns is the often underdeveloped state of the smooth endoplasmic reticulum in their hepatocytes (**neonatal hyperbilirubinemia**). The current treatment for these cases is exposure to blue light from ordinary fluorescent tubes, which transforms unconjugated bilirubin into a water-soluble photoisomer that can be excreted by the kidneys.

The hepatocyte frequently contains glycogen. This polysaccharide appears in the electron microscope as coarse, electron-dense granules that frequently collect in the cytosol close to the smooth endoplasmic reticulum (Figures 16–18 and 16–23). The amount of glycogen present in the liver conforms to a diurnal rhythm; it also depends on the nutritional state of the individual. Liver glycogen is a depot for glucose and is mobilized if the blood glucose level falls below normal. In this way, hepatocytes maintain a steady level of blood glucose, one of the main sources of energy for use by the body.

Each hepatocyte has approximately 2000 mitochondria. Another common cellular component is the lipid droplet, whose numbers vary greatly. Hepatocyte lysosomes are important in the turnover and degradation of intracellular organelles. They also play a fundamental role in the receptor-mediated endocytosis of many macromolecular ligands. These macromolecules are first transported to endosomes that later fuse with lysosomes. Catabolism of macromolecules occurs in these secondary lysosomes. Peroxisomes are abundant in hepatocytes. Golgi complexes in the liver are also numerous—up to 50 per cell. Each Golgi complex consists of flattened cisternae, small vesicles, and larger vacuoles lying near the bile canaliculi. The functions of this organelle include the formation of lysosomes and the secretion of plasma proteins (eg, albumin), glycoproteins (eg, transferrin), and lipoproteins (eg, very low-density lipoproteins).

2. FUNCTIONS

The hepatocyte is probably the most versatile cell in the body. It is a cell with both endocrine and exocrine functions; it also synthesizes and accumulates certain substances, detoxifies others, and transports still others.

Protein Synthesis

In addition to synthesizing proteins for its own maintenance, the hepatocyte produces various plasma proteins for export—among them albumin,

bosomes in these structures. Various important processes take place in the smooth endoplasmic reticulum, which is distributed diffusely throughout the cytoplasm. This organelle is responsible for the processes of oxidation, methylation, and conjugation required for inactivation or detoxification of various substances before their excretion from the body. The smooth endoplasmic reticulum is a labile system that reacts promptly to the molecules received by the hepatocyte.

One of the main processes occurring in the smooth endoplasmic reticulum is the conjugation of hydrophobic (water-insoluble) toxic bilirubin by glucuronyltransferase to form a water-soluble nontoxic bilirubin glucuronide. This conjugate is excreted by hepatocytes into the

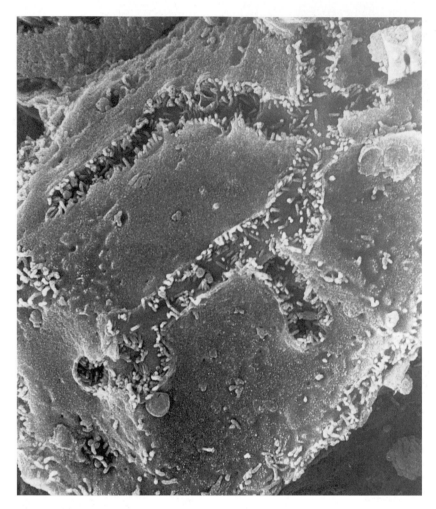

Figure 16–17. Scanning electron micrograph of branching bile canaliculi in the liver. Note the microvilli lining the internal surface. (Reproduced, with permission, from Motta P et al: *The Liver: An Atlas of Scanning Electron Microscopy.* Igaku-Shonin, 1978.)

prothrombin, fibrinogen, and lipoproteins. These proteins are synthesized on polyribosomes attached to the rough endoplasmic reticulum. Contrary to what is observed in other glandular cells, the hepatocyte does not store proteins in its cytoplasm as secretory granules but continuously releases them into the bloodstream, thus functioning as an endocrine gland (Figure 16–23). About 5% of the protein exported by the liver is produced by the cells of the macrophage system (Kupffer cells); the remainder is synthesized in the hepatocytes.

Bile Secretion

Bile secretion is an exocrine function in the sense that hepatocytes promote the uptake, transformation, and excretion of blood components into the bile canaliculi. Bile has several other essential components in addition to water and electrolytes: bile acids,

phospholipids, cholesterol, and bilirubin. The secretion of bile acids is illustrated in Figure 16–24. About 90% of these substances are derived by absorption from the distal intestinal epithelium and are transported by the hepatocyte from the blood to bile canaliculi (enterohepatic recirculation). About 10% of bile acids are synthesized in the smooth endoplasmic reticulum of the hepatocyte by conjugation of cholic acid (synthesized by the liver from cholesterol) with the amino acid glycine or taurine, producing glycocholic and taurocholic acids. Bile acids have an important function in emulsifying the lipids in the digestive tract, promoting easier digestion by lipase and subsequent absorption.

Abnormal proportions of bile acids may lead to the formation of gallstones (cholelithiasis). Gallstones can block bile flow and cause jaun-

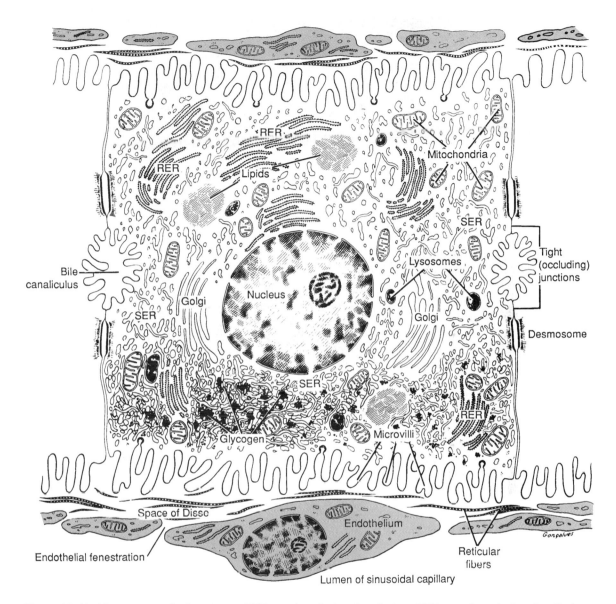

Figure 16–18. Ultrastructure of a hepatocyte. RER, rough endoplasmic reticulum; SER, smooth endoplasmic reticulum. Cells of the sinusoidal capillary are shown in color. × 10,000.

dice—the presence of bile pigments in blood—from the rupture of tight junctions around the bile canaliculi.

Bilirubin, most of which results from the breakdown of hemoglobin, is formed in the mononuclear phagocyte system (which includes the Kupffer cells of the liver sinusoids) and is transported to the hepatocytes. In the smooth endoplasmic reticulum of the hepatocyte, hydrophobic bilirubin is conjugated to glucuronic acid, forming water-soluble bilirubin glu-

curonide (Figure 16–25). In a further step, **bilirubin glucuronide** is secreted into the bile canaliculi.

Metabolite Storage

Lipids and carbohydrates are stored in the liver in the form of triglycerides and glycogen (Figure 16–23). This capacity to store metabolites is important, because it supplies the body with energy between meals. Figure 16–23 shows how carbohydrates are stored. The liver also serves as the major storage compartment for vitamins, especially vitamin A.

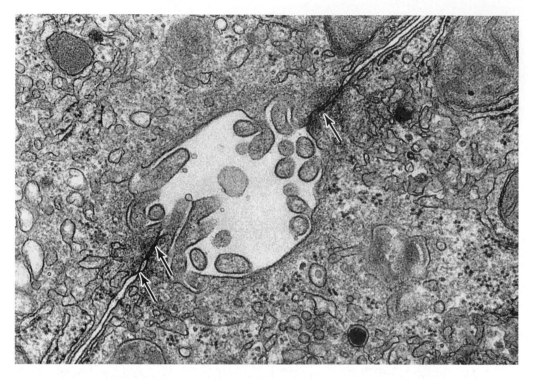

Figure 16–19. Electron micrograph of a bile canaliculus in rat liver. Note the microvilli in its lumen and the junctional complexes (arrows) that seal off this space from the remaining extracellular space. × 54,000. (Courtesy of SL Wissig.)

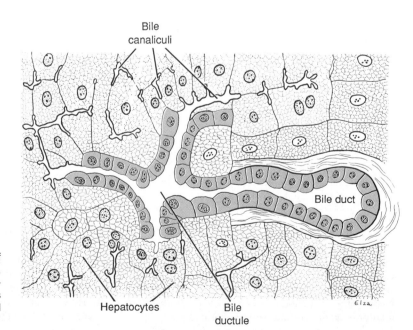

Figure 16–20. The confluence of bile canaliculi and bile ductules, which are lined by cuboidal epithelium (shown in color). The ductules merge with bile ducts in the portal spaces.

Sinusoid

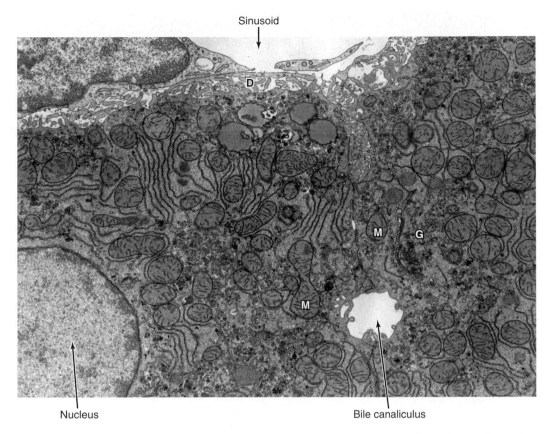

Nucleus   Bile canaliculus

Figure 16–21. Electron micrograph of the liver. Note the two adjacent hepatocytes with a bile canaliculus between them. The hepatocytes contain numerous mitochondria (M) and smooth and rough endoplasmic reticulum. A prominent Golgi complex (G) is near the bile canaliculus. The sinusoid is lined by endothelial cells with large open fenestrae. The space of Disse (D) is occupied by numerous microvilli projecting from the hepatocytes. × 9200. (Courtesy of D Schmucker.)

Metabolic Functions

The hepatocyte is responsible for converting lipids and amino acids into glucose by means of a complex enzymatic process called **gluconeogenesis** (Gr. *glykys,* sweet, + *neos,* new, + *genesis,* production). It is also the main site of amino acid deamination, resulting in the production of urea. Urea is transported through the blood to the kidney and is excreted by that organ.

Detoxification & Inactivation

Various drugs and substances can be inactivated by oxidation, methylation, or conjugation. The enzymes participating in these processes are located mainly in the smooth endoplasmic reticulum. Glucuronyltransferase, an enzyme that conjugates glucuronic acid to bilirubin, also causes conjugation of several other compounds such as steroids, barbiturates, antihistamines, and anticonvulsants.

The administration of barbiturates to laboratory animals results in rapid development of smooth endoplasmic reticulum in hepatocytes. Barbiturates can also increase synthesis of glucuronyltransferase. This finding has led to the use of barbiturates in the treatment of glucuronyltransferase deficiencies.

Liver Regeneration

Despite its slow rate of cell renewal, the liver has an extraordinary capacity for regeneration. The loss of hepatic tissue by surgical removal or from the action of toxic substances triggers a mechanism by which hepatocytes begin to divide, continuing until the original mass of tissue is restored. In rats, the liver can regenerate a loss of 75% of its weight in one month. In humans, this capacity is considerably restricted. The process of regeneration is probably controlled by circulating substances called **chalones,**

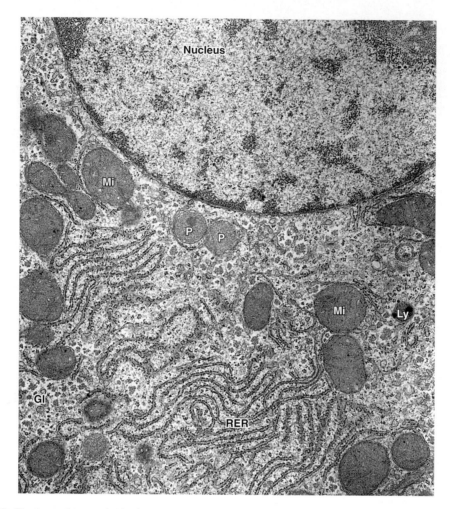

Figure 16–22. Electron micrograph of a hepatocyte. In the cytoplasm, below the nucleus, are mitochondria (Mi), rough endoplasmic reticulum (RER), glycogen (Gl), lysosomes (Ly), and peroxisomes (P). × 6600.

which inhibit the mitotic division of certain cell types.

When the liver is injured or partially removed, it produces fewer chalones; consequently, a burst of mitotic activity occurs in the tissue. As regeneration proceeds, the number of chalones increases and mitotic activity decreases. This process is self-regulating.

The regenerated liver tissue is usually similar to the injured or removed tissue. If there is continuous or repeated damage to this organ, however, connective tissue is abundantly produced along with the hepatocyte regeneration. The excess of connective tissue results in disorganization of the liver structure, a condition known as **cirrhosis.** Liver function is impaired in this condition, because the scar tissue (collagen) not only replaces functional hepatocytes but also disorganizes the liver, vascular, and bile duct systems.

BILIARY TRACT

The bile produced by the hepatocyte flows through the **bile canaliculi, bile ductules,** and **bile ducts.** These structures gradually merge, forming a network that converges to form the **hepatic duct.** The hepatic duct, after receiving the **cystic duct** from the gallbladder, continues to the duodenum as the **common bile duct** (**ductus choledochus**).

The hepatic, cystic, and common bile ducts are lined with a mucous membrane of simple columnar epithelium. The lamina propria is thin and surrounded by an inconspicuous layer of smooth mus-

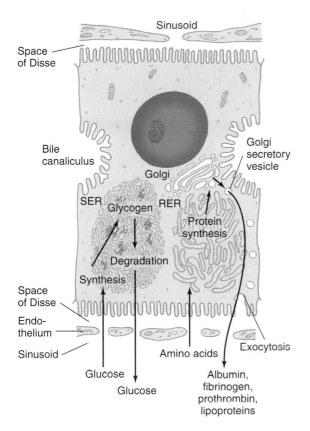

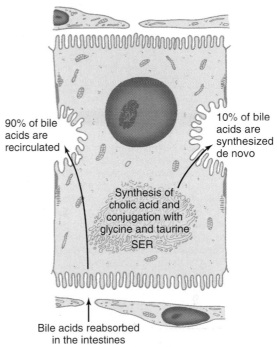

Figure 16–23. Protein synthesis and carbohydrate storage in the liver. Protein synthesis occurs in the rough endoplasmic reticulum (RER), which explains why hepatocyte lesions or starvation lead to a decrease in the amounts of albumin, fibrinogen, and prothrombin in a patient's blood. In several diseases, glycogen degradation is depressed, resulting in abnormal intracellular accumulations of glycogen. SER, smooth endoplasmic reticulum.

Figure 16–24. Mechanism of secretion of bile acids. About 90% of bile acids are derived from the intestinal epithelium and transported to the liver. The remaining 10% are synthesized in the liver by the conjugation of cholic acid with the amino acids glycine and taurine. This process occurs in the smooth endoplasmic reticulum (SER).

cle. This muscle layer becomes thicker near the duodenum and finally, in the intramural portion, forms a sphincter that regulates bile flow (sphincter of Oddi).

GALLBLADDER

The gallbladder is a hollow, pear-shaped organ attached to the lower surface of the liver. It can store 30–50 mL of bile and communicates with the hepatic duct through the cystic duct. The wall of the gallbladder consists of a mucosa composed of simple columnar epithelium and lamina propria, a layer of smooth muscle, a well-developed perimuscular connective tissue layer, and a serous membrane (Figure 16–26).

The mucosa has abundant folds that are particularly evident when the gallbladder is empty. The epithelial cells are rich in mitochondria and have their nuclei in their basal third (Figure 16–27). All these cells are capable of secreting small amounts of mucus. Microvilli are frequent at the apical surface. Near the cystic duct, the epithelium invaginates into the lamina propria, forming tubuloacinar glands with wide lumens. Cells of these glands have characteristics of mucus-secreting cells and are responsible for the production of most of the mucus present in bile.

The muscular layer is thin, with most of the smooth muscle cells oriented around the circumference of the gallbladder. A thick connective tissue layer binds the superior surface of the gallbladder to the liver. The opposite surface is covered by a typical serous layer, the peritoneum.

The main function of the gallbladder is to store bile, concentrate it by absorbing its water, and release it when necessary into the digestive tract. This process depends on an active sodium-transporting mechanism in the gallbladder's epithelium. Water absorption is an osmotic consequence of the sodium pump. Contraction of the smooth muscle of the gallbladder is induced by **cholecystokinin,** a hormone

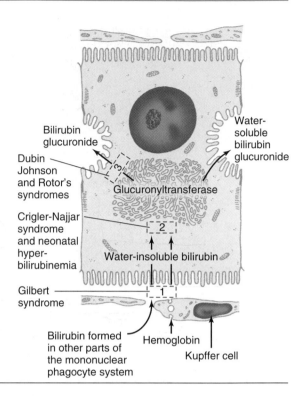

Figure 16–25. The secretion of bilirubin. The water-insoluble form of bilirubin is derived from the metabolism of hemoglobin in macrophages. Glucuronyltransferase activity in the hepatocytes causes bilirubin to be conjugated with glucuronide in the smooth endoplasmic reticulum, forming a water-soluble compound. When bile secretion is blocked, the yellow bilirubin or bilirubin glucuronide is not excreted; it accumulates in the blood, and jaundice results. Several defective processes in the hepatocytes can cause diseases that produce jaundice: a defect in the capacity of the cell to trap and absorb bilirubin (rectangle 1); the inability of the cell to conjugate bilirubin because of a deficiency in glucuronyltransferase (rectangle 2); or problems in the transfer and excretion of bilirubin glucuronide into the bile canaliculi (rectangle 3). One of the most frequent causes of jaundice, however—unrelated to hepatocyte activity—is the obstruction of bile flow as a result of gallstones or tumors of the pancreas.

produced by enteroendocrine cells (I cells) located in the epithelial lining of the small intestine. Release of cholecystokinin is, in turn, stimulated by the presence of dietary fats in the small intestine.

Tumors of the Digestive Glands

Most malignant tumors of the liver derive from hepatic parenchyma or epithelial cells of the bile duct. Liver carcinomas are often preceded by connective tissue proliferation (cirrhosis). Most tumors of the exocrine pancreas arise from ductal epithelial cells; the mortality rate from pancreatic tumors is high.

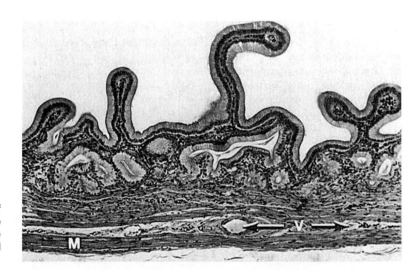

Figure 16–26. Photomicrograph of a section of gallbladder. Note the lining of columnar epithelium, the smooth muscle layer (M), and blood vessels (V). H&E stain. × 30.

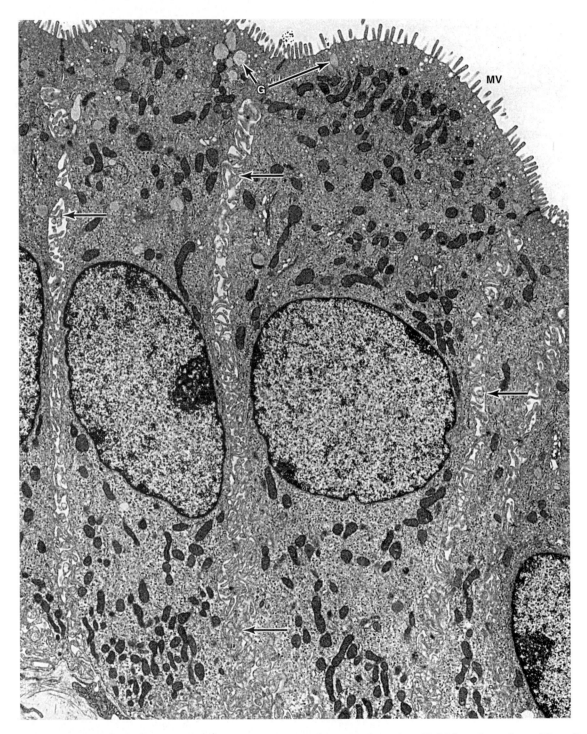

Figure 16–27. Electron micrograph of the gallbladder of a guinea pig. Note the microvilli (MV) on the surface of the cell and the secretory granules (G) containing mucus. Arrows indicate the intercellular spaces. These epithelial cells transport sodium chloride from the lumen to the subjacent connective tissue. Water follows passively, causing the bile to become concentrated. × 5600.

REFERENCES

PANCREAS & SALIVARY GLANDS

Mason DK, Chisholm DM: *Salivary Glands in Health and Disease.* Saunders, 1975.

McDaniel ML et al: Cytokines and nitric oxide in islet inflammation and diabetes. Proc Soc Exp Biol Med 1996;211:24.

Young JA, Van Lennep DW: *The Morphology of Salivary Glands.* Academic Press, 1978.

Young JA et al: A microperfusion investigation of sodium resorption and potassium secretion by the main excretory duct of the rat submaxillary gland. Pfluegers Arch 1967;295:157.

LIVER & BILIARY TRACT

Gerber MA, Swan NT: Histology of the liver. Am J Surg Pathol 1987;11:709.

Ito T, Shibasaki S: Electron microscopic study on the hepatic sinusoidal wall and the fat-storing cells in the human normal liver. Arch Histol Jpn 1968;29:137.

Jones AL, Fawcett CW: Hypertrophy of the agranular endoplasmic reticulum in hamster liver induced by phenobarbital. J Histochem Cytochem 1966;14:215.

Rouiller C (editor): *The Liver: Morphology, Biochemistry, Physiology.* 2 vols. Academic Press, 1963, 1964.

Trutman M, Sasse D: The lymphatics of the liver. Anat Embryol 1994;190:201.

The Respiratory System

17

The respiratory system includes the **lungs** and a system of tubes that link the sites of gas exchange with the external environment. A **ventilation mechanism,** consisting of the thoracic cage, intercostal muscles, diaphragm, and elastic and collagen components of the lungs, is important in the movement of air through the lungs. The respiratory system is customarily divided into two principal regions (Figure 17–1): a **conducting portion,** consisting of the nasal cavity, nasopharynx, larynx, trachea, bronchi (Gr. *bronchos,* windpipe), bronchioles, and terminal bronchioles; and a **respiratory portion** (where gas exchange takes place), consisting of respiratory bronchioles, alveolar ducts, and alveoli. **Alveoli** are specialized sac-like structures that make up the greater part of the lungs. They are the main sites for the principal function of the lungs—the exchange of O_2 and CO_2 between inspired air and blood.

The conducting portion serves two main functions: to provide a conduit through which air can travel to and from the lungs and to condition the inspired air. To ensure an uninterrupted supply of air, a combination of cartilage, elastic and collagen fibers, and smooth muscle provides the conducting portion with rigid structural support and the necessary flexibility and extensibility. The cartilages, primarily hyaline (with some elastic cartilage in the larynx), are found in the periphery of the lamina propria. They have various forms, ranging from small plaques to irregular rings and, in the trachea, C-shaped cartilages. The cartilages generally serve to support the walls of the conducting portion, preventing collapse of the lumen and thereby ensuring continuous access of air to the lungs. Both the conducting and respiratory portions are richly endowed with elastic fibers that provide these structures with flexibility and allow them to spring back after distention. In the conducting portion, the elastic fibers are found in the lamina propria; their orientation is mainly longitudinal. The concentration of elastic fiber is inversely proportionate to the diameter of the conducting tubule (ie, the smallest bronchioles have the highest proportion of elastic fibers). Bundles of smooth muscle encircle the tubes from the trachea to the alveolar ducts (a subdi-

vision of the respiratory portion). Contraction of the smooth muscle reduces the diameter of the conducting tubules and thereby regulates air flow during inspiration and expiration. The conducting portion of the respiratory system gradually undergoes a transition into the respiratory portion. The content of ciliated epithelium, goblet cells, and cartilage is gradually reduced, and the content of smooth muscle and elastic fibers gradually increases (Table 17–1).

Conditioning of Air

A major function of the conducting portion is to condition the inspired air. Before it enters the lungs, inspired air is cleansed, moistened, and warmed. To carry out these functions, the mucosa of the conducting portion is lined with a specialized **respiratory epithelium,** and there are numerous mucous and serous glands as well as a rich superficial vascular network in the lamina propria.

As the air enters the nose, large **vibrissae** (specialized hairs) remove coarse particles of dust. Once the air reaches the **nasal fossae,** particulate and gaseous impurities are trapped in a layer of mucus. This mucus, in conjunction with serous secretions, also serves to moisten the incoming air, protecting the delicate alveolar lining from desiccation. The incoming air is also warmed by a rich superficial vascular network.

Respiratory Epithelium

Most of the conducting portion is lined with ciliated pseudostratified columnar epithelium that contains a rich population of goblet cells. Deeper in the bronchial tree, this epithelial cell population is modified in a transition to simple squamous epithelium. As the bronchi subdivide into the bronchioles, the pseudostratified organization gives way to a simple columnar epithelium, which is further reduced to a simple cuboidal layer in the smallest (terminal) bronchioles. The rich goblet cell population tapers off in the smaller bronchi and is completely absent from the epithelium in the terminal bronchioles. Ciliated cells, which accompany the goblet cells, continue through the finer bronchioles without the goblet cells. The continuation

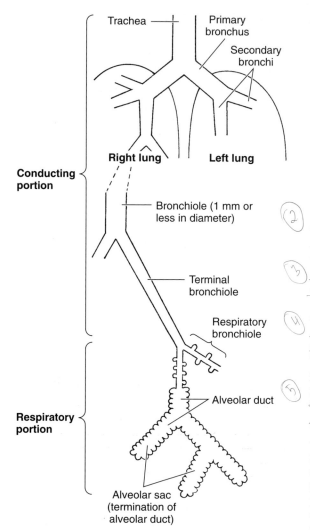

Figure 17–1. The main divisions of the respiratory tract. The natural proportions of these structures have been altered for clarity; the respiratory bronchiole, for example, is in reality a short transitional structure.

chondria. Experiments have shown that ATP is required for ciliary beating, an observation that is consistent with the apical localization of mitochondria.

Immotile cilia syndrome (Kartagener syndrome), a disorder that causes infertility in men and chronic respiratory-tract infections in both sexes, is caused by immobility of cilia and flagella induced by deficiency of **dynein,** a protein normally present in the cilia. Dynein is responsible for the sliding of the microtubules, a process that is necessary for ciliary movement (see Chapter 2).

The next most abundant cells in the respiratory epithelium are the **mucous goblet cells** (Figure 17–4). The apical portion of these cells (described in Chapter 4) contains the polysaccharide-rich mucous droplets. The remaining columnar cells are known as **brush cells** (Figures 17–3 and 17–4) because of the numerous microvilli on their apical surface. Brush cells have afferent nerve endings on their basal surfaces and are considered to be sensory receptors. **Basal (short) cells** are small rounded cells that lie on the basal lamina but do not extend to the luminal surface of the epithelium. These cells are believed to be generative cells that undergo mitosis and subsequently differentiate into the other cell types. The last cell type is the **small granule cell,** which resembles a basal cell except that it possesses numerous granules 100–300 nm in diameter with dense cores. Histochemical studies reveal that these cells constitute a population of cells of the diffuse neuroendocrine system (see Chapter 4). These endocrine-like granule cells may act as effectors in the integration of the mucous and serous secretory processes. All cells of the ciliated pseudostratified columnar epithelium touch the basement membrane (Figure 17–4, bottom).

of the ciliated cells beyond the goblet cells prevents mucus from accumulating in the respiratory portion of the system. The superficial mucus, which traps particulate matter and absorbs water-soluble gases (eg, SO_2, ozone), floats on a subjacent sol phase secreted by serous glands located in the lamina propria (see Figure 17–4). Cilia of these epithelia move the more fluid sol phase, together with the overlying mucous layer, toward the mouth. Here, the mucous layer is either swallowed or expectorated.

Typical respiratory epithelium consists of five cell types (as seen in the electron microscope). **Ciliated columnar cells** constitute the most abundant type. Each cell has about 300 cilia on its apical surface (Figures 17–2, 17–3, and 17–4); beneath the cilia, in addition to basal bodies, are numerous small mito-

From the nasal cavity through the larynx, portions of the epithelium are stratified squamous. This type of epithelium is evident in regions exposed to direct air flow or physical abrasion (eg, oropharynx, epiglottis, vocal folds); it provides more protection from attrition than does typical respiratory epithelium. If air-flow currents are altered or new abrasive sites develop, the affected areas can convert from typical ciliated pseudostratified columnar epithelium to stratified squamous epithelium. Similarly, in smokers, the proportion of ciliated cells to goblet cells is altered to aid in clearing the increased particulate and gaseous pollutants (eg, CO, SO_2). Although the greater numbers of goblet cells in a smoker's epithelium provide for a more rapid clearance of pollutants, the reduction in ciliated cells caused by excessive intake of CO results in decreased movement of the mucous layer and frequently leads to congestion of the smaller airways.

Table 17–1. Structural changes in the conducting portion of the respiratory tract.

	Nasal Fossae	Naso-pharynx	Larynx	Trachea	Bronchi Large	Bronchi Small	Bronchioles Regular	Bronchioles Terminal	Bronchioles Respiratory
Epithelium	Ciliated pseudostratified columnar[1,2]						→ Transition →		
							Ciliated pseudo- → stratified columnar	Ciliated simple → columnar	Ciliated simple cuboidal
Goblet cells	Abundant				Present	Few	Scattered	None	
Glands	Abundant			Present		Few	None		
Cartilage			Complex (hyaline and elastic)	C-shaped rings	Irregular rings	Plates and islands	None		
Smooth muscle	None			Spanning open ends of C-shaped rings	Crisscrossing spiral bundles				
Elastic fibers	None	Present					Abundant		

[1]Stratified squamous in regions of direct air flow or abrasion.
[2]The vestibule of the nose shows a transition from keratinized stratified squamous to ciliated pseudostratified columnar epithelium.

NASAL CAVITY

The nasal cavity consists of two structures: the external **vestibule** and the internal **nasal fossae.**

Vestibule

The vestibule is the most anterior and dilated portion of the nasal cavity. The outer integument of the nose enters the **nares** (nostrils) and continues partway up the vestibule. Around the inner surface of the nares are numerous sebaceous and sweat glands, in addition to the thick short hairs, or **vibrissae,** that filter out large particles from the inspired air. Within the vestibule, the epithelium loses its keratinized nature and undergoes a transition into typical respiratory epithelium before entering the nasal fossae.

Nasal Fossae

Within the skull lie two cavernous chambers separated by the osseous **nasal septum.** Extending from each lateral wall are three bony shelf-like projections known as **conchae.** Of the superior, middle, and inferior conchae, only the middle and inferior projections are covered with respiratory epithelium. The superior conchae are covered with a specialized **olfactory epithelium.** (The structure and function of olfactory epithelium are discussed in Chapter 24.) The narrow, ribbon-like passages created by the conchae improve the conditioning of the inspired air by increasing the surface area of respiratory epithelium and by creating turbulence in the air flow. The result is increased contact between air streams and the mucous layer. Within the lamina propria of the conchae are large venous plexuses known as **swell bodies.** Every 20–30 minutes, the swell bodies on one side of the nasal fossae become engorged with blood, resulting in distention of the conchal mucosa and a concomitant decrease in the flow of air. During this time, most of the air is directed through the other nasal fossa. These periodic intervals of occlusion reduce air flow, allowing the respiratory epithelium to recover from desiccation.

Allergic reactions and inflammation can cause abnormal engorgement of swell bodies in both fossae, severely restricting the air flow.

In addition to swell bodies, the nasal cavity has a rich vascular system with a complex organization. Large vessels form a close-meshed latticework next to the periosteum, from which arcading branches lead toward the surface. Smaller vessels branch from the arcading vessels and run perpendicular to the surface. These smaller vessels form a rich capillary bed beneath the epithelium. Blood flows forward from the rear to each fossa. In each arcading loop, the flow of blood counters the flow of inspired air. As a result, the incoming air is efficiently warmed by a countercurrent system.

PARANASAL SINUSES

The paranasal sinuses are closed cavities in the frontal, maxillary, ethmoid, and sphenoid bones. They are lined with a thinner respiratory epithelium that contains few goblet cells. The lamina propria contains only a few small glands and is continuous

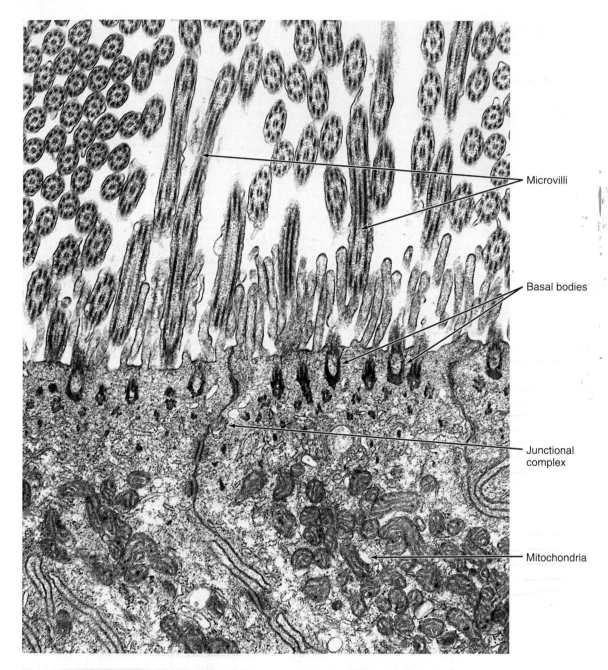

Microvilli

Basal bodies

Junctional
complex

Mitochondria

Figure 17–2. Electron micrograph of ciliated columnar epithelium in the lung, showing the ciliary microtubules in transverse and oblique section. In the cell apex are the U-shaped basal bodies that serve as the source of, and anchoring sites for, the ciliary axonemes. The local accumulation of mitochondria is related to energy production for ciliary movement. Note the junctional complex and the emergence of microvilli between the ciliary roots. × 9200.

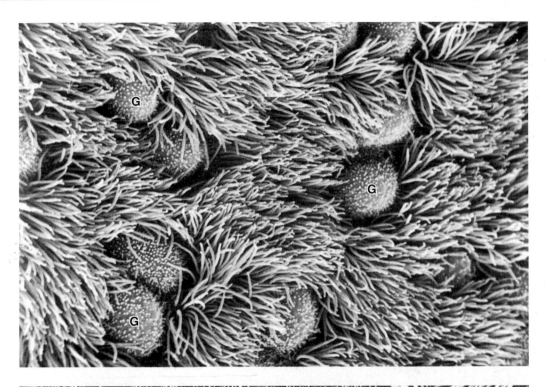

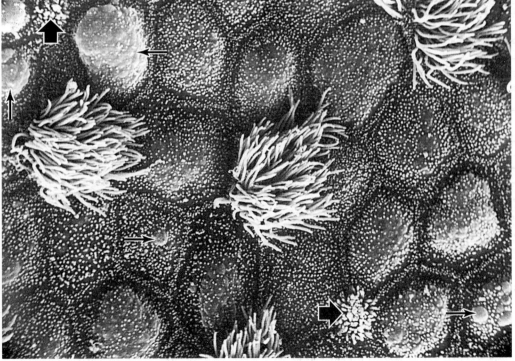

Figure 17–3. Scanning electron micrographs of the surface of rat respiratory mucosa. **Top:** Most of the surface is covered with cilia. G, goblet cells. × 2500. **Bottom:** Subsurface accumulations of mucus are evident in the goblet cells (thin arrows). Brush cells are indicated by thick arrowheads. × 3000. (Reproduced, with permission, from Andrews P: A scanning electron microscopic study of the extrapulmonary respiratory tract. Am J Anat 1974;139:421.)

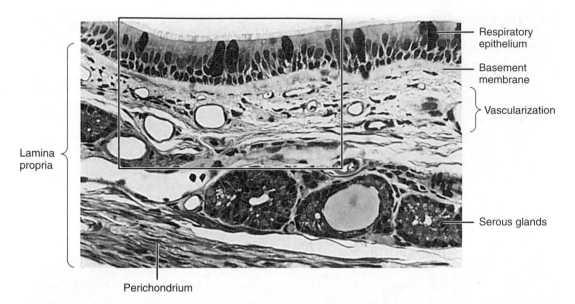

Respiratory epithelium

Basement membrane

Vascularization

Lamina propria

Serous glands

Perichondrium

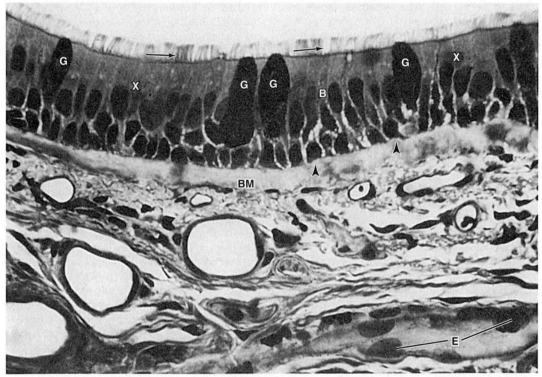

Figure 17–4. Top: Section of monkey trachea showing typical respiratory epithelium, thick basement membrane, richly vascularized connective tissue of the lamina propria, and glands containing both serous and mucous cells. Beneath the glands lies the dense connective tissue of the perichondrium, which surrounds the supporting hyaline cartilage (not visible). × 200. **Bottom:** Enlargement of the area shown in the rectangle at top. The tracheal lumen is lined with typical ciliated pseudostratified columnar epithelium with goblet cells. This epithelium plays a significant role in conditioning the inspired air. Beneath the unusually thick basement membrane (BM) lies the lamina propria, whose rich vascularity aids in warming the incoming air. G, goblet cells containing mucus; X, ciliated columnar cells; B, nonciliated brush cell. Arrowheads indicate rounded basal cells; arrows above the respiratory epithelium indicate cilia; E, *en face* of venule endothelial cells. × 500.

with the underlying periosteum. The paranasal sinuses communicate with the nasal cavity through small openings. The mucus produced in these cavities drains into the nasal passages as a result of the activity of its ciliated epithelial cells.

> **Sinusitis** is an inflammatory process of the sinuses that may persist for long periods of time, mainly because of obstruction of drainage orifices. Chronic sinusitis is a component of Kartagener syndrome, which is characterized by defective ciliary action.

NASOPHARYNX

The nasopharynx is the first part of the pharynx, continuing caudally with the oropharynx, the oral portion of this organ. It is lined with respiratory epithelium in the portion that is in contact with the soft palate.

LARYNX

The larynx is an irregular tube that connects the pharynx to the trachea. Within the lamina propria lie a number of laryngeal cartilages. The larger cartilages (thyroid, cricoid, and most of the arytenoids) are hyaline, and some are subject to calcification in the elderly. The smaller cartilages (epiglottis, cuneiform, corniculate, and the tips of the arytenoids) are elastic cartilages. Ligaments bind the cartilages together; most of the cartilages are articulated by the intrinsic muscles of the larynx, which are unusual in that they are striated skeletal muscle. In addition to their supporting role (maintenance of an open airway), these cartilages serve as a valve to prevent swallowed food or fluid from entering the trachea. They also participate in producing sounds for phonation.

The **epiglottis,** which projects from the rim of the larynx, extends into the pharynx and has both a lingual and a laryngeal surface. The entire lingual surface and the apical portion of the laryngeal surface are covered with stratified squamous epithelium. Toward the base of the epiglottis on the laryngeal surface, the epithelium undergoes a transition into ciliated pseudostratified columnar epithelium. Mixed mucous and serous glands are found beneath the epithelium.

Below the epiglottis, the mucosa forms two pairs of folds that extend into the lumen of the larynx. The upper pair constitutes the **false vocal cords** (vestibular folds), covered with typical respiratory epithelium beneath which lie numerous serous glands within the lamina propria. The lower pair of folds constitutes the **true vocal cords.** Large bundles of parallel elastic fibers that compose the **vocal ligament** lie within

the vocal folds, which are covered with a stratified squamous epithelium. Parallel to the ligaments are bundles of skeletal muscle, the **vocalis muscles,** which regulate the tension of the fold and its ligaments. As air is forced between the folds, these muscles provide the means for sounds of different frequencies to be produced.

TRACHEA

The trachea is a thin-walled tube, about 10 cm long, that extends from the base of the larynx to the point at which it bifurcates into the two primary bronchi. The trachea is lined with a typical respiratory mucosa (Figures 17–4 and 17–5). In the lamina propria are 16–20 C-shaped rings of hyaline cartilage that keep the tracheal lumen open. The open ends of these rings are located on the posterior surface of the trachea. A fibroelastic ligament and bundle of smooth muscle (trachealis muscle) bind to the perichondrium and bridge the open ends of these C-shaped cartilages. The ligament prevents overdistention of the lumen, and the muscle allows regulation of the lumen.

Contraction of the muscle and the resultant narrowing of the tracheal lumen are used in the cough reflex. The smaller bore of the trachea after contraction provides for increased velocity of expired air, which aids in clearing the air passage.

BRONCHIAL TREE

The trachea divides into two **primary bronchi** (Figure 17–1) that enter the lungs at the hilum. At each hilum, arteries enter, and veins and lymphatic vessels leave. These structures are surrounded by dense connective tissue and form a unit called the **pulmonary root.**

After entering the lungs, the primary bronchi course downward and outward, giving rise to three bronchi in the right lung and two in the left lung (Figure 17–1), each of which supplies a pulmonary lobe. These **lobar bronchi** divide repeatedly, giving rise to smaller bronchi, whose terminal branches are called **bronchioles.** Each bronchiole enters a pulmonary lobule, where it branches to form 5–7 **terminal bronchioles.**

The pulmonary lobules are pyramid-shaped, with the apex directed toward the pulmonary hilum. Each lobule is delineated by a thin connective tissue septum, best seen in the fetus. In adults, these septa are frequently incomplete, resulting in a poor delineation of the lobules.

The primary bronchi generally have the same histologic appearance as the trachea. Proceeding toward the respiratory portion, the histologic organization of both the epithelium and the underlying lamina pro-

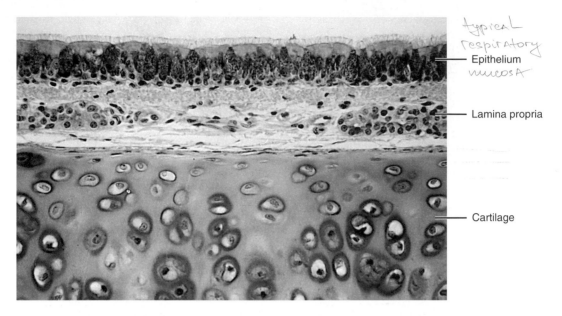

Epithelium *(handwritten: typical respiratory mucosa)*

Lamina propria

Cartilage

Figure 17–5. Photomicrograph of a section of dog trachea. × 200.

pria becomes simplified. It must be stressed that this simplification is gradual; no abrupt transition can be observed between the bronchi and bronchioles. For this reason, the division of the bronchial tree into bronchi, bronchioles, etc, is to some extent artificial—although this division has both pedagogic and practical value.

Bronchi

Each primary bronchus branches dichotomously 9–12 times, with each branch becoming progres-

sively smaller until it reaches a diameter of about 5 mm. Except for the organization of cartilage and smooth muscle, the mucosa of the bronchi is structurally similar to the mucosa of the trachea (Figures 17–6 and 17–7). The bronchial cartilages are more irregular in shape than those found in the trachea; in the larger portions of the bronchi, the cartilage rings completely encircle the lumen. As bronchial diameter decreases, the cartilage rings are replaced with isolated plates, or islands, of hyaline cartilage. Beneath the epithelium, in the bronchial lamina propria, is a

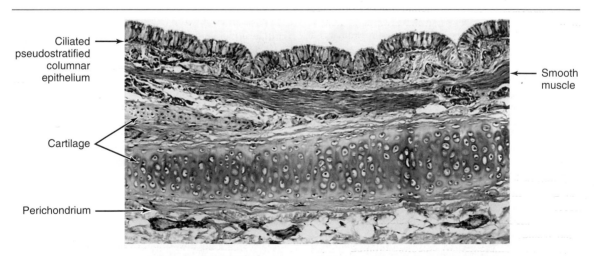

Ciliated pseudostratified columnar epithelium

Smooth muscle

Cartilage

Perichondrium

Figure 17–6. Photomicrograph of a large bronchus. Note the ciliated pseudostratified columnar epithelium with many goblet cells, two cartilaginous plates, and smooth muscle. Hematoxylin-and-eosin (H&E) stain. × 180.

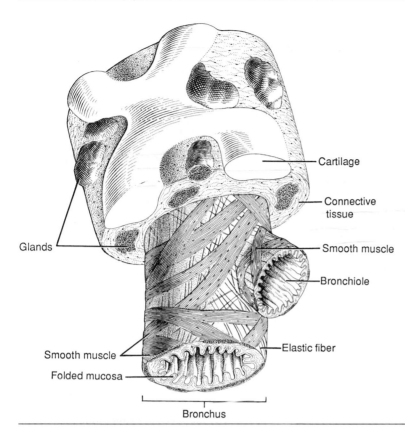

Glands

Smooth muscle

Folded mucosa

Bronchus

Cartilage

Connective tissue

Smooth muscle

Bronchiole

Elastic fiber

Figure 17–7. Structure of a bronchus. Contraction of this muscle induces folding of the mucosa. Smooth muscle is present in all of the bronchiolar tree, including the respiratory bronchiole. The elastic fibers in the bronchus continue into the bronchiole. An irregular cartilaginous plate sectioned in two regions is shown in white. The lower portion of the drawing represents a region with its connective tissue removed to show the presence of elastic fibers and smooth muscle. The adventitia is not shown.

smooth muscle layer consisting of crisscrossing bundles of spirally arranged smooth muscle (Figure 17–7) Bundles of smooth muscle become more prominent in the walls of the conducting portion near the respiratory zone. In histologic sections, this muscle layer appears to be discontinuous. Contraction of this muscle layer after death is responsible for the folded appearance of the bronchial mucosa observed in histologic section. The lamina propria is rich in elastic fibers and contains an abundance of mucous and serous glands whose ducts open into the bronchial lumen. Numerous lymphocytes are found both within the lamina propria and among the epithelial cells. Lymphatic nodules are present and are particularly numerous at the branching points of the bronchial tree.

Bronchioles

Bronchioles, intralobular airways with diameters of 5 mm or less (Figure 17–7), have neither cartilage nor glands in their mucosa; there are only scattered goblet cells within the epithelium of the initial segments. In the larger bronchioles, the epithelium is ciliated pseudostratified columnar, which decreases in height and complexity to become ciliated simple columnar or cuboidal epithelium in the smaller terminal bronchioles. The epithelium of terminal bronchi-

oles also contains **Clara cells** (Figure 17–8). These cells, which are devoid of cilia, have secretory granules in their apex and are known to secrete glycosaminoglycans that protect the bronchiolar lining. Probably, they are also a secondary source of surfactant for the bronchoalveolar fluid

The lamina propria is composed largely of smooth muscle and elastic fibers. The musculature of both the bronchi and the bronchioles is under the control of the vagus nerve and the sympathetic nervous system. Stimulation of the vagus nerve decreases the diameter of these structures; sympathetic stimulation produces the opposite effect. Bronchioles also exhibit specialized regions called **neuroepithelial bodies.** These are formed by groups of 80–100 cells that contain secretory granules and receive cholinergic nerve endings. Their function is poorly understood, but they are probably chemoreceptors that react to changes in gas composition within the airway. Their secretions are locally active.

The increase in bronchiole diameter in response to stimulation of the sympathetic nervous system explains why epinephrine and other sympathomimetic drugs are frequently used to relax smooth muscle during asthma attacks. When the thicknesses of the bronchial and bronchiolar

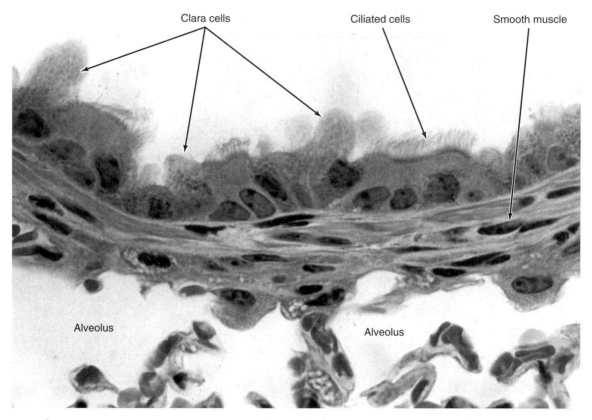

Figure 17–8. Photomicrograph of a portion of a terminal bronchiole in mouse lung. In addition to the ciliated cuboidal cells are larger secretory Clara cells. Bundles of smooth muscle cells lie beneath the epithelium, and alveoli surround the terminal bronchiole. × 800.

walls are compared, it can be seen that the bronchiolar muscle layer is more developed than that of the bronchi. Increased airway resistance in asthma is believed to be due mainly to contraction of bronchiolar smooth muscle.

Respiratory Bronchioles

Each terminal bronchiole subdivides into two or more respiratory bronchioles that serve as regions of transition between the conducting and respiratory portions of the respiratory system (Figures 17–9 and 17–10). The respiratory bronchiolar mucosa is structurally identical to that of the terminal bronchioles, except that their walls are interrupted by numerous sac-like alveoli where gas exchange occurs (Figures 17–1, 17–9, and 17–10). Portions of the respiratory bronchioles are lined with ciliated cuboidal epithelial cells and Clara cells, but at the rim of the alveolar openings the bronchiolar epithelium becomes continuous with the squamous alveolar lining cells (type I alveolar cells; see below). Proceeding distally along these bronchioles, the alveoli increase greatly in number, and the distance between them is markedly reduced. Between alveoli, the bronchiolar epithelium

consists of ciliated cuboidal epithelium; however, the cilia may be absent in more distal portions. Smooth muscle and elastic connective tissue lie beneath the epithelium of respiratory bronchioles.

Alveolar Ducts

Proceeding distally along the respiratory bronchioles, the number of alveolar openings into the bronchiolar wall becomes ever greater until the wall consists of nothing else, and the tube is now called an **alveolar duct** (Figure 17–10). Both the alveolar ducts and the alveoli are lined with extremely attenuated squamous alveolar cells. In the lamina propria surrounding the rim of the alveoli is a network of smooth muscle cells. These sphincter-like smooth muscle bundles appear as knobs between adjacent alveoli. Smooth muscle disappears at the distal ends of alveolar ducts. A rich matrix of elastic and collagen fibers provides the only support of the duct and its alveoli.

Alveolar ducts open into **atria** that communicate with **alveolar sacs,** two or more of which arise from each atrium. Elastic and reticular fibers form a complex network encircling the openings of atria, alveo-

Terminal bronchiole

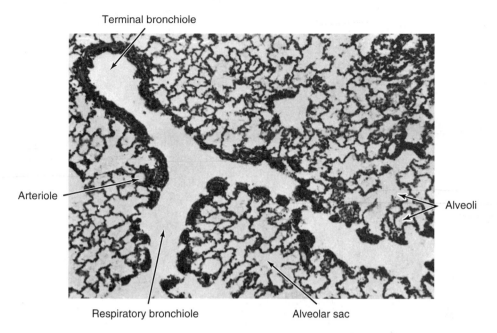

Arteriole

Alveoli

Respiratory bronchiole

Alveolar sac

Figure 17–9. Photomicrograph of a thick section of lung showing a terminal bronchiole dividing into two respiratory bronchioles, in which alveoli appear. The sponge-like appearance of the lung is due to the abundance of alveoli and alveolar sacs. H&E stain. × 80.

lar sacs, and alveoli. The elastic fibers enable the alveoli to expand with inspiration and to contract passively with expiration. The reticular fibers serve as a support that prevents overdistention and damage to the delicate capillaries and thin alveolar septa.

Alveoli

Alveoli are sac-like evaginations (about 200 μm in diameter) of the respiratory bronchioles, alveolar ducts, and alveolar sacs. Alveoli are the terminal portions of the bronchial tree and are responsible for the spongy structure of the lungs. Structurally, alveoli resemble small pockets that are open on one side, similar to the honeycombs of a beehive. Within these cup-like structures, O_2 and CO_2 are exchanged between the air and the blood. The structure of the alveolar walls is specialized for enhancing diffusion between the external and internal environments. Generally, each wall lies between two neighboring alveoli and is therefore called an **interalveolar septum,** or **wall.** An interalveolar septum consists of two thin squamous epithelial layers between which lie capillaries, fibroblasts, elastic and reticular fibers, and macrophages. The capillaries and connective tissue matrix constitute the **interstitium.** Within the interstitium of the interalveolar septum is found the richest capillary network in the body (Figure 17–11).

Air in the alveoli is separated from capillary blood by three components referred to collectively as the **blood-air barrier:** the surface lining and cytoplasm

of the alveolar cells; the fused basal laminae of the closely apposed alveolar and endothelial cells; and the cytoplasm of the endothelial cells (Figures 17–11, 17–12, and 17–13). The total thickness of these layers varies from 0.1 to 1.5 μm. Within the interalveolar septum, anastomosing pulmonary capillaries are supported by a meshwork of reticular and elastic fibers. These fibers, which are arranged to permit expansion and contraction of the interalveolar septum, are the primary means of structural support of the alveoli. The basement membrane, leukocytes, macrophages, and fibroblasts can also be found within the interstitium of the septum (Figure 17–11). The basement membrane is formed by the fusion of two basal laminae produced by the endothelial cells and the epithelial (alveolar) cells of the interalveolar septum.

O_2 from the alveolar air passes into the capillary blood through the blood-air barrier (Figure 17–13); CO_2 diffuses in the opposite direction. Liberation of CO_2 from H_2CO_3 is catalyzed by the enzyme **carbonic anhydrase** present in erythrocytes. The approximately 300 million alveoli in the lungs considerably increase their internal exchange surface, which has been calculated to be approximately 140 m².

The interalveolar septum is composed of five main cell types: capillary endothelial cells (30%); type I (squamous alveolar) epithelial cells (8%); type II (septal, great alveolar) epithelial cells (16%); intersti-

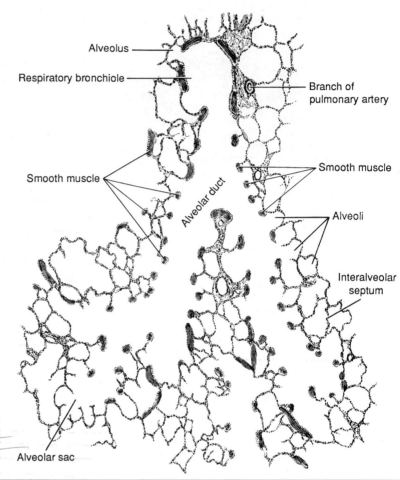

Alveolus

Respiratory bronchiole

Branch of
pulmonary artery

Smooth muscle

Smooth muscle

Alveolar duct

Alveoli

Interalveolar
septum

Figure 17–10. Diagram of a portion of the bronchial tree. Note that the smooth muscle in the alveolar duct disappears in the alveoli. (Redrawn from Baltisberger.)

Alveolar sac

tial cells, including fibroblasts and mast cells (36%); and alveolar macrophages (10%). See Figures 17–11, 17–12, and 17–14.

Capillary endothelial cells are extremely thin and can be easily confused with type I alveolar epithelial cells. The endothelial lining of the capillaries is continuous and not fenestrated (Figure 17–12). Clustering of the nuclei and other organelles allows the remaining areas of the cell to become extremely thin, increasing the efficiency of gas exchange. The most prominent feature of the cytoplasm in the flattened portions of the cell is numerous pinocytotic vesicles.

Type I cells, or **squamous alveolar cells,** are extremely attenuated cells that line the alveolar surfaces. Type I cells make up 97% of the alveolar surfaces (type II cells make up the remaining 3%). These cells are so thin (sometimes only 25 nm) that the electron microscope was needed to prove that all alveoli are covered with an epithelial lining (Figures 17–11 and 17–12). Organelles such as the Golgi complex, endoplasmic reticulum, and mitochondria

are grouped around the nucleus, reducing the thickness of the blood-air barrier and leaving large areas of cytoplasm virtually free of organelles. The cytoplasm in the thin portion contains abundant pinocytotic vesicles, which may play a role in the turnover of surfactant (described below) and the removal of small particulate contaminants from the outer surface. In addition to desmosomes, all type I epithelial cells have occluding junctions that prevent the leakage of tissue fluid into the alveolar air space (Figure 17–15). The main role of these cells is to provide a barrier of minimal thickness that is readily permeable to gases.

Type II cells, or **great alveolar cells** (also called **septal cells**), are interspersed among the type I alveolar cells with which they have occluding and desmosomal junctions (Figures 17–16 and 17–17). Type II cells are roughly cuboidal cells that are usually found in groups of two or three along the alveolar surface at points where the alveolar walls unite and form angles. These cells, which rest on the basement mem-

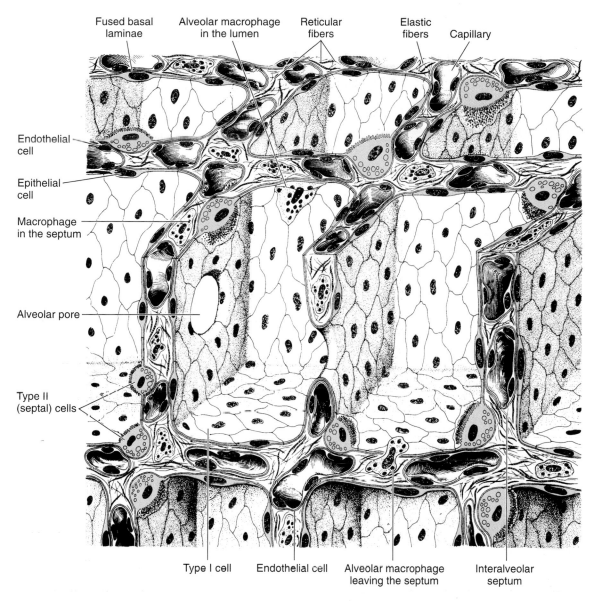

Figure 17–11. Three-dimensional schematic diagram of pulmonary alveoli showing the structure of the interalveolar septum. Note the capillaries, connective tissue, and macrophages. These cells can also be seen in—or passing into—the alveolar lumen. Alveolar pores are numerous. Type II cells are identified by their abundant apical microvilli. The alveoli are lined with a continuous epithelial layer of type I cells.

brane, are part of the epithelium, with the same origin as the type I cells that line the alveolar walls. They divide by mitosis to replace their own population and also the type I population. In histologic sections, they exhibit a characteristic vesicular or foamy cytoplasm. These vesicles are caused by the presence of **lamellar bodies** (Figures 17–16 and 17–17) that are preserved and evident in tissue prepared for electron microscopy. Lamellar bodies, which average

1–2 μm in diameter, contain concentric or parallel lamellae limited by a unit membrane. Histochemical studies show that these bodies, which contain phospholipids, glycosaminoglycans, and proteins, are continuously synthesized and released at the apical surface of the cells. The lamellar bodies give rise to a material that spreads over the alveolar surfaces, providing an extracellular alveolar coating, **pulmonary surfactant,** that lowers alveolar surface tension.

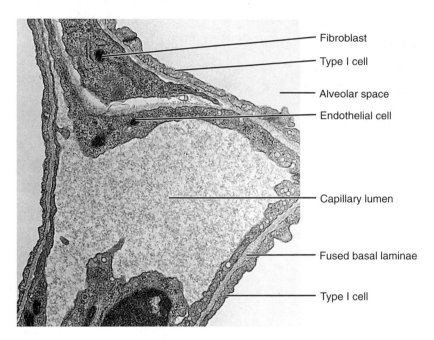

Fibroblast

Type I cell

Alveolar space

Endothelial cell

Capillary lumen

Fused basal laminae

Type I cell

Figure 17–12. Electron micrograph of the interalveolar septum. Note the capillary lumen, alveolar spaces, alveolar type I epithelial cells, fused basal laminae, and a fibroblast. × 30,000. (Courtesy of MC Williams.)

The surfactant layer consists of an aqueous, proteinaceous hypophase covered with a monomolecular phospholipid film that is primarily composed of **dipalmitoyl phosphatidylcholine** and **phosphatidylglycerol.** Surfactant also contains unique proteins, called **surfactant proteins A, B, C,** and **D.** Pulmonary surfactant serves several major functions in the economy of the lung, but it primarily aids in reducing the surface tension of the alveolar cells. The reduction of surface tension means that less inspiratory force is needed to inflate the alveoli, and thus the work of breathing in reduced. In addition, without surfactant, alveoli would tend to collapse during expiration. In fetal development, surfactant appears in the last weeks of gestation and coincides with the appearance of lamellar bodies in the type II cells.

Infants born prematurely often have the labored breathing that signifies respiratory distress. **Hyaline membrane disease** in these newborns has been shown to be the result of insufficient surfactant production—the infant has difficulty expanding the alveoli. Fortunately, synthesis of surfactant can be induced by administration of glucocorticoids, so the **respiratory distress syndrome** is usually a short-term management problem. Recently, surfactant has also been suggested to have a bactericidal effect, aiding in the removal of potentially dangerous bacteria that reach the alveoli.

The surfactant layer is not static but is constantly being turned over. The lipoproteins are gradually removed from the surface by the pinocytotic vesicles of the squamous epithelial cells, by macrophages, and by type II alveolar cells.

Alveolar lining fluids are also removed via the conducting passages as a result of ciliary activity. As the secretions pass up through the airways, they combine with bronchial mucus, forming a **bronchoalveolar fluid,** which aids in the removal of particulate and noxious components from the inspired air. The bronchoalveolar fluid contains several lytic enzymes (eg, lysozyme, collagenase, β-glucuronidase) that are probably derived from the alveolar macrophages.

Interalveolar Septum

The barrier between blood plasma and inspired air is the alveolar epithelium, a basement membrane of two fused basal laminae, and the capillary endothelium. Alveolar macrophages, also called **dust cells,** are derived from monocytes that originate in bone marrow. They are found in the interior of the interalveolar septum and are often seen on the surface of the alveolus. Numerous carbon- and dust-laden macrophages in the connective tissue around major blood vessels or in the pleura probably represent cells that have never passed through the epithelial lining. The phagocytized debris within these cells was most likely passed from the alveolar lumen into the interstitium by the pinocytotic activity of type I

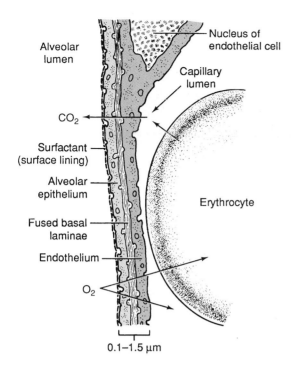

Figure 17–13. Portion of the interalveolar septum showing the blood-air barrier. To reach the erythrocyte, O_2 traverses the surface lining, the alveolar epithelium cytoplasm, and the plasma. In some locations, there is loose interstitial tissue between the epithelium and the endothelium. (Modified and reproduced, with permission, from Ganong WF: *Review of Medical Physiology,* 8th ed. Lange, 1977.)

alveolar cells. The alveolar macrophages that scavenge the outer surface of the epithelium within the surfactant layer are carried to the pharynx, where they are swallowed.

In congestive heart failure, the lungs become congested with blood, and erythrocytes pass into the alveoli, where they are phagocytized by alveolar macrophages. In such cases, these macrophages are called **heart failure cells** when present in the lung and sputum; they are identified by a positive histochemical reaction for iron pigment (hemosiderin).

In addition to the cells discussed above, the interalveolar septum contains fibroblasts, mast cells, and other connective tissue cells. Interstitial fibroblasts synthesize collagen, elastic fibers, and proteoglycans. Collagen (type III) is present mainly in the alveolar reticular fibers. Collagen and elastic fibers are important components that contribute resilience and elasticity, respectively, to the biomechanical properties of the lung.

Increased production of collagen is common, and many diseases that lead to respiratory distress are known to be associated with lung fibrosis. In these pathologic conditions the collagen present is type I.

Alveolar Pores

The interalveolar septum contains pores, 10–15 μm in diameter, that connect neighboring alveoli (Figures 17–11 and 17–18). These pores equalize air pressure in the alveoli and promote the collateral circulation of air when a bronchiole is obstructed.

Alveolar-Lining Regeneration

Inhalation of NO_2 destroys most of the cells lining the alveoli (type I and type II cells). The action of this compound or other toxic substances with the same effect is followed by an increase in the mitotic activity of the remaining type II cells. The normal turnover rate of type II cells is estimated to be 1% per day and results in a continuous renewal of both its own population and that of type I cells.

The destruction of the interalveolar septum, with subsequent reduction of the respiratory portion of the lungs, is called **emphysema.** Emphysema usually develops gradually and results in respiratory insufficiency. This leading cause of death in the industrialized world is clearly associated with smoking and environmental air pollution.

PULMONARY BLOOD VESSELS

Circulation in the lungs includes both nutrient (systemic) and functional (pulmonary) vessels. The functional circulation is represented by pulmonary arteries and veins. Pulmonary arteries are thin-walled as a result of the low pressures (25 mm Hg systolic, 5 mm Hg diastolic) encountered in the pulmonary circuit. Within the lung the pulmonary artery branches, accompanying the bronchial tree (Figure 17–19). Its branches are surrounded by adventitia of the bronchi and bronchioles. At the level of the alveolar duct, the branches of this artery form a capillary network in the interalveolar septum and in close contact with the alveolar epithelium. The lung has the best-developed capillary network in the body, with capillaries between all alveoli, including those in the respiratory bronchioles.

Venules that originate in the capillary network are found singly in the parenchyma, somewhat removed from the airways; they are supported by a thin covering of connective tissue and enter the interlobular septum (Figure 17–19). After veins leave a lobule, they follow the bronchial tree toward the hilum.

Nutrient vessels follow the bronchial tree and distribute blood to most of the lung up to the respiratory

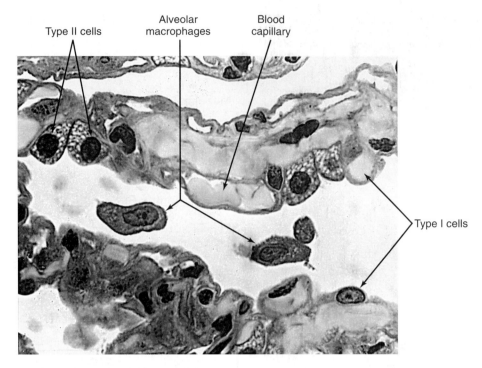

Figure 17–14. Photomicrograph of lung alveolar walls showing type I and type II cells, blood capillaries, and alveolar macrophages.

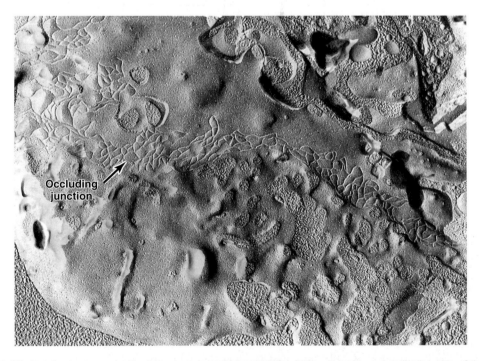

Figure 17–15. Cryofracture preparation showing an occluding junction between two type I epithelial cells of the alveolar lining. × 25,000. (Reproduced, with permission, from Schneeberger EE: *Lung Liquids.* Ciba Foundation Symposium no. 38. Elsevier/North-Holland, 1976.)

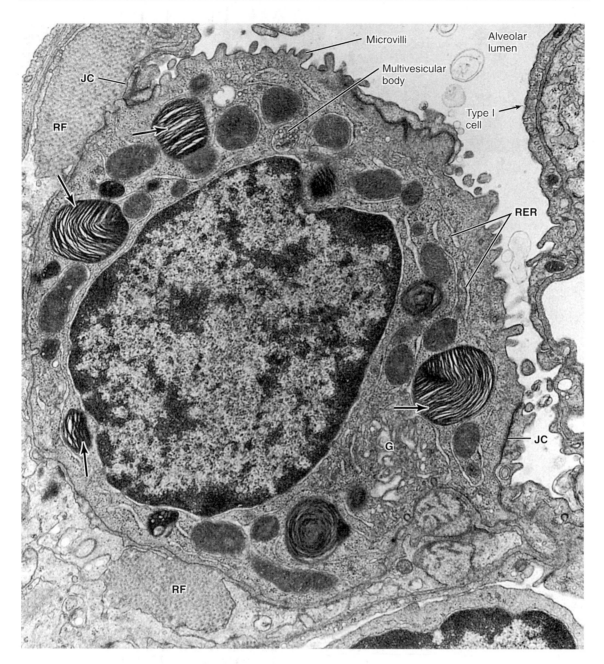

Figure 17–16. Photomicrograph of a type II cell protruding into the alveolar lumen of a rat lung. Arrows indicate lamellar bodies containing newly synthesized pulmonary surfactant. RER, rough endoplasmic reticulum; G, Golgi complex; RF, reticular fibers; A, cytoplasm of a type I epithelial cell. Note the microvilli of the type II cell and the junctional complexes (JC) with the type I epithelial cell. × 17,000. (Courtesy of MC Williams.)

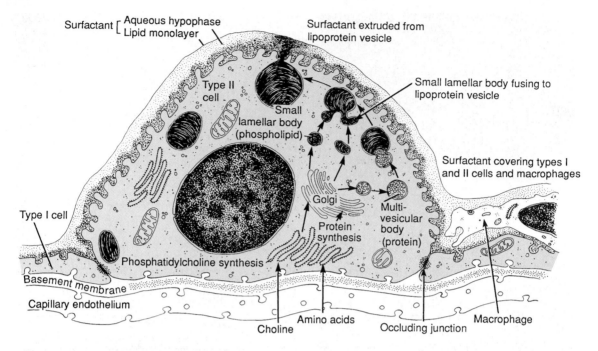

Figure 17–17. Secretion of surfactant by a type II cell. Surfactant is a protein-lipid complex synthesized in the rough endoplasmic reticulum and Golgi complex and stored in the lamellar bodies. It is continuously secreted by means of exocytosis (arrows) and forms an overlying monomolecular film of lipid covering an underlying aqueous hypophase. When macrophages are present in the alveolar lumen, they lie outside the epithelium but within the surfactant layer. Occluding junctions around the margins of the epithelial cells prevent leakage of tissue fluid into the alveolar lumen.

bronchioles, at which point they anastomose with small branches of the pulmonary artery.

PULMONARY LYMPHATIC VESSELS

The lymphatic vessels (Figure 17–19) follow the bronchi and the pulmonary vessels; they are also found in the interlobular septum, and they all drain into lymph nodes in the region of the hilum. This lymphatic network is called the **deep network** to distinguish it from the **superficial network,** which includes the lymphatic vessels in the visceral pleura. The lymphatic vessels of the superficial network drain toward the hilum. They either follow the entire length of the pleura or penetrate the lung tissue via the interlobular septum.

Lymphatic vessels are not found in the terminal portions of the bronchial tree or beyond the alveolar ducts.

NERVES

Both parasympathetic and sympathetic efferent fibers innervate the lungs; general visceral afferent fibers, carrying poorly localized pain sensations, are also present. Most of the nerves are found in the connective tissues surrounding the larger airways.

Parasympathetic stimulation, via the vagus nerve, results in bronchial constriction from smooth muscle contraction, whereas sympathetic stimulation causes bronchial dilatation. Drugs that mimic sympathetic neurotransmitters, such as isoproterenol, are used to cause bronchial dilatation during asthma attacks.

PLEURA

The pleura (Figure 17–19) is the serous membrane covering the lung. It consists of two layers, parietal and visceral, that are continuous in the region of the hilum. Both membranes are composed of mesothelial cells resting on a fine connective tissue layer that contains collagen and elastic fibers. The elastic fibers of the visceral pleura are continuous with those of the pulmonary parenchyma.

The parietal and visceral layers define a cavity entirely lined with squamous mesothelial cells. Under normal conditions, this pleural cavity contains only a

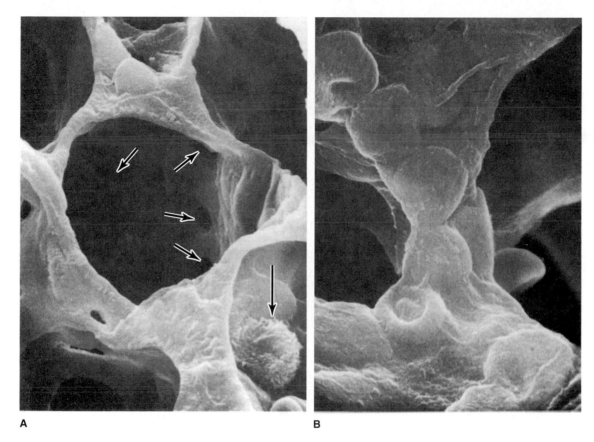

Figure 17–18. Scanning electron micrographs of mouse lung. **A:** Note the thin septa and alveolar pores (white arrows). At the black arrow, a macrophage with its typical ruffled membrane is seen. × 3200. **B:** The interalveolar septum is so thin that the shape of the erythrocytes in a capillary can be seen. × 6700. (Reprinted, with permission, from Greenwood MF, Holland P: The mammalian respiratory tract surface: a scanning electron microscope study. Lab Invest 1972;27:296.)

film of liquid that acts as a lubricant, facilitating the smooth sliding of one surface over the other during respiratory movements.

In certain pathologic states, the pleural cavity can become a real cavity, containing liquid or air. The walls of the pleural cavity, like all serosal cavities (peritoneal and pericardial), are quite permeable to water and other substances—hence the high frequency of fluid accumulation (pleural effusion) in this cavity in pathologic conditions. This fluid is derived from the blood plasma by exudation. Conversely, under certain conditions, liquids or gases in the pleural cavity can be rapidly absorbed.

RESPIRATORY MOVEMENTS

During inhalation, contraction of the intercostal muscles elevates the ribs, and contraction of the di-aphragm lowers the bottom of the thoracic cavity, increasing its diameter and resulting in pulmonary expansion. The bronchi and bronchioles increase in diameter and length during inhalation. The respiratory portion also enlarges, mainly as a result of expansion of the alveolar ducts; the alveoli enlarge only slightly. The elastic fibers of the pulmonary parenchyma are stretched by this expansion. Retraction of the lungs is passive during exhalation. Retraction is the result of muscle relaxation and the action of elastic fibers, which had been under tension.

DEFENSE MECHANISMS

The respiratory system has an exceptionally large area that is exposed to both blood and the external environment. Because it is consequently very susceptible to the invasion of airborne infective and noninfective agents, it is not surprising that the respiratory system presents an elaborate array of defense mecha-

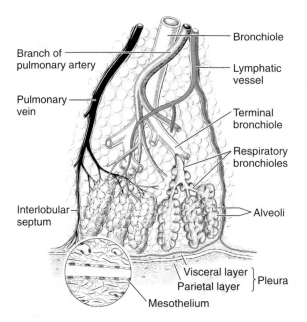

Branch of pulmonary artery

Pulmonary vein

Interlobular septum

Bronchiole

Lymphatic vessel

Terminal bronchiole

Respiratory bronchioles

Alveoli

Visceral layer
Parietal layer } Pleura

Mesothelium

Figure 17–19. Blood and lymph circulation in a pulmonary lobule. Both vessels and bronchi are enlarged out of proportion in this drawing. In the interlobular septum, only one vein (on the left) and one lymphatic vessel (on the right) are shown, although both actually coexist in both regions. At the lower left, an enlargement of the pleura shows its mesothelial lining. (Modified and reproduced, with permission, from Ham AW: *Histology,* 6th ed. Lippincott, 1969.)

nisms. Particles larger than 10 μm are retained in the nasal passages, and particles of 2 to 10 μm are trapped by the mucus-coated ciliated epithelium. The cough reflex can eliminate these particles by expectoration or swallowing. Smaller particles are removed by alveolar macrophages. In addition to these nonspecific mechanisms, elaborate immunologic processes occur in abundant lymphoid tissues of the bronchus, mainly in nodules containing T and B lymphocytes that interact with lung macrophages. This important component of the immune system is called **BALT** (bronchus-associated lymphatic tissue).

Tumors of the Lung

The incidence of lung tumors is higher in men but is increasing in women, probably because of cigarette smoking. There is conclusive evidence that squamous cell carcinoma, the principal lung tumor type, is related to the effects of cigarette smoking on the bronchial and bronchiolar epithelial lining. Chronic smoking induces the transformation of the respiratory epithelium into a stratified squamous epithelium, an initial step in its eventual differentiation into a tumor.

REFERENCES

Bouhuy SA: *Lung Cells in Disease.* Elsevier/North-Holland, 1976.
Breeze RG, Wheeldon EG: The cells of the pulmonary airways. Am Rev Respir Dis 1977;116:705.
Camner P et al: Evidence for congenital nonfunctional cilia in the tracheobronchial tract in two subjects. Am Rev Respir Dis 1975;112:807.
Cummings G (editor): *Cellular Biology of the Lung.* Ettore Majorana International Science Service, 1982.
Evans MJ: Transformation of type II cells to type I cells following exposure to NO_2. Exp Mol Pathol 1975;22:142.
Gehr P et al: The normal human lung: ultrastructure and morphometric estimation of diffusion capacity. Respir Physiol 1978;32:121.

Greenwood M, Holland P: The mammalian respiratory tract surface: a scanning electron microscope study. Lab Invest 1972;27:296.
Kikkawa Y, Smith F: Cellular and biochemical aspects of pulmonary surfactant in health and disease. Lab Invest 1983;49:122.
Kuhn C III: The cells of the lung and their organelles. In: *The Biochemical Basis of Pulmonary Function.* Crystal RG (editor). Marcel Dekker, 1976.
Takashima T: *Airway Secretion: Physiological Bases for the Control of Mucous Hypersecretion.* Marcel Dekker, 1994.
Thurlbeck WM, Abell RM (editors): *The Lung: Structure, Function, and Disease.* Williams & Wilkins, 1978.

Skin

18

The skin is the heaviest single organ of the body, accounting for about 16% of total body weight and, in adults, presenting 1.2–2.3 m² of surface to the external environment. It is composed of the **epidermis,** an epithelial layer of ectodermal origin, and the **dermis,** a layer of connective tissue of mesodermal origin. Based on the comparative thickness of the epidermis, **thick** and **thin** skin can be distinguished (Figures 18–1 and 18–2). The junction of dermis and epidermis is irregular, and projections of the dermis called **papillae** interdigitate with evaginations of the epidermis known as **epidermal ridges.** In three dimensions, these interdigitations may be of the peg-and-socket variety (thin skin) or formed of ridges and grooves (thick skin). Epidermal derivatives include hairs, nails, and sebaceous and sweat glands. Beneath the dermis lies the **hypodermis** (Gr. *hypo,* under, + *derma,* skin), or **subcutaneous tissue,** a loose connective tissue that may contain a pad of adipose cells, the **panniculus adiposus.** The hypodermis, which is not considered part of the skin, binds skin loosely to the subjacent tissues and corresponds to the superficial fascia of gross anatomy.

The external layer of the skin is relatively impermeable to water, which prevents water loss by evaporation and allows for terrestrial life. The skin functions as a receptor organ in continuous communication with the environment (see Chapter 24) and protects the organism from impact and friction injuries. **Melanin,** a pigment produced and stored in the cells of the epidermis, provides further protective action against the sun's ultraviolet rays. Glands of the skin, blood vessels, and adipose tissue participate in thermoregulation, body metabolism, and the excretion of various substances. Under the action of solar radiation, vitamin D_3 is formed from precursors synthesized by the epidermal layer. Because skin is elastic, it can expand to cover large areas in conditions associated with swelling, such as edema and pregnancy.

Upon close observation, certain portions of human skin show ridges and grooves arranged in distinctive patterns. These ridges first appear during intrauterine life—at 13 weeks in the tips of the fingers and later in the volar surfaces of the hands and feet (palm and sole). The patterns assumed by ridges and intervening sulci are known as **dermatoglyphics** (fingerprints). They are unique for each individual, appearing as loops, arches, whorls, or combinations of these forms. These configurations, which are used for personal identification, are probably determined by multiple genes; the field of dermatoglyphics has come to be of considerable medical and anthropologic as well as legal interest.

EPIDERMIS

The epidermis consists mainly of a stratified squamous keratinized epithelium, but it also contains three less abundant cell types: **melanocytes, Langerhans cells,** and **Merkel's cells.** The keratinizing epidermal cells are called **keratinocytes.** It is customary to distinguish between the **thick skin (glabrous,** or smooth and nonhairy) found on the palms and soles and the **thin skin** (hairy) found elsewhere on the body. The designations "thick" and "thin" refer to the thickness of the epidermal layer, which varies between 75 and 150 μm for thin skin and 400 and 600 μm for thick skin. Total skin thickness (epidermis plus dermis) also varies according to site. For example, skin on the back is about 4 mm thick, whereas that of the scalp is about 1.5 mm thick.

From the dermis outward, the epidermis consists of five layers of keratin-producing cells (keratinocytes).

A. Stratum Basale (Stratum Germinativum): The stratum basale consists of a single layer of basophilic columnar or cuboidal cells resting on the basal lamina at the dermal-epidermal junction. Desmosomes bind the cells of this layer together in their lateral and upper surfaces. Hemidesmosomes, found in the basal plasmalemma, help bind these cells to the basal lamina. The stratum basale is characterized by intense mitotic activity and is responsible, in conjunction with the initial portion of the next layer, for constant renewal of epidermal cells. The human epidermis is renewed about every 15–30

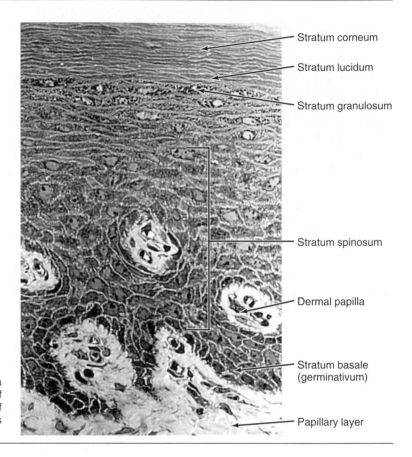

Stratum corneum

Stratum lucidum

Stratum granulosum

Stratum spinosum

Dermal papilla

Stratum basale
(germinativum)

Papillary layer

Figure 18–1. Photomicrograph of a section of thick skin from the sole of a human foot. Note the papillae of the papillary layer and the thickness of the stratum corneum.

days, depending on age, the region of the body, and other factors. All cells in the stratum basale contain intermediate keratin filaments about 10 nm in diameter. As the cells progress upward, the number of filaments increases until they represent half the total protein in the stratum corneum.

B. Stratum Spinosum: The stratum spinosum (Figure 18–1) consists of cuboidal, or slightly flattened, cells with a central nucleus and a cytoplasm whose processes are filled with bundles of keratin filaments. These bundles converge into many small cellular extensions, terminating with desmosomes located at the tips of these spiny projections (Figure 18–3). The cells of this layer are firmly bound together by the filament-filled cytoplasmic spines and desmosomes that punctuate the cell surface, giving a spine-studded appearance. These tonofilament bundles, visible under the light microscope, are called **tonofibrils;** they end at and insert into the cytoplasmic densities of the desmosomes. The filaments play an important role in maintaining cohesion among cells and resisting the effects of abrasion. The epidermis of areas subjected to continuous friction and pressure (such as the soles of the feet) has a thicker stratum spinosum with more abundant tonofibrils and desmosomes.

All mitoses are confined to what is termed the

malpighian layer, which consists of both the stratum basale and the stratum spinosum.

C. Stratum Granulosum: The stratum granulosum consists of three to five layers of flattened polygonal cells whose cytoplasm is filled with coarse basophilic granules (Figure 18–1) called **keratohyalin granules.** These granules contain a phosphorylated histidine-rich protein as well as proteins containing cystine. The numerous phosphate groups account for the intense basophilia of keratohyalin granules, which are not surrounded by a membrane.

Another characteristic structure in the cells of the granular layer of epidermis that can be seen with the electron microscope is the membrane-coated **lamellar granule,** a small (0.1–0.3 μm) ovoid or rod-like structure containing lamellar disks that are formed by lipid bilayers. These granules fuse with the cell membrane and discharge their contents into the intercellular spaces of the stratum granulosum, where they are deposited in the form of sheets containing lipid. The function of this extruded material is similar to that of an intercellular cement in that it acts as a barrier to penetration by foreign materials and provides a very important sealing effect in the skin. Studies of keratinized and nonkeratinized human oral epithelium show no penetration by peroxidase and lanthanum tracers in the regions where this material fills the ex-

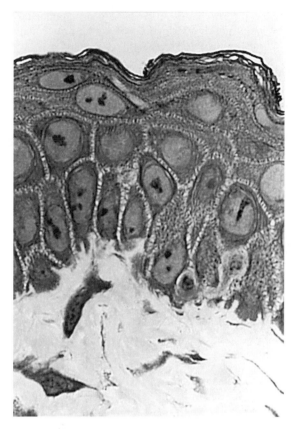

Figure 18–2. Photomicrograph of a section of thin human skin. Note the comparative reduction of cell layers in the stratum spinosum and the thinness of the stratum corneum.

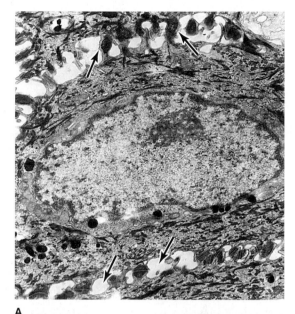

A

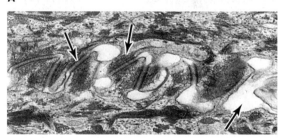

B

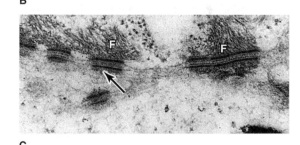

C

Figure 18–3. Electron micrograph of the stratum spinosum of human skin. **A:** A cell of the stratum spinosum with melanin granules and with its cytoplasm full of tonofibrils. The arrows show the spines, or intercellular bridges, with their desmosomes. × 8400. **B** and **C:** The desmosomes from A, in greater detail. Note that a dense substance appears between the cell membranes and that bundles of cytoplasmic filaments (tonofilaments; F) insert themselves on the desmosomes. B, × 36,000; C, × 45,000. (Courtesy of C Barros.)

tracellular space. Formation of this barrier, which appeared first in reptiles, was one of the important evolutionary events that permitted development of terrestrial life.

D. Stratum Lucidum: More apparent in thick skin, the stratum lucidum is a translucent, thin layer of extremely flattened eosinophilic cells (Figure 18–1). The organelles and nuclei are no longer evident, and the cytoplasm consists primarily of densely packed keratin filaments embedded in an electron-dense matrix. Desmosomes are still evident between adjacent cells.

E. Stratum Corneum: The stratum corneum (Figure 18–1) consists of 15–20 layers of flattened nonnucleated keratinized cells whose cytoplasm is filled with a birefringent filamentous scleroprotein, **keratin.** Keratin contains at least six different polypeptides with molecular mass ranging from 40 to 70 kDa. Three polypeptide chains coil around one another to form subunits (47 nm long) of the tonofilament. At least one of the polypeptides is different from the others in the subunit, allowing great diversity in composition. Nine of the three-chain subunits coil around each other, forming a filament about 10 nm in diameter. End-to-end aggregation of three-chain subunits increases the length of the tonofilament. The composition of tonofilaments changes as epidermal cells differentiate. Basal cells contain polypeptides of lower molecular weight, whereas more differentiated cells synthesize the higher-molecular-weight polypeptides. Tonofilaments are packed together in a matrix contributed by the keratohyalin granules.

After keratinization, the cells consist of only fibrillar and amorphous proteins and thickened plasma membranes; they are called **horny cells.** Lysosomal hydrolytic enzymes play a role in the disappearance of the cytoplasmic organelles. These cells are continuously shed at the surface of the stratum corneum.

This description of the epidermis corresponds to its most complex structure in areas where it is very thick, as on the soles of the feet. In thin skin, the stratum granulosum and the stratum lucidum are often less well developed, and the stratum corneum may be quite thin.

> In **psoriasis,** a common skin disease, there is an increase in the number of proliferating cells in the stratum basale and the stratum spinosum as well as a decrease in the cycle time of these

cells. This results in greater epidermal thickness and more rapid renewal of epidermis—7 days instead of 15–30 days.

Melanocytes

The color of the skin is the result of several factors, the most important of which are its content of **melanin** and **carotene,** the number of blood vessels in the dermis, and the color of the blood flowing in them.

Eumelanin is a dark brown pigment produced by the **melanocyte** (Figures 18–4 and 18–5), a specialized cell of the epidermis found beneath or between the cells of the stratum basale and in the hair follicles. The pigment found in red hair is called **pheomelanin** (Gr. *phaios,* dusky, + *melas,* black) and contains **cysteine** as part of its structure. Melanocytes are derived from neural crest cells. They have rounded cell bodies from which long irregular extensions branch into the epidermis, running between the cells of the strata basale and spinosum. Tips of these extensions terminate in invaginations of the cells present in the two layers. The electron microscope reveals a pale-staining cell containing numerous small mitochondria, a well-developed Golgi complex, and short cisternae of rough endoplasmic reticulum. Intermediate filaments, about 10 nm in diameter, are also present. Although melanocytes are

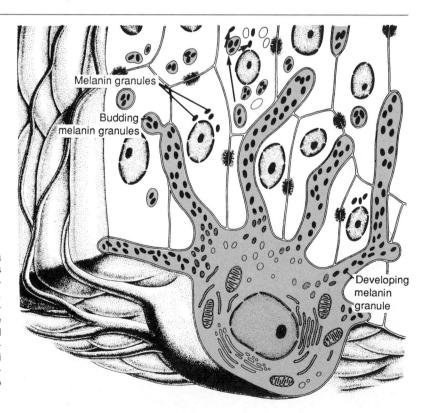

Figure 18–4. Diagram of a melanocyte (shown in color). Its arms extend upward into the interstices between keratinocytes. The melanin granules are synthesized in the melanocyte, migrate to its arms, and are transferred into the cytoplasm of keratinocytes (arrows). Ribosomes, Golgi complex, rough endoplasmic reticulum, and mitochondria are also present.

Melanin granules

Budding melanin granules

Developing melanin granule

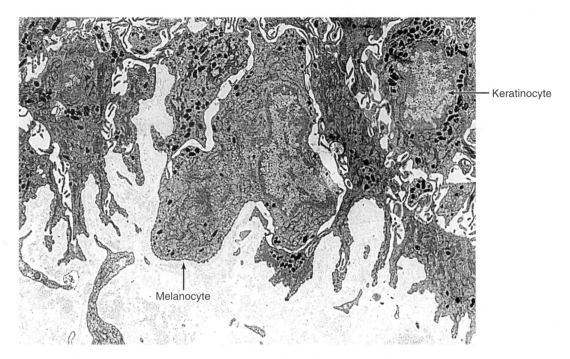

Figure 18–5. Electron micrograph of human skin containing melanocytes and keratinocytes. Note the greater abundance of melanin granules in the keratinocyte at right than in the adjacent melanocyte. The clear material at the bottom is dermal collagen. × 1800.

not attached to the adjacent keratinocytes by desmosomes, they are bound to the basal lamina by hemidesmosomes.

Melanin is synthesized in the melanocyte, with tyrosinase playing an important role in the process. As a result of tyrosinase activity, tyrosine is transformed first into **3,4-dihydroxyphenylalanine** (**dopa**) and then into **dopaquinone,** which is converted, after a series of transformations, into melanin. Tyrosinase is synthesized on ribosomes, transported in the lumen of the rough endoplasmic reticulum of melanocytes, and accumulated in vesicles formed in the Golgi complex (Figure 18–6). Four stages can be distinguished in the development of the mature melanin granule:

A.   Stage I: A vesicle is surrounded by a membrane and shows the beginning of tyrosinase activity and formation of fine granular material; at its periphery, electron-dense strands have an orderly arrangement of tyrosinase molecules on a protein matrix.

B.   Stage II: The vesicle (**melanosome**) is ovoid and shows, in its interior, parallel filaments with a periodicity of about 10 nm or cross-striations of about the same periodicity. Melanin is deposited on the protein matrix.

C.   Stage III: Increased melanin formation makes the periodic fine structure less visible.

D.   Stage IV: The mature melanin granule is visible in the light microscope, and melanin completely fills the vesicle. No ultrastructure is visible. The mature granules are ellipsoid, with a length of 1 μm and a diameter of 0.4 μm.

Once formed, melanin granules migrate within cytoplasmic extensions of the melanocyte and are transferred to cells of the strata germinativum and spinosum of the epidermis. This transfer has been directly observed in tissue cultures of skin.

Melanin granules are essentially injected into keratinocytes. Once inside the keratinocyte, melanin granules accumulate in the supranuclear region of the cytoplasm, thus protecting the nuclei from the deleterious effects of solar radiation.

Although melanocytes synthesize melanin, epithelial cells act as a depot and contain more of this pigment than do melanocytes. Within the keratinocytes, melanin granules fuse with lysosomes—the reason that melanin disappears in upper epithelial cells. In this interaction between keratinocytes and melanocytes, which creates the pigmentation of the skin, the important factors are the rate of formation of melanin granules within the melanocyte, the transfer of the granules into the keratinocytes, and their ultimate disposition by the keratinocytes. A feedback mechanism may exist between melanocytes and keratinocytes.

Melanocytes can be easily seen by incubating fragments of epidermis in dopa. This compound is converted to dark brown deposits of melanin in

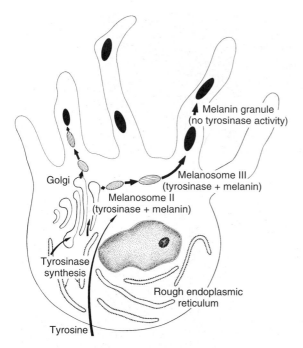

Figure 18–6. Diagram of a melanocyte, illustrating the principal process occurring during melanogenesis. Tyrosinase is synthesized in the rough endoplasmic reticulum and accumulated in vesicles of the Golgi complex. The free vesicles are now called melanosomes. Melanin synthesis begins in the stage II melanosomes, where melanin is accumulated and forms stage III melanosomes. Later, this structure loses its tyrosinase activity and becomes a melanin granule. Melanin granules migrate to the tips of the melanocyte's arms and are then transferred to the keratinocytes of the malpighian layer.

melanocytes, a reaction catalyzed by the enzyme tyrosinase. This method makes it possible to count the number of melanocytes per unit area of the epidermis. Such studies show that these cells are not distributed at random among keratinocytes; rather, there is a pattern in their distribution, called the **epidermal-melanin unit.** In humans, the ratio of dopa-positive melanocytes to keratinocytes in the stratum basale is constant within each area of the body but varies from one region to another. For example, there are about 1000 melanocytes/mm^2 in the skin of the thigh and 2000/mm^2 in the skin of the scrotum. The number of melanocytes per unit area is not influenced by sex or race; differences in skin color are due mainly to differences in the number of melanin granules in the keratinocytes.

Darkening of the skin (tanning) after exposure to solar radiation (wavelength of 290–320 nm) is the result of a two-step process. First, a physicochemical reaction darkens the preexisting melanin and releases it rapidly into the keratinocytes. Next, the rate of melanin synthesis in the melanocytes accelerates, increasing the amount of this pigment.

In humans, lack of cortisol from the adrenal cortex causes overproduction of adrenocorticotropic hormone, which increases the pigmentation of the skin. An example of this is **Addison disease,** which is caused by dysfunction of the adrenal glands.

Albinism, a hereditary inability of the melanocytes to synthesize melanin, is caused by the absence of tyrosinase activity or the inability of cells to take up tyrosine. As a result, the skin is not protected from solar radiation by melanin, and there is a greater incidence of basal and squamous cell carcinomas.

The degeneration and disappearance of entire melanocytes results in a depigmentation disorder called **vitiligo.**

Langerhans Cells

Langerhans cells, star-shaped cells found mainly in the stratum spinosum of the epidermis, represent 2–8% of the epidermal cells. They are bone marrow–derived macrophages that are capable of binding, processing, and presenting antigens to T lymphocytes, thus participating in the stimulation of these cells. Consequently, they have a significant role in immunologic skin reactions.

Merkel's Cells

Merkel's cells, generally present in the thick skin of palms and soles, somewhat resemble the epidermal epithelial cells but have small dense granules in their cytoplasm. The composition of these granules is not known. Free nerve endings that form an expanded terminal disk are present at the base of Merkel's cells. These cells may serve as sensory mechanoreceptors, although other evidence suggests that they have functions related to the diffuse neuroendocrine system.

IMMUNOLOGIC ACTIVITY IN THE SKIN

Because of its large size, the skin has an impressive number of lymphocytes and antigen-presenting cells (Langerhans cells), and because of its location it is in close contact with many antigenic molecules. For these reasons, the epidermis has an important role in some types of immune responses. Most lymphocytes found in the skin are "homed" in the epidermis. It has been shown that keratinocytes of the stratum basale produce a local messenger (thymopoietin) that promotes T cells' terminal maturation in the skin. These basal keratinocytes have three cell proteins (markers) also found in thymus epithelial reticular cells. Like thymus epithelial cells, they can produce interleukin-1 when stimulated.

DERMIS

The dermis is the connective tissue that supports the epidermis and binds it to the subcutaneous tissue (hypodermis). The thickness of the dermis varies according to the region of the body and reaches its maximum of 4 mm on the back. The surface of the dermis is very irregular and has many projections (dermal papillae) that interdigitate with projections (epidermal pegs or ridges) of the epidermis (Figure 18–1). Dermal papillae are more numerous in skin that is subjected to frequent pressure; they increase and reinforce the dermal-epidermal junction. During embryonic development, the dermis determines the developmental pattern of the overlying epidermis. Dermis obtained from the sole always induces the formation of a heavily keratinized epidermis irrespective of the site of origin of the epithelial cells.

A **basal lamina** is always found between the stratum germinativum and the papillary layer of the dermis and follows the contour of the interdigitations between these layers. Underlying the basal lamina is a delicate net of reticular fibers, the **lamina reticularis.** This composite structure is called the **basement membrane** and can be seen with the light microscope.

Abnormalities of the dermal-epidermal junction can lead to one type of blistering disorder (**bullous pemphigoid**). Another type of blistering disorder (**pemphigus**) is caused by the loss of intercellular junctions between keratinocytes.

The dermis contains two layers with rather indistinct boundaries—the outermost papillary layer and the deeper reticular layer. The thin **papillary layer** is composed of loose connective tissue; fibroblasts and other connective tissue cells, such as mast cells and macrophages, are present. Extravasated leukocytes are also seen. The papillary layer is so called because it constitutes the major part of the dermal papillae. From this layer, special collagen fibrils insert into the basal lamina and extend into the dermis. They bind the dermis to the epidermis and are called **anchoring fibrils** (see Figure 4–4). The **reticular layer** is thicker, composed of irregular dense connective tissue (mainly type I collagen), and therefore has more fibers and fewer cells than does the papillary layer. The principal glycosaminoglycan is dermatan sulfate. The dermis contains a network of fibers of the elastic system (Figure 18–7), with the thicker fibers characteristically found in the reticular layer. From this region emerge fibers that become gradually thinner and end by inserting into the basal lamina. As these fibers progress toward the basal lamina, they gradually lose their amorphous elastin component, and only the microfibrillar component inserts into the basal lamina. This elastic network is responsible for the elasticity of the skin.

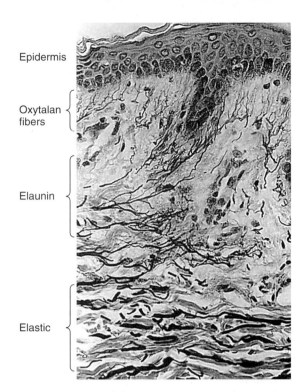

Figure 18–7. Photomicrograph of a section of human abdominal skin stained for elastic fibers. Note the gradual decrease in the diameter of fibers as they approach the epidermis. The thick fibers are the elastic fibers. Those with intermediate diameter are elaunin fibers. The very thin superficial fibers are oxytalan fibers formed by microfibrils that insert into the basal lamina.

With age, collagen fibers thicken and collagen synthesis decreases. Elastic fibers steadily increase in number and thickness, so the elastin content of human skin increases approximately fivefold from fetal to adult life. In old age, extensive cross-linking of collagen fibers, the loss of elastic fibers, and degeneration of these fibers caused by excessive exposure to the sun (**solar elastosis**) cause the skin to become more fragile, lose its suppleness, and develop wrinkles. In several disorders, such as **cutis laxa** and **Ehlers-Danlos syndrome** (Table 5–3), there is a considerable increase in skin and ligament extensibility caused by defective collagen-fibril processing.

The dermis has a rich network of blood and lymph vessels. In certain areas of the skin, blood can pass directly from arteries to veins through arteriovenous anastomoses, or shunts. These shunts play a very important role in temperature regulation.

In addition to these components, the dermis contains such epidermal derivatives as the hair follicles and sweat and sebaceous glands. There is a rich supply of nerves in the dermis, and the effector nerves to the skin are postganglionic fibers of sympathetic ganglia of the paravertebral chain. No parasympathetic innervation is present. The afferent nerve endings form a superficial dermal network with free nerve endings, a hair follicle network, and the innervation of encapsulated sensory organs (**Meissner's** and **pacinian corpuscles,** described in Chapter 24).

SUBCUTANEOUS TISSUE

The subcutaneous tissue layer consists of loose connective tissue that binds the skin loosely to the subjacent organs, making it possible for the skin to slide over them. The hypodermis often contains fat cells that vary in number according to the area of the body and vary in size according to nutritional state. This layer is also referred to as the superficial fascia and, where thick enough, the panniculus adiposus.

HAIRS

Hairs are elongated keratinized structures derived from invaginations of epidermal epithelium. Their color, size, and disposition vary according to race, age, sex, and region of the body. Hairs are found everywhere on the body except on the palms, soles, lips, glans penis, clitoris, and labia minora. The face has about 600 hairs/cm², and the remainder of the body has about 60/cm². Hairs grow discontinuously and have periods of growth followed by periods of rest. This growth does not occur synchronously in all regions of the body or even in the same area; rather, it tends to occur in patches. The duration of the growth and rest periods also varies according to the region of the body. Thus, in the scalp, the growth periods (anagen) may last for several years, whereas the rest periods (catagen and telogen) average 3 months. Hair growth in such regions of the body as the scalp, face, and pubis is strongly influenced not only by sex hormones—especially androgens—but also by adrenal and thyroid hormones.

Each hair arises from an epidermal invagination, the **hair follicle** (Figures 18–8 and 18–9), that during its growth period has a terminal dilatation called a **hair bulb.** At the base of the hair bulb, a **dermal papilla** can be observed. The dermal papilla contains a capillary network that is vital in sustaining the hair follicle. The loss of blood flow or the vitality of the dermal papilla will result in death of the follicle. The epidermal cells covering this dermal papilla form the hair root that produces and is continuous with the hair shaft, which protrudes beyond the skin.

During periods of growth, the epithelial cells that make up the hair bulb are equivalent to those in the stratum germinativum of the skin. They divide constantly and differentiate into specific cell types. In certain types of thick hairs, the cells of the central region of the root at the apex of the dermal papilla produce large, vacuolated, and moderately keratinized cells that form the **medulla** of the hair (Figure 18–8). Root cells multiply and differentiate into heavily keratinized, compactly grouped fusiform cells that form the **hair cortex.**

Farther toward the periphery are the cells that produce the **hair cuticle,** a layer of cells that are cuboidal midway up the bulb, then become tall and columnar. Higher up, they change from horizontal to vertical, at which point they form a layer of flattened, heavily keratinized, shingle-like cells covering the cortex. These cuticle cells are the last cell type in the hair follicle to differentiate.

The outermost cells give rise to the **internal root sheath,** which completely surrounds the initial part of the hair shaft. The internal sheath is a transient structure whose cells degenerate and disappear above the level of the sebaceous glands. The **external root sheath** is continuous with epidermal cells and, near the surface, shows all the layers of epidermis. Near the dermal papilla, the external root sheath is thinner and is composed of cells corresponding to the stratum germinativum of the epidermis.

Separating the hair follicle from the dermis is a noncellular hyaline layer, the **glassy membrane** (Figure 18–8), which results from a thickening of the basal lamina. The dermis that surrounds the follicle is denser, forming a sheath of connective tissue. Bound to this sheath and connecting it to the papillary layer of the dermis are bundles of smooth muscle cells, the **arrector pili** muscles (Figure 18–10). They are disposed in an oblique direction, and their contraction results in the erection of the hair shaft to a more upright position. Contraction of arrector pili muscles also causes a depression in the skin where the muscles attach to the dermis. This contraction produces the "gooseflesh" of common parlance.

Hair color is created by the activity of melanocytes located between the papilla and the epithelial cells of the hair root. The epithelial cells produce the pigment found in the medullary and cortical cells of the hair shaft (Figure 18–8). The melanocytes produce and transfer melanin to the epithelial cells by a mechanism similar to that described for the epidermis.

Although the keratinization processes in the epidermis and hair appear to be similar, they differ in several ways:

1. The epidermis produces relatively soft keratinized outer layers of dead cells that adhere slightly to the skin and desquamate continuously. The opposite occurs in the hair, which has a hard and compact keratinized structure.
2. Although keratinization in the epidermis occurs

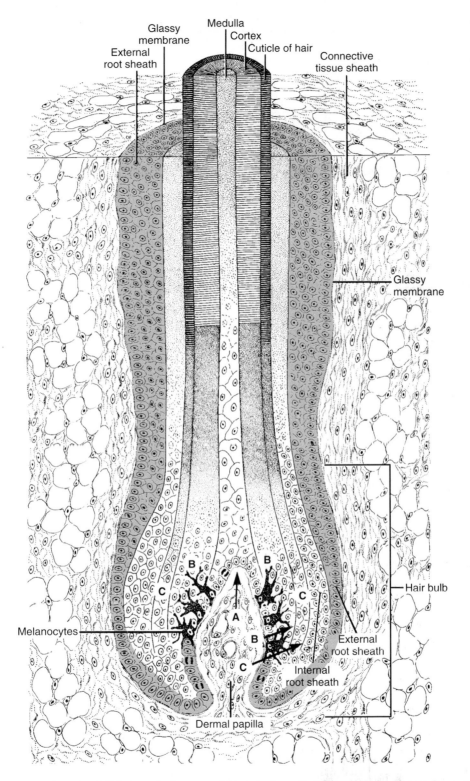

Figure 18–8. Hair follicle. The follicle has a bulbous terminal expansion with a dermal papilla. The papilla contains capillaries and is covered by cells that form the hair root and develop into the hair shaft. The central cells (A) produce large, vacuolated, moderately keratinized cells (arrow) that form the medulla of the hair. The cells that produce the cortex of the hair are located laterally (B). Cells forming the hair cuticle originate in the next layer (C). The peripheral epithelial cells develop into the internal and external root sheaths. The external root sheath (shown in color) is continuous with the epidermis, whereas the cells of the internal root sheath disappear at the level of the openings of the sebaceous gland ducts (not shown).

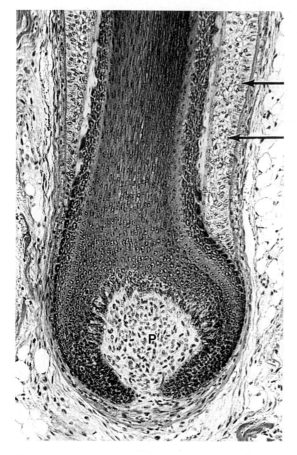

Figure 18–9. Photomicrograph of a section of hair follicle from human skin. Note the papilla (P) and the outer root sheath (arrows), surrounded by a connective tissue sheath. Hematoxylin-and-eosin (H&E stain). × 118.

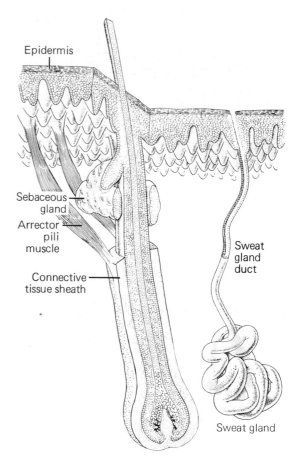

Figure 18–10. Relationships between the skin, hair follicle, arrector pili muscle, and sebaceous and sweat glands. The arrector pili muscle originates in the connective tissue sheath of the hair follicle and inserts into the papillary layer of the dermis, where it ends.

continuously and over the entire surface, it is intermittent in the hair and occurs only in the hair root. The hair papilla has an inductive action on the covering epithelial cells, promoting their proliferation and differentiation. Injuries to the dermal papillae thus result in the loss of hair.

3. Contrary to what happens in the epidermis, where the differentiation of all cells in the same direction gives rise to the final keratinized layer, cells in the hair root differentiate into various cell types that differ in ultrastructure, histochemical characteristics, and function. Mitotic activity in hair follicles is influenced by androgens.

NAILS

Nails are plates of keratinized epithelial cells on the dorsal surface of each distal phalanx (Figure 18–11). The proximal part of the nail, hidden in the

nail groove, is the **nail root.** The epithelium of the fold of skin covering the nail root consists of the usual layers of cells. The stratum corneum of this epithelium forms the **eponychium,** or **cuticle.** The **nail plate,** which corresponds to the stratum corneum of the skin, rests on a bed of epidermis called the **nail bed.** Only the stratum basale and the stratum spinosum are present in the nail bed. Nail plate epithelium arises from the **nail matrix.** The proximal end of the matrix extends deep to the nail root. Cells of the matrix divide, move distally, and eventually cornify, forming the proximal part of the nail plate. The nail plate then slides forward over the nail bed (which makes no contribution to the formation of the plate). The distal end of the plate becomes free of the nail bed and is worn away or cut off. The nearly transparent nail plate and the thin epithelium of the nail bed provide a useful window on the amount of oxygen in the blood by showing the color of blood in the dermal vessels.

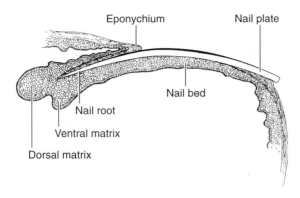

Figure 18–11. The nail and its components.

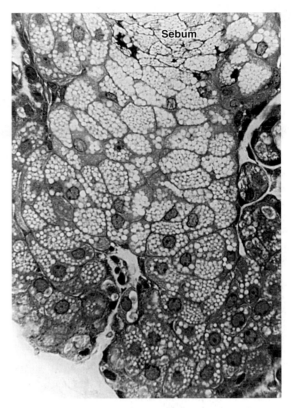

Figure 18–12. Photomicrograph of a sebaceous gland acinus. Note that the cells differentiate, accumulating lipids (light vesicles in the photograph) while they are pushed from the base to the apex of the acinus. Here the cells rupture, forming a protective fat material called sebum. H&E stain.

GLANDS OF THE SKIN

Sebaceous Glands

Sebaceous glands are embedded in the dermis over most of the body surface. There are about 100 of these glands per square centimeter over most of the body, but the frequency increases to 400–900/cm^2 in the face, forehead, and scalp. Sebaceous glands, which are not found in the glabrous skin of the palms and soles, are acinar glands that usually have several acini opening into a short duct. This duct usually ends in the upper portion of a hair follicle (Figure 18–10); in certain regions, such as the glans penis, glans clitoridis, and lips, it opens directly onto the epidermal surface. The acini consist of a basal layer of undifferentiated flattened epithelial cells that rest on the basal lamina. These cells proliferate and differentiate, filling the acini with rounded cells containing abundant fat droplets in their cytoplasm (Figure 18–12). Their nuclei gradually shrink, and the cells simultaneously become filled with fat droplets and burst. The product of this process is **sebum,** the secretion of the sebaceous gland, which is gradually moved to the surface of the skin.

The sebaceous gland is an example of a **holocrine** gland, because its product of secretion is released with remnants of dead cells. This product comprises a complex mixture of lipids that includes triglycerides, waxes, squalene, and cholesterol and its esters. Sebaceous glands begin to function at puberty. The primary controlling factor of sebaceous gland secretion in men is testosterone; in women it is a combination of ovarian and adrenal androgens.

The flow of sebum is continuous, and a disturbance in the normal secretion and flow of sebum is one of the reasons for the development of acne, a chronic inflammation of obstructed sebaceous glands. It occurs mainly during puberty.

The functions of sebum in humans are largely unknown. It may have weak antibacterial and antifungal properties. Sebum does not have any importance in preventing water loss.

Sweat Glands

Sweat glands are widely distributed in the skin except for certain regions, such as the glans penis.

The **eccrine** (**merocrine**) sweat glands are simple, coiled tubular glands whose ducts open at the skin surface (Figure 18–10). Their ducts do not divide, and their diameter is thinner than that of the secretory portion (Figure 18–13). The secretory part of the gland is embedded in the dermis; it measures approximately 0.4 mm in diameter and is surrounded by myoepithelial cells (described in Chapter 4). Contraction of these cells helps to discharge the secretion. A fairly thick basal lamina lies outside the secretory portion of the gland. Two types of cells have been described in the secretory portion of eccrine sweat glands. **Dark cells** (mucoid cells) are pyramidal cells that line most of the luminal surface of this

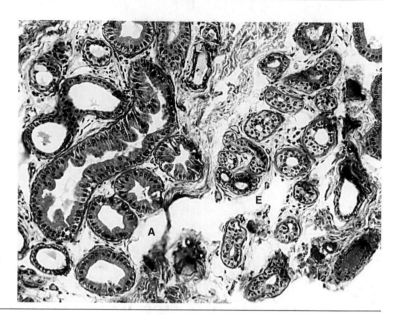

Figure 18–13. Photomicrograph of axillary human skin, showing apocrine (A) and eccrine (E) gland portions. The epidermal side is at the upper border. × 110. (Courtesy of J James.)

portion of the gland. Their basal surface does not touch the basal lamina. Secretory granules containing glycoproteins are abundant in their apical cytoplasm. **Clear cells** are devoid of secretory granules. Their basal plasmalemma has the numerous invaginations characteristic of cells involved in transepithelial salt and fluid transport. The ducts of these glands are lined by stratified cuboidal epithelium (Figure 18–13).

The fluid secreted by eccrine sweat glands is not viscous and contains little protein. Its main components are water, sodium chloride, urea, ammonia, and uric acid. Its sodium content of 85 mEq/L is distinctly below that of blood (144 mEq/L), and the cells present in the sweat ducts are responsible for sodium absorption. The fluid in the lumen of the secretory portion of the gland is an ultrafiltrate of the blood plasma. This ultrafiltrate is derived from a network of capillaries that intimately envelop the secretory region of each gland. After its release on the surface of the skin, sweat evaporates, cooling the surface.

In addition to eccrine sweat glands, another type of sweat gland—the **apocrine** gland—is present in the axillary, areolar, and anal regions. Apocrine glands are much larger (3–5 mm in diameter) than eccrine sweat glands. They are embedded in the dermis and hypodermis, and their ducts open into hair follicles. These glands produce a viscous secretion that is initially odorless but may acquire a distinctive odor as a result of bacterial decomposition. Apocrine glands are innervated by adrenergic nerve endings, whereas eccrine glands receive cholinergic fibers. The glands of Moll in the margins of the eyelids and the ceruminous glands of the ear are modified sweat glands.

VESSELS & NERVES OF THE SKIN

The arterial vessels that nourish the skin form two plexuses. One is located between the papillary and reticular layers, the other between the dermis and the subcutaneous tissue. Thin branches leave these plexuses and vascularize the dermal papillae. Each papilla has only one arterial ascending branch and one venous descending branch. Veins are disposed in three plexuses, two in the position described for arterial vessels and the third in the middle of the dermis. Arteriovenous anastomoses with glomera (see Chapter 11) are frequent in the skin. Lymphatic vessels begin as closed sacs in the papillae of the dermis and converge to form two plexuses, as described for the arterial vessels.

One of the most important functions of the skin, with its abundant sensory innervation, is to receive stimuli from the environment. In addition to free nerve endings in the epidermis and cutaneous glands, receptors are present in the dermis and subcutaneous tissue; they are more frequently found in the dermal papillae (see Chapter 24). The hair follicles possess a rich network of nerve endings that are essential in the processing of tactile impressions from the environment.

Tumors of the Skin

One third of all tumors are of the skin. Most of these tumors derive from the basal cells, the squamous cells of the stratum spinosum, and melanocytes. They produce, respectively, basal cell carcinomas, squamous cell carcinomas, and melanomas. The first two types of tumors can be diagnosed and excised early and consequently are rarely lethal. Skin tumors show an increased incidence in fair-skinned individuals residing in regions with high amounts of solar radiation. **Malignant melanoma** is an invasive tumor of melanocytes. Dividing rapidly, malignantly transformed melanocytes penetrate the basal lamina, enter the dermis, and invade the blood and lymphatic vessels to gain wide distribution throughout the body. Malignant melanoma represents approximately 1–3% of all tumors.

REFERENCES

Edelson RL, Fink JM: The immunologic function of the skin. Sci Am 1985;252:46.

Green H et al: Differentiated structural components of the keratinocyte. Cold Spring Harbor Symp Quant Biol, 1982.

Halprin KM: Epidermal turnover time: a reexamination. J Invest Dermatol 1972;86:14.

Hayward AF: Membrane coating granules. Int Rev Cytol 1979;59:97.

Millington PF, Wilkinson R: *Skin.* Cambridge Univ Press, 1983.

Montagna W: *The Structure and Function of Skin,* 3rd ed. Academic Press, 1974.

Strauss JS et al: The sebaceous glands: twenty-five years of progress. J Invest Dermatol 1976;67:90.

Winkelmann RK: The Merkel cell system and a comparison between it and the neurosecretory or APUD cell system. J Invest Dermatol 1977;69:41.

Zelickson AS: *Ultrastructure of Normal and Abnormal Skin.* Lea & Febiger, 1967.

The Urinary System

The urinary system consists of the paired kidneys and ureters and the unpaired bladder and urethra. This system contributes to the maintenance of homeostasis by producing urine, in which various metabolic waste products are eliminated. Urine produced in the kidneys passes through the ureters to the bladder, where it is temporarily stored and then released to the exterior through the urethra. The kidneys also regulate the fluid and electrolyte balance of the body and are the site of production of the hormones renin and erythropoietin. Renin participates in the regulation of blood pressure, and erythropoietin is a growth factor glycoprotein of 30 kDa that stimulates the production of erythrocytes.

KIDNEYS

1. STRUCTURE

Each kidney has a concave medial border, the **hilum**—where nerves enter, blood and lymph vessels enter and exit, and the ureter exits—and a convex lateral surface (Figure 19–1). The **renal pelvis,** the expanded upper end of the ureter, is divided into two or three **major calyces.** Several small branches, the **minor calyces,** arise from each major calyx.

The kidney can be divided into an outer **cortex** and an inner **medulla** (Figures 19–1 and 19–2). In humans, the renal medulla consists of 10–18 conical or pyramidal structures, the **medullary pyramids.** From the base of each medullary pyramid, parallel arrays of tubules, the **medullary rays,** penetrate the cortex (Figure 19–1). Each medullary ray consists of one or more collecting tubules together with the straight portions of several **nephrons.** The mass of cortical tissue surrounding each medullary pyramid is a renal lobe, and each medullary ray forms the center of a conical **renal lobule** (see Figure 19–19).

Nephrons

Each kidney is composed of 1–4 million nephrons (Gr. *nephros,* kidney). Each nephron consists of a dilated portion, the **renal corpuscle;** the **proximal convoluted tubule;** the thin and thick limbs of Henle's loop; and the **distal convoluted tubule** (Figure 19–1). The **collecting tubules** and **ducts,** whose embryologic origin differs from that of the nephron, collect the urine produced by nephrons and conduct it to the renal pelvis. The nephron and the collecting duct into which it empties constitute a **uriniferous tubule,** which can be considered the functional unit of the kidney.

Each renal corpuscle is about 200 μm in diameter and consists of a tuff of capillaries, the **glomerulus,** surrounded by a double-walled epithelial capsule called **Bowman's capsule** (Figures 19–1, 19–2, 19–3, and 19–9). The internal layer (the **visceral layer**) of the capsule envelops the capillaries of the glomerulus. The external layer forms the outer limit of the renal corpuscle and is called the **parietal layer** of Bowman's capsule (Figures 19–2 and 19–3). Between the two layers of Bowman's capsule is the **urinary space,** which receives the fluid filtered through the capillary wall and the visceral layer. Each renal corpuscle has a **vascular pole,** where the **afferent arteriole** enters and the efferent arteriole leaves (Figure 19–3), and a **urinary pole,** where the proximal convoluted tubule begins (Figure 19–3). After entering the renal corpuscle, the afferent arteriole usually divides into two to five primary branches, each subdividing into capillaries and forming the renal glomerulus.

The parietal layer of Bowman's capsule consists of a simple squamous epithelium supported by a basal lamina and a thin layer of reticular fibers (Figures 19–3 and 19–4). At the urinary pole, the epithelium changes to the simple columnar epithelium characteristic of the proximal tubule (Figure 19–3).

During embryonic development, the epithelium of the parietal layer remains relatively unchanged, whereas the internal, or visceral, layer is greatly modified. The cells of this internal layer, the **podocytes** (Figures 19–3, 19–5, 19–6, and 19–7), have a cell body from which arise several **primary processes.** Each primary process gives rise to numerous **secondary processes,** called **pedicels** (Figures 19–5, 19–6, and 19–7), that embrace the capillaries of the

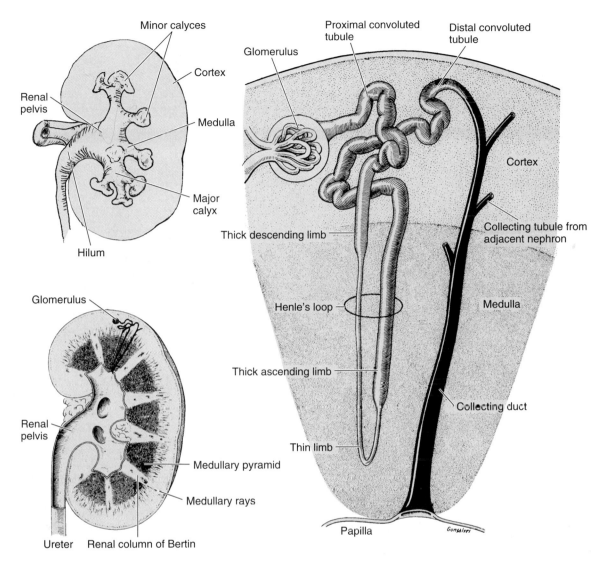

Figure 19–1. Left: General organization of the kidney. **Right:** Parts of a juxtamedullary nephron and its collecting duct and tubule (shown in black).

glomerulus. At a periodic distance of 25 nm, the secondary processes are in direct contact with the basal lamina. However, the cell bodies of podocytes and their primary processes do not touch the basal lamina (Figures 19–5 and 19–7). The pedicels from one podocyte embrace more than one capillary; on a single capillary, the pedicels of two podocytes alternate in position next to the basal lamina (Figure 19–7). Although pedicels contain few or no organelles, microfilaments and microtubules are numerous.

The secondary processes of podocytes interdigitate, defining elongated spaces about 25 nm wide—the **filtration slits.** Spanning adjacent processes (and thus bridging the filtration slits) is a diaphragm about 6 nm thick that is comparable to the diaphragm en-

countered in fenestrated endothelial cells. The cytoplasm of podocytes contains numerous free ribosomes, a few cisternae of rough endoplasmic reticulum, infrequent mitochondria, and a prominent Golgi complex. Podocytes have bundles of actin microfilaments in their cytoplasm that give them a contractile capacity (Figures 19–7 and 19–8).

Between the fenestrated endothelial cells of the glomerular capillaries and the podocytes that cover their external surfaces is a thick (~ 0.1-μm) basement membrane (Figure 19–8). This membrane is believed to be the filtration barrier that separates the urinary space and the blood in the capillaries. The basement membrane is derived from the fusion of capillary- and podocyte-produced basal laminae. With the aid of the electron microscope, one can distinguish a

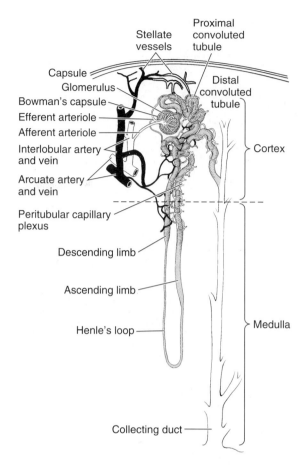

Figure 19–2. Diagram of the vascular supply of a nephron (shown in color) in the outer part of the cortex. Arteries and capillaries are white; veins are black.

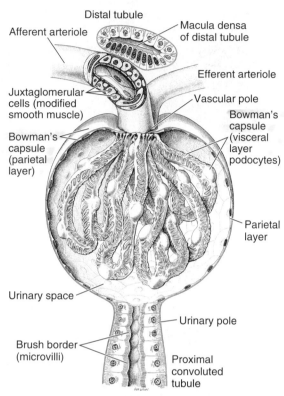

Figure 19–3. The renal corpuscle. The upper part of the drawing shows the vascular pole, with afferent and efferent arterioles and the macula densa. Note the juxtaglomerular cells in the wall of the afferent arteriole. Podocyte processes cover the outer surfaces of the glomerular capillaries; the part of the podocyte containing the nucleus protrudes into the urinary space. Note the flattened cells of the parietal layer of Bowman's capsule. The lower part of the drawing shows the urinary pole and the proximal convoluted tubule.

central electron-dense layer (**lamina densa**) and, on each side, a more electron-lucent layer (**lamina rara;** Figure 19–8). The two electron-lucent laminae rarae contain fibronectin, which may serve to bind them to the cells. The lamina densa is a meshwork of type IV collagen and laminin in a matrix containing the negatively charged proteoglycan heparan sulfate. Thus, the glomerular basal lamina is a selective macromolecular filter in which the lamina densa acts as a physical filter, whereas the anionic sites in the laminae rarae act as a charge barrier. Particles greater than 10 nm in diameter do not readily cross the basal lamina, and negatively charged proteins with a molecular mass greater than that of albumin (69 kDa) pass across only sparingly.

In diseases such as diabetes mellitus and glomerulonephritis, the glomerular filter is altered and becomes much more permeable to proteins, with the subsequent release of protein into the urine (**proteinuria**).

The endothelial cells of glomerular capillaries have a thin cytoplasm that is thicker around the nucleus, where most of the organelles are clustered. The fenestrae of these cells are larger (70–90 nm in diameter) and more numerous than those in the capillaries of other organs, and they lack the thin diaphragm commonly observed spanning the openings of other fenestrated capillaries.

Besides endothelial cells and podocytes, the glomerular capillaries have **mesangial** (Gr. *mesos,* middle, + *angeion,* vessel) cells adhering to their walls in places where the basal lamina forms a sheath that is shared by two or more capillaries (Figures 19–10 and 19–11). The cytoplasmic extensions of mesangial cells penetrate between endothelial cells to reach the capillary lumen. The cells synthesize the extracellular matrix that surrounds them and contribute to the support of the capillary walls. Little

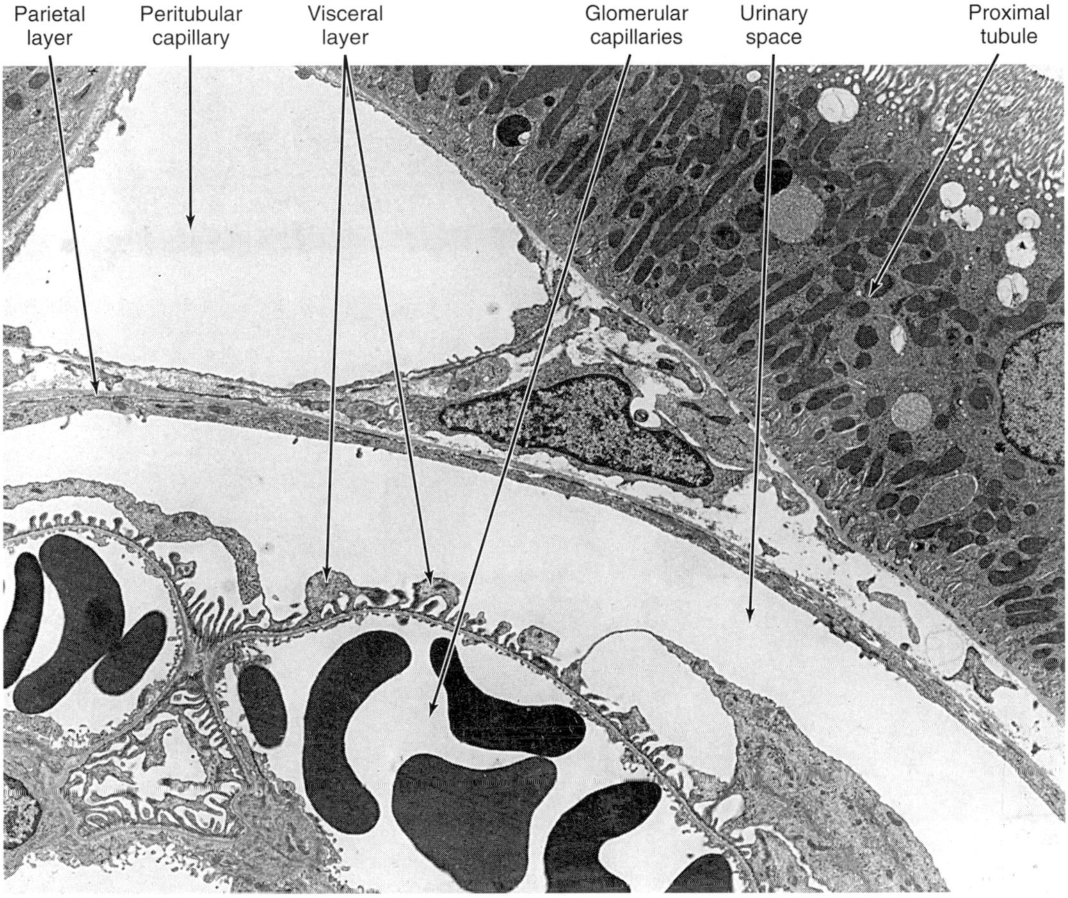

Parietal layer   Peritubular capillary   Visceral layer   Glomerular capillaries   Urinary space   Proximal tubule

Figure 19–4. Electron micrograph of a rat kidney showing part of a renal corpuscle, including the parietal layer of Bowman's capsule, the urinary space, glomerular capillaries containing erythrocytes, the visceral layer of Bowman's capsule, the peritubular capillary, and the proximal tubule. × 2850. (Courtesy of SL Wissig.)

else is known about their function: they constitute a pericyte-like population of cells. After the injection of ferritin (an electron-scattering iron-containing protein complex easily identified with the electron microscope), the cytoplasm of mesangial cells appears to be engorged with this protein. These cells may act as macrophages to clean the basal lamina of particulate material that accumulates during the filtration process.

Proximal Convoluted Tubule

At the urinary pole of the renal corpuscle, the squamous epithelium of the parietal layer of Bowman's capsule is continuous with the columnar epithelium of the proximal convoluted tubule (Figures 19–1, 19–2, and 19–9). This tubule is longer than the distal convoluted tubule and is therefore more frequently seen near renal corpuscles in the cortical labyrinth.

The proximal convoluted tubule is lined with simple cuboidal or columnar epithelium. The cells of this epithelium have an acidophilic cytoplasm that results from the presence of numerous elongated mitochondria. The cell apex has abundant microvilli about 1 μm in length, which form a **brush border** (Figures 19–3, 19–12, and 19–13). Because the cells are large, each transverse section of a proximal tubule contains only three to five spherical nuclei, usually located in the center of the cell.

In the living animal, proximal convoluted tubules have a wide lumen and are surrounded by peritubular capillaries. In routine histologic preparations, the brush border is usually disorganized and the peritubular capillary lumens are greatly reduced in size or collapsed.

The apical cytoplasm of these cells has numerous canaliculi between the bases of the microvilli; these canaliculi affect the capacity of the proximal tubule

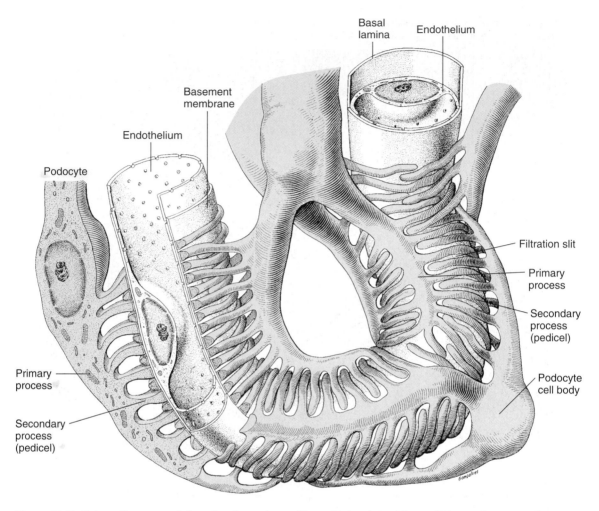

Figure 19–5. Schematic representation of a glomerular capillary with the visceral layer of Bowman's capsule (formed of podocytes; shown in color). In this capillary, endothelial cells are fenestrated, but the basal lamina on which they rest is continuous. At left is a podocyte shown in partial section. As viewed from the outside, the part of the podocyte that contains the nucleus protrudes into the urinary space. Each podocyte has many primary processes, from which arise an even greater number of secondary processes that are in contact with the basal lamina. (Modified and redrawn from Gordon. Reproduced, with permission, from Ham AW: *Histology,* 6th ed. Lippincott, 1969.)

cells to absorb macromolecules. Pinocytotic vesicles are formed by evaginations of the apical membranes and contain macromolecules (mainly proteins with a molecular mass less than 70 kDa) that have passed across the glomerular filter. The pinocytotic vesicles fuse with lysosomes, where macromolecules are degraded, and monomers are returned to the circulation. The basal portions of these cells have abundant membrane invaginations and lateral interdigitations with neighboring cells. The Na^+/K^+-ATPase (sodium pump) responsible for actively transporting sodium ions out of the cells is localized in these basolateral membranes. Mitochondria are concentrated at the base of the cell (Figure 19–14) and arranged parallel

to the long axis of the cell. This mitochondrial location and the increase in the area of the cell membrane at the base of the cell are characteristic of cells engaged in active ion transport (see Chapter 4). Because of the extensive interdigitation of the lateral membranes, no discrete cell margins can be observed (in the light microscope) between cells of the proximal tubule.

Henle's Loop

Henle's loop is a U-shaped structure consisting of a **thick descending limb,** which is very similar in structure to the proximal convoluted tubule; a **thin descending limb;** a **thin ascending limb;** and a

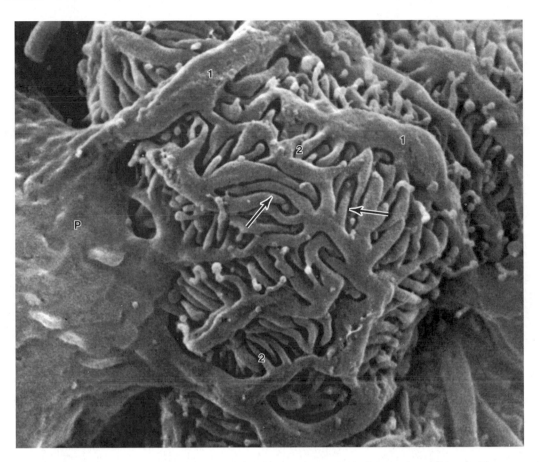

Figure 19–6. Scanning electron micrograph showing Bowman's visceral epithelial cells, or podocytes (P), surrounding capillaries of the renal glomerulus. Two orders of branching of the podocyte processes are apparent: the primary processes (1) and the secondary processes, or pedicels (2). The small spaces between adjacent processes constitute the filtration slits (arrows). × 10,700.

thick ascending limb, which is very similar in structure to the distal convoluted tubule (Figure 19–13). In the outer medulla, the thick descending limb, with an outer diameter of about 60 µm, suddenly narrows to about 12 µm and continues as the thin descending limb. The lumen of this segment of the nephron is wide because the wall consists of squamous epithelial cells whose nuclei protrude only slightly into the lumen (Figures 19–15 and 19–16).

Approximately one seventh of all nephrons are located near the corticomedullary junction and are therefore called **juxtamedullary nephrons.** The other nephrons are called **cortical nephrons.** All nephrons participate in the processes of filtration, absorption, and secretion. Juxtamedullary nephrons, however, are of prime importance in establishing the gradient of hypertonicity in the medullary interstitium—the basis of the kidneys' ability to produce hypertonic urine. Juxtamedullary nephrons have very long Henle's loops, extending deep into the medulla. These loops consist of a short thick descending limb,

long thin descending and ascending limbs, and a thick ascending limb. Cortical nephrons, on the other hand, have very short thin descending limbs and no thin ascending limbs (Figure 19–2).

Distal Convoluted Tubule

When the thick ascending limb of Henle's loop penetrates the cortex, it preserves its histologic structure (Figure 19–13) but becomes tortuous and is called the distal convoluted tubule, the last segment of the nephron. This tubule is lined with simple cuboidal epithelium (Figure 19–14).

In histologic sections, the distinction between the proximal and distal convoluted tubules, which are both found in the cortex, is based on certain characteristics. Cells of proximal tubules are larger than cells of distal tubules; they have brush borders, which distal tubule cells lack; and they are more acidophilic. The lumens of the distal tubules are larger, and because distal tubule cells are flatter and smaller than those of the proximal tubule, more cells and

Glomerular
capillary

Podocytes

Urinary
space

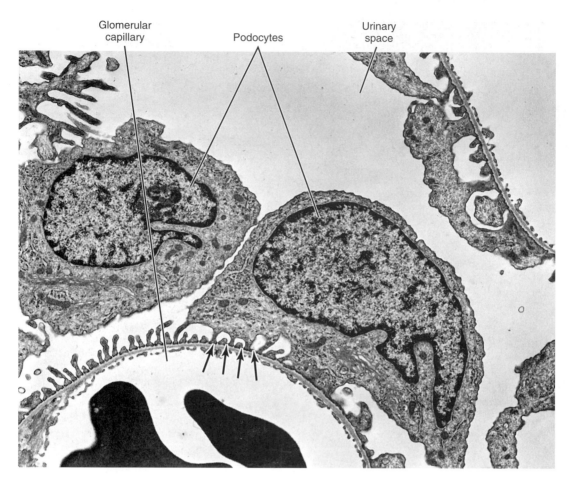

Figure 19–7. Electron micrograph showing the cell bodies of two podocytes and the alternation of secondary processes from two different cells (arrows). The urinary space and the glomerular capillary are indicated. × 9000. (Courtesy of SL Wissig.)

Figure 19–8. Electron micrograph of the filtration barrier in a renal corpuscle. Note the endothelium (E) with open fenestrae (arrowhead), the fused basal laminae (basement membrane) of epithelial and endothelial cells (BL), and the processes of podocytes (P). The basement membrane consists of a central lamina densa bounded on both sides by a light-staining lamina rara. Arrows indicate the thin diaphragms crossing the filtration slits. × 45,750. (Courtesy of SL Wissig.)

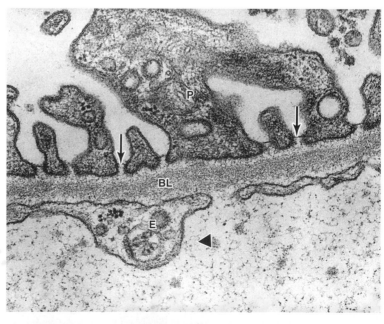

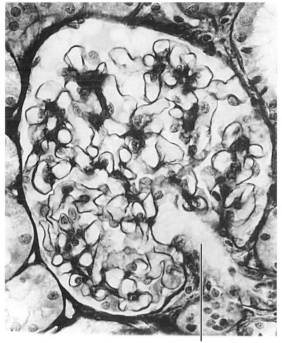

Afferent arteriole

Figure 19–9. Kidney section showing a renal corpuscle with the basement membrane of the blood capillary well stained. Picrosirius stain.

more nuclei are seen in the distal tubule than in the proximal tubule in the same histologic section. The apical canaliculi and vesicles that characterize the proximal tubule are absent in the distal tubule. Cells of the distal convoluted tubule have elaborate basal membrane invaginations and associated mitochondria indicative of their ion-transporting function.

Along its path in the cortex, the distal convoluted tubule establishes contact with the vascular pole of the renal corpuscle of its parent nephron. At this point of close contact, the distal tubule is modified, as is the afferent arteriole. In this juxtaglomerular region, cells of the distal convoluted tubule usually become columnar, and their nuclei are closely packed together. Most of the cells have a Golgi complex in the basal region. This modified segment of the wall of the distal tubule, which appears darker in microscopic preparations because of the close proximity of its nuclei, is called the **macula densa** (Figures 19–3 and 19–17). Experimental evidence suggests that cells of the macula densa are sensitive to the chloride ion content of tubular fluid, producing molecular signals that promote constriction of the glomerular afferent arteriole. This mechanism enables the macula densa to regulate the rate of glomerular filtration.

Collecting Tubules & Ducts

Urine passes from the distal convoluted tubules to collecting tubules that join each other to form larger, straight collecting ducts, the **papillary ducts of Bellini,** which widen gradually as they approach the tips of the medullary pyramids (Figure 19–1).

The smaller collecting tubules are lined with

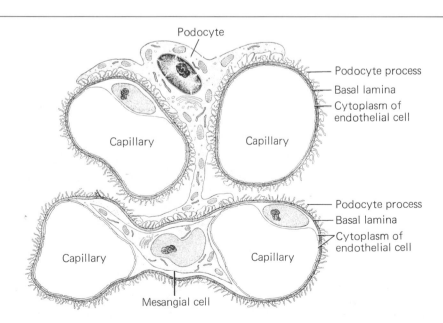

Figure 19–10. Mesangial cell of glomerular capillaries, located between two capillary lumens that are enveloped by the basal lamina.

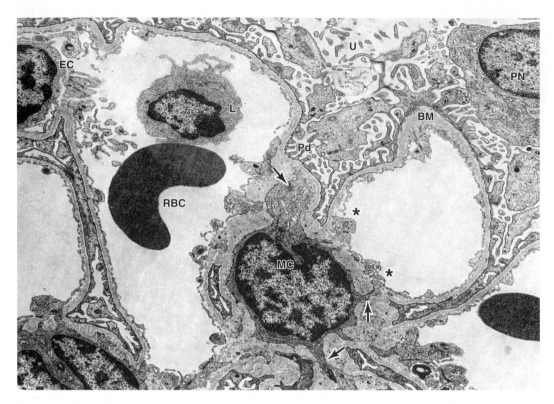

Figure 19–11. Electron micrograph showing a mesangial cell (MC) and the amorphous mesangial matrix surrounding it. The matrix helps to support the capillary loops where a basement membrane is lacking. Some of the mesangial cell's processes (arrows) reach the capillary lumen, passing between endothelial cells (asterisks). The capillary at left contains an erythrocyte (RBC) and a leukocyte (L). BM, basement membrane; EC, endothelial cell; Pd, pedicels; PN, podocyte nucleus; U, urinary space.

cuboidal epithelium and have a diameter of approximately 40 μm. As they penetrate deeper into the medulla, their cells increase in height (Figure 19–15) until they become columnar. The diameter of the collecting duct reaches 200 μm near the tips of the medullary pyramids.

Along their entire extent, collecting tubules and ducts are composed of cells that stain weakly with the usual stains. They have an electron-lucent cytoplasm with few organelles (Figure 19–18) and almost no invaginations of the basal cell membrane. In collecting tubules and cortical collecting ducts, a dark-staining intercalated cell is also seen; its significance is not understood. The intercellular limits of the collecting tubule and duct cells are clearly visible in the light microscope, because there are no interdigitations between the lateral margins of adjacent cells (Figure 19–15). Cortical collecting ducts are joined at right angles by several generations of smaller collecting tubules that drain each medullary ray. In the medulla, collecting ducts are a major component of the urine-concentrating mechanism.

Juxtaglomerular Apparatus

Adjacent to the renal corpuscle, the tunica media

of the afferent arteriole has modified smooth muscle cells. These cells, called **juxtaglomerular (JG) cells** (Figures 19–3 and 19–17), have ellipsoid nuclei and a cytoplasm full of secretory granules that stain with periodic acid–Schiff. Secretions of juxtaglomerular cells play a role in the maintenance of blood pressure. The macula densa of the distal convoluted tubule is usually located near the region of the afferent arteriole that contains the juxtaglomerular cells; together, this portion of the arteriole and the macula densa form the juxtaglomerular apparatus (Figures 19–3 and 19–17). Also a part of the juxtaglomerular apparatus are some light-staining cells whose functions are not well understood. They are variously called **extraglomerular mesangial cells, lacis cells,** or **polkissen (pole cushions)**. The internal elastic membrane of the afferent arteriole disappears in the area of the juxtaglomerular cells.

When examined with the electron microscope, juxtaglomerular cells show characteristics of protein-secreting cells, including an abundant rough endoplasmic reticulum, a highly developed Golgi complex, and secretory granules measuring approximately 10–40 nm in diameter. Juxtaglomerular cells produce the hormone **renin,** which acts on a plasma

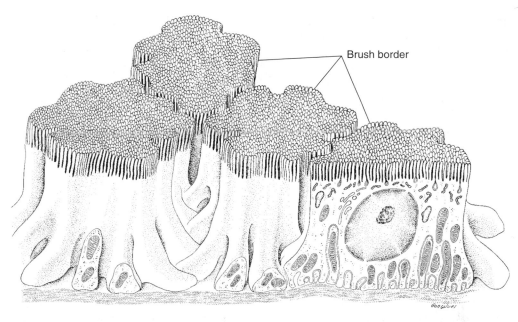

Brush border

Figure 19–12. Schematic drawing of proximal convoluted tubule cells. The apical surfaces of these cuboidal cells have abundant microvilli constituting a brush border. Note the distribution of mitochondria and associated basilar infoldings of the cell membrane. The latter processes are longer than the former and penetrate deeply among the neighboring cells. Artificial spaces between the cells are shown to make the drawing easier to understand. (Modified from Bulger R: Amer J Anat 1965;116:237.)

protein—**angiotensinogen**—to produce an inactive decapeptide, **angiotensin I.** As a result of the action of a converting enzyme present in high concentration in lung endothelial cells, this substance loses two amino acids and becomes an active octapeptide, **angiotensin II.**

After a significant hemorrhage, there is an increase in renin secretion. Angiotensin II is produced, enhancing blood pressure by both constricting arterioles and stimulating the secretion of the adrenocortical hormone **aldosterone.** Aldosterone acts on cells of the renal tubules (mostly the distal tubules) to increase the absorption of sodium and chloride ions from the glomerular apparatus. This increase in sodium and chloride ions, in turn, expands the fluid volume, leading to an increase in blood pressure.

Decreased blood pressure caused by other factors (eg, sodium depletion, dehydration) also activates the renin–angiotensin II–aldosterone mechanism that contributes to the maintenance of blood pressure.

Blood Circulation

Each kidney receives blood from its **renal artery,** which usually divides into two branches before entering the organ. One branch goes to the anterior part of the kidney, the other to the posterior part. While still in the hilum, these branches give rise to arteries that

branch again to form the **interlobar arteries** located between the renal pyramids (Figure 19–19). At the level of the corticomedullary junction, the interlobar arteries form the **arcuate arteries. Interlobular arteries** branch off at right angles from the arcuate arteries and follow a course in the cortex perpendicular to the renal capsule. Interlobular arteries form the boundaries of the renal lobules, which consist of a medullary ray and the adjacent cortical labyrinth (Figure 19–19). From the interlobular arteries arise the **afferent arterioles,** which supply blood to the capillaries of the glomeruli. Blood passes from these capillaries into the **efferent arterioles,** which at once branch again to form a **peritubular capillary network** that will nourish the proximal and distal tubules and carry away absorbed ions and low-molecular-weight materials. The efferent arterioles that are associated with juxtamedullary nephrons form long, thin capillary vessels. These vessels, which follow a straight path into the medulla and then loop back toward the corticomedullary boundary, are called **vasa recta** (straight vessels). The descending vessel is a continuous-type capillary, whereas the ascending vessel has a fenestrated endothelium. These vessels, containing blood that has been filtered through the glomeruli, provide nourishment and oxygen to the medulla. Because of their looped structure, they do not carry away the high osmotic gradient set up in the interstitium by Henle's loop.

The capillaries of the outer cortex and the capsule

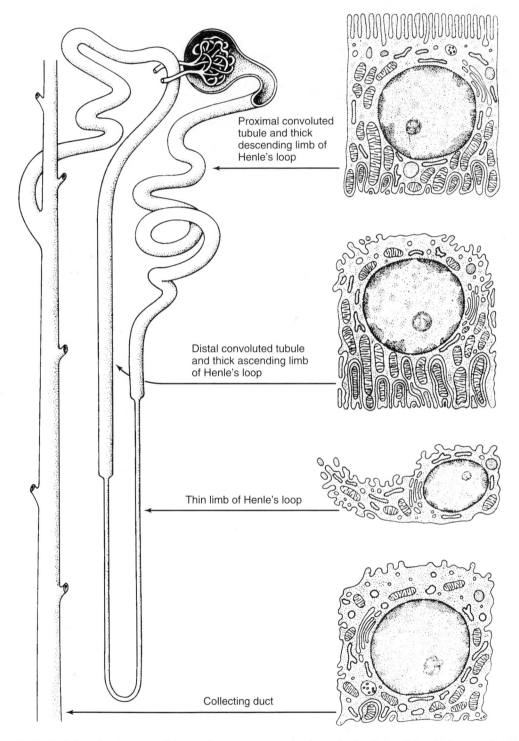

Figure 19–13. Cellular ultrastructure of the nephron, represented schematically. Cells of the thick ascending limb of Henle's loop and the distal tubule are similar in their ultrastructure but different in function.

The labels within the figure read:

Proximal convoluted tubule and thick descending limb of Henle's loop

Distal convoluted tubule and thick ascending limb of Henle's loop

Thin limb of Henle's loop

Collecting duct

Blood vessel

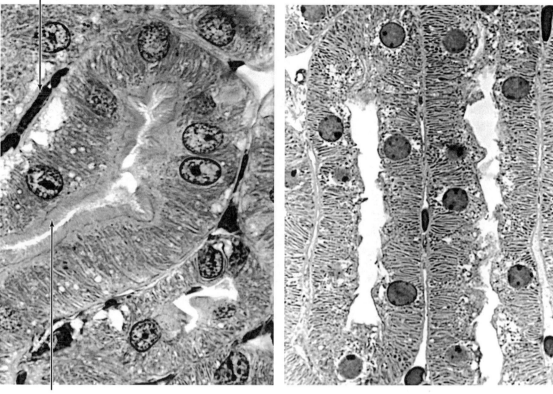

Brush border

Figure 19–14. Structural comparisons of proximal and distal convoluted tubules. Note that the thick ascending limb of Henle's loop has the same structure as the distal convoluted tubule. The proximal convoluted tubule (**left**) has higher cells, with a brush border. The distal convoluted tubule (**right**) has shorter cells and no brush border. Cells of both tubules have numerous elongated mitochondria that provide the energy needed for ion transport.

of the kidney converge to form the **stellate veins** (so called because of their configuration when seen from the surface of the kidney), which empty into the interlobular veins.

Veins follow the same course as arteries (Figure 19–19). Blood from interlobular veins flows into arcuate veins and from there to the interlobar veins. Interlobar veins converge to form the renal vein through which blood leaves the kidney.

Renal Interstitium

Both the cortex and the medulla contain specialized cells in the spaces between uriniferous tubules and the blood and lymph vessels. These **interstitial cells** are more frequent in the medulla, where cells containing cytoplasmic lipid droplets and implicated in the synthesis of a hypotensor hormone are found. These cells may be the source of medullipin I, a substance that is converted in the liver to medullipin II, a potent vasodilator that lowers blood pressure.

2. HISTOPHYSIOLOGY

The kidney regulates the chemical composition of the internal environment by a complex process that involves **filtration, active absorption, passive absorption,** and **secretion.** Filtration takes place in the glomerulus, where an ultrafiltrate of blood plasma is formed. The tubules of the nephron, primarily the proximal convoluted tubules, absorb from this filtrate the substances that are useful for body metabolism, thus maintaining the homeostasis of the internal environment. They also transfer from blood to the tubular lumen certain waste products that are eliminated with the urine. Under certain circumstances, the collecting ducts are permeable to water, contributing to the concentration of urine—which is usually hypertonic in relation to blood plasma. In this way, the organism controls its water, intercellular fluid, and osmotic balance.

The two kidneys produce about 125 mL of filtrate

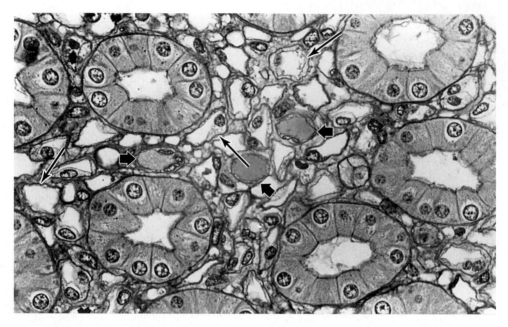

Figure 19–15. Cross section through the medulla of a rat kidney showing collecting tubules, capillary vessels of the vasa recta (arrowheads), and thin limbs of Henle's loop (arrows). × 1100.

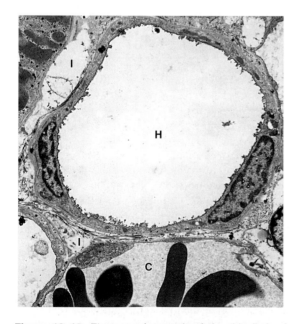

Figure 19–16. Electron micrograph of the thin limb of Henle's loop (H) composed entirely of squamous cells. Note the fenestrated capillaries with erythrocytes (C) and the interstitium (I) with bundles of collagen fibrils. × 3300. (Courtesy of J Rhodin.)

per minute; of this amount, 124 mL is absorbed and only 1 mL is released into the calyces as urine. About 1500 mL of urine is formed every 24 hours.

Filtration

The blood flow in the two kidneys of an adult amounts to 1.2–1.3 L of blood per minute. This means that all the circulating blood in the body passes through the kidneys every 4–5 minutes. The glomeruli are composed of arterial capillaries in which the hydrostatic pressure—about 45 mm Hg—is higher than that found in other capillaries.

The glomerular filtrate is formed in response to the hydrostatic pressure of blood, which is opposed by the osmotic (oncotic) pressure of plasma colloids (20 mm Hg), and the hydrostatic pressure of the fluids in Bowman's capsule (10 mm Hg). The net filtration pressure at the afferent end of glomerular capillaries is 15 mm Hg.

The glomerular filtrate has a chemical composition similar to that of blood plasma but contains almost no protein, because macromolecules do not readily cross the glomerular wall. The largest protein molecules that succeed in crossing the glomerular filter have a molecular mass of about 70 kDa, and small amounts of plasma albumin appear in the filtrate.

Because endothelial cells of glomerular capillaries are fenestrated with numerous openings (70–90 nm

Macula densa

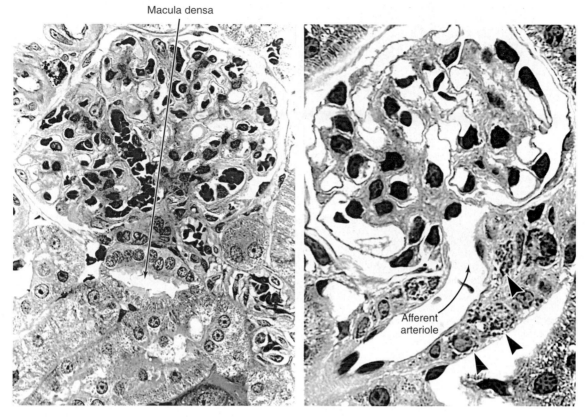

Figure 19–17. Photomicrographs of two renal corpuscles. **Left:** A macula densa with the characteristic close proximity of its nuclei. In this location, cells of the distal tubules are smaller. **Right:** A portion of a juxtaglomerular apparatus showing the wall of the afferent arteriole with cells that have secretory granules (arrowheads) containing renin.

in diameter) without diaphragms, the endothelium is easily permeated.

Proximal Convoluted Tubule

The glomerular filtrate formed in the renal corpuscle passes into the proximal convoluted tubule, where the processes of absorption and excretion begin. The proximal convoluted tubule absorbs all the glucose and amino acids and about 85% of the sodium chloride and water contained in the filtrate, in addition to phosphate and calcium. Glucose, amino acids, and sodium are absorbed by these tubular cells through an active process involving Na^+/K^+-ATPase (sodium pump) located in the basolateral cell membranes. Water diffuses passively, following the osmotic gradient. When the amount of glucose in the filtrate exceeds the absorbing capacity of the proximal tubule, urine becomes more abundant and contains glucose.

Absorption of the small amount of protein present in the filtrate takes place by pinocytosis. The proteins are digested by lysosomes, and the amino acids are reused by local cells.

In addition to these activities, the proximal convoluted tubule secretes creatinine and substances foreign to the organism, such as paraaminohippuric acid, penicillin, and iodopyracet (an iodinated organic compound used as an x-ray contrast medium), from the interstitial plasma into the filtrate. This is an active process referred to as tubular secretion. Study of the rates of secretion of these substances is useful in the clinical evaluation of kidney function.

Henle's Loop

Henle's loop is involved in water retention; only animals with such loops in their kidneys are capable of producing hypertonic urine and thus maintaining body water. Henle's loop creates a gradient of hypertonicity in the medullary interstitium that influences the concentration of the urine as it flows through the collecting ducts.

Although the thin descending limb of the loop is

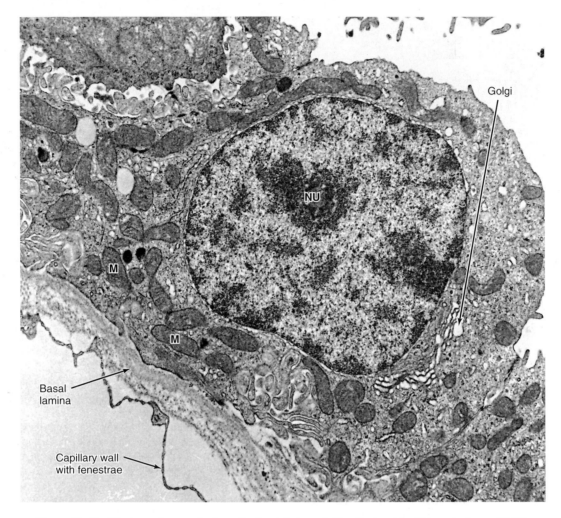

Figure 19–18. Electron micrograph of a collecting tubule wall. M, mitochondria; NU, nucleolus. × 15,000.

freely permeable to water, the entire ascending limb is impermeable to water. In the thick ascending limb, sodium chloride is actively transported out of the tubule to establish the gradient of hypertonicity in the medullary interstitium that is necessary for urine concentration. The osmolarity of the interstitium at the tips of the medullary pyramids is about four times that of blood.

Distal Convoluted Tubule

In the distal convoluted tubule, there is an ion-exchange site at which—if aldosterone is present in high enough concentration—sodium is absorbed and potassium ions are secreted. This is the site of the mechanism that controls the total salt and water content of the body. The distal tubule also secretes hydrogen and ammonium ions into tubular urine. This

activity is essential for maintenance of the acid-base balance in the blood.

Collecting Ducts

The epithelium of collecting ducts is responsive to arginine vasopressin, or antidiuretic hormone (ADH), secreted by the posterior pituitary. If water intake is limited, ADH is secreted and the epithelium of the collecting ducts becomes permeable to water, which is absorbed from the glomerular filtrate, transferred to blood capillaries, and thus retained in the body. In the presence of ADH, intramembrane particles in the luminal membrane aggregate to form what may be channels for water absorption.

Hormonal Effects

As explained above, water balance is controlled in

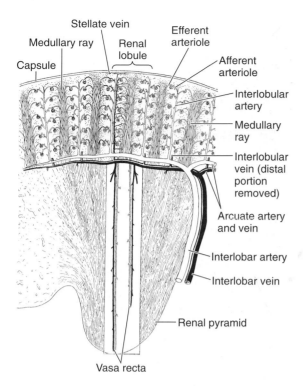

Figure 19–19. Circulation of blood in the kidney. Arcuate arteries are seen in the border between the cortex and the medulla.

part by the posterior lobe of the pituitary, which secretes ADH. A high intake of water inhibits production of ADH; the walls of the collecting ducts become impermeable to water, and water is not absorbed. The result is the formation of large amounts of hypotonic urine; water is eliminated, while the ions necessary for osmotic balance are retained. When small amounts of water are ingested or when a great loss of water occurs (eg, from excessive sweating or diarrhea), the walls of collecting ducts become permeable to water, which is absorbed, and the urine becomes hypertonic.

Steroid hormones of the adrenal cortex, mainly **aldosterone,** increase distal tubular absorption of sodium from the filtrate and thus decrease sodium loss in the urine. Aldosterone also facilitates the elimination of potassium and hydrogen ions. This hormone is crucial in maintaining electrolyte balance in the body.

Aldosterone deficiency in adrenalectomized animals and in humans with **Addison disease** results in an excessive loss of sodium in the urine.

BLADDER & URINARY PASSAGES

The bladder and the urinary passages store the urine formed in the kidneys and conduct it to the exterior. The calyces, renal pelvis, ureter, and bladder have the same basic histologic structure, with the walls of the ureters becoming gradually thicker as proximity to the bladder increases.

The mucosa of these organs consists of **transitional epithelium** (Figure 19–20) and a lamina propria of loose-to-dense connective tissue. Surrounding the lamina propria of these organs is a dense woven sheath of smooth muscle.

The transitional epithelium of the bladder in the undistended state is five or six cells in thickness; the superficial cells are rounded and bulge into the lumen. These cells are frequently polyploid or binucleate. When the epithelium is stretched, as when the bladder is full of urine, the epithelium is only three or four cells in thickness, and the superficial cells become squamous.

More than 90% of urinary bladder tumors originate in the epithelial lining.

The superficial cells of the transitional epithelium have a special membrane of thick plates separated by narrow bands of thinner membrane that are responsible for the osmotic barrier between urine and tissue fluids. When the bladder contracts, the membrane folds along the thinner regions, and the thicker plates invaginate to form fusiform cytoplasmic vesicles. These vesicles represent a reservoir of these thick plates that can be stored in the cytoplasm of the cells of the empty bladder and used to cover the increased cell surface in the full bladder (Figure 19–21). This luminal membrane is assembled in the Golgi complex and has an unusual chemical composition—cerebroside is the major component of the polar lipid fraction.

The muscular layers in the calyces, renal pelvis, and ureters have a helical arrangement. As the ureteral muscle cells reach the bladder, they become longitudinal. The muscle fibers of the bladder run in every direction (without distinct layers) until they approach the bladder neck, where three distinct layers can be identified: The internal longitudinal layer, distal to the bladder neck, becomes circular around the prostatic urethra and the prostatic parenchyma in men. It extends to the external meatus in women. Its fibers form the true involuntary urethral sphincter. The middle layer ends at the bladder neck, and the outer longitudinal layer continues to the end of the prostate in men and to the external urethral meatus in women.

The ureters pass through the wall of the bladder obliquely, forming a valve that prevents the backflow of urine. The intravesical ureter has only longitudinal muscle fibers.

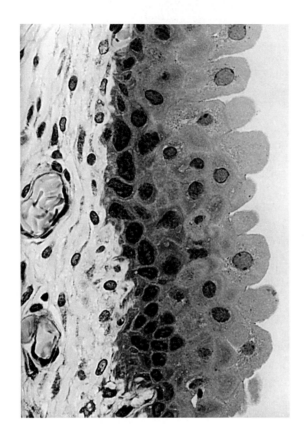

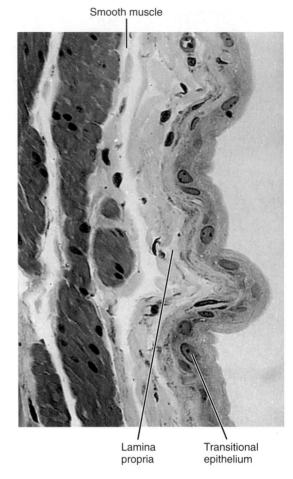

Smooth muscle

Lamina propria

Transitional epithelium

Figure 19–20. Photomicrographs of the urinary bladder wall. **Left:** Empty bladder. **Right:** Distended bladder. The transitional epithelium lies on a thin lamina propria. Hematoxylin-and-eosin stain.

The urinary passages are covered externally by an adventitial membrane—except for the upper part of the bladder, which is covered by serous peritoneum.

Urethra

The urethra is a tube that carries the urine from the bladder to the exterior. In men, sperm also pass through it during ejaculation. In women, the urethra is exclusively a urinary organ.

A. Male Urethra: The male urethra consists of four parts: **prostatic, membranous, bulbous,** and **pendulous.** The initial part of the urethra passes through the prostate (see Chapter 22), which is situated very close to the bladder, and the ducts that transport the secretions of the prostate open into the prostatic urethra.

In the dorsal and distal part of the **prostatic urethra,** there is an elevation, the **verumontanum** (from Latin, meaning mountain ridge), that protrudes into its interior. A closed tube called the prostatic utricle opens into the tip of the verumontanum; this tube has no known function. The ejaculatory ducts open on the sides of the verumontanum. The seminal fluid enters the proximal urethra through these ducts to be stored just before ejaculation. The prostatic urethra is lined with transitional epithelium.

The **membranous urethra** extends for only 1 cm and is lined with stratified or pseudostratified columnar epithelium. Surrounding this part of the urethra is a sphincter of striated muscle, the **external sphincter** of the urethra. The voluntary external striated sphincter adds further closing pressure to that exerted by the involuntary urethral sphincter. The latter is formed by the continuation of the internal longitudinal muscle of the bladder.

The **bulbous** and **pendulous** parts of the urethra are located in the **corpus spongiosum** of the penis. The urethral lumen dilates distally, forming the **fossa**

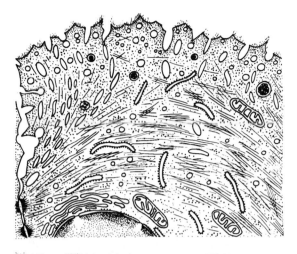

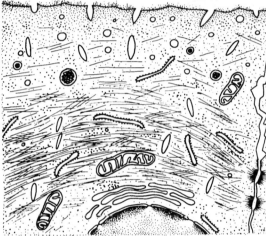

Figure 19–21. Ultrastructure of superficial cells of the bladder's transitional epithelium. **Top:** Contracted bladder. **Bottom:** Distended bladder.

navicularis. The epithelium of this portion of the urethra is mostly pseudostratified and columnar, with stratified and squamous areas.

Littre's glands are mucous glands found along the entire length of the urethra but mostly in the pendulous part. The secretory portions of some of these glands are directly linked to the epithelial lining of the urethra; others have excretory ducts.

B. Female Urethra: The female urethra is a tube 4–5 cm long, lined with stratified squamous epithelium and areas of pseudostratified columnar epithelium. The mid part of the female urethra is surrounded by an external striated voluntary sphincter.

REFERENCES

Barger AC, Herd JA: The renal circulation. N Engl J Med 1971;284:482.

Bulger RE, Dobyan DC: Recent advances in renal morphology. Annu Rev Physiol 1982;44:147.

Farquhar MG: The glomerular basement membrane: a selective macromolecular filter. In: *Cell Biology of Extracellular Matrix.* Hay ED (editor). Plenum Press, 1981.

Ganong WF: Formation and excretion of urine. In: *Review of Medical Physiology,* 18th ed. Appleton & Lange, 1997.

Hicks RM: The mammalian urinary bladder: an accommodating organ. Biol Rev 1975;50:215.

Levy BJ, Wight TN: The role of proteoglycans in bladder structure and function. Adv Exp Med Biol 1995;385: 191.

Maunsbach AB (editors): *Functional Ultrastructure of the Kidney.* Academic Press, 1981.

Staehelin LA et al: Luminal plasma membrane of the urinary bladder. 1. Three-dimensional reconstruction from freeze-etch images. J Cell Biol 1972;53:73.

The Neuroendocrine Hypothalamo-Hypophyseal System

A **hormone** is an organic chemical that is liberated—at a specific time and in small amounts—by **endocrine cells** into the tissue fluids or vascular system. In general, hormones exert their effects at a distance from the site of their secretion. The tissues and organs on which the hormones act are called **target organs.** Hormones of many endocrine glands have an effect on the nervous system, and several endocrine organs are stimulated or inhibited by neural mechanisms. Figure 20–1 illustrates several situations in which chemical messengers produced in the nervous system act either directly or via endocrine organs. This interlocking mechanism is so remarkable that its nervous system and endocrine elements are considered to constitute a single **neuroendocrine system,** the neuroendocrine hypothalamo-hypophyseal system (NHS).

The immune system also participates in the regulatory mechanisms of the body, exchanging information with the endocrine and nervous systems through chemical signals. It is well known that endocrine, nervous, and immune systems interact via hormones, neurotransmitters, and cytokines (Figure 20–2) traveling through blood and nerves. For example, stress can influence immunity, increasing susceptibility to infection and progression of cancer, and hormones can influence behavior by acting on the nervous system. modified

COMPONENTS OF THE NHS

The **hypophysis** (Gr. *hypo,* under, + *physis,* growth), or **pituitary gland,** weighs about 0.5 g, and

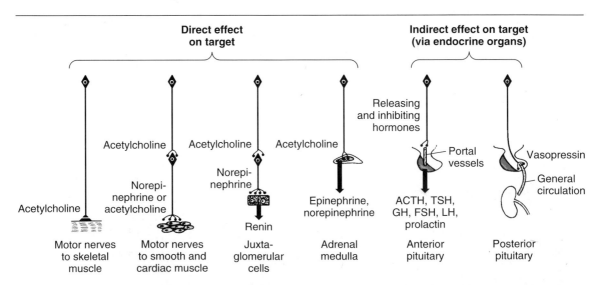

Figure 20–1. Six situations in which chemical messengers are released by neurons. The last two are examples of neurosecretion. ACTH, adrenocorticotropic hormone; TSH, thyrotropin; GH, growth hormone; FSH, follicle-stimulating hormone; LH, luteinizing hormone. (Reproduced, with permission, from Ganong WF. *Review of Medical Physiology.* 16th ed. Appleton & Lange, 1993.)

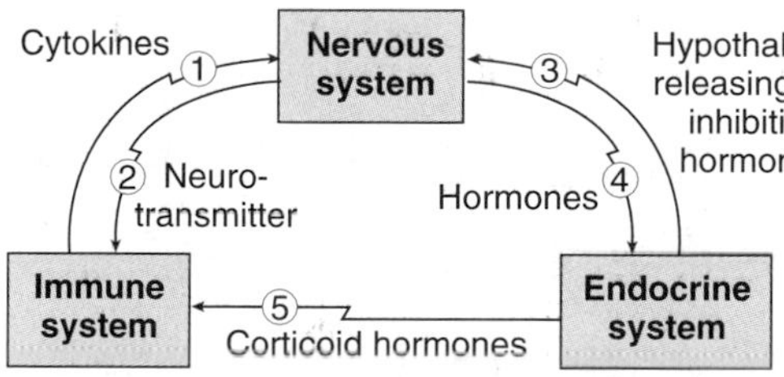

Cytokines

Neuro-
transmitter

Hormones

Corticoid hormones

Hypothalamic
releasing and
inhibiting
hormones

Figure 20–2. Interactions among the three main control systems of the body. The immune system acts on the nervous system mainly through proteins called cytokines (1) produced by its cells. Simultaneously, the immune system is influenced by neurotransmitters (2) synthesized and released by nerve cells. Information is passed through hormones (3 and 4) between the nervous and endocrine systems and between the endocrine and immune systems (5). The three systems play key roles in maintaining the state of equilibrium in the body with respect to various functions and chemical compositions of the fluids and tissues (homeostasis).

its normal dimensions in humans are about $10 \times 13 \times 6$ mm. It lies in a cavity of the sphenoid bone—**the sella turcica**—an important radiologic landmark. The hypophysis is connected to the hypothalamus at the base of the brain, with which it has important anatomic and functional relationships.

During embryogenesis, the hypophysis develops partly from oral ectoderm and partly from nerve tissue. The neural component arises as an evagination from the floor of the diencephalon and grows caudally as a stalk without detaching itself from the brain. The oral component arises as an outpocketing of ectoderm from the roof of the primitive mouth of the embryo and grows cranially, forming a structure called **Rathke's pouch.** Later, a constriction at the base of this pouch separates it from the oral cavity. Its anterior wall thickens at the same time, reducing the lumen of Rathke's pouch to a small fissure (Figure 20–3).

The **neurohypophysis,** the part of the hypophysis that develops from nerve tissue, consists of a large portion, the **pars nervosa,** and the smaller **infundibulum,** or **neural stalk** (Figure 20–4). The neural stalk is composed of the stem and median eminence. The part of the hypophysis that arises from oral ectoderm is known as the **adenohypophysis** and is subdivided into three portions: a large **pars distalis,** or **anterior lobe;** a cranial part, the **pars tuberalis,** that surrounds the neural stalk; and the **pars intermedia** (Figure 20–3).

Production & Storage of NHS Hormones

The NHS is intimately interconnected by both nerve cells and blood supply; it produces hormones that are active in providing the various levels of both nervous system and hormonal control. The hormones can be divided into two groups. The first group consists of peptides or small proteins produced by aggregates of secretory neurons (**nuclei**) in the hypothalamus. Some of these hormones are transported via neuronal axons to the median eminence, where they are stored in the dilated closed ends of the axons. Others are stored in the pars nervosa, also in the dilated ends of axons. Figure 20–4 illustrates the nuclei and the axon bundles (tracts) that produce, transport, and store these hormones.

In the second group of hormones are the secretory products of protein- and glycoprotein-synthesizing and -storing cells in the pars distalis. These hormones are stored in these endocrine epithelial cells as secretory granules (Figure 20–5). Both groups of hormones are released according to external stimuli; they constitute a delicately balanced system of neuroendocrine regulation for the organism.

Blood Supply & Innervation

The blood supply of the hypophysis derives from two groups of blood vessels that come from the internal carotid artery. From above, the right and left **superior hypophyseal arteries** supply the median eminence and the neural stalk; from below, the right and

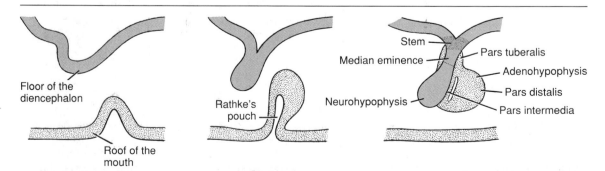

Figure 20–3. Development of the adenohypophysis and the neurohypophysis. The lower portion shows the ectoderm of the roof of the mouth and its derivatives (stippled). The upper portion shows the neural ectoderm from the floor of the diencephalon (shown in color).

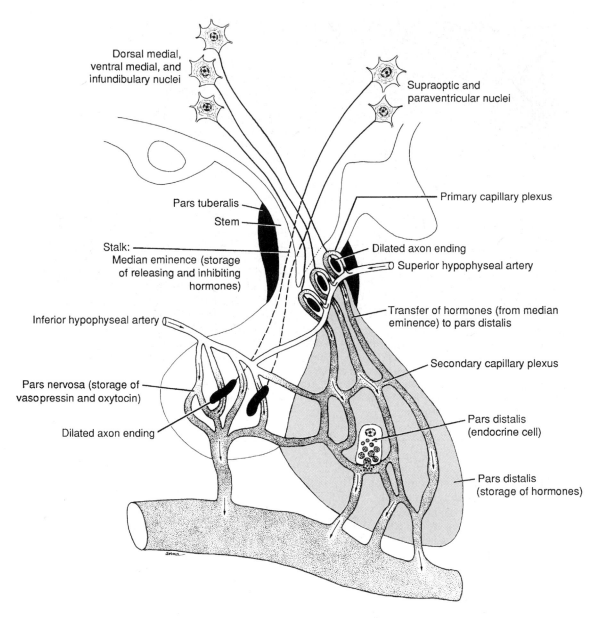

Figure 20–4. The hypothalamo-hypophyseal system, with its vascularization and sites of hormone production and storage.

left **inferior hypophyseal arteries** provide blood mainly for the neurohypophysis, with a small supply to the stalk. The superior hypophyseal arteries form a **primary capillary plexus** of fenestrated capillaries that irrigate the stalk and median eminence. They then rejoin to form veins that develop a **secondary capillary plexus** in the adenohypophysis (Figure 20–4). This **hypophyseal portal system** is of utmost importance in regulating hypophyseal function: it carries neurohormones from the median eminence to the adenohypophysis.

The nerve supply of the anterior lobe is derived from the carotid plexus, which accompanies the arteriolar branches. These nerves appear to have a vasomotor function and do not directly affect the cells of the anterior lobe. Blood from both hypophyseal lobes drains into the cavernous sinuses through a number of venous channels.

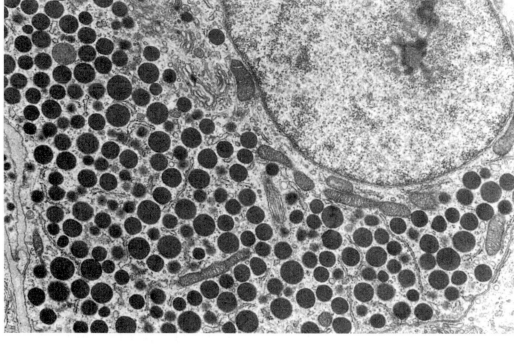

Figure 20–5. Electron micrograph of a somatotroph (growth hormone–secreting cell) of a cat anterior hypophysis. Note the numerous secretory granules, long mitochondria, cisternae of rough endoplasmic reticulum, and prominent juxtanuclear Golgi complex. × 10,270.

Table 20–1. Secretory cells of the pars distalis.

Cell Type	Stain Affinity	Hormone Produced	Main Physiologic Activity	Secretory Granules in Humans	Hypothalamic Releasing Hormones	Hypothalamic Inhibiting Hormones
Somatotropic cell	Acidophilic	Somatotropin (growth hormone)	Acts on growth of long bones via somatomedins synthesized in liver	Numerous, round or oval; 300 to 400 nm in diameter	Somatotropin-releasing hormone (SRH)	Somatostatin
Mammotropic cell	Acidophilic	Prolactin	Promotes milk secretion	200 nm; increases in size during pregnancy and lactation (600 nm in diameter)	Prolactin-releasing hormone (PRH)	Prolactin-inhibiting hormone (PIH)
Gonadotropic cell	Basophilic	Follicle-stimulating hormone (FSH) and luteinizing hormone (LH) in the same cell type	FSH promotes ovarian follicle development and estrogen secretion in women and stimulates spermatogenesis in men. LH promotes ovarian follicle maturation and progesterone secretion in women and, Leydig cell stimulation and androgen secretion in men.	250 to 400 nm diameter	Gonadotropin-releasing hormone (GnRH). May be two releasing hormones: FRH (follicle-releasing) and LRH (lutein-releasing)	
Thyrotropic cell	Basophilic	Thyrotropin (TSH)	Stimulates thyroid hormone synthesis, storage, and liberation	Small granules, 120 to 200 nm in diameter	Thyrotropin-releasing hormone (TRH)	
Corticotropic cell	Basophilic	Corticotropin (ACTH)	Stimulates secretion of adrenal cortex hormones	Large granules, 400 to 550 nm in diameter	Corticotropin-releasing hormone (CRH)	

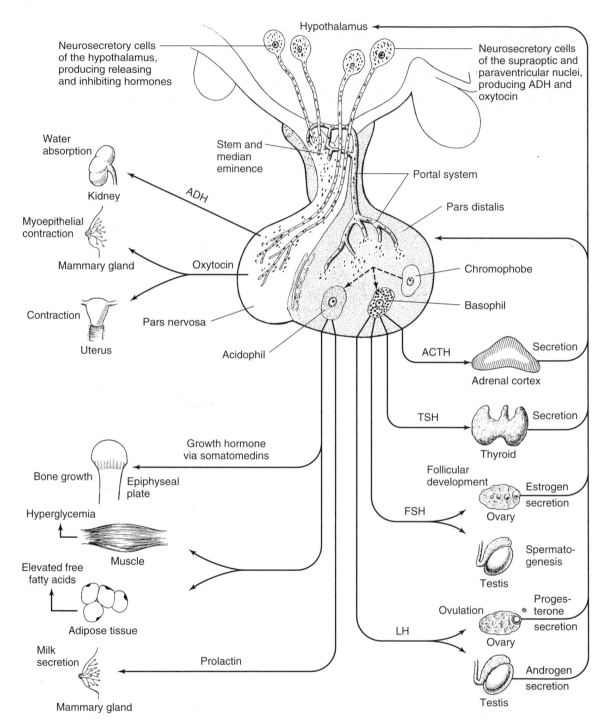

Figure 20–6. The effects of various hypophyseal hormones on target organs. Several of the hormones produced by the target organs can act on the hypophysis or the hypothalamus to regulate their activity (negative feedback; see Figure 20–8). The neurohypophysis is shown in color; the adenohypophysis is stippled. ADH, antidiuretic hormone. For definitions of other abbreviations, see the legend to Figure 20–1.

ADENOHYPOPHYSIS

Pars Distalis ANT. pit

The pars distalis is formed of cords of aggregated cells interspersed with capillaries. The few fibroblasts present produce reticular fibers that support the cords of hormone-secreting cells. The pars distalis accounts for 75% of the mass of the hypophysis. Cells of the pars distalis have been described as **chromophobes** (Gr. *chroma,* color, + *phobos,* fear) and **chromophils** (*chroma* + Gr. *philein,* to love) according to their staining affinity. Chromophobes do not stain intensely and, when observed with an electron microscope, show two populations of cells. One has few secretory granules, and the other has none. The group with no secretory granules probably contains undifferentiated cells and follicular cells. The long branching processes of follicular cells form a supporting network for the other cells. Chromophils, which can be stained with basic or acid dyes, are called basophils or acidophils according to their affinity (Table 20–1 and Figure 20–6). As shown in Table 20–1, these secretory cells are named for the hormones they produce. Most cells produce only a single hormone each, with the exception of the gonadotropic cell, which produces two hormones. These hormones have widespread physiologic activity (Figure 20–6); they regulate almost all endocrine glands, the secretion of milk, and the metabolism of muscle, bone, and adipose tissue.

Many dyes have been used in attempts to distinguish the five types of hormone-secreting cells, but with little success. Immunocytochemical methods and electron microscopy are currently the only reliable techniques to distinguish these cell types.

Control of the Pars Distalis

The activities of the cells of the pars distalis are controlled by more than one mechanism. The main mechanism uses the peptide hormones (Table 20–2) produced in the hypothalamic aggregates of neurosecretory cells and stored in the median eminence. Most of these hormones are called **hypothalamic releasing hormones;** when liberated, they go to the pars distalis through the primary and secondary capillary plexuses (see Figure 20–4). Two of these hormones, which act on specific cells of the par distalis, inhibit the release of hormones (**hypothalamic inhibiting hormones;** see Table 20–1).

A second general control mechanism is the direct effect of hormones from stimulated endocrine cells on the release of peptides from the median eminence and the pars distalis. Figure 20–7 illustrates both these mechanisms, using the thyroid as an example. It also illustrates the complex chain of events that begin with the action of neurons on neurosecretory cells of the hypothalamic nuclei and end on the effector cells with the action of the last hormone in the sequence. This mechanism participates in fine-tuning the coordination of these events and may offer insights into the effects of psychic stimulation and depression.

Pars Tuberalis

The pars tuberalis is a funnel-shaped region surrounding the infundibulum of the neurohypophysis (Figure 20–4). Most of the cells of the pars tuberalis secrete gonadotropins (follicle-stimulating hormone and luteinizing hormone) and are arranged in cords alongside the blood vessels.

Pars Intermedia

The pars intermedia, which develops from the dorsal portion of Rathke's pouch (Figure 20–3), is, in humans, a rudimentary region made up of cords and follicles of weakly basophilic cells that contain small

Table 20–2. Hormones of the neurohypophysis.

Hypothalamus		Pars Nervosa	
Hormone	Function	Hormone	Function
Thyrotropin-releasing hormone (TRH)	Stimulates release of thyrotropin and prolactin	Vasopressin	Increases water permeability of kidney collecting ducts and promotes vascular smooth muscle contraction
Gonadotropin-releasing hormone (GnRH)	Stimulates the release of both follicle-stimulating hormone and luteinizing hormone	Oxytocin	Acts on contraction of uterine smooth muscle and the myoepithelial cells of the mammary gland
Somatostatin	Inhibits release of both growth hormone and thyrotropin		
Growth hormone–releasing hormone (GRH)	Stimulates release of growth hormone		
Prolactin-inhibiting hormone (PIH) Dopamine	Inhibits release of prolactin		
Corticotropin-releasing hormone (CRH)	Stimulates release of both B lipotropin and corticotropin		

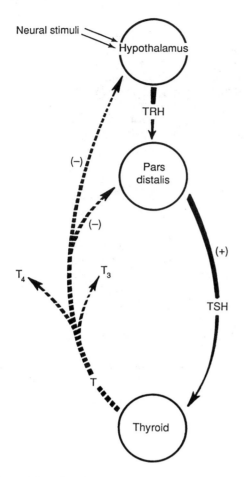

Figure 20–7. Relationship between the hypothalamus, the hypophysis, and the thyroid. Thyrotropin-releasing hormone (TRH) promotes secretion of thyrotropin (TSH), which regulates the synthesis and secretion of the hormones T_3 and T_4. In addition to their effect on peripheral tissues, these hormones regulate TSH and TRH secretion from the pars distalis and the hypothalamus by a negative-feedback mechanism. T, thyroglobulin. Solid arrows indicate stimulation; dashed arrows, inhibition.

secretory granules. The function of these cells is not known.

NEUROHYPOPHYSIS

The neurohypophysis consists of the pars nervosa and the neural stalk. The pars nervosa, which contains no secretory cells, is composed of some 100,000 unmyelinated axons of secretory neurons from the supraoptic and paraventricular nuclei (Figure 20–4). The secretory neurons have all the characteristics of typical neurons, including the ability to conduct an action potential, but have more developed

Nissl bodies related to the production of the neurosecretory material, which can be studied by specific techniques (eg, using Gomori's chrome hematoxylin stain).

The electron microscope reveals that these neurosecretory granules have a diameter of 100–200 nm, are surrounded by a membrane, and are more numerous in the dilated terminal parts of the axons that are apposed to fenestrated blood capillaries. There they form accumulations, known as **Herring bodies,** that are visible with the light microscope. The hormones contained in these stored granules are released as needed by the organism.

The **neurosecretory material** consists of hormones (either **oxytocin** or **vasopressin**) and a binding protein (**neurophysin**) specific for each hormone. The hormones are peptides of nine amino acids, with a ring structure formed by a disulfide bridge. Each hormone has a slightly different composition, which results in greatly different functions. The hormone-neurophysin complex is synthesized as a single long peptide on ribosomes of rough endoplasmic reticulum. The peptide is partly glycosylated in the lumen of the endoplasmic reticulum and then passed on to the Golgi complex, where there is further glycosylation and packaging in secretory granules. As the granules pass down axons of the hypothalamo-hypophyseal tract, proteolysis of the precursor yields the hormone and its specific binding protein. Vasopressin and oxytocin are stored in the neurohypophysis and released into the blood by impulses in the nerve fibers from the hypothalamus. Although there is some overlap, the fibers from supraoptic nuclei are mainly concerned with vasopressin secretion, whereas most of the fibers from the paraventricular nuclei are concerned with oxytocin secretion.

Neurohypophyseal Cells

Although the neurohypophysis consists mainly of axons from hypothalamic neurons, about 25% of the volume of this structure consists of a specific type of highly branched glial cell called a **pituicyte** (Figure 20–8).

Histophysiology

The neurohypophysis secretes two hormones, both cyclic peptides made up of nine amino acids. These hormones are **arginine vasopressin**—also called **antidiuretic hormone (ADH)**—and **oxytocin.** These hormones are present in different secretory granules and in different neurons. In large doses, vasopressin promotes the contraction of smooth muscle of blood vessels, raising the blood pressure. It acts mainly on the muscle layers of small arteries and arterioles. It is doubtful if the amount of endogenous vasopressin secreted is sufficient to exert any appreciable effect on blood pressure homeostasis.

Vasopressin is secreted whenever the osmotic

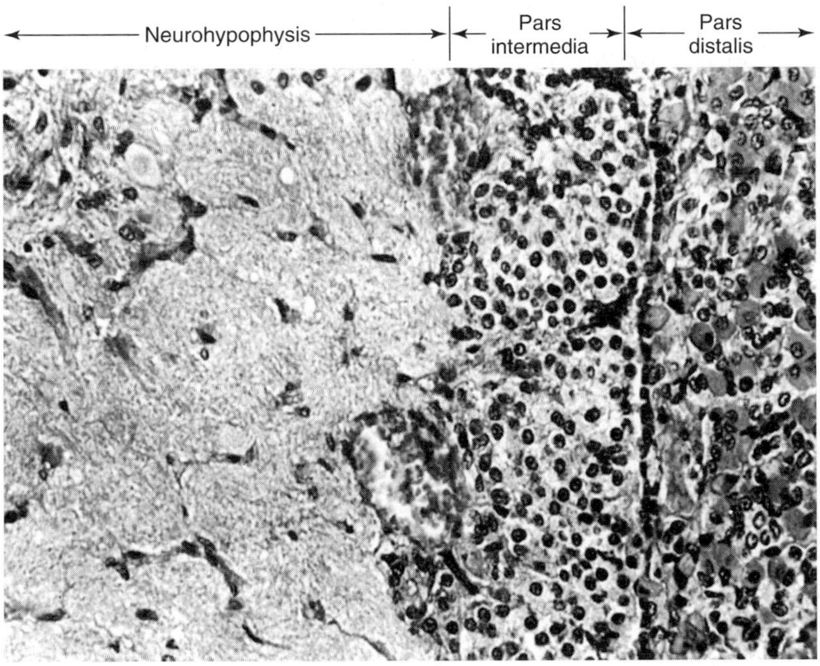

Figure 20–8. Section of the hypophysis of a rat showing (from left to right) the neurohypophysis, the pars intermedia, and the pars distalis. Chromophilic and chromophobic cells are apparent in the pars distalis. The pars intermedia consists of cords of one cell type. Nuclei of pituicytes are clearly visible in the neurohypophysis. × 340.

pressure of the blood increases. The blood then acts on osmoreceptor cells in the anterior hypothalamus, stimulating the secretion of the hormone from supraoptic neurons. Its main effect is to increase the permeability to water of the collecting tubules of the kidney. As a result, water is absorbed by these tubules and urine becomes hypertonic. Thus, vasopressin helps to regulate the osmotic balance of the internal milieu.

Oxytocin stimulates contraction of the smooth muscle of the uterine wall during copulation and childbirth and of the myoepithelial cells that surround the alveoli and ducts of the mammary glands during nursing. The secretion of oxytocin is stimulated by distention of the vagina or of the uterine cervix and by nursing. This occurs via nerve tracts that act on the hypothalamus. The neurohormonal reflex triggered by nursing is called the **milk-ejection reflex** (Figure 20–6).

Lesions of the hypothalamus, which destroy the neurosecretory cells that produce ADH, cause **diabetes insipidus,** a disease characterized by loss of renal capacity to concentrate urine. As a result, an individual suffering from this disease may excrete up to 20 liters of urine per day (polyuria) and will drink enormous quantities of liquids.

Tumors of the Hypophysis

Tumors of the hypophysis are usually benign. About two thirds of them produce hormones that cause clinical symptoms. These tumors can produce growth hormone, prolactin, adrenocorticotropin and, less frequently, thyroid-stimulating hormone. Clinical diagnosis of these tumors can be confirmed by immunocytochemical methods after surgical removal.

REFERENCES

Bhatnagar AS (editor): *The Anterior Pituitary Gland.* Raven Press, 1983.

Brownstein MJ et al: Synthesis, transport, and release of posterior pituitary hormones. Science 1980;207:373.

Cross BA, Leng G (editors): The neurohypophysis; structure, function and control. Prog Brain Res 1982;60:3.

Daniel PM: The blood supply of the hypothalamus and pituitary gland. Br Med Bull 1966;22:202.

Dietrichs E et al: Hypothalamocerebellar and cerebellohypothalamic projections: circuits for regulating nonsomatic cerebellar activity? Histol Histopathol 1994; 9:603.

Girod C: Immunocytochemistry of the vertebrate adenohypophysis. In: *Handbook of Histochemistry.* Vol 8, Suppl 5. Graumann W, Neumann K (editors). Gustav Fischer, 1983.

Pantic VR: The specificity of pituitary cells and regulation of their activities. Int Rev Cytol 1975;40:153.

Pelletier G et al: Identification of human anterior pituitary cells by immunoelectron microscopy. J Clin Endocrinol Metab 1978;46:534.

Phifer RF et al: Immunohistologic and histologic evidence that follicle-stimulating hormone and luteinizing hormone are present in the same cell type in the human pars distalis. J Clin Endocrinol Metab 1973;36:125.

Phifer RF et al: Specific demonstration of the human hypophyseal cells which produce adrenocorticotropic hormone. J Clin Endocrinol 1970;31:347.

Reichlin S (editor): *The Neurohypophysis: Physiological and Clinical Aspects.* Plenum, 1984.

Seyama S et al: Ultrastructural study of the human neurohypophysis. 1. Neurosecretory axons and their dilatations in the pars nervosa. Cell Tissue Res 1980;205:253.

Seyama S et al: Ultrastructural study of the human neurohypophysis. 3. Vascular and perivascular structures. Cell Tissue Res 1980;206:291.

Takei Y et al: Ultrastructural study of the human neurohypophysis. 2. Cellular elements of neural parenchyma, the pituicytes. Cell Tissue Res 1980;205:273.

Adrenals, Islets of Langerhans, Thyroid, Parathyroids, & Pineal Gland

21

ADRENAL (SUPRARENAL) GLANDS

The adrenal glands are paired organs that lie near the superior poles of the kidneys, embedded in adipose tissue (Figure 21–1). They are flattened structures with a half-moon shape; in the human, they are about 4–6 cm long, 1–2 cm wide, and 4–6 mm thick. Together they weigh about 8 g, but their weight and size vary with the age and physiologic condition of the individual. Examination of a fresh section of adrenal gland shows it to be covered by a capsule of dense collagenous connective tissue. The gland consists of two concentric layers: a yellow peripheral layer, the **adrenal cortex;** and a reddish-brown central layer, the **adrenal medulla** (Figures 21–2 and 21–5). Cortical and medullary tissues sometimes are found at other sites, as shown in Figure 21–1.

The adrenal cortex and the adrenal medulla can be considered two organs with distinct origins, functions, and morphologic characteristics that unite during embryonic development. They arise from different germ layers. The cortex arises from coelomic intermediate mesoderm; the medulla consists of cells derived from the neural crest, from which sympathetic ganglion cells also originate. The general histologic appearance of the adrenal gland is typical of an endocrine gland in which cells of both cortex and medulla are grouped in cords along capillaries (see Chapter 4).

The collagenous connective tissue capsule that covers the adrenal gland sends thin septa to the interior of the gland as trabeculae. The stroma consists mainly of a rich network of reticular fibers that support the secretory cells.

Blood Supply

The adrenal glands are supplied by several arteries that enter at various points around their periphery (Figure 21–2). The three main groups are the **superior suprarenal artery,** arising from the inferior phrenic artery; the **middle suprarenal artery,** arising from the aorta; and the **inferior suprarenal artery,** arising from the renal artery. The arterial

branches form a subcapsular plexus from which arise three groups of vessels: arteries of the capsule; arteries of the cortex, which branch repeatedly to form the capillary bed between the parenchymal cells (these capillaries drain into medullary capillaries); and arteries of the medulla, which pass through the cortex before breaking up to form part of the extensive capillary network of the medulla (Figure 21–2).

A dual blood supply provides the medulla with both arterial (via **medullary arteries**) and venous (via **cortical arteries**) blood. The capillary endothelium is extremely attenuated and interrupted by small fenestrae that are closed by thin diaphragms. A continuous basal lamina is present beneath the endothelium. Capillaries of the medulla, together with capillaries that supply the cortex, form the medullary veins, which join to constitute the **adrenal** or **suprarenal vein** (Figure 21–2).

Adrenal Cortex

Because of the differences in disposition and appearance of its cells, the adrenal cortex can be subdivided into three concentric layers that are usually not sharply defined in humans (Figures 21–2, 21–3, and 21–5): the **zona glomerulosa,** the **zona fasciculata,** and the **zona reticularis.** These zones occupy 15%, 65%, and 7%, respectively, of the total volume of the adrenal glands.

The layer immediately beneath the connective tissue capsule is the zona glomerulosa, in which the columnar or pyramidal cells are arranged in closely packed, rounded, or arched clusters surrounded by capillaries (Figure 21–3A and B).

The next layer of cells is known as the zona fasciculata because of the arrangement of the cells in straight cords, one or two cells thick (Figure 21–3C), that run at right angles to the surface of the organ and have capillaries between them. The cells of the zona fasciculata are polyhedral, with a great number of lipid droplets in their cytoplasm. As a result of the dissolution of the lipids during tissue preparation, the fasciculata cells appear vacuolated in common histologic preparations (Figure 21–3C).

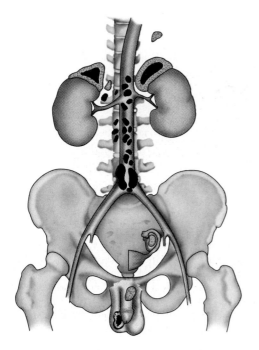

Figure 21–1. Human adrenal glands. Adrenocortical tissue is shown stippled; adrenal medullary tissue is shown black. Note the location of the adrenal glands at the superior pole of each kidney. Also shown are extra-adrenal sites where cortical and medullary tissues are sometimes found. (Reproduced, with permission, from Forsham in: *Textbook of Endocrinology,* 4th ed. Williams RH [editor]. Saunders, 1968.)

The zona reticularis (Figure 21–3D), the innermost layer of the cortex, lies between the zona fasciculata and the medulla; it contains cells disposed in irregular cords that form an anastomosing network. These cells are smaller than those of the other two layers. Lipofuscin pigment granules in the cells are large and quite numerous. Irregularly shaped cells with pyknotic nuclei—suggesting cellular degradation—are often found in this layer.

Cells of the adrenal cortex do not store their secretory products in granules; rather, they synthesize and secrete steroid hormones only upon demand. Steroids, being low-molecular-weight lipid-soluble molecules, can freely diffuse through the plasma membrane and do not require the specialized process of exocytosis for their release. Cells of the adrenal cortex (Figure 21–4) have the typical ultrastructure of steroid-secreting cells (see Chapter 4).

Histophysiology

The steroids secreted by the cortex can be divided into three groups, according to their main physiologic actions: **glucocorticoids, mineralocorticoids,**

and **androgens** (Figure 21–5). The zona glomerulosa secretes mineralocorticoids, primarily aldosterone, that maintain electrolyte (eg, sodium and potassium) and water balance. The zona fasciculata and probably the zona reticularis secrete the glucocorticoids cortisone and cortisol or, in some animals, corticosterone; these glucocorticoids regulate carbohydrate, protein, and fat metabolism. These zones also produce androgens and perhaps estrogens in small amounts.

The location of the enzymes participating in aldosterone synthesis has been determined through differential centrifugation. The synthesis of cholesterol from acetate takes place in smooth endoplasmic reticulum, and the conversion of cholesterol to pregnenolone takes place in the mitochondria. The enzymes associated with the synthesis of progesterone and deoxycorticosterone from pregnenolone are found in smooth endoplasmic reticulum; those enzymes that convert deoxycorticosterone → corticosterone → 18-hydroxycorticosterone → aldosterone are located in mitochondria—a clear example of collaboration between two cell organelles.

The **glucocorticoids,** mainly cortisol and corticosterone, exert a profound effect on the metabolism of carbohydrates, as well as on that of proteins and lipids. In the liver, glucocorticoids promote the uptake and use of fatty acids (energy source), amino acids (enzyme synthesis), and carbohydrates (glucose synthesis) that are used in gluconeogenesis and glycogenesis (glycogen assembly). These hormones can stimulate the synthesis of so much glucose that the resulting high levels in the blood produce a condition similar to diabetes mellitus. Outside the liver, however, glucocorticoids induce an opposite, or catabolic, effect on peripheral organs (eg, skin, muscle, adipose tissue). In these structures, glucocorticoids not only decrease synthetic activity but also promote protein and lipid degradation. The by-products of degradation, amino and fatty acids, are removed from the blood and used by the synthetically active hepatocytes.

Glucocorticoids also suppress the immune response by destroying circulating lymphocytes and inhibiting mitotic activity in lymphocyte-forming organs.

The **mineralocorticoids** act mainly on the distal renal tubules as well as on the gastric mucosa and the salivary and sweat glands, stimulating the absorption of sodium. They may increase the concentration of potassium and decrease the concentration of sodium in muscle and brain cells.

Dehydroepiandrosterone is the only sex hormone that is secreted in significant physiologic quantities by the adrenal cortex. It has virilizing and anabolic effects, but it is less than one-fifth as potent as testicular androgens. For this reason, and because it is secreted in small quantities, it produces a negligible physiologic effect under normal conditions.

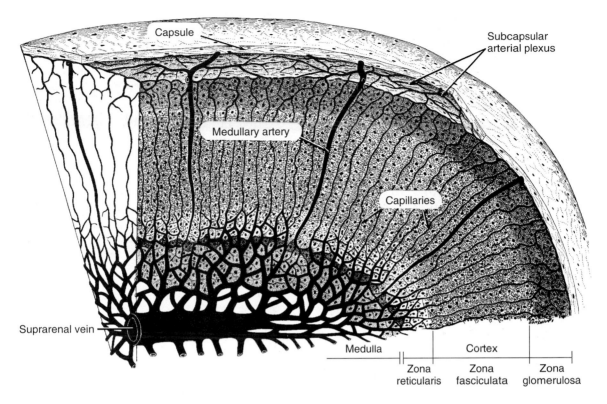

Figure 21–2. General architecture and blood circulation of the adrenal gland.

As in other endocrine glands, the adrenal cortex is controlled initially through the release of its corresponding releasing hormone stored in the median eminence. This is followed by secretion of adrenocorticotropic hormone, or corticotropin (ACTH), which stimulates the synthesis and secretion of cortical hormones (eg, glucocorticoids). Free glucocorticoids may then inhibit ACTH secretion. The degree of pituitary inhibition is proportionate to the concentration of circulating glucocorticoids; inhibition is exerted at both the pituitary and hypothalamic levels (Figures 21–6 and 21–7).

Fetal, or Provisional, Cortex

In humans and some other animals, the adrenal gland of the newborn is proportionately larger than that of the adult. At this early age, a layer known as the **fetal,** or **provisional, cortex** is present between the medulla and the thin permanent cortex. This layer is fairly thick, and its cells are disposed in cords. After birth, the provisional cortex undergoes involution while the permanent cortex—the initially thin layer—develops, differentiating into the three layers (zones) described above. A major function of the fetal cortex is the secretion of sulfate conjugates of androgens, which are converted in the placenta to ac-

tive androgens and estrogens that enter the maternal circulation.

Adrenal Medulla

The adrenal medulla is composed of polyhedral parenchymal cells arranged in cords or clumps and supported by a reticular fiber network (Figure 21–8). A profuse capillary supply intervenes between adjacent cords, and there are a few parasympathetic ganglion cells. Medullary parenchymal cells arise from neural crest cells, as do the postganglionic neurons of sympathetic and parasympathetic ganglia. Parenchymal cells of the adrenal medulla can be regarded as modified sympathetic postganglionic neurons that have lost their axons and dendrites during embryonic development and have become secretory cells.

Medullary parenchymal cells have abundant membrane-limited electron-dense secretory granules, 150–350 nm in diameter. These granules contain one or the other of the catecholamines, epinephrine or norepinephrine (Figure 21–9). The secretory granules also contain ATP, proteins called **chromogranins** (which may serve as binding proteins for catecholamines), dopamine β-hydroxylase (which converts dopamine to norepinephrine), and opiate-like peptides (enkephalins). Figure 21–10 shows the par-

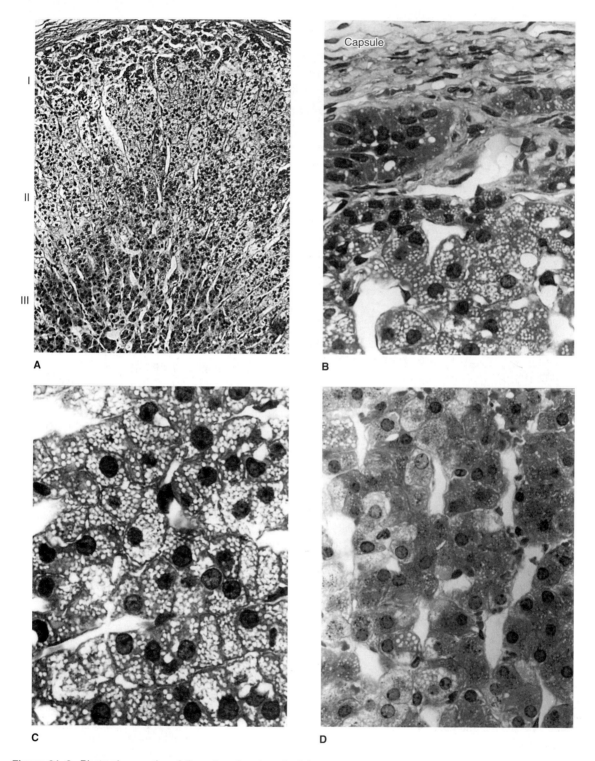

Figure 21–3. Photomicrographs of the adrenal cortex. **A:** A low-power general view. I, the zona glomerulosa; II, the zona fasciculata; III, the zona reticularis. × 80. **B:** The capsule, the zona glomerulosa, and the beginning of the zona fasciculata. × 330. **C:** The zona fasciculata, showing cells with abundant lipid droplets. × 330. **D:** The zona reticularis, showing cells with few lipid droplets. × 330. Hematoxylin-and-eosin (H&E) stain.

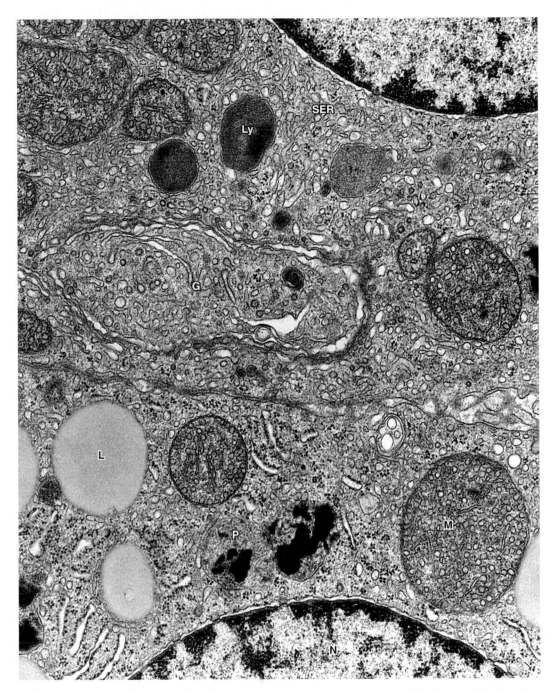

Figure 21–4. Fine structure of two steroid-secreting cells from the zona fasciculata of the human adrenal cortex. The lipid droplets (L) contain cholesterol esters. M, mitochondria with characteristic tubular and vesicular cristae; SER, smooth endoplasmic reticulum; N, nucleus; G, Golgi complex; Ly, lysosome; P, lipofuscin pigment granule. × 25,700.

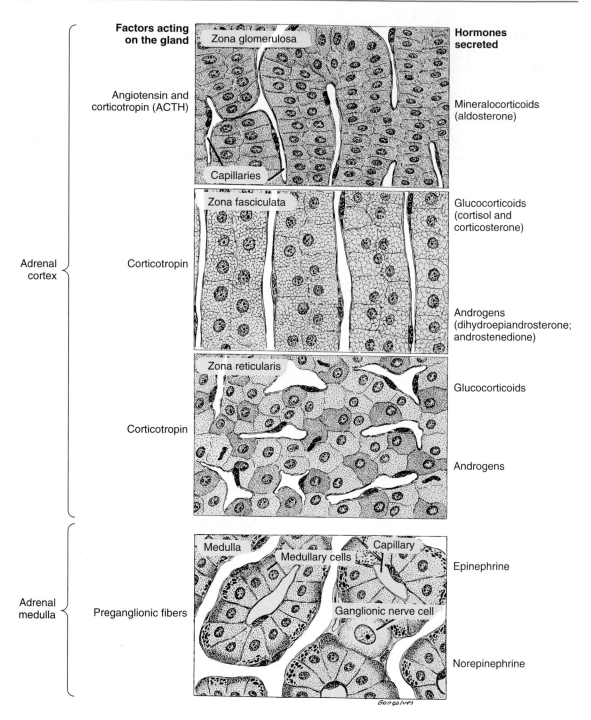

Figure 21–5. Structure and histophysiology of the adrenal gland.

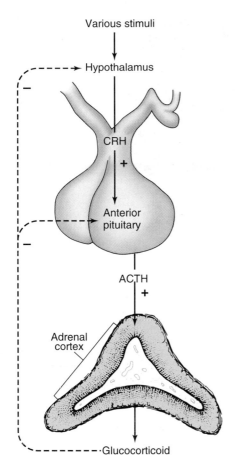

ticipation of cell organelles in the synthetic processes that lead to the formation of secretory granules in medullary cells.

A large body of evidence shows that epinephrine and norepinephrine are secreted by two different types of cells in the medulla. Epinephrine-secreting cells have smaller granules that are less electron-dense, and their contents fill the granule. Norepinephrine-secreting cells have larger granules that are more electron-dense; their contents are irregular in shape, and there is an electron-lucent layer beneath the surrounding membrane. About 80% of the catecholamine output of the adrenal vein is epinephrine.

All adrenal medullary cells are innervated by cholinergic endings of <u>preganglionic sympathetic neurons</u>. Unlike the cortex, which does not store steroids, cells of the medulla accumulate and store their hormones in granules.

> Epinephrine and norepinephrine are secreted in large quantities in response to intense emotional reactions (eg, fright). Secretion of these substances is mediated by the preganglionic fibers that innervate medullary cells. Vasoconstriction, hypertension, changes in heart rate, and metabolic effects such as elevated blood glucose result from the secretion and release of catecholamines into the bloodstream. These effects are part of the organism's defense reaction to stress (the fight-or-flight response). During normal activity, the medulla continuously secretes small quantities of these hormones.

Medullary cells are also found in the paraganglia (collections of catecholamine-secreting cells adjacent to the autonomic ganglia) as well as in various viscera. Paraganglia are a diffuse source of catecholamines.

Figure 21–6. Feedback mechanism of ACTH-glucocorticoid secretion. Solid arrows indicate stimulation; dashed arrows, inhibition. CRH, corticotropin-releasing hormone, ACTH, corticotropin.

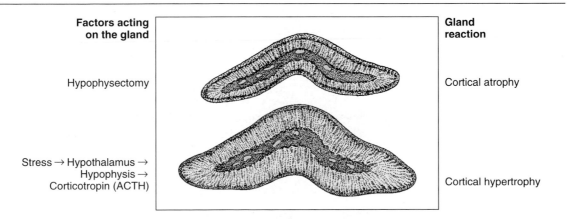

Figure 21–7. Effects of decreased or increased stimulation of the structure of the adrenal gland.

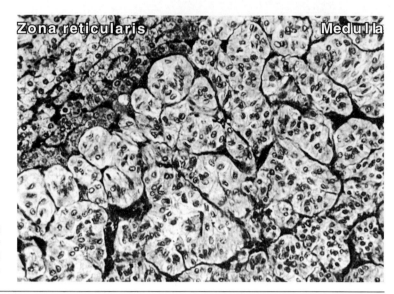

Figure 21–8. Photomicrograph of a section of the corticomedullary transition in the adrenal gland, showing cords of medullary cells. H&E stain. × 200.

Adrenal Dysfunction

A common disorder of the adrenal medulla is **pheochromocytoma,** a tumor of its cells that causes hyperglycemia and transient elevations of blood pressure. These tumors can also develop in extramedullary sites (Figure 21–1).

Disorders of the adrenal cortex can be classified as **hyperfunctional** or **hypofunctional.** Tumors of the adrenal cortex can result in excessive production of glucocorticoids (**Cushing syndrome**) or aldosterone (**Conn syndrome**). Cushing syndrome is most often (90%) due to a pituitary adenoma that results in excessive production of ACTH; it is rarely caused by adrenal hyperplasia or an adrenal tumor. Excessive production of adrenal androgens has little effect in

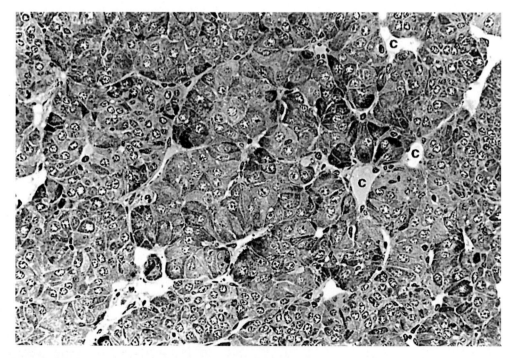

Figure 21–9. Photomicrograph of adrenal medulla showing cords of cells and interspersed capillaries (C). Most are epinephrine-producing cells; a smaller number of darker norepinephrine-producing cells are also present.

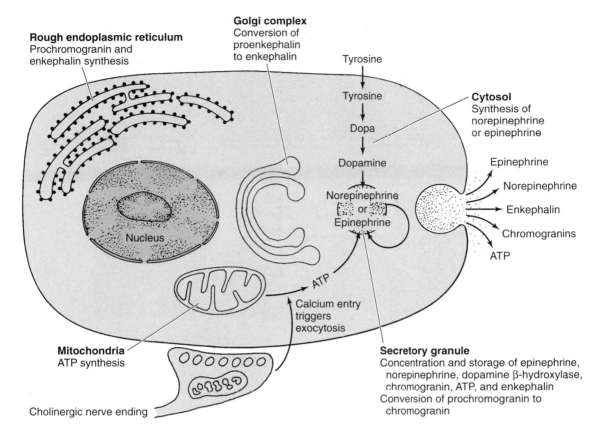

Figure 21-10. Diagram of an adrenal medullary cell showing the role of several organelles in synthesizing the constituents of secretory granules. Synthesis of norepinephrine and conversion to epinephrine take place in the cytosol.

men. Hirsutism (abnormal hair growth) is seen in women, and precocious puberty (in boys) and virilization (in girls) are encountered in prepubertal children. These adrenogenital syndromes are the result of several enzymatic defects in steroid metabolism that cause increased biosynthesis of androgens by the adrenal cortex.

Adrenocortical insufficiency (**Addison disease**) is mainly caused by autoimmune destruction of the adrenal cortex (80%), or it can be a complication of tuberculosis (20%). The signs and symptoms suggest failure of secretion of both glucocorticoids and mineralocorticoids by the adrenal cortex.

Carcinomas of the adrenal cortex are rare, but most are highly malignant. About 90% of these tumors produce steroids associated with endocrine glands.

ISLETS OF LANGERHANS

The islets of Langerhans are multihormonal endocrine microorgans of the pancreas; they appear as rounded clusters of cells embedded within exocrine pancreatic tissue.

Although most islets are 100–200 μm in diameter and contain several hundred cells, small islets of endocrine cells are also found interspersed among the pancreatic exocrine cells. There may be more than 1 million islets in the human pancreas, with a slight tendency for islets to be more abundant in the tail region.

In sections, each islet consists of lightly stained polygonal or rounded cells, arranged in cords separated by a network of fenestrated blood capillaries (Figures 21–11 and 21–12). In three-dimensional reconstructions, islets of Langerhans are round, compact masses of secretory epithelial cells pervaded by a labyrinthine network of blood capillaries. Both the parenchymal cells and the blood vessels are innervated by autonomic nerve fibers. A fine capsule of reticular fibers surrounds each islet, separating it from the adjacent exocrine pancreatic tissue.

Using immunocytochemical methods (Figures 21–13, 21–14, and 21–15), four types of cells—A, B, D, and F—have been located in the islets. The secretory granules of these cells vary according to the

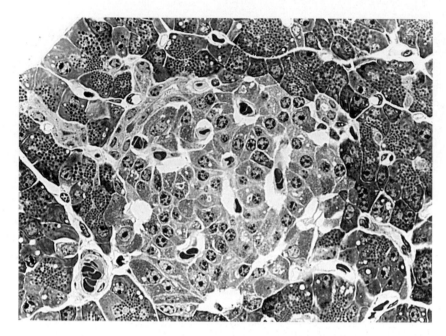

Figure 21–11. Photomicrograph of a section of the pancreas. Note the islet of Langerhans, where the A cells appear mainly in the periphery as large cells with a dark cytoplasm. The other cells are mostly B cells. The islet is formed of cell cords and capillaries and is surrounded by pancreatic acinar cells.

species studied. In humans, the A cells have regular granules with a dense core surrounded by a clear region bounded by a membrane. The B cells have irregular granules with a core formed of irregular crystals of insulin in complex with zinc (Figure 21–13). The main steps of insulin synthesis are shown in Figure 21–16.

Diabetic patients with high blood levels of proin-sulin have been reported. This condition is due to either (1) production of structurally abnormal proinsulin molecules or (2) production of normal proinsulin, but with a defect in the enzymatic process that converts proinsulin to insulin. In a strain of diabetic mice, B cells synthesize normal amounts of insulin, but this hormone is not secreted because of a deficiency of microtubules in these cells.

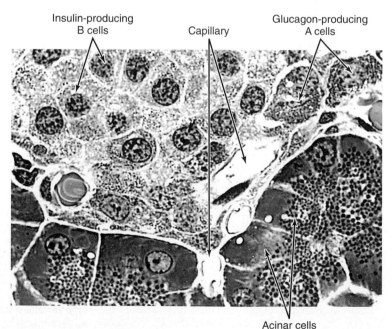

Insulin-producing
B cells

Capillary

Glucagon-producing
A cells

Acinar cells

Figure 21–12. Photomicrograph of an islet of Langerhans. The A cells have larger, darker granules than do the B cells. Note the secretory granules in the cytoplasm of the digestive enzyme–producing acinar cells. The acinar cells appear dark.

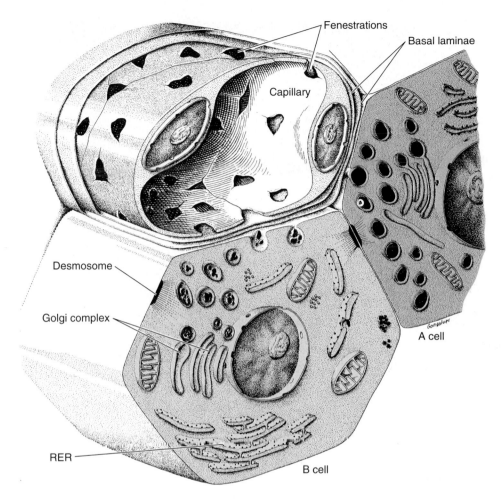

Figure 21–13. Schematic drawing of the A and B cells, showing the morphologic features of the secretory granules and their relation to blood vessels. The B cell's granules are irregular, whereas the A cell's granules are round and uniform. RER, rough endoplasmic reticulum.

The relative quantities of the four cell types found in islets are not uniform; they vary considerably with the islet's location in the pancreas. Table 21–1 summarizes the types, quantities, and functions of the hormones produced by the islet cells. The ultrastructure of these cells (Figure 21–13) resembles that of cells synthesizing polypeptides (see Chapter 4).

Terminations of nerve fibers on islet cells can be observed by light or electron microscopy. Both sympathetic and parasympathetic nerve endings have been found in close association with about 10% of the A, B, and D cells. Gap junctions presumably serve to transfer the ionic changes associated with autonomic discharge to the other cells. These nerves function as part of the insulin and glucagon control system.

Several tumor types arise from islet cells that produce such hormones as insulin, glucagon, so-matostatin, and pancreatic polypeptide. Some pancreatic tumors produce two or more of these hormones simultaneously, generating complex clinical symptoms.

One of the principal types of diabetes (type I) is an autoimmune disease in which antibodies against B cells depress the cells' activity.

THYROID

In early embryonic life, the thyroid is derived from the cephalic portion of the alimentary canal endoderm. Its function is to synthesize the hormones thyroxine (T_4) and triiodothyronine (T_3), which stimulate the rate of metabolism.

The thyroid gland, located in the cervical region anterior to the larynx, consists of two lobes united by an isthmus (Figure 21–17). Thyroid tissue is com-

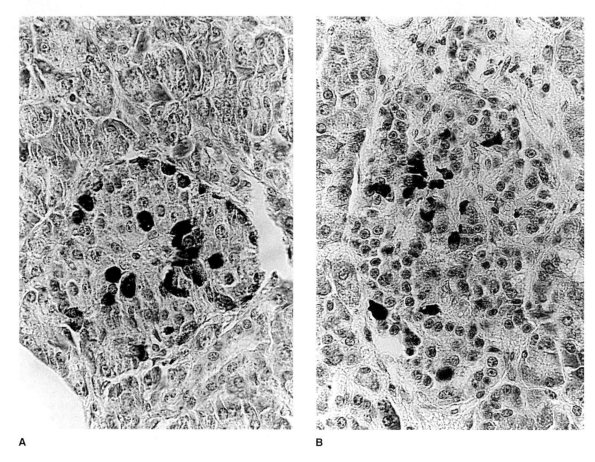

A   B

Figure 21–14. Photomicrographs of human islets of Langerhans treated by immunohistochemical methods to demonstrate glucagon-secreting A cells (**A**) and somatostatin-secreting B cells (**B**). × 250. (Courtesy of V Alberti.)

posed of **follicles** that consist of a simple epithelial sphere whose lumen contains **colloid,** a gelatinous substance (Figure 21–18). In typical sections, follicular cells range from squamous to low columnar; the follicles have a variable diameter. The gland is covered by a loose connective tissue capsule that sends septa into the parenchyma. These septa gradually become thinner; they reach all the follicles, separated from one another by fine, irregular connective tissue composed mainly of reticular fibers. The thyroid is an extremely vascularized organ, with an extensive blood and lymphatic capillary network surrounding the follicles. Endothelial cells of these capillaries are fenestrated, as they are in other endocrine glands. This configuration facilitates the passage of the hormones into the blood capillaries.

The major regulator of the anatomic and functional state of the thyroid gland is thyroid-stimulating hormone (TSH, or thyrotropin), which is secreted by the anterior pituitary.

The morphologic appearance of thyroid follicles varies according to the region of the gland and its functional activity. In the same gland, larger follicles that are full of colloid and have a cuboidal or squamous epithelium are found alongside follicles that are lined by columnar epithelium. Despite this variation, the gland is considered hypoactive when the average composition of these follicles is squamous. Thyrotropin, which is secreted by the anterior pituitary gland, stimulates the synthesis of thyroid hormone, increases the height of the follicular epithelium, and decreases the quantity of the colloid and the size of the follicles. The cell membrane of the basal portion of follicular cells is rich in receptors for thyrotropin.

The thyroid epithelium rests on a basal lamina. The follicular epithelium exhibits all the characteristics of a cell that simultaneously synthesizes, secretes, absorbs, and digests proteins (Figure 21–21). The basal part of these cells is rich in rough endoplasmic reticulum. The nucleus is generally round and situated in the center of the cell. The apical pole has a discrete Golgi complex and small secretory granules with the morphologic characteristics of follicular colloid. Abundant lysosomes, 0.5–0.6 μm in diameter, and some large phagosomes are found in

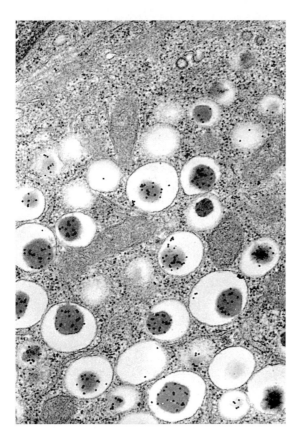

Figure 21–15. Immunocytochemical localization of insulin in a B cell of an islet of Langerhans. The black granules are gold particles used to label anti-insulin. They indicate the sites where this antibody was attached to the insulin in the secretory granules. Note also the clear zone between the secretory material and the granule membrane. × 35,000. (Courtesy of M Bendayan.)

this region. The cell membrane of the apical pole has a moderate number of microvilli. Mitochondria and cisternae of rough endoplasmic reticulum are dispersed throughout the cytoplasm.

Another type of cell, the **parafollicular,** or **C, cell,** is found as part of the follicular epithelium or as isolated clusters between thyroid follicles (Figure 21–19). Parafollicular cells are somewhat larger than thyroid follicular cells and stain less intensely. They have a small amount of rough endoplasmic reticulum, long mitochondria, and a large Golgi complex. The most striking feature of these cells is their numerous small (100–180 nm in diameter) granules containing hormone (Figure 21–20). These cells are responsible for the synthesis and secretion of **calcitonin,** a hormone whose main effect is to lower blood calcium levels by inhibiting bone resorption. Secretion of calcitonin is triggered by an elevation in blood calcium concentration.

Histophysiology

The thyroid is the only endocrine gland whose secretory product is stored in great quantity. This accumulation is also unusual in that it occurs in the extracellular colloid. In humans, there is sufficient hormone within the follicles to supply the organism for up to 3 months. Thyroid colloid is composed of a glycoprotein (thyroglobulin) of high molecular mass (660 kDa).

Control of the activity of thyroid follicular cells is summarized in Figure 20–7. This mechanism maintains an adequate quantity of T_4 and T_3 within the organism. Secretion of thyrotropin is also increased by exposure to cold and decreased by heat and stressful stimuli.

Synthesis & Accumulation of Hormones by Follicular Cells

Synthesis and accumulation of hormones take place in four stages (Figure 21–21): synthesis of thyroglobulin, uptake of iodide from the blood, activation of iodide, and iodination of the tyrosine residues of thyroglobulin.

1. The **synthesis of thyroglobulin** is similar to that in other protein-exporting cells (described in Chapter 4). Briefly, the secretory pathway consists of the synthesis of protein in the rough endoplasmic reticulum, the addition of carbohydrate in the endoplasmic reticulum and the Golgi complex, and the release of thyroglobulin from formed vesicles at the apical surface of the cell into the lumen of the follicle.

2. The **uptake of circulating iodide** is accomplished in the thyroid by a mechanism of active transport, using the iodide pump. This pump, located within the cytoplasmic membrane of the basal region of the follicular cells, is readily stimulated by thyrotropin. The uptake of iodide can be inhibited by such drugs as perchlorate and thiocyanate, which compete with iodide.

3. During the **activation of iodide,** iodide is oxidized by thyroid peroxidase to an intermediate, which in turn combines in the colloid with the tyrosine residues of thyroglobulin.

4. In contrast to the first three processes, **iodination of tyrosine residues** bound to thyroglobulin takes place, not inside the follicular cells, but in the colloid, in contact with the membrane of the apical region of the cells.

It is postulated that the union of the iodinated tyrosines is catalyzed by an enzymatic mechanism. Thyroglobulin must have the correct spatial configuration for this process to occur normally. When disease causes the production of abnormal amounts of thyroglobulin, this process is blocked, resulting in deficient synthesis of thyroid hormone. The process can also be

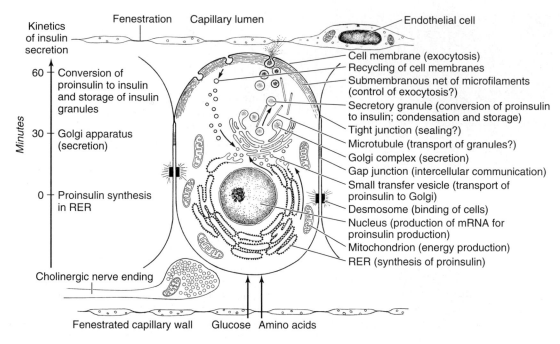

Figure 21–16. The physiology of B cells in the islets of Langerhans. Note the complex secretory process, which begins with the entrance of blood-borne amino acids into the cell, probably aided by an active amino acid pump in the cell membrane. The amino acids are polymerized to preproinsulin by the polyribosomes on the surface of the rough endoplasmic reticulum (RER), and the polypeptide chain is injected through the membrane of the RER into the cisternae. The preproinsulin undergoes a limited proteolysis and becomes proinsulin. Proinsulin is then transferred into small vesicles by a process of budding that occurs in the cisternae near the Golgi complex. (No polyribosomes cover the RER in this region.) The small vesicles are transported to the Golgi cisternae. Their contents are then packed into immature secretory granules by the Golgi complex, and the granules gradually condense to form mature secretory granules. In the secretory granules, proinsulin is cleaved enzymatically to yield insulin; microtubules play a role in the transport of these granules to the cell surface. When the cell membrane fuses with the membrane of the granule, the contents of the granule spill into the extracellular space and diffuse into a blood vessel. There is evidence to suggest that a submembranous net of microfilaments participates in mechanical inhibition of the extrusion process until the appropriate stimulus has been received.

The granule membrane is incorporated into the cell membrane and is probably recycled by the cell by means of small endocytotic vesicles (shown at upper left). The secretory processes of the B cell are regulated mainly by the blood glucose level and by autonomic nerve endings. (Based on data presented by Orci L: A portrait of the pancreatic B cell. Diabetologia 1974;10:163.)

Table 21–1. Cell types in human islets of Langerhans.

Cell Type	Quantity	Position	Hormone Produced	Hormonal Function
A	~20%	Usually in periphery	Glucagon	Acts on several tissues to make energy stored in glycogen and fat available through glycogenolysis and lipolysis; increases blood glucose content
B	~70%	Central region	Insulin	Acts on several tissues to cause storage of energy from excess nutrients; promotes decrease of blood glucose content
D	<5%	Variable	Somatostatin	Inhibits release of other islet cell hormones through local paracrine action
F	Rare	Variable	Pancreatic polypeptide	Not well established

The islets of Langerhans contain several cell types that secrete hormones that increase or decrease blood glucose. This mechanism precisely controls blood glucose concentration, an important factor in body homeostasis.

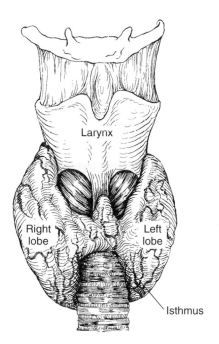

Figure 21–17. Anatomy of the human thyroid. (Reproduced, with permission, from Ganong WF: *Review of Medical Physiology,* 15th ed. Lange, 1991.)

blocked by drugs (eg, propylthiouracil, carbamazole) that inhibit the peroxidase-catalyzed iodination of thyroglobulin. Some forms of thyroid dysfunction are related to a genetic deficiency of peroxidase or the iodide pump.

Liberation of T_3 & T_4

When stimulated by thyrotropin, thyroid follicular cells take up colloid by a form of pinocytosis. Folds of apical cytoplasm (lamellipodia) encircle a portion of colloid and bring it into the follicular cell. The pinocytotic vesicles then fuse with lysosomes. The peptide bonds between the iodinated residues and the thyroglobulin molecule are broken by proteases in lysosomes, and T_4, T_3, diiodotyrosine (DIT), and monoiodotyrosine (MIT) are liberated into the cytoplasm. The free T_4 and T_3 then cross the cell membrane and are discharged into the capillaries. MIT and DIT are not secreted into the blood, because their iodine is removed as a result of the intracellular action of **iodotyrosine dehalogenase.** The products of this enzymatic reaction, iodine and tyrosine, are reused by the follicular cells. T_4 is the more abundant compound, constituting 90% of the circulating thyroid hormone, although T_3 acts more rapidly and is more potent.

Thyroxine has a gradual effect, stimulating mitochondrial respiration and oxidative phosphorylation; this effect is dependent on mRNA synthesis. T_3 and T_4 increase the numbers of both mitochondria and their cristae. Synthesis of mitochondrial proteins is increased, and degradation of the proteins is decreased.

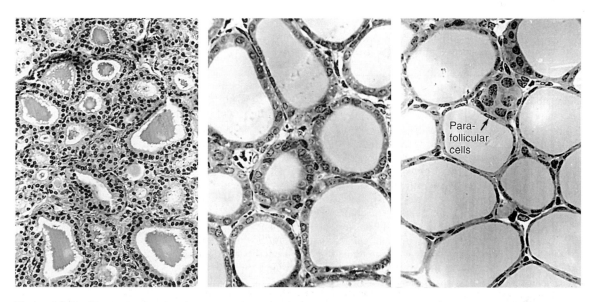

Figure 21–18. Photomicrographs of sections of thyroid gland in three stages of activity. The height of the follicular cells is directly proportional to the glandular activity. Calcitonin-producing parafollicular cells are clearly shown at the right.

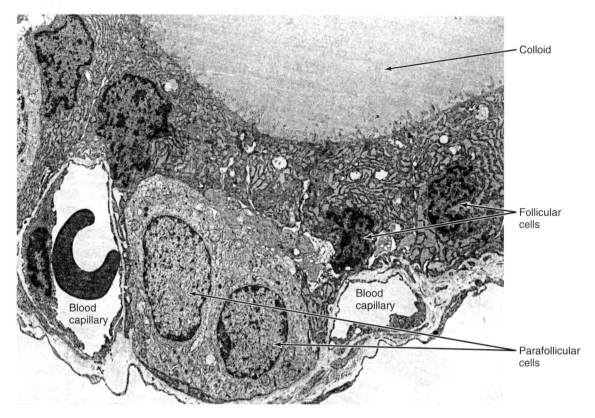

Colloid

Follicular
cells

Blood
capillary

Blood
capillary

Parafollicular
cells

Figure 21–19. Electron micrograph of thyroid showing two calcitonin-producing parafollicular cells and part of a thyroid follicle. Note two blood capillaries at both sides of the parafollicular cells.

Most of the effects of thyroid hormones are the result of their action on the basal metabolic rate; they increase the absorption of carbohydrates from the intestine and regulate lipid metabolism. Thyroid hormones also influence body growth and the development of the nervous system during fetal life.

Thyroid Disorders
& Hormone Synthesis

A diet low in iodine hinders the synthesis of thyroid hormones, causing hypothyroidism. Thyroid hypertrophy as a result of increased thyrotropin secretion causes the disorder known as **iodine deficiency goiter,** which occurs widely in some regions of the world.

The syndrome of adult hypothyroidism, **myxedema,** may be the result of a number of diseases of the thyroid gland, or it may be secondary to pituitary or hypothalamic failure. Autoimmune diseases of this gland impair its function, with consequent hypothyroidism. In Hashimoto thyroiditis it is possible to detect antibodies against thyroid tissue in the patient's blood. As with other autoimmune malfunctions, Hashimoto disease is more common in women.

Children who are hypothyroid from birth are called **cretins;** cretinism is characterized by arrested physical and mental development.

Hyperthyroidism, or thyrotoxicosis, may be caused by a variety of thyroid diseases, of which the most common form is **Graves disease,** or **exophthalmic goiter.** This thyroid hyperfunction is due to an immunologic dysfunction, with production of a circulating immunoglobulin that binds to thyrotropin receptors in thyroid follicular cells, and whose effects resemble those of thyrotropin. Patients with Graves disease exhibit decreased body weight, nervousness, eye protrusion, asthenia, and accelerated heart rate.

PARATHYROID GLANDS

The parathyroids are four small glands—3 × 6 mm—with a total weight of about 0.4 g. They are located behind the thyroid gland, one at each end of the upper and lower poles, usually in the capsule that covers the lobes of the thyroid (Figure 21–22). Sometimes they are embedded in the thyroid gland. The parathyroid glands are derived from the pharyngeal pouches—the superior glands from the fourth pouch and the inferior glands from the third pouch.

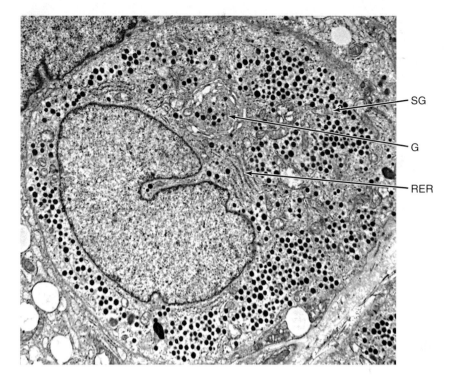

Figure 21–20. Electron micrograph of a calcitonin-producing cell. Note the small secretory granules (SG) and the scarcity of rough endoplasmic reticulum (RER). G, Golgi region. × 5000.

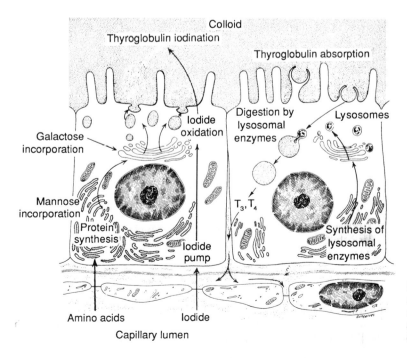

Figure 21–21. The processes of synthesis and iodination of thyroglobulin (left) and its absorption and digestion (right). These events occur in the same cell.

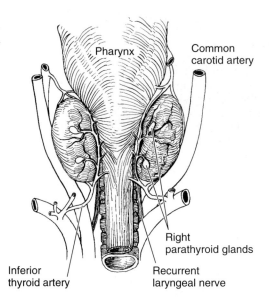

Figure 21–22. The human parathyroid glands, viewed from behind. (Redrawn and reproduced, with permission, from Nordland in: Surg Gynecol Obstet 130;51:449; and from *Gray's Anatomy of the Human Body,* 29th ed. Goss CM [editor]. Lea & Febiger, 1973.)

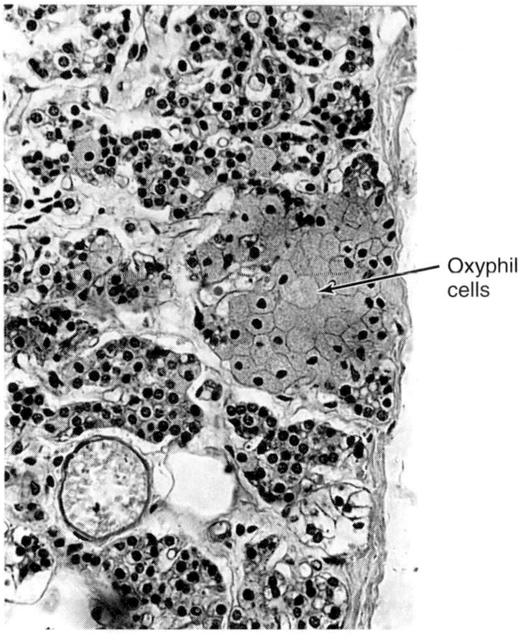

Figure 21–23. Photomicrograph of a section of a parathyroid gland. Note a group of large, acidophilic oxyphil cells at the right. × 220. (Courtesy of J James.)

They can be found in the mediastinum, lying beside the thymus, which originates from the same pharyngeal pouches.

Each parathyroid gland is contained within a connective tissue capsule. These capsules send septa into the gland, where they merge with the reticular fibers that support elongated cord-like clusters of secretory cells.

The parenchyma of the parathyroid glands consists of two types of cells: the chief, or principal, cells and the oxyphil cells (Figure 21–23).

The **chief cells** are small polygonal cells with a vesicular nucleus and a pale-staining, slightly acidophilic cytoplasm. Electron microscopy shows irregularly shaped granules (200–400 nm in diameter) in their cytoplasm. They are the secretory granules containing **parathyroid hormone,** which is a polypeptide in its active form. **Oxyphil cells** are larger polygonal cells; their cytoplasm contains many acidophilic mitochondria with abundant cristae. The function of the oxyphil cells is not known.

With increasing age, secretory cells are replaced with adipocytes. Adipose cells constitute more than 50% of the gland in older people.

Histophysiology

Parathyroid hormone binds to receptors in osteoclasts. This is a signal for these cells to produce an osteoclast-stimulating factor, which increases the number and activity of osteoclasts and thus promotes the absorption of the calcified bone matrix and the release of Ca^{2+} into the blood. The resulting increase in the concentration of Ca^{2+} in the blood suppresses the production of parathyroid hormone. Calcitonin from the thyroid gland also influences osteoclasts by inhibiting both their resorptive action on bone and the liberation of Ca^{2+}. Calcitonin thus lowers blood Ca^{2+} concentration and increases osteogenesis; its effect is opposite to that of parathyroid hormone. These hormones constitute a dual mechanism to regulate blood levels of Ca^{2+}, an important factor in homeostasis.

In addition to increasing the concentration of Ca^{2+}, parathyroid hormone reduces the concentration of phosphate in the blood. This effect is a result of the activity of parathyroid hormone on kidney tubule cells, diminishing the absorption of phosphate and causing an increase of phosphate excretion in urine. Parathyroid hormone indirectly increases the absorption of Ca^{2+} from the gastrointestinal tract by stimulating the synthesis of vitamin D, which is necessary for this absorption. The secretion of parathyroid cells is regulated by blood Ca^{2+} levels.

In **hyperparathyroidism,** concentrations of blood phosphate are decreased and concentrations of blood Ca^{2+} are increased. This condition frequently produces pathologic deposits of calcium in several organs, such as the kidneys and arteries. The bone disease caused by hyperparathyroidism, which is characterized by an increased number of osteoclasts and multiple bone cavities, is known as **osteitis fibrosa cystica.** Bones from patients with osteitis fibrosa cystica are less resistant and prone to fractures.

In **hypoparathyroidism,** concentrations of blood phosphate are increased and concentrations of blood Ca^{2+} are decreased. The bones become denser and more mineralized. This condition causes spastic contractions of the skeletal muscles and generalized convulsions called **tetany.** These symptoms are caused by the exaggerated excitability of the nervous system, which is due to the lack of Ca^{2+} in the blood. Patients with hypoparathyroidism are treated with calcium salts and vitamin D.

PINEAL GLAND

The pineal gland is also known as the **epiphysis cerebri,** or **pineal body.** In the adult, it is a flattened conical organ measuring approximately 5–8 mm in length and 3–5 mm at its greatest width and weighing about 120 mg. It is found in the posterior extremity of the third ventricle, above the roof of the diencephalon, to which it is connected by a short stalk.

The pineal gland is covered by pia mater. Connective tissue septa (containing blood vessels and unmyelinated nerve fibers) originate in the pia mater and penetrate the pineal tissue. Along with the capillaries, they surround the cellular cords and follicles, forming irregular lobules.

The pineal gland consists of several types of cells, principally pinealocytes and astrocytes. **Pinealocytes** have a slightly basophilic cytoplasm with large irregular or lobate nuclei and sharply defined nucleoli. When impregnated with silver salts, the pinealocytes appear to have long and tortuous branches reaching out to the vascular connective tissue septa, where they end as flattened dilatations. These cells produce **melatonin** and some ill-defined pineal peptides.

The **astrocytes** of the pineal gland are a specific type of cell characterized by elongated nuclei that stain more heavily than do those of parenchymal cells. They are observed between the cords of pinealocytes and in perivascular areas. These cells have long cytoplasmic processes that contain a large number of intermediate filaments 10 nm in diameter.

Innervation

Nerve fibers lose their myelin sheaths when they penetrate the pineal gland; the unmyelinated axons end among pinealocytes, with some forming synapses. A great number of small vesicles containing norepinephrine are seen in these nerve endings. Serotonin is also present, in both the pinealocytes and the sympathetic nerve terminals.

Histophysiology

The pineal gland is involved in both circadian (24-hour) and seasonal biorhythms. It responds to external visual stimuli (light) relayed to it by the sympathetic nerves by secreting melatonin and several peptides. The number of these molecules liberated into the blood increases greatly during the dark hours of the 24-hour daily cycle. In turn, these secreted molecules promote rhythmic changes in the secretory activities of the gonads and other organs. The pineal gland is therefore a neuroendocrine transducer, converting nerve input into variations in hormone output.

REFERENCES

ADRENAL GLANDS

Christy NP (editor): *The Human Adrenal Cortex.* Harper & Row, 1971.
James VHT (editor): *The Adrenal Gland.* Raven Press, 1979.
Neville AM, O'Hare MJ: *The Human Adrenal Cortex.* Springer-Verlag, 1982.

ISLETS OF LANGERHANS

Cooperstein SJ, Watkins D (editors): *The Islets of Langerhans.* Academic Press, 1981.
Gruppuso PA: Familial hyperproinsulinemia due to proposed defect in conversion of proinsulin to insulin. New Engl J Med 1984; 629:311.
Ganong WF: *Review of Medical Physiology,* 15th ed. Appleton & Lange, 1991.
Orci L et al: The insulin factory. Sci Am 1988;259:85.

THYROID GLAND

Nunez EA, Gershon MD: Cytophysiology of thyroid parafollicular cells. Int Rev Cytol 1978;52:1.

PARATHYROID GLANDS

Gaillard PJ et al (editors): *The Parathyroid Glands.* Univ of Chicago Press, 1965.

PINEAL GLAND

Sugden D: Melatonin: binding site characteristics and biochemical and cellular responses. Neurochem Int 1994;24:147.
Tapp E, Huxley M: The histological appearance of the human pineal gland from puberty to old age. J Pathol 1972;108:137.

22

The Male Reproductive System

The male reproductive system is composed of the testes, genital ducts, accessory glands, and penis. The dual function of the **testis** is to produce hormones and spermatozoa. It is surrounded by a thick capsule of collagenous connective tissue, the **tunica albuginea.** The tunica albuginea is thickened on the posterior surface of the testis to form the **mediastinum testis,** from which fibrous septa penetrate the gland, dividing it into about 250 pyramidal compartments called the **testicular lobules** (Figure 22–1). These septa are incomplete, and there is frequently intercommunication between the lobules. Each lobule is occupied by 1–4 seminiferous tubules enmeshed in a web of loose connective tissue that is rich in blood and lymphatic vessels, nerves, and interstitial (Leydig) cells. Seminiferous tubules produce male reproductive cells, the spermatozoa. Interstitial cells secrete testicular androgens (Figure 22–2).

The genital ducts and accessory glands produce secretions that, aided by smooth muscle contractions, propel spermatozoa toward the exterior. These secretions also provide nutrients for spermatozoa while they are confined to the male reproductive tract. Spermatozoa and the secretions of the genital ducts and accessory glands make up the **semen** (from Latin, meaning seed), which is introduced into the female reproductive tract through the penis.

The testes develop retroperitoneally in the dorsal wall of the abdominal cavity. They migrate during fetal development and eventually are suspended within the scrotum at the ends of the spermatic cords. Each testis carries with it a serous sac, the **tunica vaginalis** (Figure 22–1), derived from the peritoneum. The tunic consists of an outer parietal layer and an inner visceral layer, covering the tunica albuginea on the anterior and lateral sides of the testis. The scrotum has an important role in maintaining the testes at a temperature lower than the abdominal temperature.

TESTES

Seminiferous Tubules

Each seminiferous tubule is lined with a complex stratified epithelium; it is about 150–250 μm in diameter and 30–70 cm long. The combined length of the tubules of one testis is about 250 m. The convoluted tubules form a network in which individual tubules are initially closed-ended and can branch. At the termination of each tubule, the lumen narrows and continues in short segments, known as **straight tubules,** or **tubuli recti,** that connect the seminiferous tubules to an anastomosing labyrinth of epithelium-lined channels, the **rete testis.** The rete, present in the connective tissue of the mediastinum, is connected to the cephalic portion of the **epididymis** by 10–20 **ductuli efferentes** (Figure 22–1).

The seminiferous tubules consist of a tunic of fibrous connective tissue, a well-defined basal lamina, and a complex **germinal,** or **seminiferous, epithelium** (Figures 22–2, 22–3, and 22–4).

The fibrous **tunica propria** enveloping the seminiferous tubule consists of several layers of fibroblasts. The innermost layer adhering to the basal lamina consists of flattened **myoid cells,** which have characteristics of smooth muscle.

The epithelium consists of two types of cells: **Sertoli,** or **supporting, cells** and cells that constitute the **spermatogenic lineage.** The cells of the spermatogenic lineage are stacked in 4–8 layers that occupy the space between the basal lamina and the lumen of the tubule. These cells divide several times and finally differentiate, producing spermatozoa. They represent various stages in the continuous process of differentiation of the male germ cells. This phenomenon, from start to finish, is called **spermatogenesis** and can be divided into three phases: **spermatocytogenesis** (Gr. *sperma,* seed, + *kytos,* cell, + *genesis,* production), during which spermatogonia divide, producing successive generations of cells that finally give rise to **spermatocytes; meiosis,** during which the spermatocyte goes through two successive divisions, with a 50% reduction in the number of chromosomes and amount of DNA per cell, producing **spermatids;** and **spermiogenesis,** during which the spermatids go through an elaborate process of cytodifferentiation, producing **spermatozoa,** which are highly differentiated cells adapted to transport DNA to the ovum.

The process begins with a primitive germ cell, the

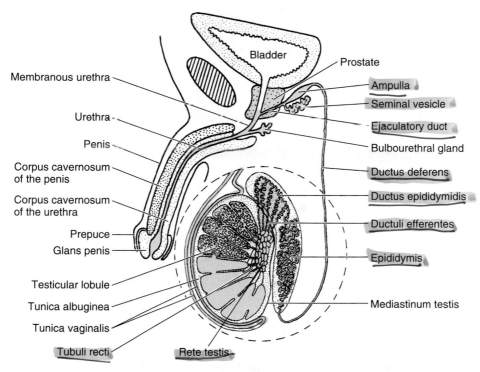

Membranous urethra

Urethra

Penis

Corpus cavernosum
of the penis

Corpus cavernosum
of the urethra

Prepuce

Glans penis

Testicular lobule

Tunica albuginea

Tunica vaginalis

Tubuli recti

Bladder

Prostate

Ampulla

Seminal vesicle

Ejaculatory duct

Bulbourethral gland

Ductus deferens

Ductus epididymidis

Ductuli efferentes

Epididymis

Mediastinum testis

Rete testis

Figure 22–1. The male genital system (shown in color). The testis and the epididymis are shown in different scales than the other parts of the reproductive system. Note the communication between the testicular lobules.

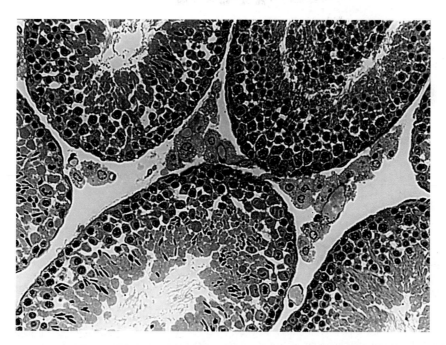

Figure 22–2. Photomicrograph of a section of testis showing several seminiferous tubules and pale-stained interstitial cells. The interstitial cells in the middle of the field contain vacuoles resulting from the dissolution of lipid droplets during histologic preparation. Hematoxylin-and-eosin (H&E) stain. × 400.

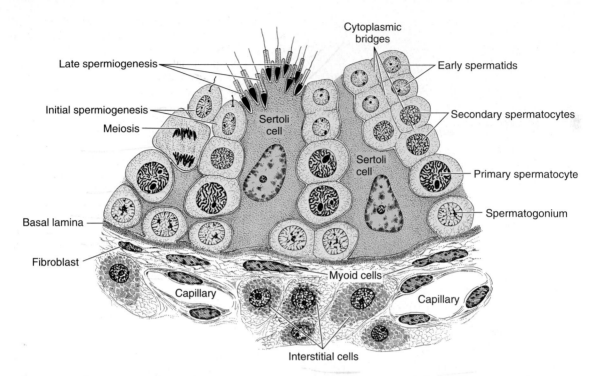

Figure 22–3. The structure of part of a seminiferous tubule and interstitial tissue. The lymphatic vessels found in the connective tissue are not shown.

spermatogonium, situated next to the basal lamina. It is a relatively small cell, about 12 μm in diameter, and its nucleus contains pale-staining chromatin (Figure 22–3). At sexual maturity, this cell undergoes a series of mitoses, and the newly formed cells can follow one of two paths: they can continue, after one or more mitotic divisions, as stem cells, or **type A spermatogonia** (Gr. *sperma* + *gone,* generation), or they can differentiate during progressive mitotic cycles to become **type B spermatogonia.**

Type A spermatogonia are the stem cells for the spermatogenic lineage, whereas type B spermatogonia are the progenitor cells that differentiate into **primary spermatocytes** (see Figure 22–8). Soon after their formation, these cells enter the prophase of the first meiotic division. At this point, the primary spermatocyte has 46 (44 + XY) chromosomes and 4N of DNA. (N denotes either the haploid set of chromosomes [23 chromosomes in humans] or the amount of DNA in this set.) In this prophase, the cell passes through four stages—leptotene, zygotene, pachytene, and diplotene—and reaches the stage of diakinesis, resulting in the separation of the chromosomes. The crossing over of genes of the chromosomes occurs during these stages of meiosis. The cell then enters the metaphase, and the chromosomes move toward each pole in the following anaphase. Since the prophase of this division takes about 22 days, the majority of cells seen in sections will be in this

phase. The primary spermatocytes are the largest cells of the spermatogenic lineage and are characterized by the presence of chromosomes in various stages of the coiling process within their nuclei.

From this first meiotic division come smaller cells called **secondary spermatocytes** (Figure 22–3) with only 23 chromosomes (22 + X or 22 + Y). This decrease in number (from 46 to 23) is accompanied by a reduction in the amount of DNA per cell (from 4N to 2N). Secondary spermatocytes are difficult to observe in sections of the testis because they are short-lived cells that remain in interphase very briefly and quickly enter into the second meiotic division. Division of the secondary spermatocytes results in spermatids—cells that contain 23 chromosomes. Because no S phase (DNA synthesis) occurs between the first and second meiotic divisions of the spermatocytes, the amount of DNA per cell in this second division is reduced by half, forming haploid (1N) cells. The meiotic process therefore results in the formation of cells with a haploid number of chromosomes. With fertilization, they return to the normal diploid number. It is the meiotic process that, because of the reductional process of cell division, guarantees a constant (fixed) number of chromosomes for the species.

Spermiogenesis

Spermatids are the cells that result from the division of secondary spermatocytes. They can be distin-

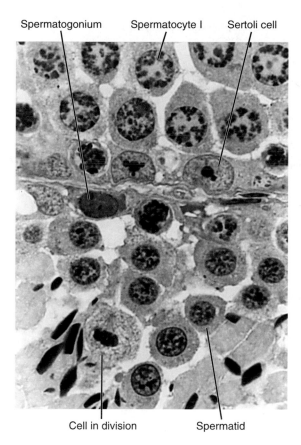

Spermatogonium Spermatocyte I Sertoli cell

Cell in division Spermatid

Figure 22–4. Photomicrograph of a section of testis showing parts of two seminiferous tubules. Primary spermatocytes, Sertoli cells, and several stages in spermiogenesis can be seen.

guished by their small size (7–8 μm in diameter), nuclei with areas of condensed chromatin, and juxtaluminal location within the seminiferous tubules (Figure 22–3). Spermatids undergo **spermiogenesis,** a complex process of differentiation that includes formation of the acrosome (Gr. *akron,* extremity, + *soma,* body), condensation and elongation of the nucleus, development of the flagellum, and the loss of much of the cytoplasm. The end result is the mature spermatozoon, which is then released into the lumen of the seminiferous tubule.

Spermiogenesis can be divided into three phases (Figures 22–5 and 22–6).

A. The Golgi Phase: The cytoplasm of spermatids contains a prominent Golgi complex near the nucleus, mitochondria, a pair of centrioles, free ribosomes, and tubules of smooth endoplasmic reticulum. Small periodic acid–Schiff (PAS)-positive proacrosomal granules accumulate in the Golgi complex and subsequently coalesce to form a single **acrosomal granule** within a membrane-limited **acrosomal vesicle.** The centrioles migrate to a posi-

tion near the cell surface and opposite the forming acrosome. The flagellar axoneme begins to form, and the centrioles migrate back toward the nucleus, spinning out the axonemal components as they move.

B. The Acrosomal Phase: The acrosomal vesicle and granule spread to cover the anterior half of the condensing nucleus and are then known as the **acrosome.** The acrosome contains several hydrolytic enzymes, such as hyaluronidase, neuraminidase, acid phosphatase, and a protease that has trypsin-like activity. The acrosome thus serves as a specialized type of lysosome. These enzymes are known to dissociate cells of the corona radiata and to digest the zona pellucida, structures that surround recently produced eggs (see Figure 23–3). When spermatozoa encounter an ovum, the outer membrane of the acrosome fuses with the plasma membrane at several sites, liberating the acrosomal enzymes. This process, the **acrosomal reaction,** is one of the first steps in fertilization.

During this phase the anterior pole of the cell, containing the acrosome, becomes oriented toward the base of the seminiferous tubule. In addition, the nucleus becomes more elongated and condensed (Figure 22–6). One of the centrioles grows concomitantly, forming the **flagellum.** Mitochondria aggregate around the proximal part of the flagellum, forming a thickened region known as the **middle piece,** the region where the movements of the spermatozoa are generated.

This disposition of mitochondria is another example of a concentration of these organelles in sites related to cell movement and high energy consumption. (Flagellar structure and function are described in Chapter 2.) Movement of the flagellum is a result of the interaction among microtubules, ATP, and **dynein,** a protein with ATPase activity.

Immotile cilia syndrome (Kartagener syndrome) is characterized by immotile spermatozoa and consequent infertility. It is due to a lack of dynein or other proteins required for flagellar motility in the spermatozoa. This disorder usually coincides with chronic respiratory infections, since a similar deficiency exists in the ciliary axonemes of respiratory epithelial cells.

C. The Maturation Phase: Residual cytoplasm is shed and phagocytized by Sertoli cells (Figures 22–4 and 22–9), and the spermatozoa are released into the lumen of the tubule. Mature spermatozoa are shown in Figures 22–5 and 22–7.

During division of the spermatogonia, the resulting cells do not separate completely but remain attached by cytoplasmic bridges (Figure 22–8). The intercellular bridges provide communication between all the primary and secondary spermatocytes and spermatids derived from a single spermatogonium. By permitting the interchange of information from

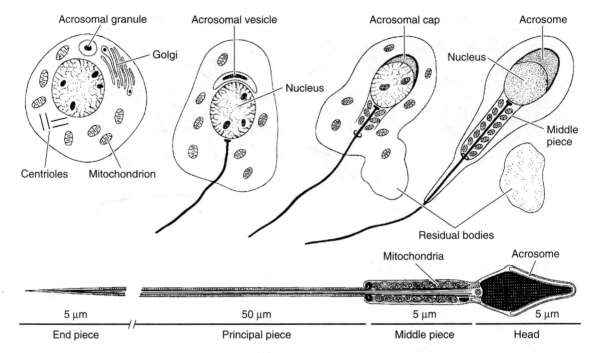

Figure 22–5. Top: The principal changes occurring in spermatids during spermiogenesis. The basic structural feature of the spermatozoon is the head, which consists primarily of condensed nuclear chromatin. The reduced volume of the nucleus affords the sperm greater mobility and may protect the genome from damage while in transit to the egg. The rest of the spermatozoon is structurally arranged to promote motility. **Bottom:** The structure of a spermatozoon.

cell to cell, these bridges play an important role in coordinating the sequence of events in spermatogenesis. This detail may be of importance in understanding the cycle of the seminiferous epithelium (described below). When the process of spermatogenesis is completed, the sloughing of the cytoplasm and cytoplasmic bridges as residual bodies leads to a separation of the spermatids.

Experimental injection of ^{3}H-thymidine into the testes of volunteers shows that, in humans, the changes that occur between the spermatogonia stage and the formation of the spermatozoa take about 64 days. Aside from the slowness of the process, spermatogenesis occurs neither simultaneously nor synchronously in all the seminiferous tubules, but occurs instead in a wave-like fashion. This explains the irregular appearance of the tubules, in which each region exhibits a different phase of spermatogenesis. It also explains why spermatozoa are encountered in some regions of the seminiferous tubules, whereas only spermatids are found in others. The **cycle of the seminiferous epithelium** refers to the sequence of maturation changes in a given area of the germinal epithelium between two successive appearances of a given cell stage. In the human, each cycle lasts 16 ±

1 days, and spermatogenesis ends about 4 cycles (64 ± 4.5 days) later.

Sertoli Cells

The **Sertoli cells** are elongated pyramidal cells that partially envelop cells of the spermatogenic lineage. The bases of the Sertoli cells adhere to the basal lamina, and their apical ends frequently extend into the lumen of the seminiferous tubule. In the light microscope, the outlines of Sertoli cells appear poorly defined because of the numerous lateral processes that surround spermatogenic cells (Figures 22–3 and 22–9). Studies with the electron microscope reveal that these cells contain abundant smooth endoplasmic reticulum, some rough endoplasmic reticulum, a well-developed Golgi complex, and numerous mitochondria and lysosomes. The elongated nucleus, which is often triangular in outline, possesses numerous infoldings and a prominent nucleolus; it exhibits little heterochromatin (Figure 22–9).

Adjacent Sertoli cells are bound together (Figure 22–10) by occluding junctions at the level of the spermatogonia, which lie in a **basal compartment** that has free access to materials found in blood. During spermatogenesis, progeny of spermatogonia some-

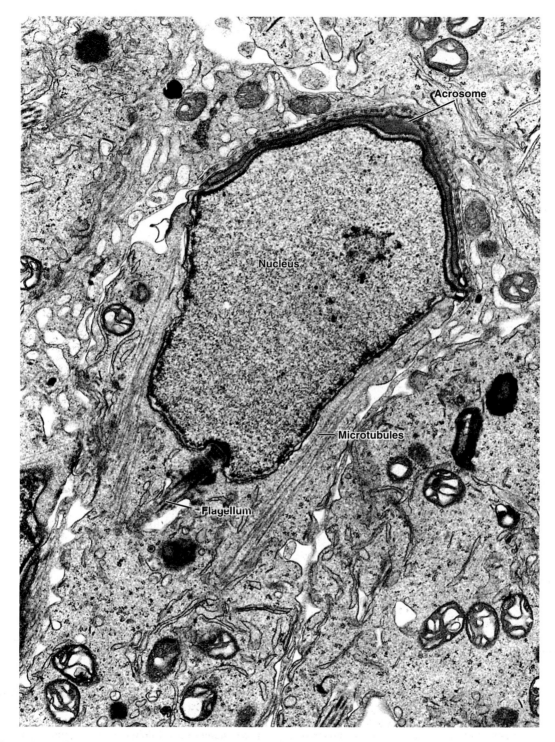

Figure 22–6. Electron micrograph of a mouse spermatid. In the center is the nucleus, covered by the acrosomal cap. The flagellum can be seen emerging in the lower region below the nucleus. A cylindrical bundle of microtubules, the manchette, limits the nucleus laterally. × 15,000. (Courtesy of KR Porter.)

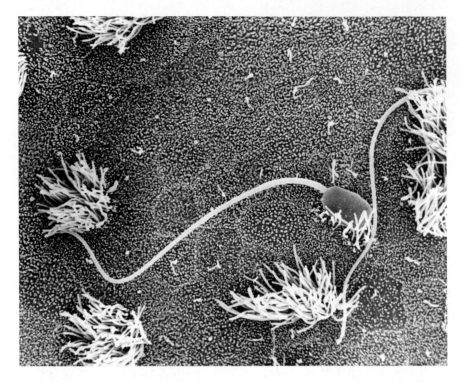

Figure 22–7. Scanning electron micrograph of a spermatozoon in the uterine cavity of a rodent. The tufts are ciliated cells. × 2000. (Reproduced, with permission, from Motta P et al: *Microanatomy of Cell and Tissue Surfaces: An Atlas of Scanning Electron Microscopy.* Lea & Febiger, 1977. Copyright (©) Societa Editrice Libraria [Milan].)

how traverse these junctions and come to lie in the **adluminal compartment.** Here, the more advanced stages of spermatogenesis are protected from blood-borne products by a **blood-testis barrier** formed by the occluding junctions between Sertoli cells. Spermatocytes and spermatids lie within deep invaginations of the lateral and apical margins of the Sertoli cells. As the flagellar tails of the spermatids develop, they appear as tufts extending from the apical ends of the Sertoli cells. Sertoli cells are also connected by gap junctions that provide ionic and chemical coupling of the cells; this may be important in coordinating the cycle of the seminiferous epithelium described above.

Sertoli cells have at least four main functions:

- **Support, protection, and nutritional regulation of the developing spermatozoa.** As mentioned above, the cells of the spermatogenic series are interconnected via cytoplasmic bridges. This network of cells is physically supported by extensive cytoplasmic ramifications of the Sertoli cells. Because spermatocytes, spermatids, and spermatozoa are isolated from the blood supply by the blood-testis barrier, these spermatogenic cells de-

pend on the Sertoli cells to mediate the exchange of nutrients and metabolites. The Sertoli cell barrier also protects the developing sperm cells from immunologic attack (discussed below).
- **Phagocytosis.** During spermiogenesis, excess spermatid cytoplasm is shed as residual bodies. These cytoplasmic fragments are phagocytized and digested by Sertoli cell lysosomes.
- **Secretion.** Sertoli cells continuously secrete into the seminiferous tubules a fluid that flows in the direction of the genital ducts and is used for sperm transport. Secretion of an androgen-binding protein by Sertoli cells is under the control of follicle-stimulating hormone (FSH) and testosterone and serves to concentrate testosterone in the seminiferous tubule, where it is necessary for spermatogenesis. Sertoli cells can convert testosterone to estradiol. They also secrete a peptide called **inhibin,** which suppresses FSH synthesis and release in the anterior pituitary gland.
- **Production of the anti-Müllerian hormone.** Anti-müllerian hormone (also called **müllerian-inhibiting hormone**) is a glycoprotein that acts during embryonic development to promote regression of the müllerian (paramesonephric) ducts

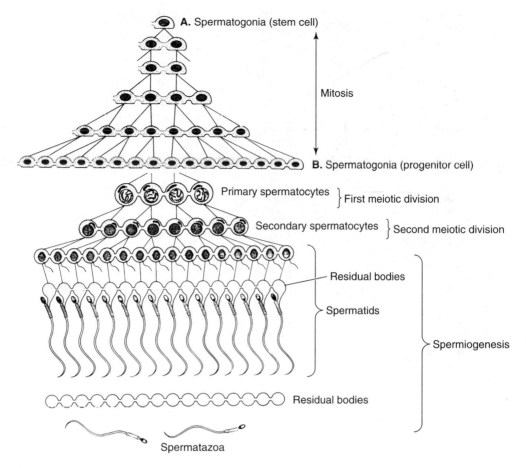

Figure 22–8. Diagram showing the clonal nature of the germ cells. Only the initial spermatogonia divide and produce separate daughter cells. Once committed to differentiation, the cells of all subsequent divisions are connected by intercellular cytoplasmic bridges. Only after they are separated from the residual bodies can the spermatozoa be considered isolated cells. The actual number of cells is greater than shown in this drawing. (Modified and reproduced, with permission, from Bloom W, Fawcett DW: *A Textbook of Histology,* 10th ed. Saunders, 1975.)

in the male fetus; testosterone fosters the development of structures derived from the Wolffian (mesonephric) ducts.

Sertoli cells in humans and other animals do not divide during the reproductive period. They are extremely resistant to such adverse conditions as infection, malnutrition, and x-irradiation and have a much better rate of survival after these insults than do cells of the spermatogenic lineage.

In mammals, spermatozoa are probably released as a result of cellular movements, with the participation of microtubules and microfilaments in the Sertoli cell apex.

Interstitial Tissue

The spaces between the seminiferous tubules in the testis are filled with accumulations of connective tissue, nerves, blood, and lymphatic vessels. Testicular capillaries are fenestrated and permit the free passage of macromolecules such as blood proteins. The extensive network of lymphatic vessels in the interstitial space explains the similarity of composition between the interstitial fluid and lymph collected from this organ. The connective tissue consists of various cell types, including fibroblasts, undifferentiated connective cells, mast cells, and macrophages. During puberty, an additional cell type becomes apparent; it is either rounded or polygonal in shape and has a central nucleus and an eosinophilic cytoplasm rich in small lipid droplets (Figures 22–3 and 22–11). These are the **interstitial,** or **Leydig,** cells of the testis, and they have the characteristics of steroid-secreting cells (described in Chapter 4). These cells

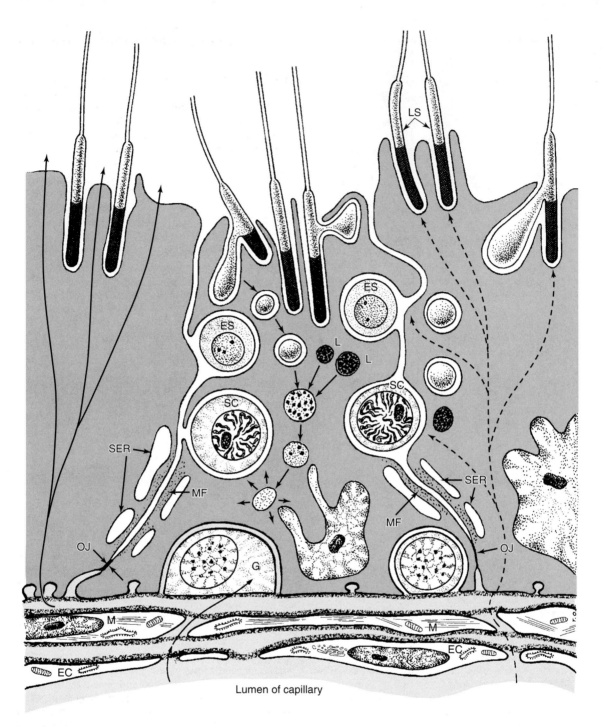

Figure 22–9. The position and functions of Sertoli cells. These cells are bounded by their lateral walls and divide the seminiferous tubules into two compartments. The lower part is the basal compartment (in color) and comprises the lumen of the blood vessels, the interstitial space, and the regions occupied by the spermatogonia (G). The upper part is the adluminal compartment of the seminiferous tubules, down to the level of the occluding junctions (OJ). The arrows pointing to the occluding junctions show the zones where the membranes converge and impede the passage of substances from the lower to the upper compartment. Above the junctional membrane, specialized regions are characterized by the presence of circularly disposed microfilaments (MF) and cisternae of the smooth endoplasmic reticulum (SER). Some functions of Sertoli cells are also portrayed. In the cell at left, the arrows indicate the secretion of testicular fluid. In the middle cell, cytoplasmic residual bodies from the forming spermatids undergo phagocytosis and are digested by lysosomes (L). In the cell at right, the dotted arrows indicate the transport of metabolites from the extracellular space to the spermatocytes (SC) and the early (ES) and late (LS) spermatids and spermatozoa. Note that the transport of material from the basal compartment to the lumen and spermatogenic cells passes through the Sertoli cells. Note also the myoid cells (M) and the endothelial cells (EC) at bottom.

Adluminal compartment

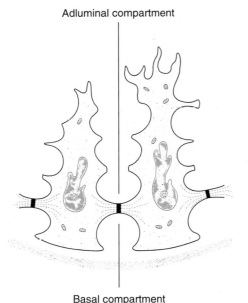

Basal compartment

Figure 22–10. Two Sertoli cells joined by occluding junctions to form the two functional compartments of the testis: the basal compartment and the adluminal compartment.

produce the male hormone **testosterone,** which is responsible for the development of the secondary male sex characteristics. Testosterone is synthesized by enzymes present in mitochondria and the smooth endoplasmic reticulum, an example of cooperation between organelles.

Both the activity and the number of the interstitial cells depend on hormonal stimuli. During human pregnancy, placental gonadotropic hormone passes from the maternal blood to the male fetus, stimulating the abundant fetal testicular interstitial cells that produce androgenic hormones. The presence of these hormones is required for the embryonic differentiation of the male genitalia. The embryonic interstitial cells remain fully differentiated up to 4 months of gestation; they then regress, with an associated decrease in testosterone synthesis. They remain quiescent throughout the rest of the pregnancy and up to the prepubertal period, when they resume testosterone synthesis in response to the stimulus of luteinizing hormone from the hypophysis.

Histophysiology

Temperature is very important in the regulation of spermatogenesis, which occurs only at temperatures below the core body temperature of 37°C. Testicular temperature is about 35°C and is controlled by several mechanisms. A rich venous plexus (the **pampiniform plexus**) surrounds each testicular artery and forms a countercurrent heat-exchange system

that is important in maintaining the testicular temperature. Other factors are evaporation of sweat from the scrotum, which contributes to heat loss, and contraction of cremaster muscles of the spermatic cords, which pull the testes into the inguinal canals, where their temperature can be increased.

Failure of descent of the testes (**cryptorchidism** [Gr. *kryptos,* hidden, + *orchis,* testis]) maintains the testes at the core temperature of 37°C, which inhibits spermatogenesis. In cases that are not too far advanced, spermatogenesis can occur normally if the testes are moved surgically to the scrotum. Although germ cell proliferation is inhibited by abdominal temperature, testosterone synthesis is not. This explains why men with cryptorchidism can be sterile but still develop secondary male characteristics and achieve erection.

Malnutrition, alcoholism, and the action of certain drugs lead to alterations in spermatogonia, with a resulting decrease in production of spermatozoa. X-irradiation and cadmium salts are quite toxic to cells of the spermatogenic lineage, causing the death of those cells and sterility in animals. The drug busulfan acts on the germinal cells; when administered to pregnant female rats, it promotes the death of the germinal cells of their male offspring. The offspring are therefore sterile, and their seminiferous tubules contain only Sertoli cells. Androgen-producing interstitial cell tumors can cause precocious puberty in males.

Without doubt, however, endocrine factors have the most important effect on spermatogenesis. Spermatogenesis depends on the action of the FSH and luteinizing (LH) hormones of the hypophysis on the testicular cells. LH acts on the interstitial cells, stimulating the production of testosterone necessary for the normal development of cells of the spermatogenic lineage. FSH is known to act on the Sertoli cells, stimulating adenylate cyclase and consequently increasing the presence of cAMP; it also promotes the synthesis and secretion of **androgen-binding protein.** This protein combines with testosterone and transports it into the lumen of the seminiferous tubules (Figure 22–12). Spermatogenesis is stimulated by testosterone and inhibited by estrogens and progestogens. The mechanisms of endocrine control are shown in Figure 22–12.

Spermatozoa are transported to the epididymis in an appropriate medium, **testicular fluid,** produced by the Sertoli cells and rete testis. This fluid contains steroids, proteins, ions, and androgen-binding protein associated with testosterone.

Blood-Testis Barrier

The existence of a barrier between the blood and

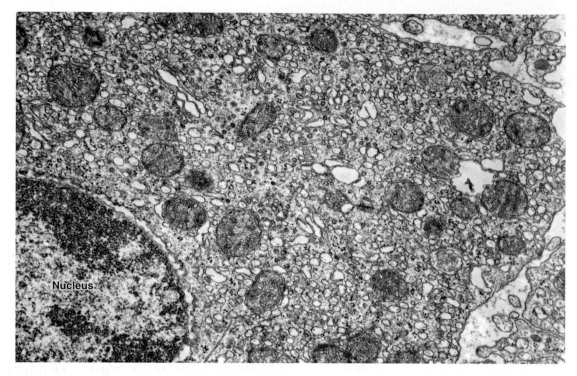

Figure 22–11. Electron micrograph of a section of an interstitial cell from a rat testis. There are abundant mitochondria and vesicles of smooth endoplasmic reticulum. × 12,000.

the interior of the seminiferous tubules accounts for the fact that few substances from the blood are found in the testicular fluid. The testicular capillaries are of the fenestrated type and permit passage of large molecules. However, occluding junctions between the Sertoli cells form a functional barrier to the transport of large molecules. This barrier is of importance in protecting male germ cells against blood-borne noxious agents.

Differentiation of spermatogonial cells leads to the appearance of sperm-specific proteins. Since sexual maturity occurs long after the development of immunocompetence, differentiating sperm cells could be recognized as foreign and provoke an immune response that would destroy the germ cells. The blood-testis barrier eliminates any interaction between developing sperm and the immune system. This barrier prevents the passage of immunoglobulins into the seminiferous tubule and accounts for the lack of impaired fertility in men whose serum contains high levels of sperm antibodies. The Sertoli cell barrier thus functions to protect the seminiferous epithelium against an autoimmune reaction.

INTRATESTICULAR GENITAL DUCTS

The intratesticular genital ducts are the **tubuli recti** (straight tubules), the **rete testis,** and the **ductuli efferentes** (Figure 22–1).

Most seminiferous tubules are in the form of loops, both ends of which join the rete testis by structures known as **tubuli recti.** These tubules are recognized by the gradual loss of spermatogenic cells, with an initial segment in which only Sertoli cells remain to form their walls, followed by a main segment consisting of cuboidal epithelium supported by a dense connective tissue sheath.

Tubuli recti empty into the **rete testis,** contained within the mediastinum, a thickening of the tunica albuginea. The rete testis is a highly anastomotic network of channels lined with cuboidal epithelium.

From the rete testis extend 10–20 **ductuli efferentes** (Figure 22–1). They have an epithelium composed of groups of nonciliated cuboidal cells alternating with ciliated cells that beat in the direction of the epididymis. This gives the epithelium a characteristic scalloped appearance. The nonciliated cells absorb much of the fluid secreted by the seminiferous tubules. The activity of ciliated cells and fluid absorption create a fluid flow that sweeps spermato-

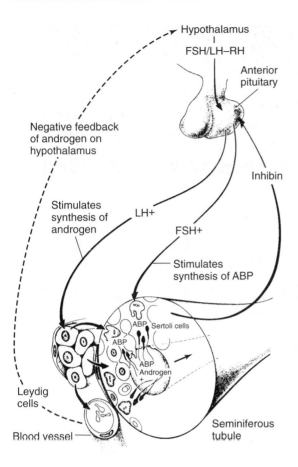

Figure 22–12. Diagram of the hypophyseal control of male reproduction. Luteinizing hormone (LH) acts on the Leydig cells, and follicle-stimulating hormone (FSH) acts on the seminiferous tubules. A testicular hormone, in hibin, inhibits FSH secretion in the pituitary. ABP, androgen-binding protein. (Modified and reproduced, with permission, from Bloom W, Fawcett DW: *A Textbook of Histology,* 10th ed. Saunders, 1975.)

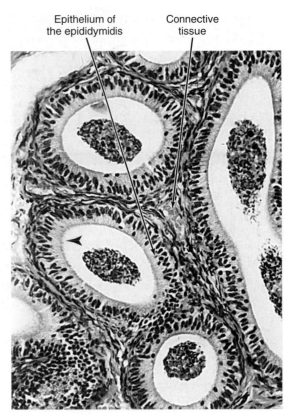

Figure 22–13. Photomicrograph of a section of epididymis showing its structure. Note the epithelium of the ductus epididymis, the connective tissue, and the stereocilia (arrow head). Note aggregates of spermatozoa in the lumen of the duct. H&E stain. × 200.

zoa toward the epididymis. A thin layer of circularly oriented smooth muscle cells is seen outside the basal lamina of the epithelium. The ductuli efferentes gradually fuse to form the **ductus epididymidis** of the epididymis (Figure 22–1).

EXCRETORY GENITAL DUCTS

The ducts that transport the spermatozoa produced in the testis toward the penile meatus are the **ductus epididymidis,** the **ductus (vas) deferens,** and the **urethra.**

The **ductus epididymidis** is a single highly coiled tube (Figure 22–13) about 4–6 m in length. With sur-

rounding connective tissue and blood vessels, this long canal forms the body and tail of the **epididymis.** It is lined with pseudostratified columnar epithelium composed of rounded basal cells and columnar cells. These cells are supported on a basal lamina surrounded by smooth muscle cells whose peristaltic contractions help to move the sperm along the duct and by loose connective tissue rich in blood capillaries. Their surface is covered by long, branched, irregular microvilli called **stereocilia.** The epithelium of the ductus epididymidis participates in the uptake and digestion of residual bodies that are eliminated during spermatogenesis.

From the epididymis the **ductus (vas) deferens,** a straight tube with a thick, muscular wall, continues toward the prostatic urethra and empties into it (Figure 22–1). It is characterized by a narrow lumen and a thick layer of smooth muscle (Figure 22–14). Its mucosa forms longitudinal folds and is covered along most of its extent by pseudostratified columnar epithelium with stereocilia. The lamina propria is a

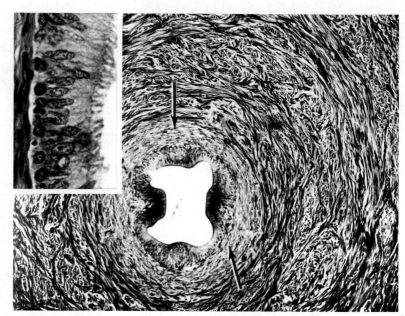

Figure 22–14. Photomicrograph of a section of ductus deferens. The duct has a thick wall formed by smooth muscle cells (SM). The arrows indicate the thin lamina propria. × 16. **Inset:** Details of the pseudostratified columnar epithelium with aggregated stereocilia. × 400.

layer of connective tissue rich in elastic fibers, and the thick muscular layer consists of longitudinal inner and outer layers separated by a circular layer. The ductus deferens forms part of the spermatic cord, which includes the testicular artery, the pampiniform plexus, and nerves. Before it enters the prostate, the ductus deferens dilates, forming a region called the **ampulla.** In this area, the epithelium becomes thicker and extensively folded. At the final portion of the ampulla, the seminal vesicles join the duct. From there on, the ductus deferens enters the prostate, opening into the prostatic **urethra.** The segment entering the prostate is called the **ejaculatory duct.** The mucous layer of the ductus deferens continues through the ampulla into the ejaculatory duct, but the muscle layer ends after the ampulla.

ACCESSORY GENITAL GLANDS

The accessory genital glands are the **seminal vesicles,** the **prostate,** and the **bulbourethral glands.**

The **seminal vesicles,** which are not reservoirs for spermatozoa, consist of two highly tortuous tubes 15 cm in length. When the organ is sectioned, the same tube is observed in different orientations. It has a folded mucosa that is lined with pseudostratified columnar epithelium rich in secretory granules. These granules have ultrastructural characteristics similar to those found in protein-synthesizing cells (see Chapter 4). The lamina propria of the seminal vesicles is rich in elastic fibers and surrounded by a thin layer of smooth muscle (Figure 22–15). The viscid, yellowish secretion of the seminal vesicles con-

tains spermatozoa-activating substances such as fructose, citrate, inositol, prostaglandins, and several proteins. Carbohydrates produced by the glands associated with the male reproductive system and secreted in the seminal fluid are the source of energy for sperm motility. The monosaccharide **fructose** is the most abundant of these carbohydrates. Seventy percent of human ejaculate originates in the seminal vesicles. The height of the epithelial cells of the seminal vesicles and the degree of activity of the secretory processes are dependent on testosterone levels.

The **prostate** is a collection of 30–50 branched tubuloalveolar glands whose ducts empty into the prostatic urethra. This gland produces prostatic fluid and stores it in its interior for expulsion during ejaculation. The prostate is surrounded by a fibroelastic capsule rich in smooth muscle. Septa from this capsule penetrate the gland and divide it into lobes that are indistinct in adult men. An exceptionally rich fibromuscular stroma surrounds the glands.

The prostate has three distinct zones: The **central zone** has a pseudostratified epithelium and occupies 25% of the gland's volume. Seventy percent of the gland is formed by the **peripheral zone,** which has a more regular epithelium and is the major site of prostatic cancer. The **transition zone** is of medical importance because it is the site where most benign prostatic hyperplasia originates.

Benign prostatic hypertrophy is present in 50% of men more than 50 years of age and in 95% of men more than 70 years of age. It leads to obstruction of the urethra with clinical symptoms in only 5–10% of cases. Malignant prosta-

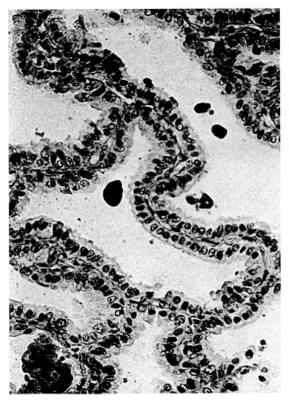

Figure 22–15. Photomicrograph of a section of human seminal vesicle. Masson's trichrome stain. × 300.

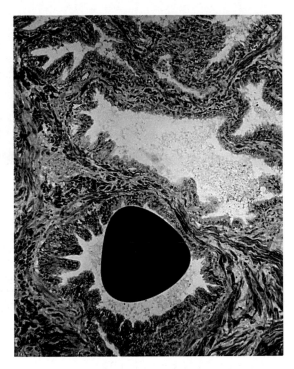

Figure 22–16. Section of a prostate, showing its epithelium, smooth muscle fibers, and a typical prostatic concretion (corpus amylaceum). H&E stain. × 300.

tic tumor is the second most common form of cancer in men and the third leading cause of cancer deaths.

Small spherical bodies of glycoproteins, 0.2–2 mm in diameter and often calcified, are frequently observed in the lumen of prostatic glands. They are called **prostatic concretions,** or **corpora amylacea** (Figure 22–16). Their significance is not understood, but their number increases with age.

The **bulbourethral glands (Cowper's glands),** 3–5 mm in diameter, are located proximal to the membranous portion of the urethra and empty into it. They are tubuloalveolar glands lined with mucus-secreting simple cuboidal epithelium. Skeletal and smooth muscle cells are present in the septa that divide each gland into lobes. The secreted mucus is clear and acts as a lubricant.

PENIS

The penis consists mainly of three cylindrical masses of erectile tissue, plus the urethra, surrounded by skin. Two of these cylinders—the **corpora cavernosa of the penis**—are placed dorsally. The other, ventrally located, is called the **corpus cavernosum** of the urethra, or **corpus spongiosum,** and surrounds the urethra. At its end it dilates, forming the **glans penis** (Figure 22–1). The corpora cavernosa are covered by a resistant layer of dense connective tissue, the **tunica albuginea** (Figure 22–17). The corpora cavernosa of the penis and the urethra are composed of erectile tissue with venous spaces lined with unfenestrated endothelial cells and separated by trabeculae that consist of connective tissue fibers and smooth muscle cells.

The prepuce is a retractile fold of skin that contains connective tissue with smooth muscle in its interior. Sebaceous glands are present in the internal fold and in the skin that covers the glans.

Most of the penile urethra is lined with pseudostratified columnar epithelium; in the glans penis, it becomes stratified squamous epithelium. Mucus-secreting **glands of Littre** are found throughout the length of the penile urethra.

The arterial supply of the penis derives from the internal pudendal arteries, which give rise to the deep arteries and the dorsal arteries of the penis. The deep arteries branch to form nutritive and helicine arteries. Nutritive arteries supply oxygen and nutrients to the trabeculae, and helicine arteries empty directly into the cavernous spaces (erectile tissue). There are arteriovenous shunts between the helicine arteries and the deep dorsal vein.

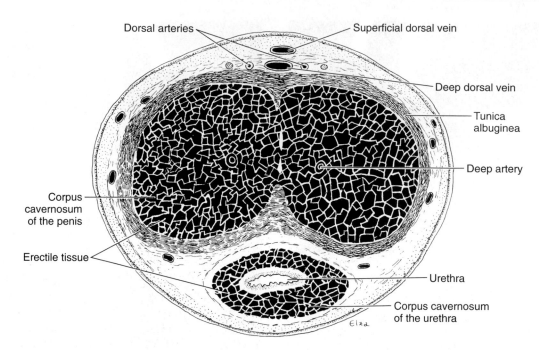

Figure 22–17. Transverse section of the penis. (Redrawn and reproduced, with permission, from Leeson TS, Leeson CR: *Histology,* 2nd ed. Saunders, 1970.)

Penile erection is a hemodynamic event that is controlled by neural input to both arterial muscle and smooth muscle in the walls of the vascular spaces in the penis; in the flaccid state, there is minimal blood flow in the penis. The nonerect state is maintained by both the intrinsic tone of penile smooth muscle and the tone induced by continuous sympathetic input. Erection occurs when vasodilator impulses of parasympathetic origin cause relaxation of the penile vessels and cavernous smooth muscle. Vasodilatation also involves the concomitant inhibition of sympathetic vasoconstrictor impulses to penile tissues. Opening of the penile arteries and cavernous spaces accounts for the increase in blood flow, filling of the cavernous spaces, and the resulting rigidity of the penis.

After ejaculation and orgasm, parasympathetic activity declines, and the penis returns to its flaccid state.

Testicular tumors are derived mainly from germ cells, Leydig (interstitial) cells, or Sertoli cells. Interstitial cell tumors can secrete steroid hormones (androgens and estrogens) that produce characteristic symptoms associated with endocrine dysfunction.

REFERENCES

Afzelius BA et al: Lack of dynein arms in immotile human spermatozoa. J Cell Biol 1975;66:225.

Bonkhoff H, Remberger K: Morphogenetic aspects of normal and abnormal prostatic growth. Pathol Res Pract 1995;191:833.

Dail WG: Autonomic control of penile erectile tissue. In: *Experimental Brain Research.* Series 16. Springer-Verlag, 1987.

Fawcett DW: The mammalian spermatozoon. Dev Biol 1975;44:394.

Hafez ESE, Spring-Mills E (editors): *Accessory Glands of the Male Reproductive Tract.* Ann Arbor Science Publishers, 1979.

Johnson AD, Gomes WR (editors): *The Testis.* Vols 1–4. Academic Press, 1970–1977.

McNeal JE: Normal histology of the prostate. Am J Surg Pathol 1988;12:619.

Oliver RT: Germ cell cancer of the testes. Curr Opin Oncol 1995;7:292.

Stambough R, Buckley J: Identification and subcellular localization of the enzymes affecting penetration of the zona pellucida of rabbit spermatozoa. J Reprod Fertil 1969;19:423.

Tindall DJ et al: Structure and biochemistry of the Sertoli cell. Int Rev Cytol 1985;94:127.

Trainer TD: Histology of the normal testis. Am J Surg Pathol 1987;11:797.

The Female Reproductive System

23

The female reproductive system (Figure 23–1) consists of two ovaries, two oviducts (uterine tubes), the uterus, the vagina, and the external genitalia. Between menarche and menopause, the system undergoes cyclic changes in structure and functional activity. These modifications are controlled by neurohumoral mechanisms. **Menarche** is the time when the first menses occurs; **menopause** is a variable period during which the cyclic changes become irregular and eventually disappear. In the postmenopausal period there is a slow involution of the reproductive system. Although the mammary glands do not belong to the genital system, we shall study them also, because they undergo changes directly connected to the functional state of the reproductive system.

OVARIES

Ovaries are almond-shaped bodies approximately 3 cm long, 1.5 cm wide, and 1 cm thick. They consist of a **medullary region,** containing a rich vascular bed within a cellular loose connective tissue; and a **cortical region,** where ovarian follicles, containing the oocytes, predominate. There are no sharp limits between the cortical and medullary regions (Figure 23–2). After about the first month of embryonic life, primordial germ cells (**oogonia**) can be identified in the endodermal yolk sac. They divide mitotically several times while migrating to the genital ridges. Oogonia populate the cortex of the future ovary, and mitotic divisions continue until about the fifth month of fetal life. At this time, each ovary contains more than 3 million oogonia. Beginning in the third fetal month, some oogonia enter the prophase of the first meiotic division and become **primary oocytes** (Gr. *oon,* egg, + *kytos,* cell). In the human, this process is completed by the end of the seventh month of gestation. During this time, many primary oocytes are lost through a degenerative process called **atresia.**

The stroma of the cortical region is composed of characteristic spindle-shaped fibroblasts that respond in a different way to hormonal stimuli than do fibroblasts of other organs. The surface of the ovary is covered by a simple squamous or cuboidal epithelium, the **germinal epithelium.** Under the germinal epithelium, the stroma forms the **tunica albuginea,** a poorly delineated layer of dense connective tissue. The tunica albuginea is responsible for the whitish color of the ovary (Figure 23–2).

Ovarian Follicles

Ovarian follicles are embedded in the stroma of the cortex. A follicle consists of an oocyte (Figure 23–3) surrounded by one or more layers of follicular cells, the **granulosa cells.** There are several stages of follicular development (described below). The total number of follicles in the two ovaries of a normal young adult woman is estimated to be 400,000, but most of them will disappear through atresia during the reproductive years. This follicular regression begins before birth and continues over the entire span of reproductive life. After menopause, only a small number of follicles remain. Since generally only one ovum is liberated by the ovaries in each menstrual cycle (average duration, 28 days) and the reproductive life of a woman lasts about 30–40 years, only about 450 ova are liberated. All the other follicles, with their oocytes, fail to mature; they become atretic and degenerate.

A. Primordial Follicles: The primordial follicles are most numerous before birth. Each consists of a primary oocyte enveloped by a single layer of flattened follicular cells (Figures 23–3 and 23–4).

The oocyte in the primordial follicle is a spherical cell about 25 μm in diameter. Its slightly eccentrically situated nucleus is large and has a large nucleolus. The chromosomes are mostly uncoiled and do not stain intensely. The organelles in the cytoplasm tend to form a clump adjacent to the nucleus. There are numerous mitochondria, several Golgi complexes, and cisternae of endoplasmic reticulum. The squamous follicular cells are joined to one another by desmosomes. A basal lamina underlies the follicular cells and marks the boundary between the avascular follicle and the surrounding stroma.

B. Growing Follicles: Follicular growth involves mainly the follicular cells but also the primary oocyte and the stroma surrounding the follicle (Fig-

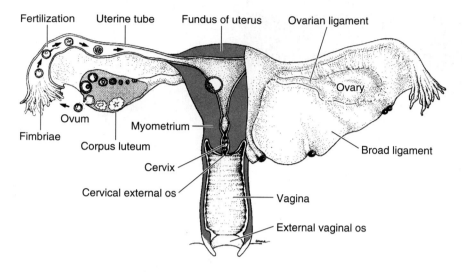

Figure 23–1. Internal organs of the female reproductive system.

ures 23–2, 23–4, and 23–5). Oocyte growth is most rapid during the first part of follicular growth, with the oocyte reaching a maximum diameter of 125–150 μm. The nucleus enlarges and is then called a **germinal vesicle.** Mitochondria increase in number and become uniformly distributed throughout the cytoplasm; the endoplasmic reticulum hypertrophies, and the Golgi complexes migrate to just beneath the cell surface. Follicular cells form a single layer of cuboidal cells, and the follicle is then called a **uni-laminar primary follicle** (Figure 23–4). Follicular cells proliferate by mitosis and form a stratified follicular epithelium, or **granulosa layer.** The follicle is then called a **multilaminar primary follicle** (Figure 23–4), and gap junctions are found between follicular cells. A thick coat, the **zona pellucida,** composed of at least three glycoproteins, surrounds the oocyte (Figures 23–5, 23–6, and 23–7). Both the oocyte and follicular cells are believed to contribute to the synthesis of the zona pellucida. Filopodia of follicular

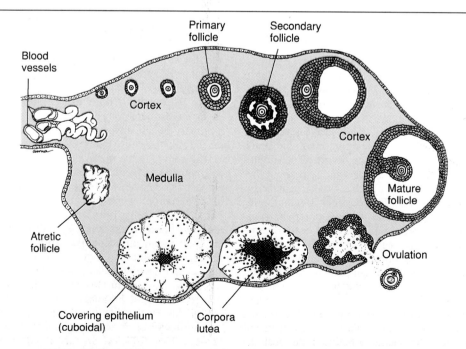

Figure 23–2. Ovarian structures and their changes during the menstrual cycle.

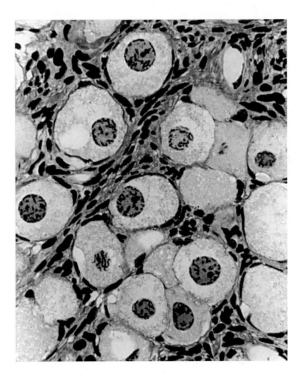

Figure 23–3. Photomicrograph of oocytes. The chromosomes can be seen because the primary oocytes stopped in the metaphase of the first meiotic division.

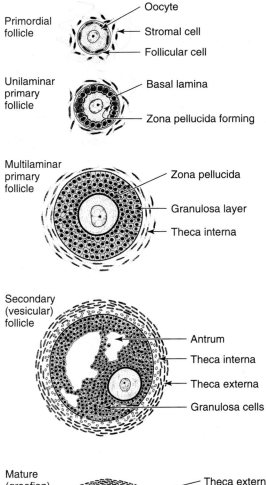

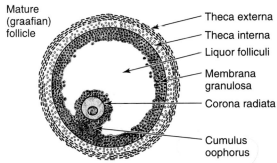

Figure 23–4. Ovarian follicles, from primordial to mature.

cells and microvilli of the oocyte penetrate the zona pellucida and make contact with one another via gap junctions (Figure 23–6).

While these modifications are taking place, the stroma immediately around the follicle differentiates to form the **theca folliculi.** This layer subsequently differentiates into the **theca interna** and the **theca externa** (Figures 23–4, 23–8, and 23–9). The cells of the theca (from Greek, meaning box) interna, when completely differentiated, have the same ultrastructural characteristics as cells that produce steroids. These characteristics include abundant profiles of smooth endoplasmic reticulum, mitochondria with tubular cristae, and numerous lipid droplets. Evidence suggests that these cells synthesize **androstenedione,** which is converted into estradiol by cells of the granulosa. Like all organs of endocrine function, the theca interna is richly vascularized. The theca externa consists mainly of connective tissue. Small vessels penetrate it and supply a rich capillary plexus around the secretory cells of the theca interna. There are no blood vessels in the granulosa cell layer during the stage of follicular growth. The boundary between the two thecas is not clear; neither is there a clear boundary between the theca externa and the ovarian stroma. The boundary between the theca interna and the granulosa layer is well defined, since

their cells are morphologically different and there is a thick basement membrane between them (Figure 23–9).

As the follicle grows—owing mainly to the increase in size and number of granulosa cells—follicular fluid (**liquor folliculi**) accumulates between the cells. The cavities that contain this fluid coalesce and form a larger cavity, the **antrum** (Figures 23–4 and 23–5). The follicles are then called **secondary (vesicular) follicles** (Figure 23–4). Follicular fluid

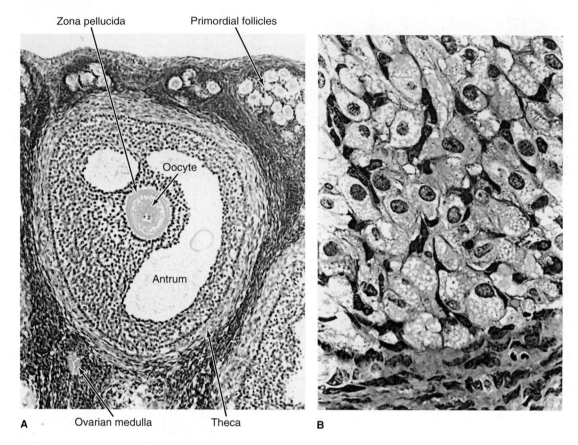

Zona pellucida   Primordial follicles

Oocyte

Antrum

A   Ovarian medulla   Theca   B

Figure 23–5. A: Photomicrograph of a developing ovarian follicle, showing the oocyte, zona pellucida, surrounding granulosa cells, theca cells, and the antrum. **B:** Corpus luteum containing lutein cells interspersed with capillaries. A portion of ovarian stroma is seen in the lower right.

Figure 23–6. Ultrastructure of the ovum, zona pellucida, and follicular cells. The zona pellucida is composed of glycoproteins penetrated by oocyte microvilli and by longer processes from follicular cells (shown in color). In the cytoplasm of the ovum are annulate lamellae, arrays of parallel layers of membranes perforated by pores that resemble the nuclear envelope.

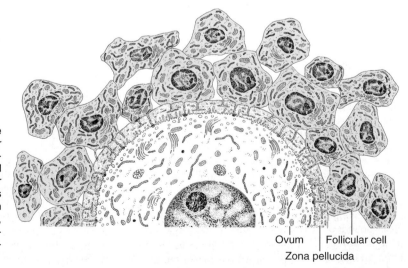

Ovum   Follicular cell
Zona pellucida

Oocyte   Follicular cells

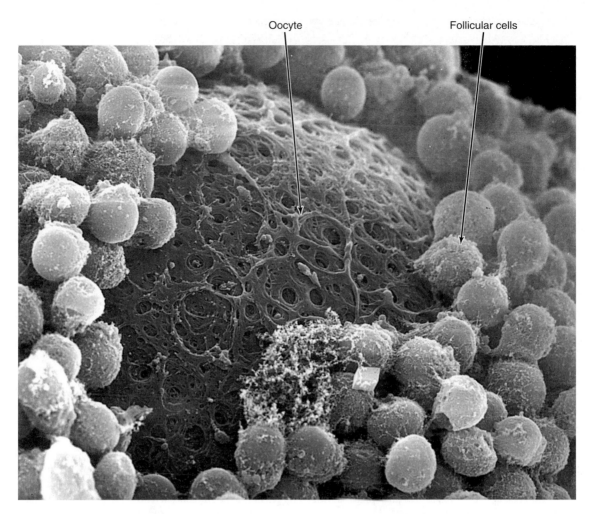

Figure 23–7. Scanning electron micrograph of an ovary, showing an oocyte surrounded by follicular cells. The structure covering the oocyte is the zona pellucida, which appears as an irregular meshwork. × 2950. (Courtesy of C Barros.)

contains transudates of plasma and products secreted by follicular cells. Glycosaminoglycans, several proteins (including steroid-binding proteins), and high concentrations of steroids (progesterone, androgens, and estrogens) are also present. The cells of the granulosa layer are more numerous at a certain point on the follicular wall, forming a small hillock of cells, the **cumulus oophorus,** which contains the oocyte. The cumulus oophorus protrudes toward the interior of the antrum (Figure 23–4). The oocyte grows no more.

C. Mature Follicles: The **mature (graafian) follicle** is about 2.5 cm in diameter and can be seen as a transparent vesicle that bulges from the surface of the ovary. As a result of the accumulation of liquid, the follicular cavity increases in size, and the oocyte adheres to the wall of the follicle through a pedicle formed by granulosa cells. Since the granulosa cells do not multiply in proportion to the accu-

mulation of liquid, the granulosa layer becomes thinner.

The granulosa cells that form the first layer around the ovum—and are, therefore, in close contact with the zona pellucida—become elongated and form the **corona radiata,** which accompanies the ovum when it leaves the ovary. The corona radiata is still present when the spermatozoon fertilizes the ovum; it is retained for some time during the passage of the ovum through the oviduct.

Follicular Atresia

Most ovarian follicles undergo atresia, in which follicular cells and oocytes die and are disposed of by phagocytic cells. This process is characterized by cessation of mitosis in the granulosa cells, detachment of granulosa cells from the basal lamina, and death of the oocyte. Although follicular atresia takes place from before birth until a few years after

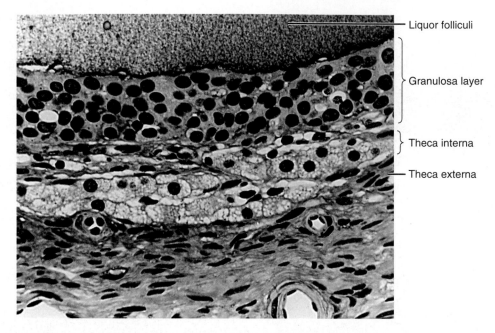

Figure 23–8. Photomicrograph showing the theca interna and the theca externa, which merges with the stroma of the ovary. The theca interna produces estrogen. The cells appear light-stained because they contain lipid droplets, a characteristic of steroid-producing cells.

menopause, there are times at which it is particularly intense. Atresia is greatly accentuated just after birth, when the effect of maternal hormones ceases, and during puberty and pregnancy, when marked qualitative and quantitative hormonal modifications take place. The process of atresia can take place during any stage in the development of a follicle.

Interstitial Glands

Although granulosa cells and the oocytes undergo degeneration during follicular atresia, the theca interna cells frequently persist and become active steroid secretors. These active thecal cells are called **interstitial cells.** Present from childhood through menopause, interstitial cells secrete small amounts of androgens.

Ovulation

The process of ovulation consists of rupture of the mature follicle and liberation of the ovum, which will be caught by the dilated extremity of the oviduct. In the human, usually only one ovum is liberated by the ovary at a time, but two or more can be expelled at the same time. In the latter case, if two or more of the liberated ova are fertilized, there may be more than one fetus (fraternal twins).

Ovulation takes place in approximately the middle of the menstrual cycle, ie, around the fourteenth day of a 28-day cycle. The stimulus is a surge of luteinizing hormone (LH) secreted by the anterior pituitary gland. Within minutes after the increase in blood LH, there is an increase in blood flow through the ovary, and plasma proteins leak through capillaries and postcapillary venules, resulting in edema. There is a local release of prostaglandins, histamine, vasopressin, and collagenase. The granulosa cells produce more hyaluronic acid and become loose. Collagen degradation, ischemia, and the death of some overlying cells cause a weakness of the outer follicular wall. This weakness, combined with an increased pressure of the antral fluid and possibly the contraction of smooth muscle cells, leads to the rupture of the outer follicular wall—and ovulation. The ovum, with its zona pellucida, covering cells, and some antral fluid, leaves the ovary and enters the uterine tube.

Before ovulation, the ovum—together with the cells of the corona radiata—detaches itself from the wall of the follicle and floats in the follicular fluid. An indication of impending ovulation is the appearance on the surface of the follicle of the **stigma,** in which the flow of blood ceases, resulting in a local change in color and translucence of the follicular wall.

The extremity of the oviduct that faces the ovary is funnel-shaped and fringed with numerous finger-like processes called **fimbriae.** At the moment of ovulation, this extremity is very close to the surface of the ovary and receives the ovum. Promoted by muscle contraction and activity of ciliated cells, the ovum

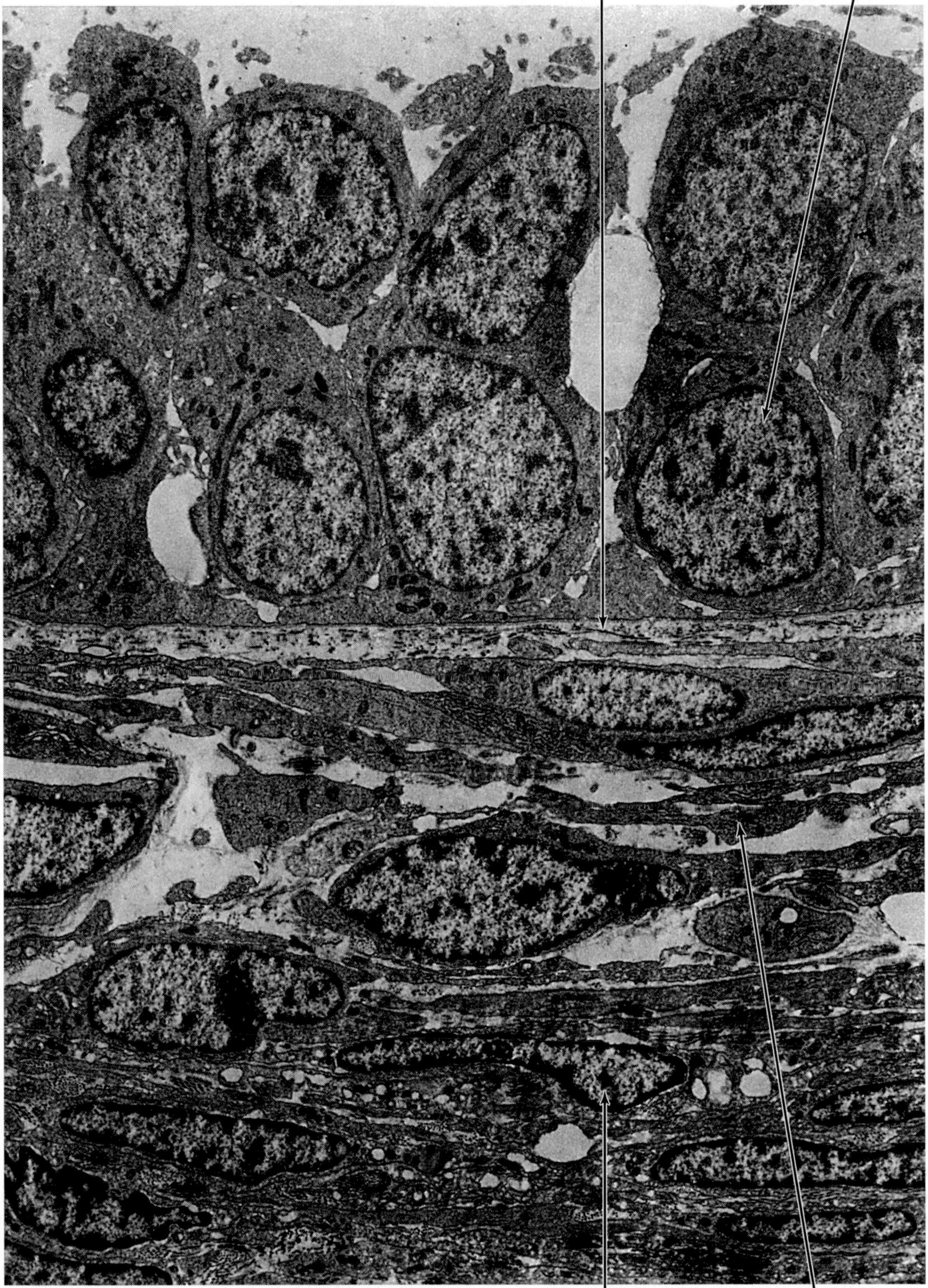

Figure 23–9. Electron micrograph of the wall of a growing ovarian follicle. In the upper part of the figure are several cuboidal follicular cells. A basement membrane separates these cells from the flattened cells of the theca interna. × 6400.

enters the infundibulum of the oviduct, where it may be fertilized. Once fertilized, the ovum, now called the zygote (Gr. *zygotos,* yolked), begins to undergo cleavage and is transported to the uterus, a process that lasts about 5 days. If the ovum is not fertilized within the first 24 hours after ovulation, it degenerates and is phagocytized.

Origin & Maturation of Oocytes

Oocytes are formed during intrauterine life, and their number does not increase after birth. The cells that are precursors of the oocytes, the **primordial germ cells,** originate in the endoderm of the yolk sac. They migrate to the genital ridge and then into the developing ovary.

Primordial and growing follicles contain primary oocytes that are the equivalent of primary spermatocytes of the seminiferous tubules (see Chapter 22). These oocytes are in the prophase of the first meiotic division.

The first meiotic division is completed just before ovulation. The chromosomes are equally divided between the daughter cells, but one of the secondary oocytes retains almost all of the cytoplasm. The other becomes the **first polar body,** a very small cell containing the nucleus and a minimal amount of cytoplasm.

Immediately after expulsion of the first polar body, and while it is still in the cortical region of the ovary, the nucleus of the ovum starts the second meiotic division, which stops in metaphase and will be completed only when fertilization has taken place. Fertilization consists of penetration of the ovum by the spermatozoon.

The ovum remains viable for an estimated maximum of 24 hours. Penetration by the sperm cell reconstitutes the diploid number of chromosomes typical of the species and serves as a stimulus for the ovum to complete the second meiotic division and cast off the second polar body. When fertilization does not take place, the ovum undergoes autolysis in the oviduct without completing the second maturation division.

Corpus Luteum

After ovulation, the granulosa cells and the cells of the theca interna (Figures 23–8 and 23–9) that remain in the ovary form a temporary endocrine gland called the corpus luteum (Figure 23–10). The corpus luteum, which is localized in the cortical region of the ovary, secretes progesterone and estrogens. Progesterone prevents the development of new ovarian follicles and thus prevents ovulation.

Release of the follicular fluid results in collapse of the follicle's wall so that it becomes folded. Some blood flows into the follicular cavity, where it coagulates and is later invaded by connective tissue. This connective tissue, with remnants of blood clots that are gradually removed, remains as the most central part of the corpus luteum.

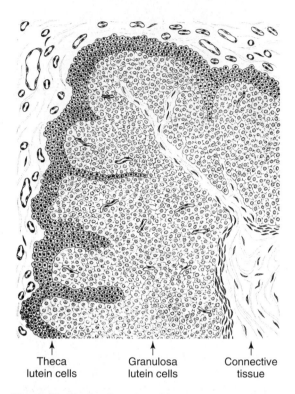

Theca lutein cells   Granulosa lutein cells   Connective tissue

Figure 23–10. Small portion of a corpus luteum. Granulosa lutein cells derived from the granulosa layer are larger and less darkly stained than the theca lutein cells, which derive from the theca interna.

Although the granulosa cells do not divide after ovulation, they increase greatly in size (20–35 µm in diameter). They make up about 80% of the parenchyma of the corpus luteum and are then called **granulosa lutein cells** (Figure 23–10), with the characteristics of steroid-secreting cells (Figure 23–5). This is in contrast to their structure in the preovulatory follicle, where they appear to be protein-secreting cells (Figure 23–9).

Cells of the theca interna also contribute to the formation of the corpus luteum by giving rise to **theca lutein cells** (Figure 23–10). These cells are similar in structure to granulosa lutein cells but are smaller (about 15 µm in diameter) and stain more intensely. They are located in the folds of the wall of the corpus luteum.

The blood capillaries and lymphatics of the theca interna grow into the interior of the corpus luteum and form the rich vascular network of this structure.

The corpus luteum is formed as a result of the stimulus provided by LH, the luteinizing hormone synthesized by the pars distalis of the pituitary under hypothalamic control. Since the progesterone produced by the corpus luteum has an inhibitory effect on the production of LH, the corpus luteum will soon degenerate unless it receives a stimulus from another

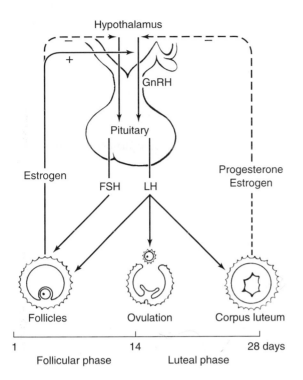

Figure 23–11. The relationships of the hypothalamus, hypophysis, and ovaries. A feedback mechanism regulates the secretion of hormones produced during the menstrual cycle. GnRH, gonadotropin-releasing hormone; FSH, follicle-stimulating hormone; LH, luteinizing hormone. Solid arrows, stimulation; broken arrows, inhibition.

phages. The site is occupied by a scar of dense connective tissue, forming a **corpus albicans.** The corpus albicans remains for a variable period and is gradually absorbed by macrophages of the stroma.

OVIDUCTS

The oviduct is a muscular tube (Figure 23–1) of great mobility, measuring about 12 cm in length. One of its extremities opens into the peritoneal cavity next to the ovary; the other passes through the wall of the uterus and opens into the interior of this organ. The free extremity of the oviduct has a fringe of finger-like extensions called **fimbriae** (Figure 23–1).

The wall of the oviduct is composed of three layers: a mucosa, a muscularis, and a serosa composed of visceral peritoneum.

The mucosa has longitudinal folds that are most numerous in the ampulla. In cross sections, the lumen of the ampulla resembles a labyrinth (Figure 23–12). These folds become smaller in the segments of the tube that are closer to the uterus. In the intra-

source. This inhibitory effect of progesterone on LH production is indirect; it is mediated through the hypothalamus (Figure 23–11).

When pregnancy does not occur, the corpus luteum lasts only 10–14 days; ie, it persists only during the second half of the menstrual cycle. This is the **corpus luteum of menstruation.** After this time, the lack of LH causes it to degenerate and disappear.

When pregnancy occurs, **human chorionic gonadotropin (HCG)** produced by the placenta will stimulate the corpus luteum, which is maintained for about 6 months and then gradually declines. It does not disappear completely, however, and continues to secrete progesterone until the end of pregnancy. This is the **corpus luteum of pregnancy.** The corpus luteum of pregnancy also secretes **relaxin,** a polypeptide hormone that softens the connective tissue of the symphysis pubica, facilitating parturition. The corpus luteum of pregnancy is larger than the corpus luteum of menstruation, sometimes reaching a diameter of 5 cm.

The cells of the corpus luteum of menstruation or pregnancy undergo degeneration by apoptosis, and their cellular remnants are phagocytized by macro-

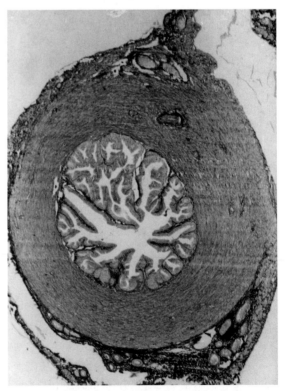

Figure 23–12. Low-power photomicrograph of a section of the oviduct. This tube provides a favorable environment and conducts the ovum or the conceptus from the ovary to the uterus. The mucosa layer is highly folded. Note the thick layer of smooth muscle.

mural portion, the folds are reduced to small bulges in the lumen, so its internal surface is almost smooth.

The epithelium lining the mucosa is simple columnar and contains two types of cells. One has cilia; the other is secretory (Figures 23–13 and 23–14). The cilia beat toward the uterus, causing movement of the viscous liquid film that covers its surface. This liquid consists mainly of products of the secretory cells interspersed between ciliated cells. This secretion has nutrient and protective functions for the ovum and promotes activation (**capacitation**) of spermatozoa. Movement of the film that covers the mucosa of the tube, in conjunction with contractions of the muscle layer, helps to transport the ovum or the conceptus toward the uterus. This movement also hampers the passage of microorganisms from the uterus to the peritoneal cavity. Transport of the ovum or conceptus to the uterus, however, is normal in females with **immotile cilia syndrome,** showing that ciliary activity is not essential for transport.

The lamina propria of the mucosa is composed of loose connective tissue. The muscularis consists of smooth muscle fibers disposed as an inner circular or spiral layer and an outer longitudinal layer.

The oviduct captures the ovum expelled by the ovary and carries it toward the uterus. Its lumen is an environment adequate for fertilization, and its secretions contribute to the nutrition of the embryo during the early phases of development.

At the time of ovulation, the oviduct exhibits active movement. The fimbriae of the infundibulum move closer to the surface of the ovary, and the funnel shape of the infundibulum facilitates the recovery of the liberated ovum.

The wall of the oviduct is richly vascularized, and its vessels become dilated at the time of ovulation. This dilatation gives rigidity and distention to the organ, facilitating its approximation to the ovary. Fertilization usually takes place in the lateral third of the oviduct.

In cases of abnormal nidation, in which the embryo implants itself in the tube (**ectopic pregnancy**), the lamina propria reacts like the endometrium, forming numerous decidual cells. Because of its small diameter, the oviduct cannot contain these new cells and bursts, causing extensive hemorrhage that can be fatal if not treated immediately.

UTERUS

The uterus is a pear-shaped organ that consists of a **body** (**corpus**), which lies above a narrowing of the uterine cavity (**the internal os**), and a lower cylindrical structure, the **cervix,** which lies below the internal os. The part of the body of the uterus that lies above the points of entrance of the uterine tubes is called the **fundus** (Figure 23–1).

The wall of the uterus is relatively thick and is formed of three layers. Depending on the part of the uterus, there is either an outer **serosa** (connective tissue and mesothelium) or **adventitia** (connective tissue). The other uterine layers are the **myometrium,** a thick tunic of smooth muscle, and the **endometrium,** or mucosa of the uterus.

Myometrium

The myometrium (Gr. *mys,* muscle, + *metra,* uterus), the thickest tunic of the uterus, is composed of bundles of smooth muscle fibers separated by connective tissue. The bundles of smooth muscle form four poorly defined layers. The first and fourth layers are composed mainly of fibers disposed longitudinally, ie, parallel to the long axis of the organ. The middle layers contain the larger blood vessels.

During pregnancy, the myometrium goes through a period of great growth as a result of both **hyperplasia** (an increase in the number of smooth muscle

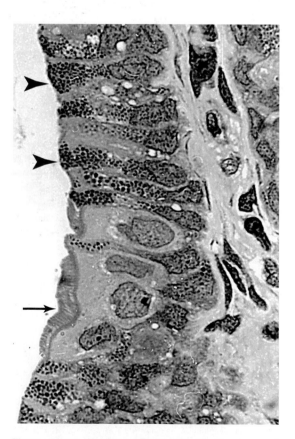

Figure 23–13. Photomicrograph showing the two main cell types of the oviduct's mucosa epithelium. Ciliated cells (arrow) contribute to the movement of the ovum or conceptus to the uterus, and secretory cells (arrowheads) produce a nutrient and protective fluid.

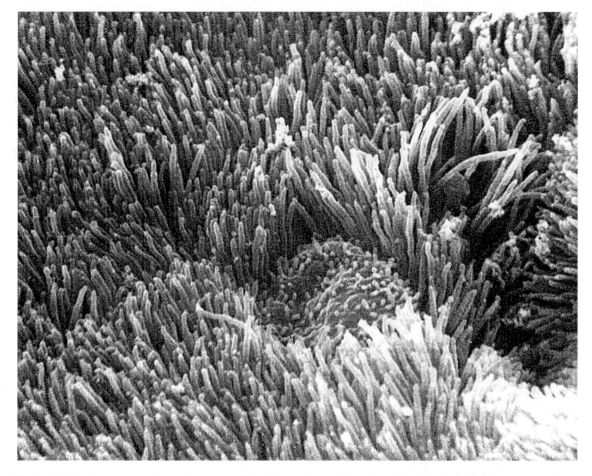

Figure 23–14. Scanning electron micrograph of the lining of an oviduct. Note the abundant cilia. In the center is the apex of a secretory cell covered by short microvilli. × 8000. (Courtesy of KR Porter.)

cells) and **hypertrophy** (an increase in cell size). During pregnancy, many smooth muscle cells have ultrastructural characteristics of protein-secreting cells and actively synthesize collagen, promoting a significant increase in uterine collagen content.

After pregnancy, there is destruction of some smooth muscle cells, reduction in the size of others, and enzymatic degradation of the collagen. The uterus is reduced in size almost to its prepregnancy dimensions.

Endometrium

The endometrium consists of epithelium and lamina propria containing simple tubular glands that sometimes branch in their deeper portions (near the myometrium). Its covering epithelial cells are a mixture of ciliated and secretory simple columnar cells. The epithelium of the uterine glands is similar to the superficial epithelium, but ciliated cells are rare within the glands.

The connective tissue of the lamina propria is rich in fibroblasts and contains abundant ground substance. Connective tissue fibers are mostly reticular.

The endometrial layer can be subdivided into two zones: the **functionalis,** which constitutes the portions sloughed off at menstruation and replaced during each menstrual cycle; and the **basalis,** the portion retained after menstruation that subsequently proliferates and provides a new epithelium and lamina propria for the renewal of the endometrium. The bases of the uterine glands, which lie deep within the basalis, are the source of the cells that divide and migrate over the exposed connective tissue of the menstrual-phase endometrium, thereby providing for the new epithelial lining of the uterus after menstruation.

The blood vessels supplying the endometrium are of special significance in the periodic sloughing of most of this layer. **Arcuate arteries** are circumferentially oriented in the middle layers of the myometrium. From these vessels, two sets of arteries arise to supply blood to the endometrium: **straight arteries,** which supply the basalis; and **coiled arteries,** which bring blood to the functionalis.

Uterine Cervix

The **cervix** is the lower, cylindrical part of the uterus (Figure 23–1). This portion differs in histologic structure from the rest of the uterus. The lining consists of a mucus-secreting simple columnar epithelium. The cervix has few smooth muscle fibers and consists mainly (85%) of dense connective tissue. The external aspect of the cervix that bulges into the lumen of the vagina (from Latin, meaning sheath) is covered with stratified squamous epithelium.

The mucosa of the cervix contains the mucous **cervical glands,** which are extensively branched. This mucosa does not desquamate during menstruation, although its glands undergo small structural variations during the menstrual cycle. When the ducts of these glands are blocked, the retained secretion causes a dilatation that gives rise to **nabothian cysts.** During pregnancy, the cervical mucous glands proliferate and secrete a more viscous and abundant mucus.

Cervical secretions play a significant role in fertilization of the ovum. At the time of ovulation, the mucous secretions are watery and allow penetration of the uterus by sperm. In the luteal phase or in pregnancy, the progesterone levels alter the mucous secretions so that they become more viscous and prevent the passage of the microorganisms, as well as sperm, into the body of the uterus. The dilatation of the cervix that precedes parturition is due to intense collagenolysis, which promotes its softening.

Cancer of the cervix (**cervical carcinoma**) is derived from its stratified squamous epithelium. Although it is frequently observed, the mortality rate is low (8 per 100,000). This low rate is due to the usual discovery of the carcinoma in its early stages, made possible by yearly physical observation of the cervix and by cytologic analysis of smears of the cervical epithelium (Papanicolaou test).

1. THE MENSTRUAL CYCLE

The action of ovarian hormones (estrogens and progesterone) under the stimulus of the anterior lobe of the pituitary causes the endometrium to undergo cyclic structural modifications during the menstrual cycle. The duration of the menstrual cycle is variable but averages 28 days (Figure 23–22).

Menstrual cycles usually start between 12 and 15 years of age and continue until about age 45–50. Since menstrual cycles are a consequence of ovarian modifications related to the production of ova, the female is fertile only during the years when she is having menstrual cycles. This does not mean that sexual activity is terminated by menopause—only that fertility ceases.

For practical purposes, the beginning of the menstrual cycle is taken as the day when menstrual bleeding appears. The menstrual discharge consists of degenerating endometrium mixed with blood from the ruptured blood vessels. The **menstrual phase** is defined as the first to the fourth days of the cycle; the **proliferative phase** is the fifth to the fourteenth days; and the **secretory,** or **luteal, phase** is the fifteenth to the twenty-eighth days. The duration of each phase is variable, and the intervals given are only averages.

Although the menstrual cycle can be described as having a proliferative phase, a secretory or luteal phase, and a menstrual phase, the structural changes that occur during the cycle are gradual; the clear division of the phases implied here is mainly for teaching value.

A. The Proliferative Phase: After the menstrual phase, the uterine mucosa is reduced to a small band of connective tissue (lamina propria) containing the basal portions of the glands. The proliferative phase is also known as the **follicular phase** because it coincides with the development of ovarian follicles and the production of estrogens.

Cells continue to proliferate during the entire proliferative phase and reconstitute both the glands and the surface epithelium lining the endometrium (Figure 23–15). Proliferation of the connective cells and deposition of the ground substance in the lamina propria also contribute to the growth of the endometrium as a whole.

At the end of the proliferative phase, the endometrium is 2–3 mm thick, and the glands, which consist of simple columnar epithelial cells, are straight tubules with narrow lumens. During this phase, these cells gradually accumulate more cisternae of rough endoplasmic reticulum, and the Golgi complex increases in size in preparation for secretory activity. Coiled arteries grow into the regenerating stroma.

B. The Secretory, or Luteal, Phase: The secretory phase starts after ovulation and depends on progesterone secreted by the corpus luteum. Acting on glands already developed by the action of estrogen, progesterone stimulates the gland cells to secrete glycoproteins that will be the major source of embryonic nutrition before implantation occurs.

The glands become highly coiled (Figure 23–16), and the epithelial cells begin to accumulate glycogen below their nuclei. Later, the amount of glycogen diminishes, and glycoprotein secretory products dilate the lumens of the glands. In this phase, the endometrium reaches its maximum thickness (5 mm) as a result of the accumulation of secretions and the edema of the stroma. Mitoses are rare during the secretory phase. The elongation and convolution of the coiled arteries continue, and they extend into the su-

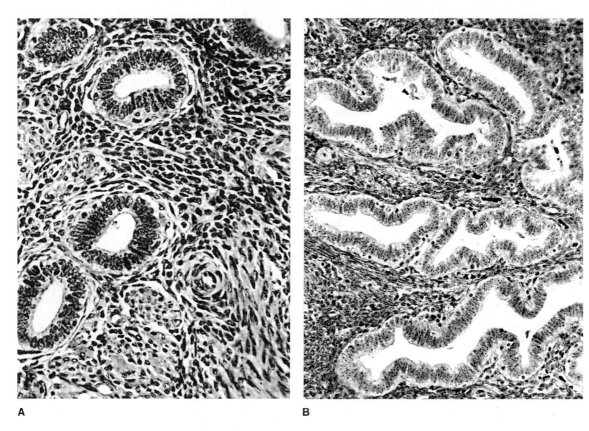

Figure 23–15. A: Endometrium in the proliferative phase. The epithelial cells of the uterine glands are organized as a simple columnar lining, although the close proximity of the nuclei may give the epithelium a pseudostratified appearance during the proliferative phase. **B:** Endometrium in the secretory phase (twenty-first day of the menstrual cycle). The uterine glands have broad lumens, dilated by the accumulation of secretions.

perficial portion of the endometrium. Progesterone inhibits the contractions of smooth muscle cells of the myometrium that might otherwise interfere with the implantation of the embryo.

C. The Menstrual Phase: When fertilization and implantation of the ovum released by the ovary fail to occur, the corpus luteum spontaneously ceases functioning after about 14 days. The levels of progesterone and estrogens in the blood drop rapidly, and the endometrium developed in response to these hormones undergoes involution and is partially shed. (If implantation occurs, HCG begins to be synthesized by the developing embryo. This sustains the life of the corpus luteum, and menstruation does not occur.)

At the end of the secretory phase, the walls of the coiled arteries contract, closing off the blood flow and producing ischemia, which leads to death (necrosis) of their walls and of the functionalis layer of the endometrium. At this time, blood vessels above the constrictions rupture, and bleeding begins.

The endometrium becomes partially detached. The amount lost varies between women and even in the same woman at different times. At the end of the

menstrual phase, the endometrium is almost always reduced to nothing but the basal layer, containing the basal ends of the endometrial glands. Proliferation of the gland cells and their migration to the surface initiate the proliferative phase, restarting the cycle.

2. PREGNANCY & IMPLANTATION

The human ovum is fertilized in the lateral third of the uterine tube, and the zygote is cleaved as it is moved passively toward the uterus. Through successive mitoses, a compact collection of cells, the **morula,** is formed. The morula, covered by the zona pellucida, is about the same size as the fertilized ovum. The cells that result from segmentation of the zygote are called **blastomeres** (Gr. *blastos,* germ, + *meros,* part). They do not grow in size at this time but divide the zygote into smaller cells that will subsequently differentiate along several pathways.

A cavity at the center of the morula appears as a result of the gradual accumulation of liquid transferred from the lumen of the oviduct by the activity

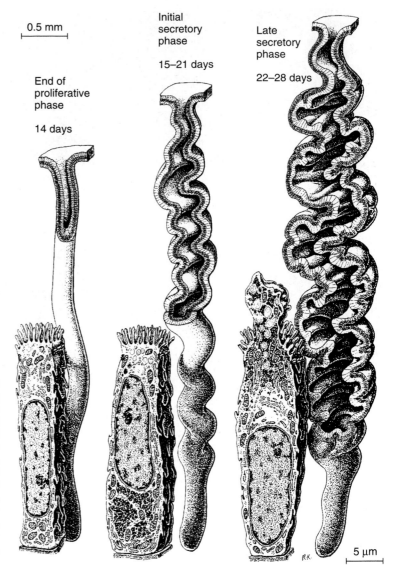

0.5 mm

End of
proliferative
phase

14 days

Initial
secretory
phase

15–21 days

Late
secretory
phase

22–28 days

5 μm

Figure 23–16. Changes in the uterine glands and in the gland cells during the phases of the menstrual cycle. In the proliferative stage the glands are straight tubules, and their cells show no secretory activity. In the initial secretory phase the glands begin to coil, and their cells accumulate glycogen in the basal region. In the late secretory phase the glands are highly coiled, and their cells present secretory activity at their apical portion. (Reproduced, with permission, from Krstić RV: *Human Microscopic Anatomy,* Springer, 1991.)

of the peripheral blastomeres. The embryo is then a fluid-filled sphere called a **blastocyst.** The blastomeres arrange themselves in a peripheral layer (**trophoblast**) that is thickened at the point where a collection of cells (**inner cell mass**) remains and bulges into the cavity. The cells in the peripheral layer are held together by tight junctions, but the cells of the inner cell mass show gap junctions that enable small molecules and ions to pass between them. This stage of development corresponds approximately to the fourth or fifth day after ovulation. The embryo arrives in the uterus at this time. The blastocyst remains in the lumen of the uterus for 2 or 3 days and comes into contact with the surface of the endometrium, immersed in the secretion of the endometrial glands.

The blastocyst separates from the zona pellucida by enzymatically degrading it, allowing cells of the trophoblast to interact with the endometrium. Immediately thereafter, the cells of the trophoblast begin to multiply, ensuring, with the help of the endometrium, the nourishment of the embryo. The inner cell mass, from which the body of the embryo will originate, grows slightly during this phase.

Implantation, or nidation (Figure 23–17), involves penetration through the uterine epithelium, with little sign of necrosis. This type of **interstitial** implantation occurs in humans and a few other mammals. Implantation takes place when the endometrium is in the secretory phase. The uterine glands secrete glycoproteins; the vessels dilate; and the lamina propria swells slightly. The process starts around the seventh

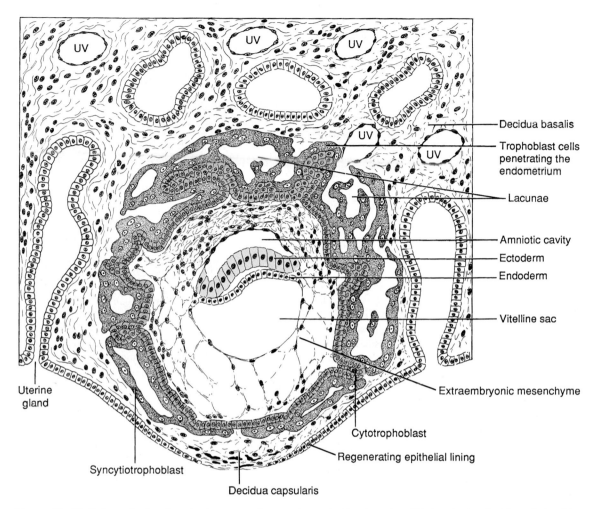

Figure 23–17. Schematic drawing of a human embryo at the end of implantation (12 days), showing the relationships between the embryo and the endometrium (called the decidua) after implantation. UV, uterine vessels, one of which opens into a lacuna, filling its spaces with blood. Darker color shows the cytotrophoblast; lighter color highlights the ectoderm and amnion.

day, and on about the ninth day after ovulation the embryo is totally submerged in the endometrium, from which it will receive protection and nourishment during pregnancy.

During implantation, the trophoblast differentiates into two layers, the **syncytiotrophoblast** and the **cytotrophoblast** (Figure 23–17). The syncytiotrophoblast, a multinucleated syncytial external layer, arises from the fusion of mononucleated cytotrophoblasts. The cytotrophoblast (*kytos* + Gr. *trophe,* nutrition, + *blastos*) consists of an irregular layer of mononucleated ovoid cells immediately under the syncytiotrophoblast.

The surface of the syncytiotrophoblast has irregular microvilli, and the superficial cytoplasm contains vesicles covered by smooth membranes. This sug-

gests an intense pinocytotic process in the syncytiotrophoblast, possibly related to the transfer of material from the maternal circulation to the fetus. Below that level, the cytoplasm of the syncytiotrophoblast shows an abundance of both rough and smooth endoplasmic reticulum, a well-developed Golgi complex, and numerous mitochondria. These ultrastructural characteristics are consistent with the role attributed to the syncytiotrophoblast in the secretion of HCG (a glycoprotein hormone), placental lactogen (a protein hormone), and estrogen and progesterone (steroids). The syncytiotrophoblast contains lipid droplets whose composition (as determined by cytochemical methods) is compatible with the presence of cholesterol, the immediate precursor of steroid hormones.

The syncytiotrophoblasts delineate extracytoplasmic cavities. These cavities increase in size and communicate with one another, resulting in a spongy structure (Figure 23–17). Thus, lacunae lined with syncytiotrophoblast are formed. The lytic activity of the syncytiotrophoblast causes the rupture of both arterial and venous maternal blood vessels, with overflow of blood into these lacunar spaces. Blood flows from the arterial vessels to the lacunae and from there to the veins.

After implantation of the embryo, the endometrium goes through profound changes and is called the **decidua.** Cells of the stroma become enlarged and polygonal and are called decidual cells. The decidua can be divided into the **decidua basalis,** situated between the embryo and the myometrium; **decidua capsularis,** between the embryo and the lumen of the uterus; and **decidua parietalis,** the remainder of the decidua (Figure 23–18).

The trophoblast in contact with the decidua capsularis develops only to a slight extent, since its nutrition is deficient. Growth of the trophoblast in the part of the embryo facing the myometrium is ensured by the maternal blood, and its growth is rapid. From this part of the trophoblast, elongated projections, **primary villi,** are formed. Their main characteristic is that they are composed of only cytotrophoblasts and an external syncytiotrophoblastic covering. During this stage of embryonic development, an extraembryonic mesenchyme appears before the intraembryonic mesenchyme and contributes to the formation of the placenta and the fetal membranes. The extraembryonic mesenchyme and the trophoblast form the **chorion** (Gr. *choreon,* fetal membrane). On the side

of the **decidua capsularis,** the chorion develops very slightly (**smooth chorion,** or **chorion laeve**); on the side of the decidua basalis, the chorion grows extensively and forms the **chorion frondosum.** The layers of the chorion (beginning at the surface) are the syncytiotrophoblast, cytotrophoblast, and extraembryonic mesenchyme.

When the mesenchyme invades the primary villi, it transforms them into **secondary villi** (Figure 23–19). Within the villi, vessels are formed gradually and later will join those formed in the body of the embryo, establishing a circulation and thus allowing exchange of substances and gases between the fetal and maternal blood.

Placenta

The placenta is a temporary organ and is the site of physiologic exchanges between the mother and the fetus. It consists of a fetal part (chorion) and a maternal part (decidua basalis).

The placenta is the only organ composed of cells derived from two distinct individuals. Since the embryo and the mother are of different genetic constitution, there should be an immunologic attack by the maternal organism against the foreign implanting embryo. Why this does not occur remains an active area of investigation.

A. Fetal Part: The fetal part of the placenta, the chorion, has a **chorionic plate** at the point where the **chorionic villi** arise—the secondary villi already described. These villi consist of a connective tissue core derived from the extraembryonic mesenchyme, surrounded by the syncytiotrophoblast and the cytotrophoblast (Figure 23–20). The syncytiotropho-

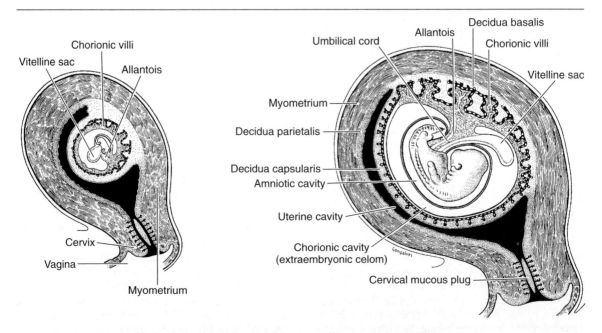

Figure 23–18. Formation of the three regions of the decidua and the chorionic villi.

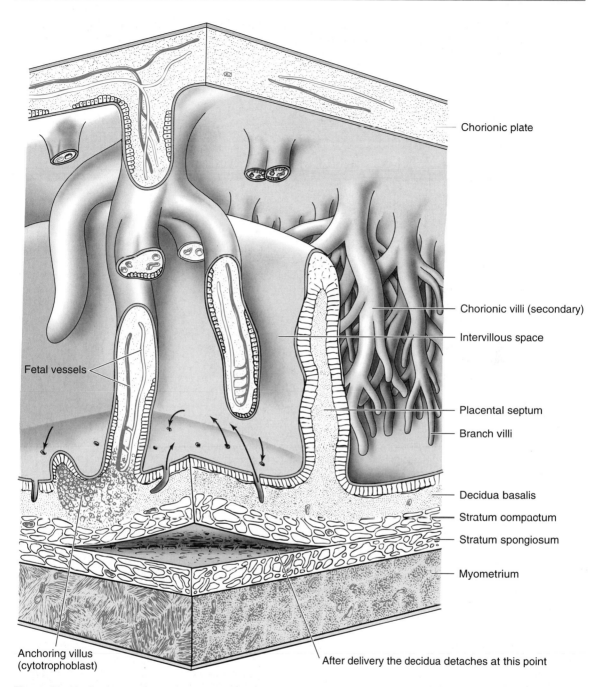

Chorionic plate

Chorionic villi (secondary)

Intervillous space

Fetal vessels

Placental septum

Branch villi

Decidua basalis

Stratum compactum

Stratum spongiosum

Myometrium

Anchoring villus
(cytotrophoblast)

After delivery the decidua detaches at this point

Figure 23–19. Structure of the placenta. Arrows indicate the blood flow from decidual arteries to intervillous space and back to decidual veins. This direction is determined by the difference in pressure between arterial and venous blood. Note the free and anchored chorionic villi. (Redrawn and reproduced, with permission, from Duplessis GDT, Haegel P: *Embryologie,* Masson, 1971 [English edition, Springer-Verlag, 1972].)

blast remains until the end of pregnancy, but the cytotrophoblast disappears gradually during the second half. Although the cytotrophoblast undergoes extensive proliferation and concomitant cell fusion during early placentation, proliferation slows in the second half of pregnancy, while the fusion continues. This results in a loss of the cytotrophoblast cells, which become incorporated into the growing **syncytium.**

The chorionic villi may be either free or anchored to the decidua basalis. Both villi have the same structure, but the free villi do not reach the decidua, whereas the anchored villi become embedded within the decidua basalis. The surfaces of the villi are

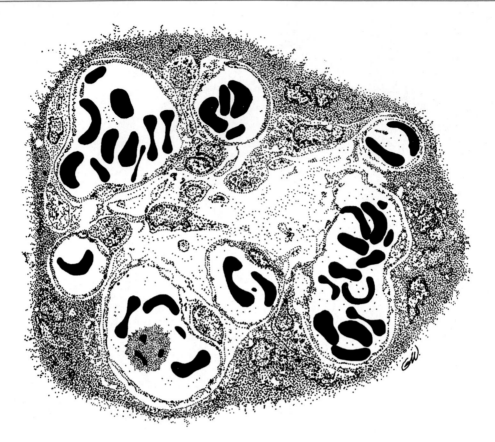

Figure 23–20. A chorionic villus in the second half of pregnancy. The syncytiotrophoblast is a continuous layer at the surface with dark nuclei. Cytotrophoblast cells form a discontinuous layer of cells with lighter and larger nuclei just beneath the syncytiotrophoblast. Note several erythrocytes and one leukocyte inside the sectioned capillaries.

bathed with blood from the lacunae of the basal decidua and are the site of the exchange of substances between fetal and maternal blood.

B. Maternal Part: The maternal part of the placenta—the decidua basalis—supplies arterial blood to, and receives venous blood from, the lacunae situated between the secondary villi. Although the maternal blood vessels are open during implantation, the fetal vessels contained in the secondary villi remain intact. Fetal blood and maternal blood do not mix except, on rare occasions, at the end of pregnancy. Some substances (see below) are, however, transferred between the two. During this period, the cytotrophoblast is no longer continuous, and the capillaries of the villi are close to the surface; a very slight exchange of blood cells may occur. At that time, the walls of the fetal capillaries are separated from the maternal blood only by the syncytiotrophoblast.

During pregnancy, cells from the connective tissue stroma of the decidua basalis and a lesser number of cells from the decidua parietalis and decidua capsularis form the **decidual cells.** These cells are large and exhibit the characteristics of protein-synthesizing cells; they produce prolactin and other biologically active substances.

At the end of a full-term pregnancy, the placenta has the shape of a disk. The umbilical cord usually arises at the center of the placenta and forms a connection between the fetal and placental circulations.

C. Histophysiology: Fetal venous blood reaches the placenta through the two umbilical arteries, which branch and ultimately give rise to the vessels of the chorionic villi. In these villi, the fetal blood receives oxygen, loses its CO_2, and returns to the fetus through the umbilical vein.

Since the chorionic villi are submerged in maternal blood, the fetal blood remains isolated by the structures that form the **placental barrier:** the endothelium of the fetal capillaries and the basal lamina of these capillaries, the mesenchyme in the interior of the villus, the basal lamina of the trophoblast, the cytotrophoblast (during the first half of pregnancy), and the syncytiotrophoblast.

The placenta is permeable to several substances; it normally transfers oxygen, water, electrolytes, carbohydrates, lipids, proteins, vitamins, hormones, some antibodies, and some drugs from maternal blood to fetal blood. CO_2, water, hormones, and residual products of metabolism are transferred from fetal blood to maternal blood.

The placenta is also an endocrine organ, producing such hormones as HCG, chorionic thyrotropin, chorionic corticotropin, estrogens, and progesterone. It also secretes a protein hormone called human chorionic somatomammotropin, which has lactogenic and growth-stimulating activity. All these hormones are synthesized by the syncytiotrophoblast.

Autoradiographic studies after injection of ^{3}H-thymidine show that the cells of the cytotrophoblast multiply actively and incorporate themselves into the syncytiotrophoblast. This indicates that the syncytiotrophoblast grows as a result of the growth and mitotic activity of the cytotrophoblast.

VAGINA

The wall of the vagina is devoid of glands and consists of three layers: a **mucosa,** a **muscular layer,** and an **adventitia.** The mucus found in the lumen of the vagina comes from the glands of the uterine cervix.

The epithelium of the mucosa is stratified squamous and has a thickness of 150–200 μm. Its cells may contain a small amount of keratohyalin. Intense keratinization, however, with the cells changing into keratin plates, as in typical keratinized epithelia, does not occur (Figure 23–21). Under the stimulus of estrogen, the vaginal epithelium synthesizes and accumulates a large quantity of glycogen, which is deposited in the lumen of the vagina when the vaginal cells desquamate. Bacteria in the vagina metabolize

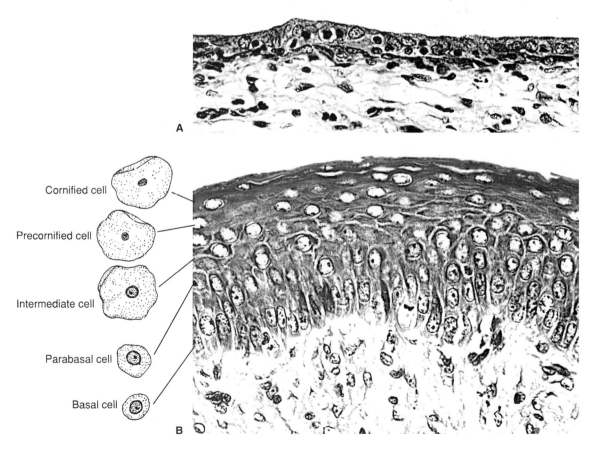

Figure 23–21. Photomicrograph of rat vaginal mucosa in the absence (**A**) and presence (**B**) of estrogen stimulation. Estrogen stimulates epithelial cell proliferation and differentiation. The appearance of exfoliated vaginal epithelium varies according to the intensity of such stimulation; cells become gradually flattened and eosinophilic, and there is progressive nuclear condensation (shown at left).

glycogen and form lactic acid, which is responsible for the usually low pH of the vagina. The acidic vaginal environment provides a protective action against some pathogenic microorganisms.

The lamina propria of the vaginal mucosa is composed of loose connective tissue that is very rich in elastic fibers. Among the cells present are lymphocytes and neutrophils in relatively large quantities. During certain phases of the menstrual cycle, these two types of leukocytes invade the epithelium and pass into the lumen of the vagina. Although the lamina propria lacks glands, it exhibits a rich vascularization that is the source of the fluid exudate that seeps through the squamous epithelium during sexual stimulation. The vaginal mucosa is virtually devoid of sensory nerve endings, and the few naked nerve endings that do exist are probably pain fibers.

The muscular layer of the vagina is composed mainly of longitudinal bundles of smooth muscle fibers. There are some circular bundles, especially in the innermost part (next to the mucosa).

Outside the muscular layer, a coat of dense connective tissue, the adventitia, rich in thick elastic fibers, unites the vagina with the surrounding tissues. The great elasticity of the vagina is related to the large number of elastic fibers in the connective tissues of its wall. In this connective tissue are an extensive venous plexus, nerve bundles, and groups of nerve cells.

EXFOLIATIVE CYTOLOGY

Exfoliative cytology is the study of the characteristics of cells that normally desquamate from various surfaces of the body. Cytologic examination of cells collected from the vagina gives information of clinical importance.

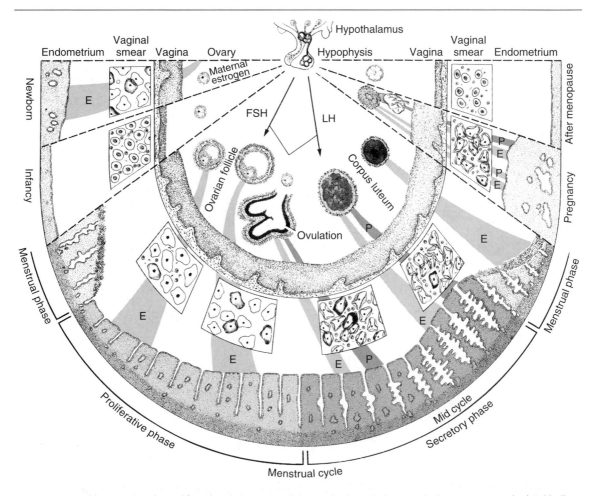

Figure 23–22. Menstrual cycle and functional changes relating to the hypothalamus, pituitary, ovary, vaginal epithelium, and endometrium. E, estrogen (gray); P, progesterone (dark gray); FSH, follicle-stimulating hormone; LH, luteinizing hormone. (Modified and redrawn from FH Netter.)

In fully mature vaginal mucosa, five types of cells are easily identified: cells of the internal portion of the basal layer (basal cells), cells of the external portion of the basal layer (parabasal cells), cells of the intermediate layers, precornified cells, and cornified cells (Figure 23–21). Based on the numbers of cell types that appear in a vaginal smear, valuable information can be obtained on the hormonal status of the patient (action of estrogen and progesterone). The vaginal smear is also useful in the early detection of cervical cancer.

EXTERNAL GENITALIA

The female external genitalia, or vulva, consists of the **clitoris, labia minora, labia majora,** and some glands that open into the vestibulum, a space enclosed by the labia minora.

The urethra and the ducts of the vestibular glands open into the vestibulum. The two **glandulae vestibulares majores,** or **glands of Bartholin,** are situated with one on each side of the vestibulum. These glands are homologous to the bulbourethral glands in the male. The more numerous **glandulae vestibulares minores** are scattered, found with greater frequency around the urethra and clitoris. All the glandulae vestibulares secrete mucus.

The clitoris and the penis are homologous in embryonic origin and histologic structure. The clitoris is formed by two erectile bodies ending in a rudimentary **glans clitoridis** and a prepuce. The clitoris is covered with stratified squamous epithelium.

The labia minora are folds of skin with a core of spongy connective tissue permeated by elastic fibers. The stratified squamous epithelium that covers them has a thin layer of keratinized cells on the surface. Sebaceous and sweat glands are present on the inner and outer surfaces of the labia minora.

The labia majora are folds of skin that contain a large quantity of adipose tissue and a thin layer of smooth muscle. Their inner surface has a histologic structure similar to that of the labia minora. The external surface is covered by skin and coarse, curly hair. Sebaceous and sweat glands are numerous on both surfaces.

The external genitalia are abundantly supplied with sensory tactile nerve endings, including Meissner's and pacinian corpuscles, which contribute to the physiology of sexual arousal.

ENDOCRINE INTERRELATIONSHIPS

Female reproductive function is regulated through certain nuclei of the hypothalamus. Nerve cells in the hypothalamus produce and introduce into the portal blood vessels specific polypeptides that act on the pars distalis of the hypophysis to liberate gonadotropins; these gonadotropins in turn stimulate the secretion of ovarian hormones (estrogens and progesterone; Figure 23–22). The hypothalamic localization of the ovarian hormone control mechanism might explain why strong, nonspecific cerebral stimuli occasionally affect reproductive function, resulting in **false pregnancy** (**pseudocyesis**) or the phenomenon of women who live or work together menstruating at virtually the same time.

The developing ovarian follicle synthesizes **estrogens,** and the corpus luteum synthesizes estrogens and **progesterone.** The main source of estrogens in the human ovarian follicle seems to be granulosa cells that have all the enzymes necessary to convert cholesterol to **estradiol-17β.** Estradiol found in blood is produced mainly by the theca interna cells of the follicle and is rapidly converted to **estrone,** which is further metabolized to **estriol,** probably in the liver. Estradiol is the most potent of the three estrogen compounds.

The hypophyseal gonadotropins, follicle-stimulating hormone (FSH) and LH, are produced under the

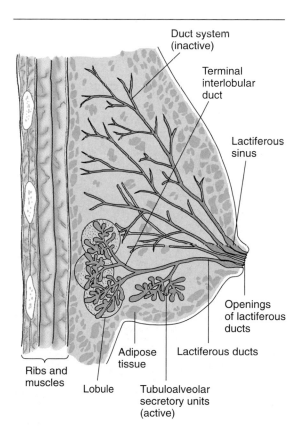

Figure 23–23. Schematic drawing of the female breast showing the mammary glands with ducts that open into the nipple. The outlines of the lobules do not exist in vivo but are shown for instructional purposes. The stippling indicates the loose intralobular connective tissue.

control of a single gonadotropin-releasing hormone (GnRH) liberated by the hypothalamus. FSH stimulates the growth of the ovarian follicles and the formation of estrogens. It is important to note that at any particular time in the cycle, the ovary possesses follicles in all stages of growth. The release of FSH does not promote the formation of a graafian follicle from a primordial follicle during one cycle. The most immediate effect of FSH is probably the maturation of existing late primary or secondary follicles. LH promotes ovulation and the formation of the corpus luteum (Figure 23–22).

The ovary also acts on the hypophysis, both directly and through the hypothalamus. Estrogen inhibits the secretion of FSH and stimulates the secretion of LH, whose production is inhibited by progesterone. Just before mid cycle, estrogen secretion reaches a peak and causes a brief surge of LH secretion. LH promotes ovulation, maturation of the oocyte, and formation of the corpus luteum. Since the secretion of LH is inhibited by progesterone produced by the corpus luteum, this structure is soon deprived of the hypophyseal stimulus (i.e., LH) necessary for its functioning, and it consequently degenerates.

During fertilization and implantation, syncytiotrophoblast cells synthesize the chorionic gonadotropins that stimulate and maintain the function of the corpus luteum during pregnancy.

In humans, prolactin initiates and maintains milk secretion by mammary glands that are already stimulated by estrogens and progesterone.

MAMMARY GLANDS

Each mammary gland consists of 15–25 lobules of the compound tubuloalveolar type whose function is to secrete milk to nourish newborns (Figure 23–23). Each lobe, separated from the others by dense connective tissue and much adipose tissue, is really a gland in itself with its own **excretory lactiferous duct.** These ducts, 2–4.5 cm long, emerge independently in the **nipple,** which has 15–25 openings, each about 0.5 mm in diameter. The histologic structure of the mammary glands varies according to sex, age, and physiologic status.

Breast Structure During Puberty & in the Adult

Before puberty, the mammary glands are composed of **lactiferous sinuses** and several branches of these sinuses, the **lactiferous ducts** (Figure 23–23).

The development of mammary glands in girls during puberty constitutes one of the secondary sex characteristics. During this period, the breasts increase in size and develop a prominent nipple. In boys, the breasts normally remain flattened.

Breast enlargement during puberty is the result of the accumulation of adipose tissue and collagenous connective tissue, with increased growth and branching of lactiferous ducts. The proliferation of the lactiferous ducts and accumulation of fat are due to an increase in the amount of ovarian estrogens during puberty.

The characteristic structure of the gland—the lob-

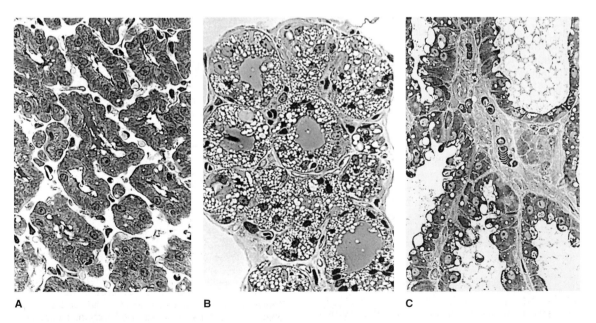

A **B** **C**

Figure 23–24. Photomicrographs of mammary tissues during pregnancy (**A**), prepartum (**B**), and during lactation (**C**). During pregnancy, the glandular epithelium is proliferating. Secretory processes begin prepartum and reach their maximum during lactation, with the accumulation of milk in the distended alveoli.

ule—in the adult woman is developed at the tips of the smallest ducts (**terminal interlobular ducts;** Figure 23–23). A lobule consists of several **intralobular** ducts that empty into one terminal interlobular duct. Each lobule is embedded in loose, cellular intralobular connective tissue. A denser, less cellular interlobular connective tissue separates the lobules.

Near the opening of the nipple, the lactiferous ducts dilate to form the lactiferous sinuses (Figure 23–23). The lactiferous sinuses are lined with stratified squamous epithelium at their external openings. This epithelium very quickly changes to stratified columnar or cuboidal epithelium. The lining of the lactiferous ducts and terminal interlobular ducts is formed of simple cuboidal epithelium covered by closely packed myoepithelial cells.

In the intralobular connective tissue surrounding the alveoli are lymphocytes and plasma cells. The plasma cell population increases significantly toward the end of pregnancy; it is responsible for the secretion of immunoglobulins (secretory IgA) that confer passive immunity on the newborn.

The histologic structure of these glands undergoes small alterations during the menstrual cycle, eg, proliferation of cells of the ducts at about the time of ovulation. These changes coincide with the time at which circulating estrogen is at its peak. Greater hydration of connective tissue in the premenstrual phase produces breast enlargement.

The **nipple** has a conical shape and may be pink, light brown, or dark brown. Externally, it is covered by keratinized stratified squamous epithelium continuous with that of the adjacent skin. The skin around the nipple constitutes the **areola.** The color of the areola darkens during pregnancy, as a result of the local accumulation of melanin. After delivery, the areola may become lighter in color but rarely returns to its original shade. The epithelium of the nipple rests on a layer of connective tissue rich in smooth muscle fibers. These fibers are disposed in circles around the deeper lactiferous ducts and parallel to them where they enter the nipple. The nipple is abundantly supplied with sensory nerve endings.

The Breasts During Pregnancy & Lactation

The mammary glands undergo intense growth during pregnancy as a result of the proliferation of **alveoli** at the ends of the terminal interlobular ducts. Alveoli are spherical collections of epithelial cells that become the active milk-secreting structures in lactation (Figure 23–24). A few fat droplets and membrane-limited secretory vacuoles containing from one to several dense aggregates of milk proteins can be seen in the apical cytoplasm of alveolar cells. The number of secretory vacuoles and fat droplets greatly increases in lactation (see below). Four to six stellate myoepithelial cells encompass each alveolus; they are found between the alveolar epithelial cells

and the basal lamina. The amounts of connective tissue stroma and adipose tissue, relative to the parenchyma, decrease considerably during lactation.

Growth of the mammary glands during pregnancy is the result of the synergistic action of several hormones, mainly estrogen, progesterone, prolactin, and human placental lactogen. These hormones stimulate the growth of the secretory parts (alveoli) of the mammary glands. The mammary gland is the only

A. Nonpregnant

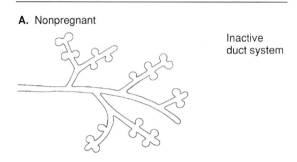

Inactive
duct system

B. During pregnancy

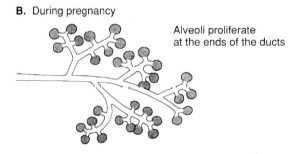

Alveoli proliferate
at the ends of the ducts

C. Lactating

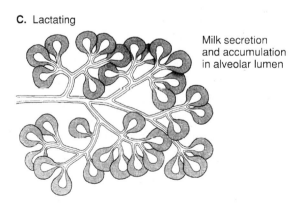

Milk secretion
and accumulation
in alveolar lumen

Figure 23–25. Changes in the mammary gland. **A:** In nonpregnant women, the gland has an inactive duct system. **B:** During pregnancy, alveoli proliferate at the ends of the ducts and prepare for the secretion of milk. **C:** During lactation, alveoli are fully differentiated, and milk secretion is abundant. Once lactation is completed, the gland reverts to the nonpregnant condition. The gland is normally quiescent and undifferentiated, undergoing this differentiation and secretion only during the cycle of pregnancy and lactation.

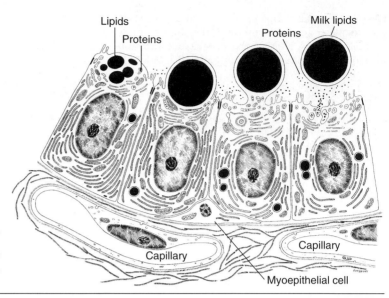

Figure 23–26. Alveolar cells from the mammary gland. From left to right, note the accumulation and extrusion of lipids and proteins. The proteins are released through exocytosis.

structure in the body that undergoes such a striking structural and physiologic change during the hormonal cycles of pregnancy (Figure 23–25).

During lactation, milk is produced by the epithelial cells of the alveoli (Figure 23–26) and accumulates in their lumens and inside the lactiferous ducts. The secretory cells become small and low cuboidal, and their cytoplasm contains spherical droplets of various sizes containing mainly neutral triglycerides. These lipid droplets pass out of the cells into the lumen and in the process are enveloped with a portion of the apical cell membrane. Lipids constitute 4% of human milk.

In addition to the lipid droplets, which are at the apical pole of the secretory cell, there are a large number of membrane-limited vacuoles that contain granules composed of caseins and other milk proteins (Figure 23–26). Milk proteins include several caseins, α-lactalbumin, and IgA, which are released by exocytosis. Proteins constitute approximately 1.5% of human milk. Lactose, the sugar of milk, is synthesized from glucose and galactose and constitutes about 7% of human milk.

The first secretion from the mammary glands to appear after birth is called **colostrum.** It contains less fat and more protein than regular milk and is rich in antibodies (predominantly secretory IgA) that provide some degree of passive immunity to the newborn, especially within the gut lumen.

When a woman is breast-feeding, the nursing action of the child stimulates tactile receptors in the nipple, resulting in liberation of the posterior pituitary hormone **oxytocin.** This hormone causes contraction of myoepithelial cells in

alveoli and ducts, resulting in ejection of milk (**milk-ejection reflex**). Negative emotional stimuli, such as frustration, anxiety, or anger, can inhibit the liberation of oxytocin and thus prevent the reflex.

Postlactational Regression of the Breasts

With cessation of breast-feeding (weaning), most alveoli that develop during pregnancy undergo degeneration. This includes sloughing of whole cells as well as autophagic absorption of cellular components. Dead cells and debris are removed by macrophages. Myoepithelial cells and the basal lamina persist and are reused in the next pregnancy.

Senile Involution of the Breasts

After menopause, involution of the mammary glands is characterized by a reduction in size and the atrophy of their secretory portions and, to a certain extent, the ducts. Atrophic changes also take place in the interlobular connective tissue.

Cancer of the Breast

About 9% of all women born in the United States will develop breast cancer at some time during their lives. Most of these cancers (carcinomas) arise from epithelial cells of the lactiferous ducts. If these cells metastasize to the lungs, brain, or bone, breast carcinoma becomes a major cause of death. Early detection (eg, through self-examination, mammography, ultrasound, and other techniques) and consequent early treatment have significantly reduced the mortality rate from breast cancer.

REFERENCES

Beaconsfield P et al: The placenta. Sci Am 1980;243:94.

Clement PB: Histology of the ovary. Am J Surg Pathol 1987;11:277.

Gulyas BJ: Fine structure of the luteal tissue. In: *Ultrastructure of Endocrine Cells and Tissues.* Motta PM (editor). Martinus Nijhoff, 1984.

Mathieu P et al: Localization of relaxin in human gestational corpus luteum. Cell Tissue Res 1981; 219:213.

Motta PM, Hafez ESE (editors): *Biology of the Ovary.* Martinus Nijhoff, 1980.

Page DL, Dupont WD: Anatomic indicators (histologic and cytologic) of increased breast cancer risk. Breast Cancer Res Treat 1993;28:157.

Peters H, McNatty KP: *The Ovary: A Correlation of Structure and Function in Mammals.* Granada Publishing, 1980.

Pitelka DR, Hamamoto ST: Ultrastructure of the mammary secretory cell. In: *Biochemistry of Lactation.* Mepham TB (editor). Elsevier, 1983.

Segal SJ: The physiology of human reproduction. Sci Am 1974;231:52.

Tersakis J: The ultrastructure of normal human first trimester placenta. J Ultrastruct Res 1963;9:268.

Vorherr H: *The Breast: Morphology, Physiology and Lactation.* Academic Press, 1974.

Wynn RM (editor): *Biology of the Uterus.* Plenum Press, 1977.

Yoshida Y: Ultrastructure and secretory function of the syncytial trophoblast of human placenta in early pregnancy. Exp Cell Res 1964;34:305.

Zuckerman S, Weir BJ (editors): *The Ovary,* 2nd ed. Vol. 1. *General Aspects.* Academic Press, 1977.

The Sense Organs

Information about the external world is conveyed to the central nervous system by sensory units called **receptors.** These structures transduce stimuli (heat, pressure, light, sound, etc) into signals that are capable of triggering action potentials in sensory nerves. The receptors are grouped into the following systems: somatic and visceral receptor, proprioceptor, chemoreceptor, photoreceptor, and audioreceptor.

SUPERFICIAL & DEEP SENSATION: THE SOMATIC & VISCERAL RECEPTOR SYSTEM

Somatic and visceral receptors can be divided into free and encapsulated nerve terminals, according to the absence or presence of a connective tissue capsule. The receptors consist of dendritic nerve endings or specialized nonneuronal cells and are responsible for the senses discussed below.

Touch & Pressure

The sense of touch and pressure is detected by both encapsulated and free nerve endings (mechanoreceptors). Encapsulated nerve endings are covered by connective tissue capsules of varied structure (Figure 24–1). They are especially numerous in the dermis of the digits (but are not restricted to the skin) and are also present in the mesenteries and peritoneum. The best-known corpuscle is the **pacinian corpuscle,** composed of 20–70 layers of flattened fibroblasts alternating with thin collagen fibers; in histologic sections it resembles a sliced onion (Figure 24–2).

Hair follicles have both circumferential and longitudinal arrays of free unmyelinated fibers around most of the length of the follicle. When a hair is bent, the sensation of touch is elicited.

Warmth, Cold, & Pain

The sensations of warmth, cold, and pain are mainly mediated by free nerve endings that branch in the dermis, penetrate the basement membrane, and extend into the lower cell layers of the epidermis (Figure 24–1).

DETECTION OF BODY POSITION IN SPACE: THE PROPRIOCEPTOR SYSTEM

All human striated muscles contain encapsulated proprioceptors (L. *proprius,* one's own, + *capio,* to take) known as **muscle spindles** (Figure 24–3). These structures consist of a connective tissue capsule surrounding a fluid-filled space that contains a few long, thick muscle fibers and some short, thinner fibers (collectively called **intrafusal fibers**). Several sensory nerve fibers penetrate the muscle spindles, where they detect changes in the length of extrafusal muscle fibers and relay this information to the spinal cord. Here, reflexes of varying complexity are activated to maintain posture and to regulate the activity of opposing muscle groups involved in motor activities such as walking.

In tendons, near the insertion sites of muscle fibers, a connective tissue sheath encapsulates several large bundles of collagen fibers that are continuous with the collagen fibers that make up the myotendinous junction. Sensory nerves penetrate the connective tissue capsule. These structures, known as **Golgi tendon organs,** contribute to proprioception by detecting tensional differences in tendons (Figure 24–1).

Because these structures are sensitive to increases in tension, they permit blind persons to know the exact position of their limbs and thereby regulate the amount of effort required to perform movements that call for variable amounts of muscular force.

TASTE & SMELL: THE CHEMORECEPTOR SYSTEM

Taste

Taste is a sensation perceived by **taste buds,** receptors located principally on the tongue (there are about 10,000 taste buds on the human tongue) and in smaller numbers on the soft palate and laryngeal surface of the epiglottis. Lingual taste buds are embedded within the stratified epithelium of the **circumval-**

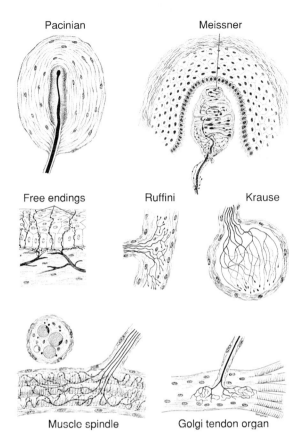

Pacinian

Meissner

Free endings

Ruffini

Krause

Muscle spindle

Golgi tendon organ

Figure 24–1. Several types of sensory endings of nerves (not drawn to the same scale). (Modified and reproduced, with permission, from Ham AW: *Histology,* 6th ed. Lippincott, 1969.)

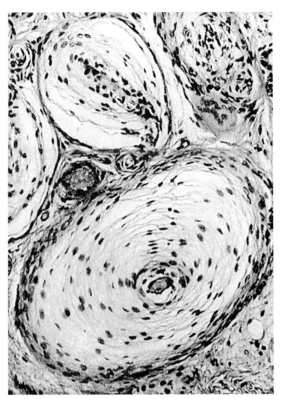

Figure 24–2. Photomicrograph of transverse and oblique sections of human pacinian corpuscles. Note the concentric layers of connective tissue surrounding the centrally disposed unmyelinated nerve. Hematoxylin-and-eosin (H&E) stain. × 320.

late, foliate, and **fungiform papillae.** Chemicals enter through the **taste pore,** a small aperture providing access to the receptor cells (Figures 24–4 and 24–5).

Taste buds are composed of at least four types of cells, which can be distinguished with the electron microscope. **Type I** and **type II** cells are tall, with microvilli at their surface. Although their function is unknown, they may support the activity of type III cells. **Type III** cells are also tall and are characterized by the presence of numerous vesicles that resemble synaptic vesicles. The close proximity of dendritic processes of sensory nerves to these accumulations of synaptic vesicles (Figure 24–5) is the basis for assigning taste reception to type III cells. A fourth cell type is a relatively undifferentiated basal cell that may be the precursor of more specialized cells in the taste buds.

Smell (Olfaction)

The olfactory chemoreceptors are located in the **olfactory epithelium,** a specialized area of the mucous membrane in the roof of the nasal cavity. In hu-

mans, it is about 10 cm^2 in area and up to 100 μm in thickness. It is a pseudostratified columnar epithelium composed of three types of cells:

The **supporting cells** have broad, cylindrical apexes and narrower bases. On their free surface are microvilli submerged in a fluid layer consisting of both serous and mucous secretions and covering the entire epithelial surface. Well-developed junctional complexes bind the supporting cells to the adjacent olfactory cells. The cells contain a light yellow pigment that is responsible for the color of the olfactory mucosa (Figure 24–6).

The **basal cells** are small; they are spherical or cone-shaped and form a single layer at the base of the epithelium.

Between the basal cells and the supporting cells are the **olfactory cells**—bipolar neurons distinguished from the supporting cells by the position of their nuclei, which lie below the nuclei of the supporting cells. Their apexes possess dilated areas from which arise 6–20 cilia. These cilia are long and nonmotile (Figure 24–7) and respond to odoriferous substances by generating a receptor potential. They in-

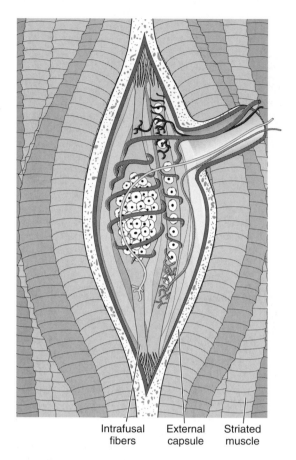

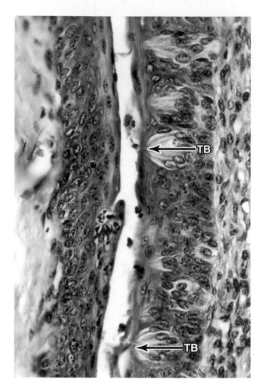

Figure 24–4. Photomicrograph of a section of a circumvallate papilla of the tongue, showing the taste buds (TB) embedded in the epithelium. H&E stain. × 400.

Intrafusal   External   Striated
fibers   capsule   muscle

Figure 24–3. Muscle spindle showing afferent and efferent nerve fibers (blue) that make synapses with the intrafusal fibers (modified muscle fibers). Note the complex nerve terminals on the intrafusal fibers. The two types of intrafusal fibers, one with a small diameter and the other with a dilatation filled with nuclei, are shown.

crease the receptor surface considerably. The afferent axons of these bipolar neurons unite in small bundles directed toward the central nervous system. Olfactory receptor cells can regenerate, which is a rare example of nerve cell replacement.

VISION: THE PHOTORECEPTOR SYSTEM

1. THE EYE

The eye (Figure 24–8) is a complex and highly developed photosensitive organ that permits an accurate analysis of the form, light intensity, and color reflected from objects. The eyes are located in protective bony structures of the skull—the **orbits.** Each eye includes a tough, fibrous globe to maintain its shape, a lens system to focus the image, a layer of photosensitive cells, and a system of cells and nerves

whose function it is to collect, process, and transmit visual information to the brain. Each eye (Figure 24–9) is composed of three concentric layers: an external layer that consists of the **sclera** and the **cornea;** a middle layer—also called the **vascular layer,** or **uveal tract**—consisting of the **choroid, ciliary body,** and **iris;** and an inner layer of nerve tissue, the **retina,** which consists of an outer pigment epithelium and an inner retina proper. The photosensitive retina proper communicates with the cerebrum through the **optic nerve** (Figures 24–8 and 24–9) and extends forward to the **ora serrata.** The optic nerve arises in the embryo as an evagination of the prosencephalon. Consequently, it is not considered a true peripheral nerve like the other cranial nerves. Since it is a tract of the central nervous system, the myelin of its nerve fibers is produced by oligodendrocytes, not by Schwann cells. This may explain the visual dysfunction often associated with multiple sclerosis, a demyelinating disorder of the central nervous system.

The **lens** of the eye is a biconvex transparent structure held in place by a circular system of fibers, the **zonule,** which extends from the lens into a thickening of the middle layer, the **ciliary body,** and, by close apposition, to the vitreous body on its posterior side (Figures 24–8 and 24–9). Partly covering the anterior surface of the lens is an opaque pigmented ex-

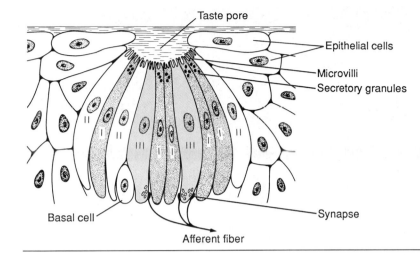

Taste pore
Epithelial cells
Microvilli
Secretory granules
Basal cell
Synapse
Afferent fiber

Figure 24–5. Structure and innervation of a taste bud. Four types of cells are shown. Type I cells (dark) contain apical secretory granules. The function of the type II cells (light) is not known. The sensory cells are type III (shown in color), with basally located synaptic vesicles and associated afferent nerve endings. Basal cells, which proliferate and give rise to the other cells, are the fourth cell type. Although only one afferent fiber is shown, about 50 fibers innervate a single taste bud.

pansion of the middle layer called the **iris.** The round hole in the middle of the iris is the **pupil** (Figure 24–8).

The eye contains three compartments: the **anterior chamber,** which occupies the space between the cornea and the iris and lens; the **posterior chamber,** between the iris, ciliary process, zonular attachments, and lens; and the **vitreous space,** which lies behind the lens and zonular attachments and is surrounded by the retina (Figures 24–8 and 24–9). Both the anterior and posterior chambers contain a protein-poor fluid called **aqueous humor.** The vitreous space is filled with a gelatinous substance called the **vitreous body.**

Note that the terms **outer (external)** and **inner (internal)** refer to the gross structure of the eye. Inner denotes a structure closer to the center of the globe, while outer means closer to the surface of the eyeball.

External Layer, or Tunica Fibrosa

The opaque white posterior five sixths of the external layer of the eye is the **sclera;** in the human, this forms a segment of a sphere approximately 22 mm in diameter (Figures 24–8 and 24–9). The sclera consists of tough, dense connective tissue made up mainly of flat collagen bundles intersecting in various directions while remaining parallel to the surface of the organ, a moderate amount of ground substance, and a few fibroblasts. The external surface of the sclera—the **episclera**—is connected by a loose system of thin collagen fibers to a dense layer of connective tissue called Tenon's capsule. Tenon's capsule comes into contact with the loose conjunctival stroma at the junction of the cornea with the sclera. Between Tenon's capsule and the sclera is **Tenon's space.** Because of this loose space, the eyeball can make rotating movements. Between the sclera and the choroid is the **suprachoroidal lamina,** a thin layer of loose connective tissue rich in melanocytes, fibroblasts, and elastic fibers. The sclera is relatively avascular.

In contrast to the posterior five sixths of the eye, the anterior one sixth—the **cornea**—is colorless and transparent (Figures 24–8 and 24–9). A transverse section of the cornea shows that it consists of five layers: epithelium, Bowman's membrane, stroma, Descemet's membrane, and endothelium (Figure 24–10). The corneal epithelium is stratified, squamous, and nonkeratinized and consists of five or six layers of cells. In the basal part of the epithelium are numerous mitotic figures that are responsible for the cornea's remarkable regenerative capacity: The turnover time for these cells is approximately 7 days. The surface corneal cells show microvilli protruding into the space filled by the precorneal tear film, a

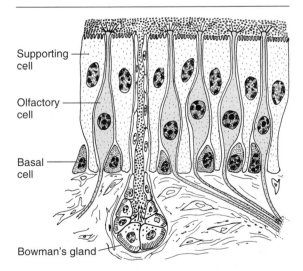

Supporting cell
Olfactory cell
Basal cell
Bowman's gland

Figure 24–6. Olfactory mucosa showing the three cell types (supporting, olfactory, and basal) and Bowman's gland.

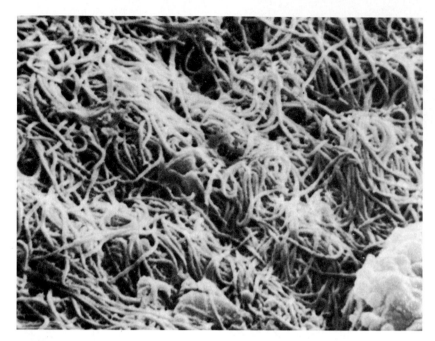

Figure 24–7. Scanning electron micrograph of the surface of the olfactory mucosa of a turtle. Note the dense net of cilia covering its surface. × 6600. (Courtesy of PP Graziadei.)

protective layer of lipid and glycoprotein, about 7 μm thick. The cornea has one of the richest sensory nerve supplies of any eye tissue.

Beneath the corneal epithelium lies a thick homogeneous layer 7–12 μm thick. This layer, **Bowman's membrane,** consists of collagen fibers crossing at random, a condensation of the intercellular substance, and no cells (Figure 24–11). Bowman's membrane contributes greatly to the stability and strength of the cornea.

The **stroma** is formed of many layers of parallel collagen bundles that cross at approximately right angles to each other. The collagen fibrils within each lamella are parallel to each other and run the full width of the cornea. Between the several layers, the cytoplasmic extensions of fibroblasts are flattened like the wings of a butterfly. Both cells and fibers of the stroma are immersed in a metachromatic glycoprotein substance rich in chondroitin sulfate. Although the stroma is avascular, migrating lymphoid cells are normally present in the cornea.

Descemet's membrane is a thick (5–10 μm) homogeneous structure composed of fine collagenous filaments organized in a three-dimensional network (Figure 24–10).

The **endothelium** of the cornea is a simple squamous epithelium. These cells possess organelles for secretion that are characteristic of cells engaged in active transport and protein synthesis and that may be related to the synthesis and maintenance of Descemet's membrane. The corneal endothelium and

epithelium are responsible for maintaining the transparency of the cornea. Both layers are capable of transporting sodium ions toward their apical surfaces. Chloride ions and water follow passively, maintaining the corneal stroma in a relatively dehydrated state. This state, along with the regular orientation of the very thin collagen fibrils of the stroma, accounts for the transparency of the cornea.

The **corneoscleral junction,** or **limbus,** is an area of transition from the transparent collagen bundles of the cornea to the white opaque fibers of the sclera. It is highly vascularized, and its blood vessels assume an important role in corneal inflammatory processes. The cornea—an avascular structure—receives its metabolites by diffusion from adjacent vessels and from the fluid of the anterior chamber of the eye. In the region of the limbus in the stromal layer, irregular endothelium-lined channels, the trabecular meshwork, merge to form **Schlemm's canal** (Figures 24–8 and 24–9), which drains fluid from the anterior chamber of the eye. Schlemm's canal communicates externally with the venous system.

Middle, or Vascular, Layer

The middle (vascular) layer of the eye consists of three parts: choroid, ciliary body, and iris (Figure 24–8), known collectively as the uveal tract.

A. Choroid: The choroid is a highly vascularized coat, with loose connective tissue between its blood vessels that is rich in fibroblasts, macrophages, lymphocytes, mast cells, plasma cells, collagen fibers,

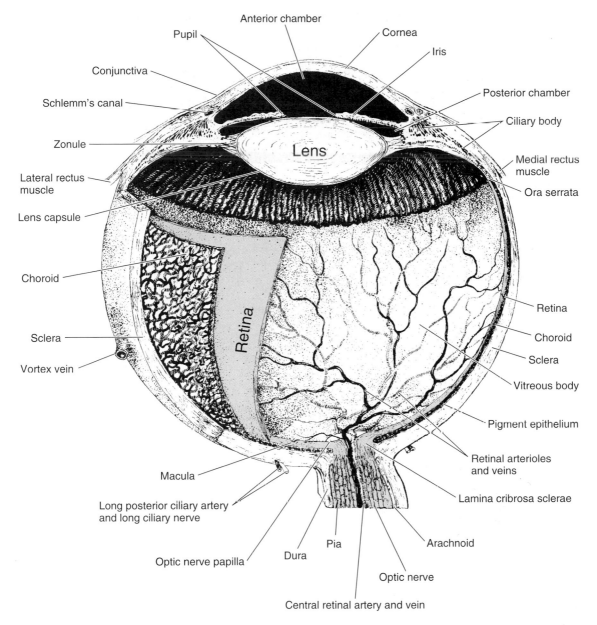

Figure 24-8. Internal structures of the human eye. The retina and optic nerve are shown in color. (Redrawn from an original drawing by Paul Peck and reproduced, with permission, from *The Anatomy of the Eye.* [Courtesy of Lederle Laboratories].)

and elastic fibers. Melanocytes are abundant in this layer and give it its characteristic black color. The inner layer of the choroid is richer than the outer layer in small vessels and is called the **choriocapillary layer.** It has an important function in nutrition of the retina, and damage to this tissue causes serious damage to the retina. A thin (3–4 μm) hyaline membrane separates the choriocapillary layer from the retina. This is known as **Bruch's membrane** and extends from the **optic disk** to the ora serrata. The optic

disk, also called the **optic papilla,** is the region where the optic nerve enters the eyeball (Figure 24–9).

Bruch's membrane is formed of five layers. The central layer is composed of a network of elastic fibers. This network is lined on its two surfaces with layers of collagen fibers that are covered by the basal lamina of the capillaries of the choriocapillary layer on one side and the basal lamina of the pigment epithelium on the other side. (See Retina, below, for a

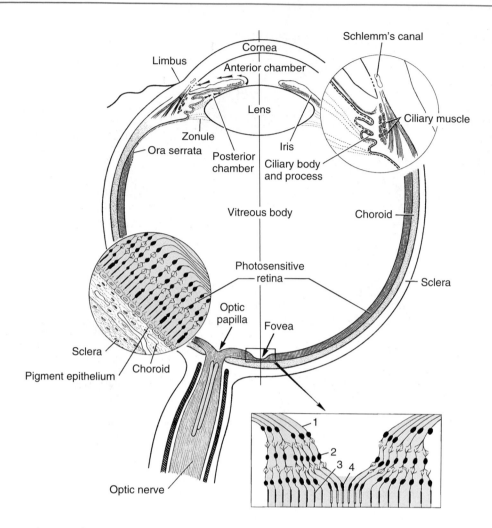

Figure 24–9. Diagram of the right eye, seen from above, showing the structure of the eye, retina, fovea, and ciliary body. Arrows in the anterior chamber show the direction of flow of aqueous humor. An enlarged diagram of the fovea is shown at lower right: (**1**) axons of ganglion cells; (**2**) bipolar cells; (**3**) rods; (**4**) cones. Enlarged diagrams of the ciliary body (upper right) and retina (lower left) are also shown. (Modified and reproduced, with permission, from Ham AW: *Histology,* 6th ed. Lippincott, 1969.)

description of the pigment epithelium.) The choroid is bound to the sclera by the **suprachoroidal lamina,** a loose layer of connective tissue rich in melanocytes.

B. Ciliary Body: The ciliary body, an anterior expansion of the choroid at the level of the lens (Figures 24–8 and 24–9), is a continuous thickened ring that lies at the inner surface of the anterior portion of the sclera; in transverse section, it forms a triangle. One of its faces is in contact with the vitreous body, one with the sclera, and the third with the lens and the posterior chamber of the eye. The histologic structure of the ciliary body is basically loose connective tissue (rich in elastic fibers, vessels, and melanocytes) surrounding the **ciliary muscle** (Figure 24–9). This structure consists of two bundles of

smooth muscle fibers that insert on the sclera anteriorly and on different regions of the ciliary body posteriorly. One of these bundles has the function of stretching the choroid; another bundle, when contracted, relaxes the tension on the lens. These muscular movements are important in visual accommodation (see Lens, below). The surfaces of the ciliary body that face the vitreous body, posterior chamber, and lens are covered by the anterior extension of the retina (Figure 24–9). In this region, the retina consists of only two cell layers. The layer directly adjacent to the ciliary body consists of simple columnar cells rich in melanin and corresponds to the forward projection of the pigment layer of the retina. The second layer, which covers the first, is derived from the sensory layer of the retina and consists of

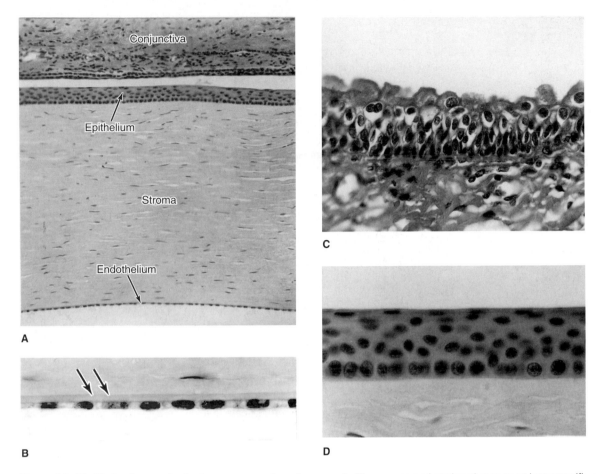

Figure 24–10. Photomicrograph of a transverse section of cornea. **A:** The cornea and conjunctiva seen at low magnification. × 80. **B:** The posterior corneal epithelium—also called endothelium. Arrows indicate Descemet's membrane. × 400. **C:** conjunctival epithelium. × 300. **D:** Anterior corneal epithelium. Note the smooth contour of the surface. × 400.

simple nonpigmented columnar epithelium (Figure 24–12A).

C. Ciliary Processes: The ciliary processes are ridge-like extensions of the ciliary body. They have a loose connective tissue core and numerous fenestrated capillaries (see Chapter 11) and are covered by the two simple epithelial layers described above (Figure 24–12B). From the ciliary processes emerge oxytalan fibers (**zonule fibers**) that insert into the capsule of the lens and anchor it in place (oxytalan fibers are described in Chapter 5). The apical ends of the epithelial cells are found at the junction between pigmented and nonpigmented cells, and the cells thus meet each other head-to-head. The basement membrane of the outer, pigmented cells is adjacent to the main mass of the ciliary body, whereas the basement membrane of the inner, nonpigmented cells is adjacent to the posterior chamber. The zonular fibers have their origin in the basement membrane of the inner cells. The apical ends of the

epithelial cells are joined by desmosomes, and elaborate tight junctions are found around the apical surfaces of epithelial cells of both layers. The nonpigmented inner layer of cells has extensive basal infoldings and interdigitations characteristic of ion-transporting cells (see Chapter 4). These cells actively transport certain constituents of plasma into the posterior chamber, thus forming the **aqueous humor.** This fluid has an inorganic ion composition similar to that of plasma but contains less than 0.1% protein (plasma has about 7% protein). Aqueous humor flows toward the lens and passes between it and the iris, reaching the anterior chamber of the eye (see Figure 24–9). Once in the anterior chamber, the humor proceeds to the angle formed by the cornea with the basal part of the iris. It penetrates the tissue of the limbus in a series of labyrinthine spaces (the trabecular meshwork) and finally reaches the irregular Schlemm's canal, lined with endothelial cells (Figures 24–8 and 24–9). This structure communicates

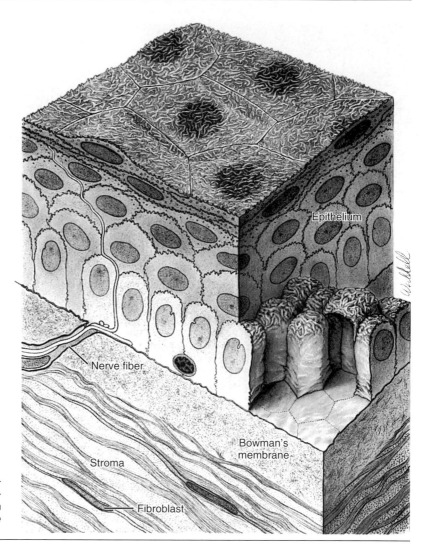

Figure 24–11. Three-dimensional drawing of the cornea. (Reproduced, with permission, from Hogan MJ et al: *Histology of the Human Eye.* Saunders, 1971.)

with small veins of the sclera, through which the aqueous humor escapes.

> Any impediment to the drainage of aqueous humor caused by an obstruction in the outflow channels results in an increase in intraocular pressure, causing **glaucoma.**

D. Iris: The iris is an extension of the choroid that partially covers the lens, leaving a round opening in the center called the **pupil** (Figure 24–8). The anterior surface of the iris is irregular and rough, with grooves and ridges. It is formed of a discontinuous layer of pigment cells and fibroblasts. Beneath this layer is a poorly vascularized connective tissue with few fibers and many fibroblasts and melanocytes. The next layer is rich in blood vessels embedded in loose connective tissue. The smooth posterior surface

of the iris is covered by two layers of epithelium, which also cover the ciliary body and its processes. The inner epithelium, in contact with the posterior chamber, is heavily pigmented with melanin granules. The outer epithelial cells have radially directed tongue-like extensions of their basal region; they are filled with overlapping myofilaments, creating the **dilator pupillae muscle** of the iris. The heavy pigmentation prevents the passage of light into the interior of the eye except through the pupil.

The function of the abundant melanocytes or pigment cells containing melanin in several regions of the eye is to keep stray light rays from interfering with image formation. The melanocytes of the stroma of the iris are responsible for the color of the eyes. If the layer of pigment in the interior region of the iris consists of only a few cells, the light reflected from the black pigment epithelium in the posterior

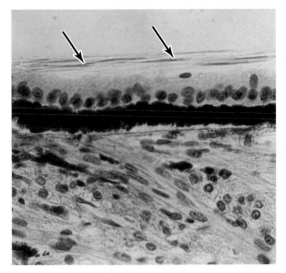

A

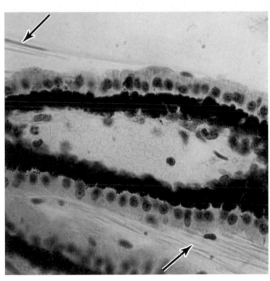

B

Figure 24–12. Photomicrographs of a ciliary body. **A:** Note the double layer, one of which consists of pigmented cells. **B:** The ciliary process is covered with epithelium on both sides. Arrows indicate zonular fibers. H&E stain. × 400.

surface of the iris will be blue. As the amount of pigment increases, the iris assumes various shades of greenish-blue, gray, and finally brown. Albinos have almost no pigment, and the pink color of their irises is due to the reflection of incident light from the blood vessels of the iris.

The iris contains smooth muscle bundles disposed in circles concentric with the pupillary margin, forming the **sphincter pupillae muscle** of the iris. The dilator and sphincter muscles have sympathetic and parasympathetic innervation, respectively.

Lens

The lens is a biconvex structure characterized by great elasticity, a feature that is lost with age as the lens hardens. The lens has three principal components:

A. Lens Capsule: The lens is enveloped by a thick (10–20 μm), homogeneous, refractile, carbohydrate-rich capsule coating the outer surface of the epithelial cells. It is a very thick basement membrane and consists mainly of collagen type IV and glycoprotein.

B. Subcapsular Epithelium: Subcapsular epithelium consists of a single layer of cuboidal epithelial cells that are present only on the anterior surface of the lens. The lens increases in size and grows throughout life as new lens fibers develop from cells located at the equator of the lens. The cells of this epithelium exhibit many interdigitations with the lens fibers.

C. Lens Fibers: Lens fibers are elongated and appear as thin, flattened structures. They are highly differentiated cells derived from cells of the subcapsular epithelium. Lens fibers eventually lose their nuclei and other organelles and become greatly elongated, attaining dimensions of 7–10 mm in length, 8–10 μm in width, and 2 μm in thickness. These cells are filled with a group of proteins called **crystallins.** Lens fibers are produced throughout life, at an ever-decreasing rate.

The lens is held in place by a radially oriented group of fibers, the **zonule,** that inserts on one side on the lens capsule and on the other on the ciliary body (Figure 24–13). Zonular fibers are similar to the microfibrils of elastic fibers. This system is important in the process known as **accommodation,** which permits focusing on near and far objects by changing the curvature of the lens. When the eye is at rest or gazing at distant objects, the lens is kept stretched by the zonule in a plane perpendicular to the optical axis. To focus on a near object, the ciliary muscles contract, causing forward displacement of the choroid and ciliary body. The tension exerted by the zonule is relieved, and the lens becomes thicker, keeping the object in focus.

Advancing age reduces the elasticity of the lens, making accommodation for near objects difficult. This is a normal aging process (**presbyopia**), which can be corrected by wearing glasses with convex lenses. In older individuals, a brownish pigment accumulates in lens fibers, making them less transparent. When the lens becomes opaque, the condition is termed **cataract,** which may also be caused by excessive exposure to ultraviolet radiation. In diabetes mellitus,

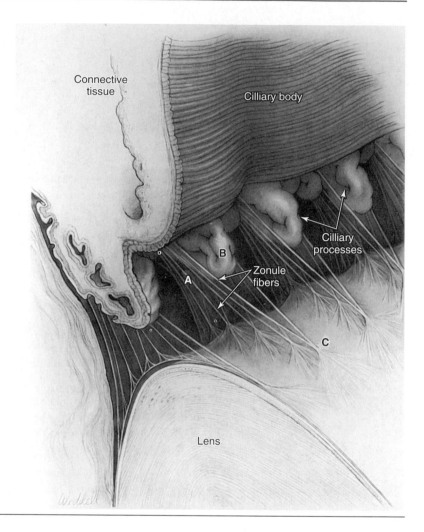

Figure 24–13. Anterior view of the ciliary processes showing the zonules attaching to the lens. Zonule fibers are bundles of microfilaments (oxytalan fibers) from the elastic fiber system. The zonules form columns (A) on either side of the ciliary processes (B), which meet on a single site (C) as they attach to the lens. (Reproduced, with permission, from Hogan MJ et al: *Histology of the Human Eye.* Saunders, 1971.)

the high levels of glucose are believed to produce cataract.

Vitreous Body

The vitreous body occupies the region of the eye behind the lens. It is a transparent gel that consists of water (about 99%), a small amount of collagen, and heavily hydrated hyaluronic acid molecules. The vitreous body contains very few cells, named **hyalocytes,** which synthesize collagen and hyaluronic acid.

Retina

The retina, the inner layer of the globe, consists of two portions. The posterior portion is photosensitive; the anterior part, which is not photosensitive, constitutes the inner lining of the ciliary body and the posterior part of the iris (Figures 24–9 and 24–14). The retina derives from an evagination of the anterior cephalic vesicle, or prosencephalon. As this **optic vesicle** comes into contact with the surface ectoderm,

it gradually invaginates in its central region, forming a double-walled **optic cup.** In adults, the outer wall gives rise to a thin membrane called the **pigment epithelium;** the optical or functioning part of the retina—the **neural retina**—is derived from the inner layer.

The pigment epithelium consists of columnar cells with a basal nucleus. The basal regions of the cells adhere firmly to Bruch's membrane, and the cell membranes have numerous basal invaginations (Figure 24–20). Mitochondria are more abundant in the region of the cytoplasm near these invaginations. These characteristics suggest an ion-transporting activity for this region.

The lateral cell membranes show cell junctions with conspicuous zonulae occludentes and zonulae adherentes at their apexes; there are also desmosomes and gap junctions. These morphologic characteristics indicate that the apical and basal regions of this epithelial sheet are sealed off and that there is intercellular communication. These junctional special-

Epithelium   Choroid   Sclera

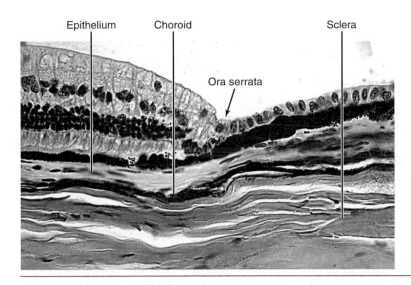

Ora serrata

Figure 24–14. Photomicrograph of a section of retina in the transition (ora serrata) between the photosensitive part (at left) and the blind (devoid of receptors) part (at right). Note the pigment epithelium, the choroid, and the sclera. H&E stain. × 200.

izations account for the electrical potential difference that results from ion transport between the two surfaces of this epithelium.

The cell apex has abundant extensions of two types: slender microvilli and cylindrical sheaths that envelop the tips of the photoreceptors.

> Because neither type of extension is anatomically joined to the photoreceptors, these regions can become separated, as in **detachment of the retina.** This common and serious disorder in humans can be treated effectively with laser surgery.

The cytoplasm of pigment epithelial cells has abundant smooth endoplasmic reticulum, believed to be a site of vitamin A esterification and transport to the photoreceptors. Melanin granules are numerous in the apical cytoplasm and microvilli. Melanin is synthesized in these cells by a mechanism similar to that described for the melanocytes in the skin (see Chapter 18). This dark pigment has the function of absorbing light after the photoreceptors have been stimulated.

The cell apex has numerous dense vesicles of variable shape that represent various stages in the phagocytosis and digestion of the tips of photoreceptor outer segments. Pigment cell structure and functions are shown in Figure 24–20.

The optical part of the retina—the posterior, or photosensitive, part—is a complex structure containing at least 15 types of neurons, and these cells form at least 38 distinct kinds of synapses with one another. The optical retina consists of an outer layer of photosensitive cells, the **rods** and **cones** (Figures 24–9, 24–15, and 24–16); an intermediate layer of **bipolar neurons,** which connect the rods and cones to the **ganglion cells;** and an internal layer of gan-

glion cells, which establish contact with the bipolar cells through their dendrites and send axons to the brain. These axons converge at the optic papilla, forming the **optic nerve.**

Between the layer of rods and cones and the bipolar cells is a region called the **external plexiform,** or **synaptic, layer,** where synapses between these two types of cells occur. The region where the synapses between the bipolar and ganglion cells are established is called the **internal plexiform layer** (Figure 24–16). The retina has an inverted structure, for the light will first cross the ganglion layer and then the bipolar layer to reach the rods and cones. The structure of the retina will now be examined in greater detail.

The rods and cones, named for the forms they assume, are polarized neurons; at one pole is a single photosensitive dendrite, and at the other are synapses with cells of the bipolar layer (Figures 24–16 and 24–17). The rod and cone cells can be divided into outer and inner segments, a nuclear region, and a synaptic region. The outer segments are modified cilia and contain stacks of membrane-limited saccules with a flattened, disk-like shape. The photosensitive pigment of the retina is in the membranes of these saccules. Both rod and cone cells pass through a thin layer, the **external limiting membrane,** that is a series of junctional complexes between the photoreceptors and glial cells of the retina (Müller cells; see Figure 24–21). The nuclei of the cones are generally disposed near the limiting membrane, whereas the nuclei of the rods lie near the center of the inner segment.

A. Rod Cells: Rod cells are thin, elongated cells (50 × 3 μm) composed of two portions (Figures 24–16 and 24–17). The external photosensitive rod-shaped portion is composed mainly of numerous (600–1000) flattened membranous disks stacked up

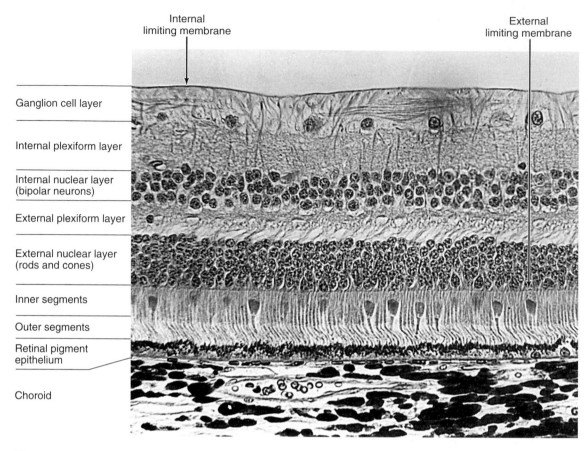

Figure 24–15. Section of the retina of a monkey. The retina is composed of three layers of cells: photoreceptor cells (rods and cones), bipolar neurons, and ganglion cells. Light enters from the top and traverses the layers shown in the figure. The internal nuclear layer contains bipolar neurons, and the external nuclear layer contains the nuclei of rods and cones. Note the inner segments of rods (narrow lines) and cones (triangular dark structures) as well as their outer segments. × 655.

like coins. The disks in rods are not continuous with the plasma membrane; the **outer segment** is separated from the **inner segment** by a constriction. Just below this constriction is a basal segment from which a cilium arises and passes to the outer segment. The inner segment is rich in glycogen and has a remarkable accumulation of mitochondria, most of which lie near the constriction (Figures 24–17 and 24–18). This local accumulation of mitochondria is related to the production of energy necessary for the visual process and protein synthesis. Polyribosomes, present in large numbers below the mitochondrial region of the inner segment, are involved in protein synthesis. Some of these proteins migrate to the outer segment of the rod cells, where they are incorporated into membranous disks. The flattened disks of the rod cells contain the pigment **visual purple,** or **rhodopsin,** which is bleached by light and initiates the visual stimulus. This substance is globular and is located in the outer surface of the lipid bilayer of the flattened membranous disks.

The human retina has approximately 120 million rods. They are extremely sensitive to light and are considered the receptors used when low levels of light are encountered, such as at dusk or nighttime. The outer segment is the site of photosensitivity; the inner segment contains the metabolic machinery necessary for the biosynthetic and energy-producing processes of these cells.

Autoradiographic studies show that proteins of the rod vesicles are synthesized in the polyribosome-rich inner segments of these cells. From there, they migrate to the outer segment and aggregate at its basal region, where they are incorporated into membranes formed by a double layer of phospholipids, producing flattened disks (Figures 24–17 and 24–18). These structures gradually migrate to the cell apex, where they are shed, phagocytized, and digested by the cells of the pigment epithelium (Figures 24–19 and 24–20). It has been calculated that, in the monkey, approximately 90 vesicles per cell are produced daily. The whole process of migration, from assem-

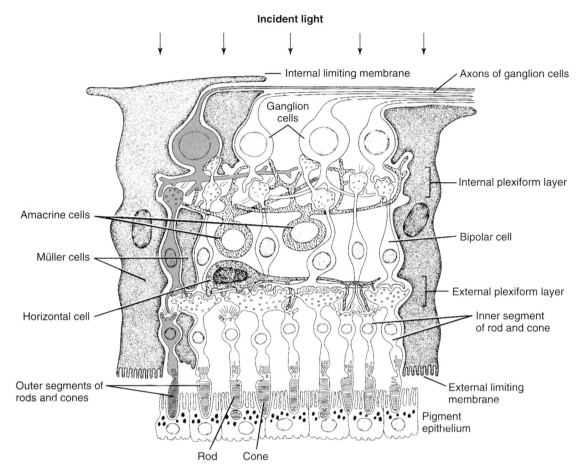

Figure 24–16. The three layers of retinal neurons. The arrows indicate the direction of the light path. The stimulation generated by the incident light on rods and cones proceeds in the opposite direction. (Redrawn and reproduced, with permission, from Boycott and Dowling: Proc R Soc Lond [Biol] 1966;166:80.)

bly at the basal cell region to apical shedding, takes from 9 to 13 days.

> In **hereditary retinal dystrophy** in the rat, the vesicles shed from the rods are not phagocytized, probably because of a dysfunction of the pigment epithelium. They are instead deposited at the surface of the pigment layer.

B. Cone Cells: Cone cells (Figure 24–17) are also elongated (60×1.5 μm) neurons. Each human retina has about 6 million cone cells. The structure is similar to that of rods, with outer and inner segments, a basal body with cilium, and an accumulation of mitochondria and polyribosomes. Cones differ from rods in their form (conical) and the structure of their outer segments. As in rods, this region is composed of stacked membranous disks; however, they are not independent of the outer plasma membrane but arise as invaginations of this structure (Figure 24–17). In cones, newly synthesized protein is not concentrated

in recently assembled disks, as it is in rods, but is distributed uniformly throughout the outer segment.

There are at least three functional types of cones that cannot be distinguished by their morphologic characteristics. Each type contains a variety of the cone photopigment called **iodopsin,** and its maximum sensitivity is in the red, green, or blue region of the visible spectrum. Cones, sensitive only to light of a higher intensity than that required to stimulate rods, are believed to permit better visual acuity than do rods.

C. Other Cells: The layer of bipolar cells consists of two types of cells (Figure 24–16): **diffuse bipolar cells,** which have synapses with two or more photoreceptors; and **monosynaptic bipolar cells,** which establish contact with the axon of only one cone photoreceptor and only one ganglion cell. A certain number of cones therefore transmit their impulses directly to the brain.

In addition to establishing contact with the bipolar cells, the cells of the ganglion layer project their ax-

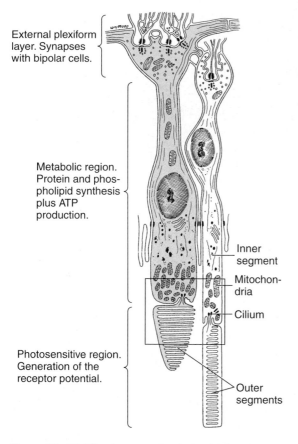

External plexiform layer. Synapses with bipolar cells.

Metabolic region. Protein and phospholipid synthesis plus ATP production.

Inner segment

Mitochondria

Cilium

Photosensitive region. Generation of the receptor potential.

Outer segments

Figure 24–17. Ultrastructure of rods (at right) and cones (at left). The rectangular outlined region is shown in the electron micrograph in Figure 24–18. (Redrawn and reproduced, with permission, from Chevremont M: *Notions de Cytologie et Histologie.* S.A. Desoer Editions [Liege], 1966.)

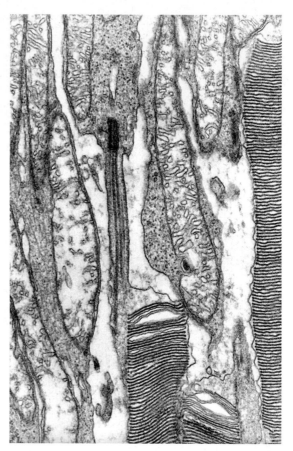

Figure 24–18. Electron micrograph of a section of the retina. In the upper part of the figure are the inner segments. This photosensitive region consists of parallel membranous flat disks. Accumulation of mitochondria takes place in the inner segment (see Figure 24–17). In the middle of the figure is a basal body giving rise to a cilium that is further modified into an outer segment.

ons to a specific region of the retina, where they come together to form the **optic nerve** (Figure 24–16). This region, which is devoid of receptors, is known as the **blind spot** of the retina, the **papilla of the optic nerve,** or the **optic nerve head** (Figure 24–9). The **ganglion cells** are typical nerve cells, containing a large euchromatic nucleus, basophilic Nissl substance, etc. These cells, like the bipolar cells, are classified as diffuse or monosynaptic in their connections with other cells.

In addition to these three main types of cells (photoreceptor, bipolar, and ganglion cells), there are other types of cells that are distributed more diffusely in the layers of the retina.

1. **Horizontal cells** (Figure 24–16) establish contact between different photoreceptors. Their exact function is not known, but they may act to integrate stimuli.
2. **Amacrine cells** are various types of neurons that

establish contact between the ganglion cells. Their function is also obscure.

3. **Supporting cells** are neuroglia that possess, in addition to the astrocyte and microglial cell types, some large, extensively ramified cells (**Müller cells**). The processes of these cells bind the neural cells of the retina and extend from the internal to the external limiting membranes of the retina (Figure 24–16). The external limiting membrane is a zone of adhesion (tight junctions) between photoreceptors and Müller cells. Müller cells are functionally analogous to neuroglia in that they support, nourish, and insulate the retinal neurons and fibers (Figure 24–21).

Retinal Histophysiology

Light passes through the layers of the retina to the rods and cones, where it is absorbed, initiating a se-

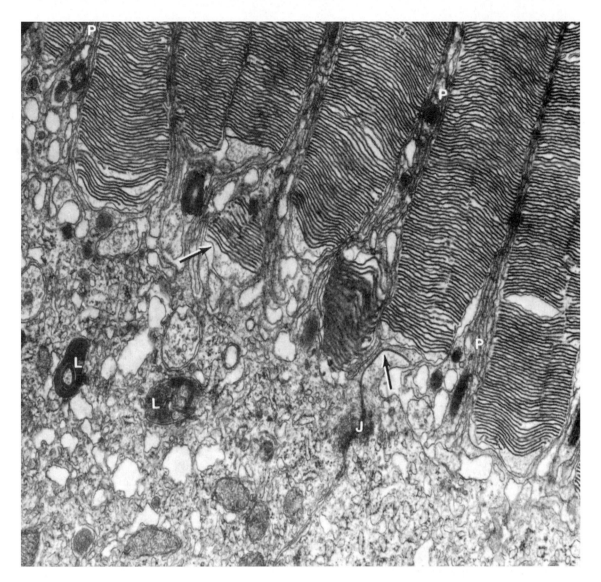

Figure 24–19. Electron micrograph of the interface between the photosensitive and pigmented layers in the rat retina. In the lower portion are parts of two pigment epithelium cells, revealing specialized junctions (J) between their lateral plasmalemmas. Above the pigment cells are the tips of several outer segments of rod cells that interdigitate with apical processes of the pigment epithelium (P). The large vacuoles containing flattened membranes (arrows) have been shed from the tips of the rods. L, lysosomal vesicles.

ries of reactions that result in vision—an extraordinarily sensitive process. Experimental evidence suggests that a single photon is enough to trigger the production of a receptor potential in a rod. Light acts to bleach the visual pigments, a photochemical process amplified by mechanisms that cause the local production of responses that are subsequently transmitted to the brain.

The visual pigment of rods, **rhodopsin,** is composed of an aldehyde of vitamin A (retinaldehyde) bound to specific proteins called **opsins.** Because rods have a low resolution, they form images without clear details; they are not sensitive to colors. Cones,

on the other hand, have a higher threshold and are responsible for sharp images and color vision. In humans, they contain three incompletely characterized pigments (**iodopsins**), which may provide a chemical basis for the classic tricolor theory of color vision.

When light strikes rhodopsin molecules, retinaldehyde undergoes isomerization from the all-*cis* form to the all-*trans* form. This change results in the dissociation of retinaldehyde from opsin, a reaction called **bleaching.** Bleaching of the visual pigment incorporated in the membrane disks increases the calcium conductance of the disk membranes and promotes the diffusion of calcium to the intracellular space of the

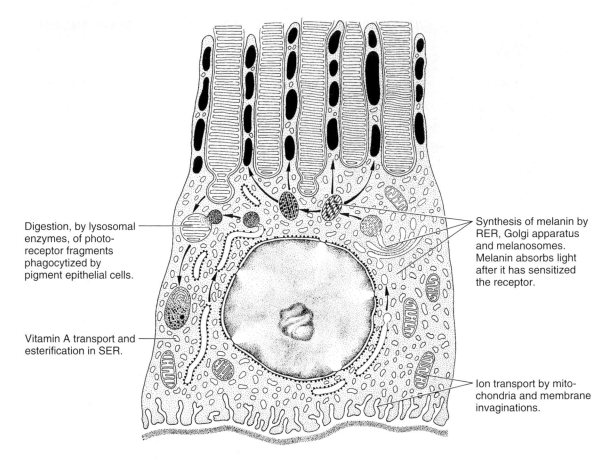

Digestion, by lysosomal enzymes, of photoreceptor fragments phagocytized by pigment epithelial cells.

Synthesis of melanin by RER, Golgi apparatus and melanosomes. Melanin absorbs light after it has sensitized the receptor.

Vitamin A transport and esterification in SER.

Ion transport by mitochondria and membrane invaginations.

Figure 24–20. Four functions of a retinal pigment epithelial cell. Note that the apical portion has abundant cell processes that fill the spaces between the outer segments of the photosensitive cells, and the membrane of the basal region has invaginations into the cytoplasm. This is a cell type with several functions, including the synthesis of melanin granules (by a process described in Chapter 18) that absorb stray light in the eye chamber. This is depicted on the right side of the figure, which shows the organelles that participate in melanin synthesis. On the left side of the figure, lysosomes containing enzymes synthesized in the rough endoplasmic reticulum (RER) coalesce with the phagocytized apical parts of the photoreceptor, digesting them. In addition to these activities, pigment cells are probably active in ion transport, since they maintain an electrical potential between the two surfaces of the epithelium membrane. The relatively well developed smooth endoplasmic reticulum (SER) participates in the processes of vitamin A esterification.

outer segment of the photoreceptor. Calcium acts on the cell membrane, reducing its permeability to sodium ions and promoting cell hyperpolarization. The electrical signals produced by closing these sodium channels spread to the inner segment and through gap junctions to neighboring cells.

In a second step, the visual pigment is reassembled, and the calcium ions are transported back into the disks in an energy-consuming process. The high energy requirement would seem to account for the abundance of mitochondria near the photosensitive site of rods and cones. Contrary to what happens in other receptors where action potentials are generated through cell depolarization, the rods and cones are hyperpolarized by light. This signal is transmitted to the bipolar, amacrine, and horizontal cells and then to the ganglion cells. Only the ganglion cells generate action potentials along their axons, which relay the information to the brain.

The clinical observation that the retina is damaged when it becomes detached suggests that the photosensitive cells derive their metabolites from the choriocapillary layer. The superficial localization of the vessels of the retina provides for their easy observation with an ophthalmoscope. This examination is of great value in the diagnosis and evaluation of disorders that affect blood vessels, such as diabetes mellitus and hypertension.

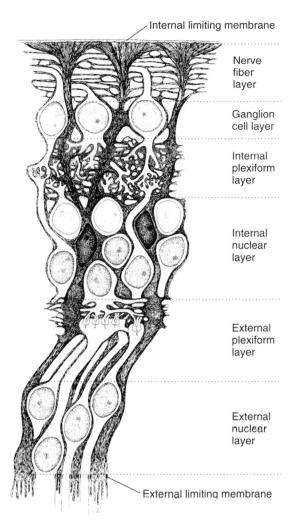

Internal limiting membrane

Nerve fiber layer

Ganglion cell layer

Internal plexiform layer

Internal nuclear layer

External plexiform layer

External nuclear layer

External limiting membrane

Figure 24–21. The close association of Müller cells with neural elements in the sensory retina. Müller cells (dark fibrous cells) appear to be structurally and functionally equivalent to the astrocytes of the central nervous system, in that they envelop and support the neurons and nerve processes of the retina. (Reproduced, with permission, from Hogan MJ et al: *Histology of the Human Eye.* Saunders, 1971.)

At the posterior pole of the optical axis lies the **fovea,** a shallow depression with very thin retina in the center. This is because the bipolar and ganglion cells accumulate in the periphery of this depression, so that its center consists only of cone cells (Figure 24–9). Cone cells in the fovea are long and narrow, resembling rod cells. This is an adaptation to permit closer packing of cones and thereby increase visual acuity. In this area, blood vessels do not cross over the photosensitive cells. Light falls directly on the cones in the central part of the fovea, which helps account for the extremely precise visual acuity of this region.

2. ACCESSORY STRUCTURES OF THE EYE

Conjunctiva

The conjunctiva (Figure 24–10A) is a thin, transparent mucous membrane that covers the anterior portion of the eye up to the cornea and the internal surface of the eyelids. It has a stratified columnar epithelium with numerous goblet cells, and its lamina propria is composed of loose connective tissue.

Eyelids

Eyelids (Figure 24–22) are movable folds of tissue that protect the eye. The skin of the lids is loose and elastic, permitting extreme swelling and subsequent return to normal shape and size.

The three types of glands in the lid are the Meibomian glands and the glands of Moll and Zeis. The Meibomian glands are long sebaceous glands in the tarsal plate. They do not communicate with the hair follicles. The Meibomian glands produce a sebaceous substance that creates an oily layer on the surface of the tear film, helping to prevent rapid evaporation of the normal tear layer. The glands of Zeis are smaller, modified sebaceous glands connected with the follicles of the eyelashes. The sweat glands of Moll are unbranched sinuous tubules that begin in a simple

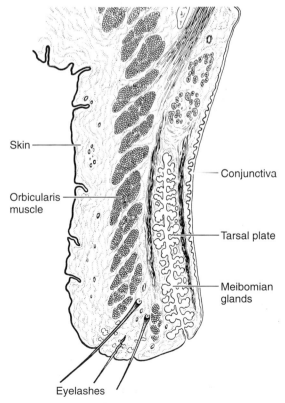

Skin

Conjunctiva

Orbicularis muscle

Tarsal plate

Meibomian glands

Eyelashes

Figure 24–22. Structure of the eyelid.

spiral and not in a glomerulus like ordinary sweat glands. They empty their secretion into the follicles of the eyelashes.

Lacrimal Apparatus

The lacrimal apparatus consists of the lacrimal gland, canaliculi, lacrimal sac, and nasolacrimal duct. The **lacrimal gland** (Figure 24–23) is a tear-secreting gland located in the anterior superior temporal portion of the orbit. It consists of several separate glandular lobes with 6–12 excretory ducts that connect the gland to the superior conjunctival fornix. (Fornices are the conjunctiva-lined recesses between the lids and the eyeball.) The lacrimal gland is a tubuloalveolar gland that usually has distended lumens and is composed of column-shaped cells of the serous type, resembling the parotid acinar cells. These cells show lightly stained secretory granules, and a basal lamina separates them from the surrounding connective tissue.

Well-developed myoepithelial cells surround the secretory portions of the lacrimal gland. The secretion of the gland passes down over the cornea and the bulbar and palpebral conjunctiva, moistening the surfaces of these structures. It drains into the **lacrimal canaliculi** through the **lacrimal puncta,** which are round apertures about 0.5 mm in diameter on the medial aspect of both the upper and lower lid margins. The canaliculi, which are about 1 mm in diameter and 8 mm long and join to form a common canaliculus just before opening into the lacrimal sac, are lined with a thick stratified squamous epithelium. Diverticuli of the common canaliculus, which may be part of the normal structure, are frequently susceptible to fungal infections.

The **lacrimal sac** is the dilated portion of the lacrimal drainage system that lies in the bony lacrimal fossa. The **nasolacrimal duct** is the downward continuation of the lacrimal sac. It opens into the inferior meatus lateral to the inferior turbinate. Both the lacrimal sac and the nasolacrimal duct are lined with ciliated pseudostratified epithelium. The lacrimal glands secrete a fluid rich in the enzyme lysozyme. Lysozyme's main functions are to moisten the surface of the eye and to hydrolyze the cell walls of certain species of bacteria.

HEARING: THE AUDIORECEPTOR SYSTEM

The Ear (Vestibulocochlear Apparatus)

The functions of the vestibulocochlear apparatus (Figure 24–24) are related to equilibrium and hearing. The organ consists of three parts: the **external ear,** which receives sound waves; the **middle ear,** where sound waves are transmitted from air to bone and by bone to the internal ear; and the **internal ear,** where these vibrations are transduced to specific nerve impulses that pass via the acoustic nerve to the central nervous system. The internal ear also contains the vestibular organ, which maintains equilibrium.

External Ear

The **auricle** (**pinna**) consists of an irregularly shaped plate of elastic cartilage covered by tightly adherent skin on all sides.

The **external auditory meatus** is a somewhat flattened canal extending from the surface into the temporal bone. Its internal limit is the tympanic membrane. A stratified squamous epithelium continuous with the skin lines the canal. Hair follicles, sebaceous glands, and the **ceruminous glands** (a type of modified sweat gland) are found in the submucosa. Ceruminous glands are coiled tubular glands that produce the cerumen—or earwax—a brownish, semisolid mixture of fats and waxes. Hairs and cerumen probably have a protective function. The wall of the external auditory meatus is supported by elastic cartilage in its outer third, whereas the temporal bone provides support for the inner part of the canal.

Across the deep end of the external auditory meatus lies an oval membrane, the tympanic membrane (eardrum). Its external surface is covered with a thin layer of epidermis, and its inner surface is covered

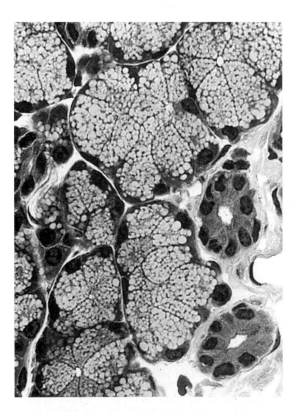

Figure 24–23. Photomicrograph of a section of a lacrimal gland. Ducts are shown at the right, the secretory portion in the center. H&E stain. × 350.

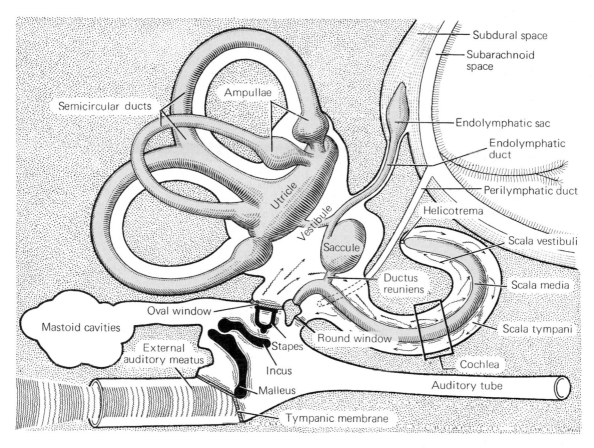

Figure 24–24. The vestibulocochlear organ and the path of sound waves in the external, middle, and internal ear. Components of the internal ear are shown in color. A cross section of the cochlea, as in the rectangular outline, is illustrated in Figure 24–28. (Redrawn and reproduced, with permission, from Best CH, Taylor NB: *The Physiological Basis of Medical Practice,* 8th ed. Williams & Wilkins, 1966.)

with simple cuboidal epithelium continuous with the lining of the tympanic cavity (see below). Between the two epithelial coverings is a tough connective tissue layer composed of collagen and elastic fibers and fibroblasts. The anterior upper quadrant of the tympanic membrane is flaccid and more transparent, since the connective tissue layer is much thinner there. This region is known as **Shrapnell's membrane.** The tympanic membrane is the structure that transmits sound waves to the ossicles of the middle ear (Figure 24–24).

Middle Ear

The middle ear, or tympanic cavity, is an irregular space that lies in the interior of the temporal bone between the tympanic membrane and the bony surface of the internal ear. It communicates anteriorly with the pharynx via the **auditory tube (eustachian tube)** and posteriorly with the air-filled cavities of the mastoid process of the temporal bone. The middle ear is lined with simple squamous epithelium resting on a thin lamina propria that is strongly adherent to the subjacent periosteum. Near the auditory tube and in its interior, the simple epithelium that lines the middle ear is gradually transformed into ciliated pseudostratified columnar epithelium. Although the walls of the tube are usually collapsed, the tube opens during the process of swallowing, balancing the pressure of the air in the middle ear with atmospheric pressure. In the medial bony wall of the middle ear are two membrane-covered oblong regions devoid of bone; these are the **oval** and **round windows** (Figure 24–24).

The tympanic membrane is connected to the oval window by a series of three small bones—the **auditory ossicles: the malleus, incus,** and **stapes** (Figure 24–24)—that transmit the mechanical vibrations generated in the tympanic membrane to the internal ear. The malleus inserts itself into the tympanic membrane and the stapes into the membrane of the oval window. These bones are articulated by synovial joints and, like all structures of this cavity, are covered with simple squamous epithelium. In the middle ear are two small muscles that insert themselves into the malleus and stapes. They have a function in regulating sound conduction.

Internal Ear

The internal ear is composed of two **labyrinths.** The **bony labyrinth** consists of a series of spaces within the petrous portion of the temporal bone that house the **membranous labyrinth** (Figure 24–24). The membranous labyrinth is a continuous epithelium-lined series of cavities of ectodermal origin. It derives from the auditory vesicle that is developed from the ectoderm of the lateral part of the embryo's head. During embryonic development, this vesicle invaginates into the subjacent connective tissue, loses contact with the cephalic ectoderm, and moves deeply into the rudiments of the future temporal bone. During this process, it undergoes a complex series of changes in form, giving rise to two specialized regions of the membranous labyrinth: the **utricle** and the **saccule.** The **semicircular ducts** take their origin from the utricle, whereas the elaborate **cochlear duct** is formed from the saccule. In each of these areas, the epithelial lining becomes specialized to form such sensory structures as the **maculae** of the utricle and saccule, the **cristae** of the semicircular ducts, and the **organ of Corti** of the cochlear duct.

The **bony labyrinth** consists of spaces in the temporal bone. There is an irregular central cavity, the **vestibule,** housing the saccule and the utricle. Behind this, three **semicircular canals** enclose the semicircular ducts; the anterolateral **cochlea** contains the cochlear duct (Figure 24–24).

The cochlea, about 35 mm in total length, makes two-and-one-half turns around a bony core known as the **modiolus.** The modiolus has spaces containing blood vessels and the cell bodies and processes of the acoustic branch of the eighth cranial nerve (spiral ganglion). Extending laterally from the modiolus is a thin bony ridge, the **osseous spiral lamina.** This structure extends farther across the cochlea in the basal region than it does at the apex (see Figure 24–28).

The bony walls of the vestibule and semicircular canals are lined with several layers of flattened connective tissue cells that form a mesothelium. From this layer, thin trabeculae, consisting of fine fibrils and fibroblasts, extend to the outer walls of the utricle, saccule, and semicircular ducts and support these parts of the membranous labyrinth. Blood vessels are also found in this connective tissue.

The bony labyrinth is filled with **perilymph,** which is similar in ionic composition to extracellular fluids elsewhere but has a very low protein content. The membranous labyrinth contains **endolymph,** which is characterized by its low sodium and high potassium content. The protein concentration in endolymph is low.

Histology of the Membranous Labyrinth

A. Saccule and Utricle: The saccule and the utricle are composed of a thin sheath of connective tissue lined with simple squamous epithelium. The membranous labyrinth is bound to the periosteum of the osseous labyrinth by thin strands of connective tissue that also contain blood vessels supplying the epithelia of the membranous labyrinth. In the wall of the saccule and utricle, one can observe small regions, called **maculae,** of differentiated neuroepithelial cells that are innervated by branches of the vestibular nerve (Figure 24–25). The macula of the saccule lies in its floor, whereas the macula of the utricle occupies the lateral wall so the maculae are perpendicular to one another. Maculae in both locations have the same basic histologic structure. They consist of a thickening of the wall and possess two types of receptor cells, some supporting cells, and the afferent and efferent nerve endings.

Receptor cells (**hair cells**) are characterized by the presence of 40–80 long, rigid stereocilia, which are actually highly specialized microvilli, and one cilium (Figure 24–25). Stereocilia are arranged in rows of increasing length, with the longest—about 100 µm—located adjacent to a cilium. The cilium has a basal body and the usual 9 + 2 arrangement of microtubules in its proximal portion, but the two central microtubules soon disappear. This cilium is usually called a kinocilium, but it probably is immotile. There are two types of hair cells, distinguished by the form of their afferent innervation. Type I cells have a large, cup-shaped ending surrounding most of the base of the cell, whereas type II cells have many afferent endings. Both cell types have efferent nerve endings that are probably inhibitory.

The supporting cells disposed between the hair cells are columnar in shape, with the nucleus at the

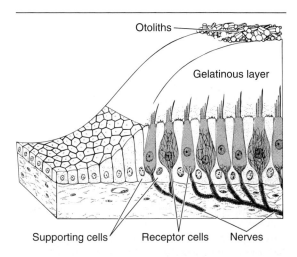

Figure 24–25. Structure of maculae.

base of the cell and microvilli on the apical surface (Figure 24–25). Covering this neuroepithelium is a thick, gelatinous glycoprotein layer, probably secreted by the supporting cells, with surface deposits of crystals composed mainly of calcium carbonate and called **otoliths,** or **otoconia** (Figures 24–25 and 24–26).

B. Semicircular Ducts: Semicircular ducts have the same general form as the corresponding parts of the bony labyrinth. The receptor areas in their **ampullae** (Figure 24–24) have an elongated ridge-like form and are called **cristae ampullares.** The ridge is perpendicular to the long axis of the duct. Cristae are structurally similar to maculae, but their glycoprotein layer is thicker; this layer has a conical form called a **cupula** and is not covered with otoliths. The cupula extends across the ampullae, establishing contact with its opposite wall (Figure 24–27).

C. Endolymphatic Duct and Sac: The endolymphatic duct initially has a simple squamous epithelial lining. As it nears the endolymphatic sac, it gradually changes to tall columnar epithelium composed of two cell types; one of these cell types has microvilli on its apical surface and abundant pinocytotic vesicles and vacuoles. It has been suggested that these cells are responsible for the absorption of endolymph and for the endocytosis of foreign material

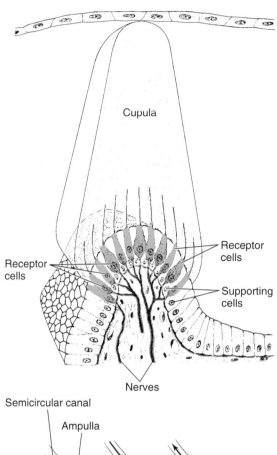

Figure 24–27. Crista ampullaris. **Top:** Structure of the crista ampullaris. **Bottom:** Movements of the cupula in a crista ampullaris during rotational acceleration. Arrows indicate the direction of fluid movement. (Redrawn and reproduced, with permission, from Wersall J: Studies of the structure and innervation of the sensory epithelium of the cristae ampullares in the guinea pig. Acta Otolaryngol [Stockh] Suppl 1956;126:1.)

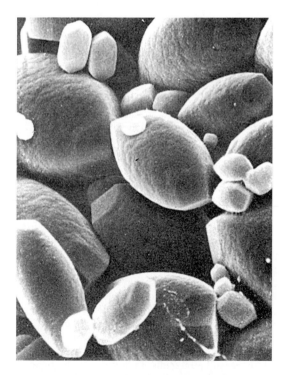

Figure 24–26. Scanning electron micrograph of the surface of a pigeon's macula showing the otoliths. (Courtesy of DJ Lim.)

and cellular remnants that may be present in endolymph.

D. Cochlear Duct: The cochlear duct, a diverticulum of the saccule, is highly specialized as a sound receptor. It is about 35 mm long and is surrounded by specialized perilymphatic spaces. When observed in histologic sections, the cochlea (in the bony labyrinth) appears to be divided into three spaces: the **scala vestibuli** (above), the **scala media** (cochlear duct) in the middle, and the **scala tympani** (below) (Figure 24–28). The cochlear duct, which

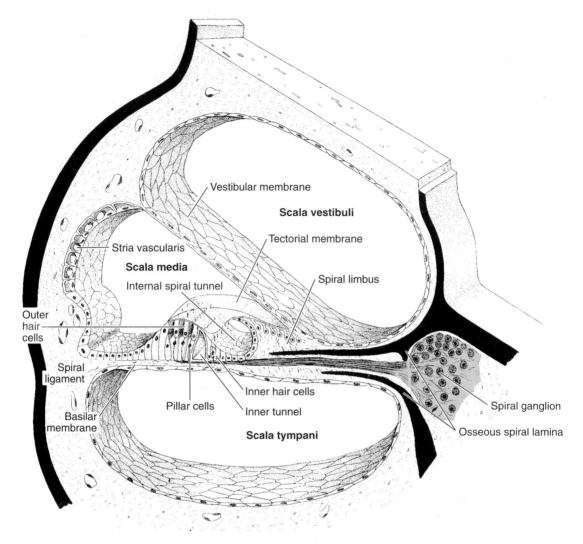

Figure 24–28. Structure of the cochlea. (Redrawn and reproduced, with permission, from Bloom W, Fawcett DW: *A Textbook of Histology,* 9th ed. Saunders, 1968.)

contains endolymph, ends at the apex of the cochlea. The other two scalae contain perilymph and are in reality one long tube, beginning at the **oval window** and terminating at the **round window** (Figure 24–24). They communicate at the apex of the cochlea via an opening known as the **helicotrema.**

The cochlear duct has the following histologic structure (Figure 24–28). The **vestibular (Reissner's) membrane** consists of two layers of squamous epithelium, one derived from the scala media and the other from the lining of the scala vestibuli. Cells of both layers are joined by means of extensive tight junctions that help preserve the very high ionic gradients across this membrane. The **stria vascularis** is an unusual vascularized epithelium located in the lateral wall of the cochlear duct. It consists of three types of cells: marginal, intermediate, and basal.

Marginal cells have many deep infoldings of their basal plasma membranes, where numerous mitochondria are located. These characteristics indicate that marginal cells are ion- and water-transporting cells, and it is generally believed that they are responsible for the characteristic ionic composition of endolymph.

The structure of the internal ear that contains special auditory receptors is called the **organ of Corti;** it contains hair cells that respond to different sound frequencies. It rests on a thick layer of ground substance—the **basilar membrane**—that contains keratin-like fibrils formed of cells of the organ of Corti and of mesothelial cells lining the scala tympani. Many types of supporting cells and two types of hair cells can be distinguished. Three to five rows of **outer hair cells** can be seen, depending on the distance from the base of the organ, and there is a single row of **inner hair cells.** Both types of hair cells are columnar, with basally located nuclei, numerous mitochondria, and distinctive cisternae of smooth endoplasmic reticulum aligned beneath the lateral plasma membranes. The most characteristic feature of these cells is the W-shaped (outer hair cells) or linear (inner hair cells) array of stereocilia (Figure 24–29), which increases in height from one side of the array to the other. A basal body is found in the cytoplasm adjacent to the tallest stereocilia. In contrast to vestibular receptors, no kinocilium is present. This absence of a kinocilium imparts a symmetry to the hair cell that is important in sensory transduction.

The tips of the tallest stereocilia of the outer hair cells are embedded in the **tectorial membrane,** a glycoprotein-rich secretion of certain cells of the spiral limbus (Figure 24–28).

Of the supporting cells, the **pillar cells** should be singled out for special mention. Pillar cells contain a large number of microtubules that seem to impart stiffness to these cells. They outline a triangular

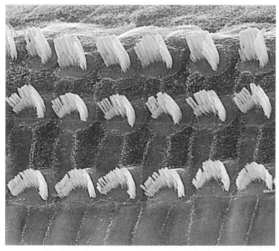

A

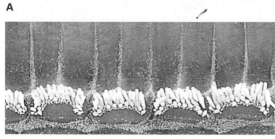

B

Figure 24–29. Scanning electron micrograph of three rows of outer hair cells (**A**) and a single row of inner hair cells (**B**) in the middle turn of a cat cochlear duct. × 2700. (Courtesy of P Leake.)

space between the outer and inner hair cells—the **inner tunnel** (Figure 24–28). This structure is of importance in sound transduction.

Both outer and inner hair cells have afferent and efferent nerve endings. Although the inner hair cells have by far the greater afferent innervation, the functional significance of this difference is not understood. The cell bodies of the bipolar afferent neurons of the organ of Corti are located in a bony core in the modiolus and constitute the spiral ganglion (Figure 24–28).

Histophysiology of the Internal Ear

A. Vestibular Functions: An increase or decrease in the velocity of circular movement—angular acceleration or deceleration—results in a flow of fluid in the semicircular ducts as a consequence of the inertia of the endolymph. This induces a corresponding movement of the cupula over the crista ampullaris and results in the bending of the stereocilia on the sensory cells. Measurement of electrical impulses along vestibular nerve fibers indicates that movement of the cupula in the direction of the kinocilium results in excitation of the receptors, accompanied by the action potentials in the vestibular nerve fibers. Movement in the opposite direction inhibits neuronal activity. When uniform movement returns, acceleration ceases; the cupula returns to its normal position; and excitation or inhibition of the receptors no longer occurs (Figure 24–27).

The semicircular ducts respond to fluid displacement and therefore body position after angular acceleration. The maculae of the saccules and the utricles respond to linear acceleration. Because of their greater density, the otoliths are displaced when there is a change in the position of the head. This displacement is transferred to the underlying hair cells via the gelatinous otolithic membrane. Deformation of stereocilia of the hair cells results in action potentials that are carried to the central nervous system by the vestibular branch of the eighth cranial nerve. Maculae are thus sensitive to the force of gravity on the otoliths. The vestibular apparatus is important for perceiving movement and orientation in space and for maintaining equilibrium or balance.

B. Auditory Functions: Sound waves impinging on the tympanic membrane set the auditory ossicles into motion. The large difference in area of the tympanic membrane and the footplate of the stapes ensures the efficient transmission of mechanical motion from air to the fluids of the internal ear. Two striated skeletal muscles are found in the middle ear—the **tensor tympani** muscle (attached to the malleus) and the **stapedius** muscle (attached to the stapes). Loud sounds cause reflex contractions of these muscles, which limit excursions of the tympanic membrane and the stapes; this helps prevent damage to the internal ear. These reflexes are too slow, however, to guard against sudden loud sounds, such as gunshots.

The following is a step-by-step explanation of how sound waves are converted to electrical impulses in the internal ear (Figure 24–24). Sound waves are longitudinal waves, with **compression** and **rarefaction** phases. The compression phase causes the stapes to move inward. Since the fluids of the internal ear are almost incompressible, the pressure change is transmitted across the vestibular membrane and the basilar membrane, causing them to be deflected downward toward the scala tympani. This pressure change also causes the covering of the round window to bulge outward, thereby relieving the pressure. Because the tips of the pillar cells form a pivot, downward deflection of the basilar membrane is converted into lateral shearing of the stereocilia of hair cells against the tectorial membrane. The tips of the stereocilia are deflected toward the modiolus and away from the basal body.

During the rarefaction phase of the sound wave, everything is reversed—the stapes move outward, the basilar membrane moves upward toward the scala vestibuli, and the stereocilia of the hair cells bend toward the stria vascularis and the basal body. Deflection in this direction sets up depolarizing generator potentials in the hair cells, resulting in the release of a neurotransmitter (whose chemical nature is unknown) that causes the production of action potentials in bipolar neurons of the spiral ganglion (**excitation**).

Discrimination between sound frequencies is based on the response of the basilar membrane. The membrane responds to the frequency of sound with maximal displacement at different points along its length. High frequencies are detected at the basal end of the membrane, whereas low frequencies are detected in the apex of the organ of Corti. This **tonotopic** localization can be correlated with the width and stiffness of the basilar membrane—the narrow basilar membrane, with greater stiffness at the base, responds best to high-frequency sounds. Maximal displacement of the basilar membrane at the threshold of hearing is very small, about 0.1 nm for a 3000-Hz tone.

REFERENCES

CUTANEOUS & OTHER SENSORY MECHANISMS

Beidler LM (editor): Olfaction. In: *Handbook of Sensory Physiology.* Vol 4. Springer, 1971.

Beidler LM (editor): Taste. In: *Handbook of Sensory Physiology.* Vol 4. Springer, 1971.

Farbman AI: The cellular basis of olfaction. Endeavour 1994;18:2.

Graziadei PPC: The olfactory mucosa of vertebrates. In: *Handbook of Sensory Physiology.* Vol 4. Beidler LM (editor). Springer, 1971.

Iggo A, Andres KH: Morphology of cutaneous receptors. Annu Rev Neurosci 1985;5:1.

Keverne EB: Chemical senses: smell. In: *The Senses.* Barlow HB, Mollon JD (editors). Cambridge Univ Press, 1982.

Margolskee RF: The molecular biology of taste transduction. Bioessays 1993;15:645.

More K, Yoshihara Y: Molecular recognition and olfactory processing in the mammalian olfactory system. Prog Neurobiol 1995;45:585.

Moulton DG: Dynamics of cell populations in the olfactory epithelium. Trans NY Acad Sci 1974;237:52.

Schmidt RF (editor): *Fundamentals of Sensory Physiology.* Springer-Verlag, 1978.

THE EYE

Bok D, Hall MO: The role of the retinal pigment epithelium in the etiology of inherited retinal dystrophy in the rat. J Cell Biol 1971;49:664.

Botelho SY: Tears and the lacrimal gland. Sci Am 1964;211:78.

Dowling JE: Organization of vertebrate retinas. Invest Ophthalmol 1970;9:665.

Hogan MJ et al: *Histology of the Human Eye.* Saunders, 1971.

McDevitt D (editor): *Cell Biology of the Eye.* Academic Press, 1982.

Young RW: Visual cells and the concept of renewal. Invest Ophthalmol 1976;15:700.

THE EAR

Dallos P: The active cochlea. J Neurosci 1992;12:4575.

Hudspeth AJ: The hair cells of the inner ear. Sci Am 1983;248:54.

Kimura RS: The ultrastructure of the organ of Corti. Int Rev Cytol 1975;42:173.

Lim DJ: Functional structure of the organ of Corti: a review. Hear Res 1986;22:117.

Index

Cerebrospinal fluid, 169
  choroid plexus elaborating, 169
Cerebrum (cerebral cortex), 164, 165,
  165*f*
Ceruminous glands, 464
Cervical carcinoma, 432
Cervical glands, 432
Cervical loop, in tooth development,
  278*f*, 279
Cervix (uterine), 422*f*, 430, 432
  cancer of, 432
CFC. *See* Colony-forming cells/units
CFU. *See* Colony-forming cells/units
Chagas disease, 273
Chalones, 61
  in liver regeneration, 321–322
Chemical messengers
  in glandular control, 78–81, 78*f*
  movement of through gap junctions,
    68
  in signal reception, 26, 28*f*, 28*t*
  in synaptic transmission, 158, 158*f*,
    158*t*
Chemical synapses, 158
  events during transmission at, 158*f*,
    159–160
Chemoreceptors/chemoreceptor system,
  204, 212, **446–448**, 449*f*, 450*f*
Chemotaxis, 118
Chief cells
  gastric, 286*f*, 288
  parathyroid, 404
Cholecystokinin (CCK), 161*f*, 308–309
  actions of, 296*t*, 308–309, 323–324
  cells producing, 86*t*, 296*t*, 324
  gallbladder affected by, 323–324
  gastrointestinal distribution of, 295*f*
Cholelithiasis (gallstones), 318–319
Cholesterol, membrane, 22, 22*f*
Cholinergic nerves, 175
Chondroblasts, 130*f*, 131
  functions of, 107*t*
  origins of, 106*f*, 131, 131*f*
Chondrocytes, 127
  elastic cartilage, 132
  fibrocartilage, 132, 133*f*
  functions of, 131
  hyaline cartilage, 128*f*, 129, 130*f*
  origins of, 106*f*, 131, 131*f*
  tumors of, 131
Chondroitin sulfate, 90, 91*t*
  in cartilage proteoglycans, 129, 129*f*
Chondroma, 131
Chondronectin, 92
  in cartilage, 129
Chondrosarcoma, 131
Choriocapillary layer, 451
Chorion, 435, 436–438, 437*f*, 438*f*
  frondosum, 436
  laeve, 436
Chorionic gonadotropin, human, 442
  corpus luteum affected by, 429
Chorionic plate, 436, 437*f*
Chorionic villi, 436, 436–438, 436*f*, 437*f*,
  438*f*
Choroid, 448, 450–452, 451*f*, 452*f*
Choroid plexus, **169**, 169*f*
Chromatids, sister, 55

Chromatin, 51–53, 52*f*, 53*f*, 56*f*
  fibrous lamina-associated, 51
  nucleolus-associated, 52*f*, 53*f*, 54, 57*f*
  sex, 52, 56*f*
Chromatolysis, 178
Chromogranins, 389
Chromosomes, 52–53, 57*f*
  in mitosis, 55, 58*f*, 59*f*
Chylomicrons
  in adipose cells, 122, 123*f*
  transport of to liver, 309
Chyme, 283
  pancreatic enzymes affecting, 308
Chymotrypsinogen, 308
Cigarette smoking, respiratory epithelium
  affected by, 328
  cancer and, 346
Cilia, 44, 45*f*, 71–72, 73*f*
  immotile (Kartagener syndrome), 44,
    49*t*, 328, 409, 430
    sinusitis and, 333
  olfactory cell, 447–448, 450*f*
  in respiratory epithelium, 327–328
Ciliary body, 448, 451*f*, 452–453, 452*f*,
  455*f*
Ciliary muscle, 452, 452*f*
Ciliary processes, 452*f*, 453–454, 455*f*,
  456*f*
Ciliated columnar cells, in respiratory
  epithelium, 328, 330*f*, 331*f*, 332*f*
Circadian biorhythm, pineal gland
  involved in, 405
Circuits, 152
Circulating compartment, neutrophil,
  241, 242, 245*f*
Circulatory system, **202–217**. *See also*
  Blood vessels; Heart; Lymphatic
  vascular system
Circumvallate papillae, 274*f*, 275,
  446–447, 448*f*
Cirrhosis of liver, 313, 321
cis face, of Golgi complex, 34, 37*f*
Cisternae
  Golgi complex, 34, 36*f*
  perinuclear, 51
  rough endoplasmic reticulum, 32
  smooth endoplasmic reticulum, 33
Clara cells, 335, 336*f*
Class I/class II major histocompatibility
  complex molecules, 253
  in antigen processing, 252–253
Class switching, immunoglobulin, 251
Classic liver lobules, 309, 314, 317*f*
Clathrin, in receptor-mediated
  endocytosis, 24–25
Clear cells, sweat gland, 358
Clear zone, 135
Clearing, for tissue embedding, 2
Clitoris, 441
Closed circulation, splenic, 267, 267*f*,
  268*f*
Clot removal, 232
Clot retraction, 231
Clotting, blood, platelets in, 229, 231
Clotting cascade, 231
Coagulation, blood, platelets in, 229, 231
Coated pits, 24
Cochlea, 465*f*, 466, 468*f*

Cochlear duct, 466, 467–469, 468*f*
Coiled arteries, uterine, 432
Colchicine, microtubules affected by,
  42, 43
Cold, sensation of, 446, 447*f*
Collagen, 97*t*
  in arterial structure, 211–212
  in basal lamina, 64
  in bone matrix, 137
  in cartilage, 127
  dermatan sulfate in, 90
  diseases associated with, 99–100, 102*t*
  in elastic cartilage, 132
  evolution of, 95–98
  in fibrocartilage, 132–133
  in hyaline cartilage, 129, 129*f*
  in interalveolar septum, 341
  renewal/turnover rate of, 120
  synthesis of, 96, 97*t*, 98–100, 101*f*
    insufficiencies/abnormalities of,
      99–100, 102*t*
  types of, 95–98, 97*t*
Collagen bundles, 99*f*, 100
Collagen fibers, 96, 100, 102*f*, 103*f*, 104*f*
  in fibrocartilage, 132–133, 133*f*
Collagen fibrils, 96–98, 98*f*, 99, 99*f*, 100*f*
Collagenases, 100
Collateral branches, axon, 157
Collecting ducts, 360, 361*f*, 362*f*,
  367–368, 370*f*
  functions of, 374
Collecting tubules, 360, 361*f*, 367–368,
  374*f*
Colloid, thyroid, 398
Colon. *See* Large intestine
Colony-forming cells/units, 235*f*, 236
Colony-stimulating factors
  (hematopoietic growth factors),
  234–235, 235*f*, 237*t*, 254
Colostrum, 444
Columnar epithelium, 63, 64*f*, 65*f*
  ciliated, in respiratory epithelium, 328,
    330*f*, 331*f*, 332*f*
  pseudostratified, 65*f*
  simple, 64, 72, 74*f*, 74*t*
  stratified, 67*f*, 73, 74*t*
Combined immunodeficiency, lymph
  node pathology in, 263*f*
Common adipose tissue
  (unilocular/yellow adipose
  tissue), **121–124**, 122*f*
  histogenesis of, 123–124, 124*f*
  histologic structure of, 121–122, 122*f*
  histophysiology of, 122–123
  tumors of, 125
Common bile duct (ductus choledochus),
  322
Communicating junctions, 69. *See also*
  Gap junctions
Compact bone, 138, 139, 139*f*, 140*f*
Complement, 250
  in hematopoiesis, 237
Compound glands, 76, 77*f*
Compression phase, of sound wave, 470
Conchae, 329
Condenser, of light microscope, 3, 3*f*
Condensing vacuoles, 34, 42*f*, 82*f*, 83
Conducting arteries, 211

Medical Epidemiology, 2/e
Greenberg, Daniels, Flanders, Eley, & Boring
1996, ISBN 0-8385-6206-X, A6206-5

Basic & Clinical Endocrinology, 5/e
Greenspan & Strewler
1997, ISBN 0-8385-0588-0, A0588-2

Occupational & Environmental Medicine, 2/e
LaDou
1997, ISBN 0-8385-7216-2, A7216-3

Primary Care of Women
Lemcke, Marshall, Pattison, & Cowley
1995, ISBN 0-8385-9813-7, A9813-5

Clinical Anesthesiology, 2/e
Morgan & Mikhail
1996, ISBN 0-8385-1381-6, A1381-1

Fundamentals of Surgery
Niederhuber
1998, ISBN 0-8385-0509-0, A0509-8

Dermatology
Orkin, Maibach, & Dahl
1991, ISBN 0-8385-1288-7, A1288-8

Rudolph's Fundamentals of Pediatrics, 2/e
Rudolph & Kamei
1998, ISBN 0-8385-8236-2, A8236-0

Genetics in Primary Care & Clinical Medicine
Seashore
1995, ISBN 0-8385-3128-8, A3128-4

The Principles and Practice of Medicine, 23/e
Stobo, Hellman, Ladenson, Petty, & Traill
1996, ISBN 0-8385-7963-9, A7963-0

Smith's General Urology, 14/e
Tanagho & McAninch
1995, ISBN 0-8385-8612-0, A8612-2

General Ophthalmology, 14/e
Vaughan, Asbury, & Riordan-Eva
1995, ISBN 0-8385-3127-X, A3127-6

Clinical Oncology
Weiss
1993, ISBN 0-8385-1325-5, A1325-8

CURRENT Clinical References

CURRENT Critical Care Diagnosis & Treatment, 2/e
Bongard & Sue
1999, ISBN 0-8385-1454-5, A1454-6

CURRENT Diagnosis & Treatment in Cardiology
Crawford
1995, ISBN 0-8385-1444-8, A1444-7

CURRENT Diagnosis & Treatment in Vascular Surgery
Dean, Yao, & Brewster
1995, ISBN 0-8385-1351-4, A1351-4

CURRENT Obstetric & Gynecologic Diagnosis & Treatment, 9/e
DeCherney
1999, ISBN 0-8385-1401-4, A1401-7

CURRENT Diagnosis and Treatment in Psychiatry
Ebert, Loosen, & Nurcombe
1999, ISBN 0-8385-1462-6, A1462-9

CURRENT Diagnosis & Treatment in Gastroenterology
Grendell, McQuaid, & Friedman
1996, ISBN 0-8385-1448-0, A1448-8

CURRENT Pediatric Diagnosis & Treatment, 13/e
Hay, Groothius, Hayward, & Levin
1997, ISBN 0-8385-1400-6, A1400-9

CURRENT Emergency Diagnosis & Treatment, 4/e
Saunders & Ho
1992, ISBN 0-8385-1347-6, A1347-2

CURRENT Diagnosis & Treatment in Orthopedics
Skinner
1995, ISBN 0-8385-1009-4, A1009-8

CURRENT Medical Diagnosis & Treatment 1998, 37/e
Tierney, McPhee, & Papadakis
1998, ISBN 0-8385-1524-X, A1524-6

CURRENT Surgical Diagnosis & Treatment, 11/e
Way
1999, ISBN 0-8385-1456-1, A1456-1

LANGE Clinical Manuals

Dermatology
Diagnosis and Therapy
Bondi, Jegasothy, & Lazarus
1991, ISBN 0-8385-1274-7, A1274-8

Manual for Human Dissection
Callas
1994, ISBN 0-8385-6133-0, A6133-1

Practical Oncology
Cameron
1994, ISBN 0-8385-1326-3, A1326-6

Office & Bedside Procedures
Chesnutt, Dewar, & Locksley
1993, ISBN 0-8385-1095-7, A1095-7

Psychiatry
Diagnosis & Treatment, 2/e
Flaherty, Davis, & Janicak
1993, ISBN 0-8385-1267-4, A1267-2

Practical Gynecology
Jacobs & Gast
1991, ISBN 0-8385-1336-0, A1336-5

Geriatrics
Lonergan
1996, ISBN 0-8385-1094-9, A1094-0

Ambulatory Medicine
The Primary Care of Families, 2/e
Mengel & Schwiebert
1996, ISBN 0-8385-1466-9, A1466-0

Poisoning & Drug Overdose, 3/e
Olson
1999, ISBN 0-8385-0260-1, A0260-8

Internal Medicine
Diagnosis and Therapy, 3/e
Stein
1993, ISBN 0-8385-1112-0, A1112-0

Surgery
Diagnosis and Therapy
Stillman
1989, ISBN 0-8385-1283-6, A1283-9

Medical Perioperative Management
Wolfsthal
1989, ISBN 0-8385-1298-4, A1298-7

LANGE Handbooks

Handbook of Gynecology & Obstetrics
Brown & Crombleholme
1993, ISBN 0-8385-3608-5, A3608-5

HIV/AIDS Primary Care Handbook, 2/e
Carmichael, Carmichael, & Fischl
1999, ISBN 0-8385-3777-4, A3777-8

Clinician's Pocket Reference, 8/e
Gomella
1997, ISBN 0-8385-1476-6, A1476-9

Neonatology
Management, Procedures, On-Call Problems, Diseases, and Drugs, 3/e
Gomella
1995, ISBN 0-8385-1331-X, A1331-6

Surgery on Call, 2/e
Gomella & Lefor
1996, ISBN 0-8385-8746-1, A8746-8

Internal Medicine On Call, 2/e
Haist, Robbins, & Gomella
1997, ISBN 0-8385-4056-2, A4056-6

Obstetrics & Gynecology On Call
Horowitz & Gomella
1993, ISBN 0-8385-7174-3, A7174-4

Pocket Guide to Commonly Prescribed Drugs, 2/e
Levine
1996, ISBN 0-8385-8099-8, A8099-2

Handbook of Pediatrics, 18/e
Merenstein, Kaplan, & Rosenberg
1997, ISBN 0-8385-3625-5, A3625-9

Pocket Guide to Diagnostic Tests, 2/e
Nicoll, McPhee, Chou, & Detmer
1997, ISBN 0-8385-8100-5, A8100-8

Quick Medical Spanish, 2/e
Rogers
1997, ISBN 0-8385-8258-3, A8258-4

How to Examine the Nervous System, 3/e
Ross
1998, ISBN 0-8385-3852-5, A3852-9

Pocket Guide to the Essentials of Diagnosis & Treatment
Tierney
1997, ISBN 0-8385-3605-0, A3605-1

 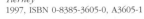 **Appleton & Lange • P.O. Box 120041 • Stamford, CT • 06912-0041 • 1-800-423-1359**